Current Progress in Reproductive Biology and Endocrinology

Current Progress in Reproductive Biology and Endocrinology

Edited by Gabriel Austin

hayle medical

New York

Hayle Medical,
750 Third Avenue, 9th Floor,
New York, NY 10017, USA

Visit us on the World Wide Web at:
www.haylemedical.com

ISBN: 978-1-63241-759-6

Cataloging-in-Publication Data

Current progress in reproductive biology and endocrinology / edited by Gabriel Austin.
    p. cm.
Includes bibliographical references and index.
ISBN 978-1-63241-759-6
1. Reproduction. 2. Human reproduction. 3. Reproduction--Endocrine aspects.
4. Human biology. 5. Reproductive health. I. Austin, Gabriel.
QP251 .C87 2019
612.6--dc23

Table of Contents

Preface

Reproductive biology is the field of biology, which delves into both sexual and asexual reproduction. It includes several other fields like, sexual development, sexual maturity, endocrinology, fertility and reproduction. Endocrinology is an area of reproductive biology, which deals with the endocrine system, and the diseases related to it. It is a system of glands, which is responsible for the secretion of hormones. They are the major drivers of human reproduction. They are responsible for controlling the menstrual cycle and for sexual reproduction. The main reproductive hormones are testosterone and estrogen. While testosterone stimulates sperm production in men, estrogen causes eggs to mature in the ovaries after a girl reaches puberty. The topics included in this book on reproductive biology and endocrinology are of utmost significance and bound to provide incredible insights to readers. It traces the progress of these fields and highlights some of their key concepts and applications. Those in search of information to further their knowledge will be greatly assisted by this book.

After months of intensive research and writing, this book is the end result of all who devoted their time and efforts in the initiation and progress of this book. It will surely be a source of reference in enhancing the required knowledge of the new developments in the area. During the course of developing this book, certain measures such as accuracy, authenticity and research focused analytical studies were given preference in order to produce a comprehensive book in the area of study.

This book would not have been possible without the efforts of the authors and the publisher. I extend my sincere thanks to them. Secondly, I express my gratitude to my family and well-wishers. And most importantly, I thank my students for constantly expressing their willingness and curiosity in enhancing their knowledge in the field, which encourages me to take up further research projects for the advancement of the area.

Editor

Age-related morphometrical peculiarities of Lithuanian women's primordial ovarian follicles

Kristina Lasiene[1*], Donatas Gasiliunas[2], Nomeda Juodziukyniene[3] and Aleksandras Vitkus[1]

Abstract

Background: For the first time, thorough morphometrical measurements of primordial ovarian follicles were performed and their age-related changes were investigated in Lithuanian women of the reproductive age.

Methods: Ovaries of dead women ($n = 30$) were divided into six age groups: 15–20 years old, 21–25 years old, 26–30 years old, 31–35 years old, 36–40 years old and 41–46 years old. Histological slides of left and right ovaries were stained using haematoxylin-eosin and periodic acid–Schiff (PAS) staining methods. The morphometrical measurements of 10 primordial ovarian follicles of the left and right ovary of each woman were made from microphotographs.

Results: The diameter of primordial ovarian follicles increased in groups of women from 15 years old to 35 years old and decreased in the groups from 36 years old to 46 years old. The area of primordial ovarian follicles increased in the groups of women until 35 years old. It decreased in the groups of women older than 36 years. The follicular basement membrane thickened from 1.29 ± 0.11 μm to 1.43 ± 0.18 μm with increasing age of women. The diameter of primary oocytes enlarged until 35 years and then began to decrease. The area of primary oocytes increased in women until 35 years. It decreased in groups of women aged 36–40 and 41–46 years old. The diameter and the area of primary oocytes nuclei increased in women aged 15–30 years old; later, it began to decrease. The length of follicular cells varied from 8.56 ± 0.43 μm to 8.72 ± 0.27 μm ($p > 0.05$). The height of follicular cells varied from 2.59 ± 0.27 μm to 2.7 ± 0.21 μm ($p > 0.05$). The diameter, the area and the basement membrane thickness of primordial ovarian follicles and the diameter and the area of primary oocytes and their nuclei differed insignificantly in left and right ovaries in all age groups of women ($p > 0.5$). The length and height of follicular cells were similar in left and right ovaries of the same age group ($p > 0.5$).

Conclusions: The age decreasing of morphometrical parameters begins in primordial ovarian follicles and their primary oocytes in Lithuanian women older than 35 years. The thickness of the follicular basement membrane increased with increasing age of women. No significant differences were found in the morphometrical parameters in primordial follicles of left and right ovaries in the same age group of women.

Keywords: Morphometrical, Primary oocyte, Primordial ovarian follicle, Women

* Correspondence: kristina.lasiene@lsmuni.lt
[1]Department of Histology and Embryology, Medical Academy, Lithuanian University of Health Sciences, A. Mickeviciaus str. 9, LT-44307 Kaunas, Lithuania
Full list of author information is available at the end of the article

Background

When ovarian follicles are formed, they enter the primordial ("resting") stage, which persists for a period of time that varies from follicle to follicle. They can develop to primary follicles or become atretic [1]. The mechanisms responsible for the initiation of follicular growth (primordial follicle activation) or atresia and the mechanisms that permit variable timing of growth initiation are completely unknown. The non-growing primordial follicles are a resource that could be utilized or manipulated to alleviate infertility, produce contraception or delay menopause [2].

Reproductive methods, such as IVF, ICSI and embryo transfer, have a limited impact on a lack of fertilizable oocytes for women. Superovulation can increase the number of oocytes ovulated by an individual, but the response is variable and large numbers are not generally obtained. In-vitro maturation of immature oocytes from antral follicles and earlier follicle stages would increase the number of fertilizable oocytes [3].

Frozen (cryopreserved) ovarian biopsies would also provide an important source of self- and donated oocytes for the many women who do not respond well to superovulation, women with primary ovarian insufficiency, damaged ovaries due to inflammation or endometriosis, and women with premature menopause, such as young cancer patients who require fertility treatment after chemotherapy and radiotherapy [3–7].

Cryopreservation of human ovarian tissue containing immature follicles and retransplantation of cryopreserved tissue after cancer treatment can be performed successfully and healthy babies can be delivered [8–12].

Primordial follicles constitute the largest part of the ovarian follicular population. The number of primordial follicles in an ovary decreases with age [13].

A lot of scientists focus their attention on the structure and ultrastructure and changes of the ultrastructure in primordial, primary, secondary (preantral) and antral (Graafian) follicles and their oocytes in women [1, 14–18].

However, we missed detailed measurements of the size of follicles, oocytes and follicular cells and their age-related changes in all stages of human ovarian follicles.

The aim of this study was to measure primordial ovarian follicles and to determine how morphometrical parameters varied in relation with women's age.

Methods

Study design

The pairs of ovaries from 30 women aged 15–46 years were obtained from Kaunas Division of State Forensic Medicine Service after autopsy at least 24 h post mortem. Left ovaries were marked using the cotton thread. The material was placed into a 10% formaldehyde solution for 24 h. Women were subdivided into six age groups: 15–20 years old ($n = 5$; 15, 16, 16, 19 and 20 years old), 21–25 years old ($n = 5$; 21, 21, 23, 24 and 25 years old), 26–30 years old ($n = 5$; 26, 27, 28, 29 and 30 years old), 31–35 years old ($n = 5$; 31, 32, 32, 34 and 35 years old), 36–40 years old ($n = 5$; 36, 36, 38, 39 and 40 years old) and 41–46 years old ($n = 5$; 41, 43, 43, 43 and 46 years old). Only ovaries without morphological pathologies, dominant follicle, corpus luteum and follicular cysts were selected as suitable for this investigation. Each ovary was cut into 3 pieces. Only the middle piece was used for the preparation of histological slides, dehydrated in the graded ethanol series and embedded to paraffin blocks. In order to avoid the re-measurement of the same follicle, sections (4 μm of thickness) were obtained at 100 μm intervals. Histological slides were prepared according to standard methods and stained with haematoxylin-eosin (Fig. 1a). In brief, deparaffinised and rehydrated sections were immersed in Mayer's haematoxylin solution for 7 min, and then washed in running tap water for 1 min, ammonia water for 30 s and tap water for 1 min again. The sections were stained in a 2% eosin solution for 1 min and 30 s, rinsed in tap water for 1 min, dehydrated and covered with cover glass (according to [19, 20] with our small modifications).

The periodic acid–Schiff (PAS) staining method was used for the emphasis of the follicular basement membrane (Fig. 1b) [21]. Briefly, after deparaffinisation and rehydration, the sections were immersed in a 0.5% periodic acid solution for 5 min. Then they were rinsed in distilled water and dried in a thermostat at 60 °C for 5 min. They were steeped in Schiff's reagent (Merck) for 20 min and then rinsed in running tap water. Then the sections were stained with Mayer's haematoxylin for 5 min, rinsed in distilled water for 5 min, and dehydrated and covered with cover glass ([19, 20] with our small modifications).

Microphotographs of primordial ovarian follicles were made from histological slides using microscope Olympus BX40 (camera Olympus XC30). Only follicles surrounded by flattened follicular cells, cut through the middle and presenting approximately equal size, rounded shape and clearly visible oocytes nuclei were selected for morphometrical analysis. Ten primordial ovarian follicles were selected from each ovary for measurement (in total, 20 follicles from each woman). Morphometrical analysis was done manually using an image analysis programme (UTHSCSA Image Tool for Windows Version 3.0) by the same person. The diameter, the area and the basement membrane thickness of primordial ovarian follicles, the diameter and the area of primary oocytes, the diameter and the area of their nuclei and the length and the height of flattened follicular cells were measured and compared in women of six age groups. Because the shape of primordial ovarian follicles, primary oocytes and their nuclei is

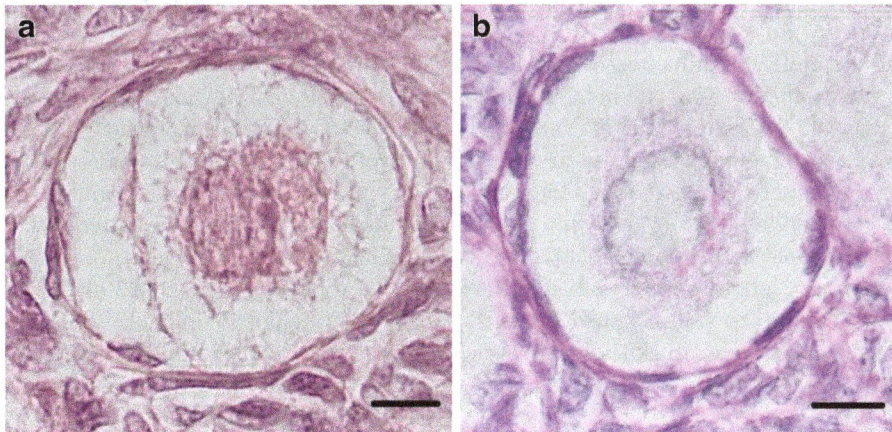

Fig. 1 Primordial ovarian follicles in a 21 year old woman. **a** – stained with haematoxylin-eosin. **b** - stained with periodic acid–Schiff (PAS). Bar = 10 μm

not perfectly round, these structures were measured in three places: the widest, the narrowest and between them, and the average was calculated. The length and the height of follicular cells were measured in three cells and the average of these parameters was calculated. The basement membrane thickness was measured at five places of the same follicle and the average was calculated too. All obtained data were tabled in the Microsoft Excel 2003 programme. Using this programme, the ratios of oocyte to follicle area, nucleus to oocyte area and follicular cell height to length were calculated.

Statistical analysis

The Statistica programme (Statistica Version 5, StatSoft inc.) Basic statistics was used for the calculation of the mean and the standard deviation. One-way ANOVA Tukey HSD post-hoc was used for statistical comparison of age groups (p values). The data were expressed as mean ± standard deviation (SD), and $p < 0.05$ was taken as significant.

Results

The study of 15–46–year-old women's primordial ovarian follicles showed that the age had a significant influence on their diameter (Fig. 2, Additional file 1: Table S1). It increased in women groups of 15–20, 21–25, 26–30 and 31–35 years old (43.55 ± 0.44 μm, 44.56 ± 0.34 μm, 44.63 ± 0.36 μm and 44.72 ± 0.38 μm, respectively). The diameter began to decrease in

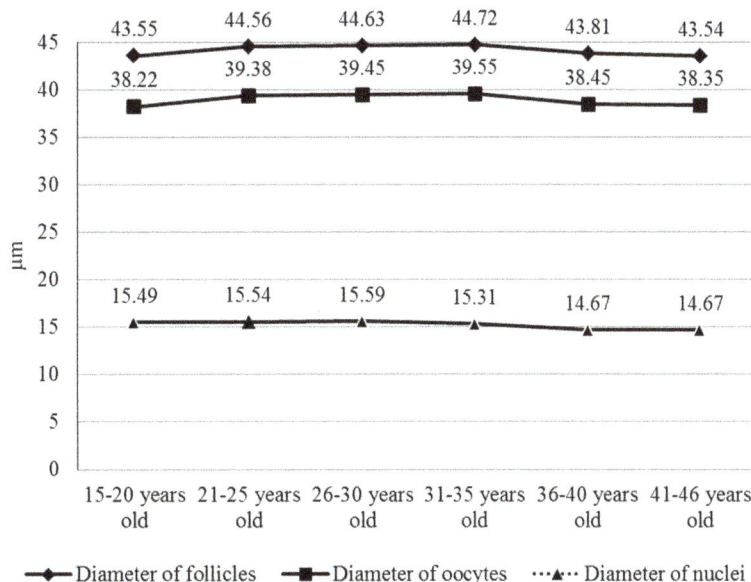

Fig. 2 The diameter of primordial ovarian follicles, primary oocytes and their nuclei

women of 36–40 and 41–46 years old (43.81 ± 0.56 μm and 43.54 ± 0.46 μm).

Women's age had a significant influence on the area of primordial ovarian follicles, too. It increased in women younger than 35 years old (from 1487.8 ± 32.14 μm^2 to 1569.2 ± 28.32 μm^2). Also, the area decreased in women groups of 36–40 and 41–46 years old (1506.3 ± 41.3 μm^2 and 1487.9 ± 36.84 μm^2, respectively) (Fig. 3, Additional file 1: Table S1).

The basement membrane of primordial follicles was broken and clearly visible only on slides stained by PAS. The follicular basement membrane thickness increased from 1.29 ± 0.11 μm to 1.43 ± 0.18 μm according to women's age (Table 1).

The diameter of primary oocytes in primordial follicles was smallest in the group of women aged 15–20 years (38.22 ± 0.39 μm). It enlarged until 35 years (to 39.55 ± 0.45 μm) and then began to decrease (to 38.35 ± 0.41 μm) (Fig. 2, Additional file 1: Table S1).

The area of primary oocytes of primordial follicles increased in women until 35 years old (from 1145.55 ± 25.75 μm^2 to 1226.75 ± 29.67 μm^2), too. It decreased in women groups of 36–40 and 41–46 years old (1159.55 ± 22.91 μm^2 and 1153.25 ± 26.71 μm^2, respectively) (Fig. 3, Additional file 1). However, the oocyte to follicle area ratio remained almost the same (0.77–0.78; $p > 0.5$) (Table 1).

The age had influence on the diameter and the area of nuclei of primary oocytes in primordial ovarian follicles in 15–36-year old women. The diameter and the area of nuclei increased fractionally in 15–30-year old women (from 15.49 ± 0.2 μm to 15.59 ± 0.14 μm, and from 187.16 ± 4.84 μm^2 to 189.55 ± 3.57 μm^2, respectively). Later, it began to decrease significantly (to 14.67 ± 0.5 μm and 168.19 ± 13.23 μm^2, respectively, Figs. 2 and 3, Additional file 1: Table S1). However, the nucleus to oocyte area ratio remained almost the same in the follicles of women of all ages (0.15–0.16; $p > 0.5$) (Table 1).

In primordial follicles, primary oocytes were surrounded by one layer of flattened follicular cells. The length of follicular cells did not differ significantly with age. It varied from 8.56 ± 0.43 μm to 8.72 ± 0.27 μm ($p > 0.05$). The height of follicular cells ranged from 2.59 ± 0.27 μm to 2.7 ± 0.21 μm ($p > 0.05$, Table 1).

Table 2 shows the comparison of morphometrical data of left and right ovaries in the group of women of the same age. The diameter, the area and the basement membrane thickness of primordial ovarian follicles differed insignificantly in left and right ovaries in all age groups of women ($p > 0.5$). Also, the diameter and the area of primary oocytes and their nuclei were similar in left and right ovaries ($p > 0.5$). The length and the height of follicular cells differed insignificantly in left and right ovaries, too ($p > 0.5$). The oocyte to follicle area, the nucleus to oocyte area and the follicular cell height to length ratios were the same in left and right ovaries in the same age group (0.77–0.78, 0.15–0.16 and 0.3–0.31, respectively; $p > 0.5$).

Discussion

In this study, we wanted to measure primordial ovarian follicles and their primary oocytes and to compare how the morphometrical parameters varied in relation to

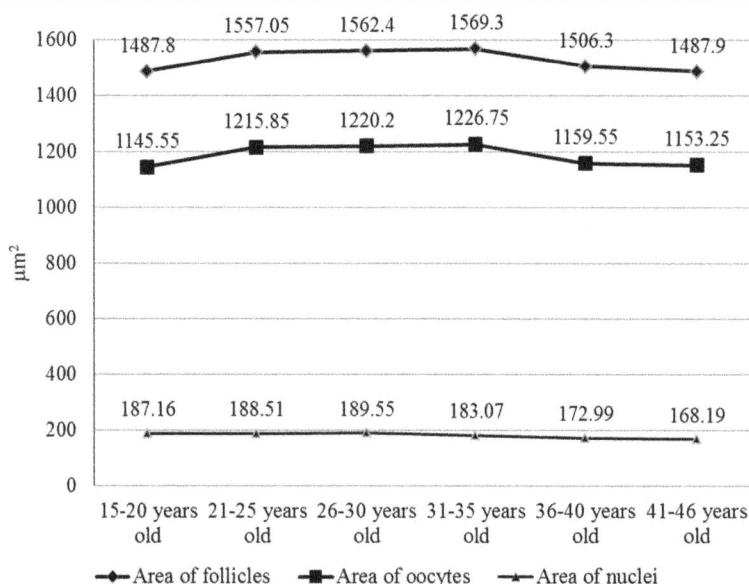

Fig. 3 The area of primordial ovarian follicles, primary oocytes and their nuclei

Table 1 The morphometric parameters of primordial follicles in the ovaries of 15–46 year old women (mean ± SD)

Parameter	15–20 years old	21–25 years old	26–30 years old	31–35 years old	36–40 years old	41–46 years old	p values
Basement membrane thickness, μm	1.29 ± 0.11 a	1.34 ± 0.06	1.38 ± 0.07	1.39 ± 0.08 b	1.43 ± 0.15 c	1.43 ± 0.18 d	a:b, a:c, a:d; $p < 0.05$
Oocyte:follicle area ratio	0.77	0.78	0.78	0.78	0.77	0.78	$p > 0.5$
Nucleus:oocyte area ratio	0.16	0.16	0.16	0.15	0.15	0.15	$p > 0.5$
Follicular cells							
Length, μm	8.69 ± 0.13	8.7 ± 0.15	8.71 ± 0.12	8.72 ± 0.27	8.62 ± 0.26	8.56 ± 0.43	$p > 0.05$
Height, μm	2.62 ± 0.12	2.66 ± 0.09	2.68 ± 0.11	2.7 ± 0.21	2.59 ± 0.27	2.62 ± 0.39	$p > 0.05$
Height:length ratio	0.3	0.31	0.31	0.31	0.3	0.31	$p > 0.5$

women's age in Lithuania. Starting this research, we *confronted with* the lack of research material. Within 10 years, we received ovaries from 49 dead women (15–46 years old only). Therefore, our study was very extended. Only ovaries from 30 women were suitable for our research (without corpus luteum, dominant follicle or follicular cysts). Also, there were cases when we received only one ovary. Therefore, we could not compare the morphometrical parameters of primordial follicles of left and right ovaries in the same women. Besides, the investigation was impeded by post mortem changes in the ovaries.

We aimed at comparing morphometrical parameters of follicles in women of different countries. However, in the literature, we found scarce data on morphometrical characteristics of primordial ovarian follicles in women from various countries.

In the USA, Griffin with co-authors [22] maintained that the mean diameter of human primordial ovarian follicles and primary oocytes was 44 μm and 36 μm, respectively. In the Netherlands, the area of oocytes was 850 ± 244 μm^2 in primordial follicles of young women's (26–32 years old) ovaries and 927 ± 258 μm^2 in those of advanced-age women (39–45 years old). The area of oocytes nuclei was 199 ± 97.7 μm^2 and 197 ± 94 μm^2, respectively. The mean nucleus to oocyte ratios were 0.23 ± 0.09 and 0.21 ± 0.08, respectively [15, 16].

In France, the diameter of human primordial ovarian follicles was 35.4 ± 6.2 μm, the diameter of oocytes was 32.1 ± 6.0 μm and the diameter of oocytes nuclei was 16.1 ± 6.1 μm [13].

We found only one source of literature which in detail compared morphometrical parameters of follicles in the ovaries of women of the reproductive age. Westergaard and co-authors [23] from Denmark proposed that the diameter of primordial ovarian follicle and its oocytes increased in women of 13–27 years old (from 39.0 ± 0.4 μm to 41.9 ± 03 μm and from 34.3 ± 0.4 μm to 37.0 ± 0.3 μm, respectively); then it began to decline (to 39.4 ± 0.3 μm and 35.1 ± 0.4 μm, respectively). The maximal diameter of oocytes nuclei was found in 13–20-year

old women's oocytes (18.9 ± 0.2 μm). The oocytes of < 13-year old girls had the smallest nuclei (17.8 ± 0.2 μm).

The results of our study correspond partially to Westergard et al.'s [23] results. The diameter and the area of primordial ovarian follicles, the diameter and the area of primary oocytes and their nuclei increased in Lithuanian women from 15 to 35 years, and then these parameters declined with age.

According to our study, the hypothesis can be made that the negative changes of aging begin in primordial ovarian follicles and their primary oocytes in Lithuanian women older than 35 years. Therefore, it can be recommended that women should plan pregnancy up to 35 years of age. Subsequently, negative changes begin in oocytes, and this may be one of the causes of decreased fertility and increased birth defects.

In results of our study, the morphometrical parameters of Lithuanian women's primordial ovarian follicles were similar to those of women in the USA, but different than those of women in France and Denmark. Primary oocytes in Lithuanian women's primordial ovarian follicles had a larger diameter and area in comparison with these parameters in women from the USA, France and Denmark. Primary oocytes in Lithuanian women had smaller nuclei than in French, Danish and Dutch women.

It can be concluded that morphometrical parameters of primordial follicles and their primary oocytes can vary according to the country and the region in which women live.

Conclusions

1. The diameter and the area of primordial ovarian follicles, the diameter and the area of primary oocytes and their nuclei increased in Lithuanian women from 15 to 35 years; then these parameters began to decrease.
2. The thickness of the follicular basement membrane increased in primordial ovarian follicles of 15–46-year old Lithuanian women with age.

Table 2 The morphometric parameters of primordial follicles of left and right ovaries in 15–46 year old women (mean ± SD)

Age	Ovary	Follicles		Basement membrane thickness, µm	Oocytes			Oocytes nuclei			Follicular cells			p values between the same parameter of left and right ovaries
		Diameter, µm	Area, µm²		Diameter, µm	Area, µm²	Oocyte:follicle area ratio	Diameter, µm	Area, µm²	Nucleus:oocyte area ratio	Length, µm	Height, µm	Height:lengh ratio	
15–20 years	Left	43.54 ± 0.54	1486.6 ± 38.45	1.28 ± 0.12	15.5 ± 0.21	187.27 ± 5.02	0.77	15.5 ± 0.21	187.27 ± 5.02	0.16	8.62 ± 0.13	2.6 ± 0.11	0.3	p > 0.5
	Right	43.57 ± 0.35	1489 ± 26.45	1.3 ± 0.11	15.49 ± 0.2	187.05 ± 4.93	0.77	15.49 ± 0.2	187.05 ± 4.93	0.16	8.67 ± 0.14	2.63 ± 0.14	0.3	
21–25 years	Left	44.59 ± 0.34	1554.7 ± 24.16	1.34 ± 0.07	15.54 ± 0.15	188.48 ± 3.67	0.78	15.54 ± 0.15	188.48 ± 3.67	0.16	8.67 ± 0.17	2.65 ± 0.07	0.31	p > 0.5
	Right	44.52 ± 0.35	1559.4 ± 24.06	1.33 ± 0.04	15.54 ± 0.16	188.55 ± 3.85	0.78	15.54 ± 0.16	188.55 ± 3.85	0.16	8.73 ± 0.12	2.67 ± 0.11	0.31	
26–30 years	Left	44.61 ± 0.37	1560.5 ± 25.51	1.37 ± 0.07	15.59 ± 0.15	189.54 ± 3.77	0.78	15.59 ± 0.15	189.54 ± 3.77	0.16	8.71 ± 0.14	2.69 ± 0.08	0.31	p > 0.5
	Right	44.66 ± 0.36	1564.3 ± 25.36	1.38 ± 0.08	15.59 ± 0.14	189.56 ± 3.56	0.78	15.59 ± 0.14	189.56 ± 3.56	0.16	8.72 ± 0.09	2.67 ± 0.13	0.31	
31–35 years	Left	44.7 ± 0.4	1569 ± 30.23	1.39 ± 0.08	15.32 ± 0.4	183.33 ± 12.2	0.78	15.32 ± 0.4	183.33 ± 12.2	0.15	8.72 ± 0.3	2.7 ± 0.24	0.31	p > 0.5
	Right	44.73 ± 0.37	1569.6 ± 27.91	1.4 ± 0.09	15.3 ± 0.41	182.81 ± 11.56	0.78	15.3 ± 0.41	182.81 ± 11.56	0.15	8.73 ± 0.24	2.69 ± 0.19	0.31	
36–40 years	Left	43.8 ± 0.66	1505.1 ± 48.6	1.42 ± 0.13	14.82 ± 0.37	171.78 ± 10.12	0.77	14.82 ± 0.37	171.78 ± 10.12	0.15	8.6 ± 0.25	2.6 ± 0.3	0.3	p > 0.5
	Right	43.83 ± 0.48	1507.5 ± 35.15	1.44 ± 0.17	14.92 ± 0.48	174.2 ± 12.96	0.77	14.92 ± 0.48	174.2 ± 12.96	0.15	8.62 ± 0.27	2.58 ± 0.26	0.3	
41–46 years	Left	43.52 ± 0.55	1485.5 ± 39.29	1.45 ± 0.18	14.65 ± 0.4	167.38 ± 10.99	0.78	14.65 ± 0.4	167.38 ± 10.99	0.15	8.54 ± 0.37	2.61 ± 0.37	0.31	p > 0.5
	Right	43.57 ± 0.38	1490.3 ± 36.18	1.41 ± 0.19	14.69 ± 0.6	169.0 ± 15.74	0.78	14.69 ± 0.6	169.0 ± 15.74	0.15	8.58 ± 0.49	2.62 ± 0.42	0.31	

3. The length and the height of follicular cells differed insignificantly in different age groups of Lithuanian women ($p > 0.05$).

4. No differences were observed in the morphometrical parameters of primordial follicles, primary oocytes and their nuclei and follicular cells of left and right ovaries in women of all age groups ($p > 0.5$).

Acknowledgements
We would like to thank the technical staff of the Department of Histology and Embryology for the help with histological slides making.

Funding
Lithuanian University of Health Sciences financially supported this work.

Authors' contributions
KL designed the study, interpreted the data and wrote the draft of the manuscript. DG provided the material (ovaries) for this study. NJ and AV revised the manuscript. All the authors approved the final version of the manuscript.

Competing interests
The authors declare that they have no competing interests.

Author details
[1]Department of Histology and Embryology, Medical Academy, Lithuanian University of Health Sciences, A. Mickevicius str. 9, LT-44307 Kaunas, Lithuania. [2]Kaunas Division of State Forensic Medicine Service, Perlojos str. 28, LT-45305 Kaunas, Lithuania. [3]Department of Veterinary Pathobiology, Veterinary Academy, Lithuanian University of Health Sciences, Tilzes str. 18, LT-47181 Kaunas, Lithuania.

References
1. Stanková J, Cech S. Ultrastructural changes during atresia in human ovarian follicles. I. Primordial follicles. Z Für Mikrosk-Anat Forsch. 1983;97:915–28.
2. Fortune JE, Cushman RA, Wahl CM, Kito S. The primordial to primary follicle transition. Mol Cell Endocrinol. 2000;163:53–60.
3. Hurk RV, Abir R, Telfer EE, Bevers MM. Primate and bovine immature oocytes and follicles as sources of fertilizable oocytes. Hum Reprod Update. 2000;6:457–74.
4. Andersen CY, Kristensen SG, Greve T, Schmidt KT. Cryopreservation of ovarian tissue for fertility preservation in young female oncological patients. Future Oncol. 2012;8:595–608.
5. Sørensen SD, Greve T, Wielenga VT, Wallace WHB, Andersen CY. Safety considerations for transplanting cryopreserved ovarian tissue to restore fertility in female patients who have recovered from Ewing's sarcoma. Future Oncol. 2014;10:277–83.
6. Bastings L, Beerendonk CCM, Westphal JR, Massuger LF a G, Kaal SEJ, van Leeuwen FE, et al. Autotransplantation of cryopreserved ovarian tissue in cancer survivors and the risk of reintroducing malignancy: a systematic review. Hum Reprod Update. 2013;19:483–506.
7. Suzuki N, Yoshioka N, Takae S, Sugishita Y, Tamura M, Hashimoto S, et al. Successful fertility preservation following ovarian tissue vitrification in patients with primary ovarian insufficiency. Hum Reprod Oxf Engl. 2015;30:608–15.
8. Dittrich R, Hackl J, Lotz L, Hoffmann I, Beckmann MW. Pregnancies and live births after 20 transplantations of cryopreserved ovarian tissue in a single center. Fertil Steril. 2015;103:462–8.
9. Dittrich R, Lotz L, Keck G, Hoffmann I, Mueller A, Beckmann MW, et al. Live birth after ovarian tissue autotransplantation following overnight transportation before cryopreservation. Fertil Steril. 2012;97:387–90.
10. Müller A, Keller K, Wacker J, Dittrich R, Keck G, Montag M, et al. Retransplantation of cryopreserved ovarian tissue: the first live birth in Germany. Dtsch Ärztebl Int. 2012;109:8–13.
11. Donnez J, Silber S, Andersen CY, Demeestere I, Piver P, Meirow D, et al. Children born after autotransplantation of cryopreserved ovarian tissue. A review of 13 live births. Ann Med. 2011;43:437–50.
12. Revelli A, Marchino G, Dolfin E, Molinari E, Delle Piane L, Salvagno F, et al. Live birth after orthotopic grafting of autologous cryopreserved ovarian tissue and spontaneous conception in Italy. Fertil Steril. 2013;99:227–30.
13. Gougeon A, Chainy GBN. Morphometric studies of small follicles in ovaries of women at different ages. J Reprod Fertil. 1987;81:433–42.
14. Sathananthan AH, Selvaraj K, Girijashankar ML, Ganesh V, Selvaraj P, Trounson AO. From oogonia to mature oocytes: inactivation of the maternal centrosome in humans. Microsc Res Tech. 2006;69:396–407.
15. Bruin JP, de Dorland M, Spek ER, Posthuma G, van Haaften M, CWN L, et al. Age-related changes in the ultrastructure of the resting follicle pool in human ovaries. Biol Reprod. 2004;70:419–24.
16. Bruin JP, de Dorland M, Spek ER, Posthuma G, van Haaften M, CWN L, et al. Ultrastructure of the resting ovarian follicle pool in healthy young women. Biol Reprod. 2002;66:1151–60.
17. Hertig AT, Adams EC. Studies on the human oocyte and its follicle. I. Ultrastructural and histochemical observations on the primordial follicle stage. J Cell Biol. 1967;34:647–75.
18. Paulini F, Silva RC, de Paula Rôlo JLJ, Lucci CM. Ultrastructural changes in oocytes during folliculogenesis in domestic mammals. J Ovarian Res. 2014;7:102.
19. Bancroft JD, Gamble M. Theory and practice of histological techniques. 5th ed: Churchill Livingstone Elsevier; 2002.
20. Suvarna K, Layton C, Bancroft JD. Bancroft's theory and practice of histological techniques. 7th ed: Churchill Livingstone Elsevier; 2012.
21. Pujar A, Pereira T, Tamgadge A, Bhalerao S, Tamgadge S. Comparing the efficacy of hematoxylin and eosin, periodic acid schiff and fluorescent periodic acid schiff-acriflavine techniques for demonstration of basement membrane in oral lichen planus: a histochemical study. Indian J Dermatol. 2015;60:450–6.
22. Griffin J, Emery BR, Huang I, Peterson CM, Carrell DT. Comparative analysis of follicle morphology and oocyte diameter in four mammalian species (mouse, hamster, pig, and human). J Exp Clin Assist Reprod. 2006;3:2.
23. Westergaard CG, Byskov AG, Andersen CY. Morphometric characteristics of the primordial to primary follicle transition in the human ovary in relation to age. Hum Reprod. 2007;22:2225–31.

2

Influencing factors of pregnancy loss and survival probability of clinical pregnancies conceived through assisted reproductive technology

Lingmin Hu[1,3†], Jiangbo Du[2,3†], Hong Lv[2,3†], Jing Zhao[3,4], Mengxi Chen[3,4], Yifeng Wang[2,3], Fang Wu[2,3], Feng Liu[2,3], Xiaojiao Chen[3,4], Junqiang Zhang[3,4], Hongxia Ma[2,3], Guangfu Jin[2,3], Hongbing Shen[2,3], Li Chen[1,3*], Xiufeng Ling[3,4*] and Zhibin Hu[2,3*]

Abstract

Background: Pregnancies following assisted reproductive technology (ART) may have elevated potential risk of pregnancy loss (PL) when compared to natural conception. However, rare studies comprehensively analyzed the IVF/ICSI cycle-dependent factors for loss of clinical pregnancy. Therefore, we aimed to determine the ART subgroup-specific risks of PL throughout pregnancy and explore different risk factors for early miscarriage and late miscarriage among pregnancies conceived through ART.

Methods: A retrospective cohort study was launched in two infertility treatment centers in Nanjing and Changzhou including 5485 IVF/ICSI embryo transfer cycles with known outcomes after clinical pregnancy by the end of 2015. Cox proportional hazards regression analysis was performed to estimate the hazard ratios and their 95% confidence intervals. The associations between survival time during pregnancy and demographics and clinical characteristics of clinical pregnancies were estimated using the Kaplan-Meier method and the Log-rank test.

Results: The overall PL rate in current ART population was 12.5%. Among the 685 pregnancy loss cycles, a total of 460 ended as early miscarriage, 191 as late miscarriage. We found couples in ART pregnancies demonstrated a significantly increased risk of PL as maternal age (HR = 1.31, P_{trend} < 0.001) grows. Pregnancies received controlled ovarian hyperstimulation (COH) protocol like GnRH antagonist protocol (HR = 3.49, P < 0.001) and minimal stimulation protocol (HR = 1.83, P < 0.001) had higher risk of PL than GnRH-a long protocol. Notably, in contrast to fresh cycle, women who received frozen cycle embryo had a significant increased risk of early miscarriage (P < 0.001), while frozen cycle was linked with lower risk of late miscarriage (P = 0.045). In addition, four factors (maternal age, COH protocol, cycle type and serum hCG level 14 days after transfer) had independent impact on miscarriage mainly before 12 weeks of gestational age.

(Continued on next page)

* Correspondence: zhibin_hu@njmu.edu.cn; lingxiufeng_njfy@163.com; shaoshan686@163.com

†Lingmin Hu, Jiangbo Du and Hong Lv contributed equally to this work.
[1]Department of Reproduction, the Affiliated Changzhou Maternity and Child Health Care, Hospital of Nanjing Medical University, Changzhou 213003, Jiangsu, China
[3]State Key Laboratory of Reproductive Medicine, Nanjing Medical University, Nanjing 211166, China
[2]Department of Epidemiology, School of Public Health, Nanjing Medical University, Nanjing 211166, China
Full list of author information is available at the end of the article

(Continued from previous page)

Conclusions: With these findings in this study, clinicians may make it better to evaluate a patient's risk of PL based on the maternal age at the time of treatment, COH protocol, cycle type and serum hCG level 14 days after transfer and the gestational week of the fetus, and we hope that it contributes to future study on its etiology and guide the clinical prevention and treatment.

Keywords: Abortion, Spontaneous, Reproductive techniques, Assisted, Kaplan-Meier estimate

Background

Nearly one in six couples will encounter with fertility problems, defined as failure to achieve a clinical pregnancy for 12-month delay [1]. Steadily increasing numbers of couples are turning to assisted reproductive technology (ART) for help, such as in vitro fertilization (IVF) or intracytoplasmic sperm injection (ICSI), conceiving and ultimately giving birth to a healthy live baby of their own. Although the clinical pregnancy rate was gradually improved over the past decade, up to 46.9% reported to Centers for Disease Control (CDC) in the United States by the end of 2012, but the rate of live birth was still low, only 38.1% [2]. Therefore, pregnancy loss (PL), including the loss of a desired pregnancy by miscarriage, stillbirth or termination for genetic indications [3], significantly threatens the rate of live-birth delivery.

The PL rate in natural conception was reported 10%-16% [4–6], while ART pregnancies might have increased potential probability of loss [2, 5, 7]. Data on 148,494 ART pregnancies in United States conceived from 1999 through 2002 had indicated that the PL rate in ART was up to 29% [7]. The potential risk of pregnancy loss in natural conceived conception was mainly determined by elder maternal age (≥35 years) [8], overweight or obese [9], history of abortion [4], microbial infections [10] and elevated reproductive hormones [11]. As for ART population, the elevated potential risk of loss had also been related to some potentially factors specific to women with infertility, such as fresh or frozen cycle type, uterine factor [12], polycystic ovary syndrome (PCOS) status [13]. However, additional unknown barriers may affect the efficiency of ART treatment and require further research. Therefore, it is essential to determine IVF/ICSI cycle-dependent factors for miscarriage and stillbirth, which has important clinical implications for the ART success rates elevation and may help understand possible mechanisms of abortion, thereby improving assisted reproduction technology and strategy.

Miscarriage or spontaneous abortion (SA) is defined as the spontaneous loss of a pregnancy during the first 24 completed weeks of gestational age and it accounted for 80% of fetal losses. Early miscarriage refers to pregnancy loss before 12 weeks of gestational age, while late miscarriage occurs between 12 weeks and 24 weeks [10]. Previous studies revealed that causative factors differed in early miscarriages and late miscarriages, and most early miscarriages resulted from aneuploidy that was greatly influenced by total parental age [14], while late miscarriages were attributed to antiphospholipid syndrome, congenital uterine anomalies, cervical weakness, infection and placental insufficiency [15]. Although many studies have assessed risk factors for early miscarriage in ART pregnancies [12, 16, 17], rare large scale studies have explored the risk factor differences between early SA and late SA among pregnancies conceived through ART. This led us to investigate different risk factors between them, which may be applied to counsel ART pregnant women about their risk time period of SA and help clarify the pathogenesis of miscarriage in order to guide the clinical prevention and ART effective treatment. In addition, previous studies utilizing cross-sectional data only discussed the relation of risk factors and miscarriages, but these studies did not explain the effect of time on ART outcomes.

Therefore, the objectives of current study were to examine PL rates and IVF/ICSI cycle-dependent factors influencing live birth probability as pregnancy progresses on specific subgroups by survival analysis method and investigate the different risks of early miscarriage and late miscarriage after following IVF/ICSI treatment.

Methods

By the end of 2015, a total of 5856 embryo transfer (ET) cycles carried out and resulted in clinical pregnancies in Reproductive Medicine Center of the Affiliated Nanjing Maternity and Child Health Hospital of Nanjing Medical University (Nanjing) and Reproductive Medicine Center of the Affiliated Changzhou Maternity and Child Health Care Hospital of Nanjing Medical University (Changzhou). We restricted the analysis to cycles with records about final pregnancy outcome (pregnancy loss or live-birth). We excluded donor/preimplantation genetic diagnosis (PGD)/preimplantation genetic screening (PGS) cycles ($N = 2$) and natural ET cycles ($N = 18$). In addition, cycles were excluded if patients were diagnosed with abnormal karyotypes ($N = 23$) or uterine anomalies like fibroids, persistent müllerian duct syndrome or asherman syndrome ($N = 87$). 241 cycles were excluded because of missing data of gestational weeks. After all exclusions, 4165 cycles in Nanjing and 1320 in Changzhou were available for analysis.

Detailed information on maternal and paternal characteristics, ART treatment procedures were collected from the electronic medical records of the two reproductive centers. The pregnancy outcomes were obtained from the follow-up database. Pregnancy was defined as positive serum human chorionic gonadotropin (hCG) level on day 14 after oocyte retrieval, and clinical pregnancy referred to visualization of a gestational sac on ultrasound 3-4weeks after positive hCG test. The gestational week was equal to survival months during pregnancy.

The risk factors for pregnancy loss investigated in this study were maternal age, maternal BMI (body mass index, kg/m^2), paternal BMI, infertility type, controlled ovarian hyperstimulation (COH) protocol, the total gonadotropin (Gn) dose, fertilization methods, cycle type, no. of embryos transferred, cleavage-stage embryo or blastocyst, serum hCG level 14 days after transfer (IU/L).

Maternal age, maternal BMI, paternal BMI and no. of embryos transferred were categorized for the clarity of data analysis. Maternal age was divided into four subgroups (<30 years, 30-35 years, 36-40 years, >40years). Maternal BMI and paternal BMI subgroups were: <18.5 kg/m^2, 18.5-24.9 kg/m^2, 25-28 kg/m^2, >28 kg/m^2. Primary infertility was defined as the inability to achieve a clinical pregnancy after 12 months of unprotected and regular sexual intercourse when a woman has never conceived, while secondary infertility was the incapability to conceive in a couple who have had at least one successful clinical pregnancy previously. Three subgroups of no. of embryos transferred were: Group 1(1 embryo transferred), Group 2 (2 embryos transferred) and Group 3 (3 embryos transferred). Depending on the usage of a gonadotropin-releasing hormone agonist (GnRH-a) versus antagonist analogue, GnRH analogue ART protocols are classified as GnRH-a or GnRH antagonist protocols. Among the various GnRH-a protocols, including long, short and rolonged protocol, GnRH-a long protocol is the most conventional protocol. Another protocol utilizes the usage of clomiphene citrate (CC) in combination with Gn, which is termed minimal stimulation protocol. Thus, COH protocols were divided into six categories in this study, including GnRH-a long protocol, GnRH-a short protocol, GnRH antagonist protocol, minimal stimulation protocol, GnRH-a rolonged protocol and other protocol. Besides among them, GnRH antagonist protocol was not utilized in Changzhou, and they only transferred cleavage-stage embryos. 2 days and 3 days embryo before transfer belong to cleavage-stage embryo, while 5 days and 6 days embryo before transfer belong to blastocyst.

Statistical methods

Demographics and clinical characteristics of pregnancies conceived through ART were calculated by chi-square test. The distributions of continuous variables were evaluated by using Wilcox-test. The associations between survival time during pregnancy and demographics and clinical characteristics of clinical pregnancies were estimated using the Kaplan-Meier method and the Log-rank test. Cox proportional hazards regression analysis was performed to estimate the hazard ratio (HR) and 95% confidence interval (CI). P values were given for two-sided tests and statistical significance was defined by $P < 0.05$. Superscript asterisk (*) was added after P values with significnce in Tables. Pregnancy survival curves were constructed by the Kaplan-Meier method [18]. Pregnancies were right-censored at completion of the 26th week, because above 98% pregnancy loss were occurred before the 26th week while all of live births occurred between 26 and 42 weeks' gestation. All the statistical analyses were carried out by R software (Version 3.0.2, 2013-09-25; R Foundation for Statistical Computing, http://www.cran.r-project.org/).

Results

Demographics and clinical characteristics of clinical pregnancies

Table 1 summarized demographics and clinical characteristics of clinical pregnancies conceived through ART and compared the differences of these demographics and clinical characteristics between Nanjing and Changzhou. We found that compared with clinical pregnancies in Nanjing, those in Changzhou had significantly higher maternal age (30.42±4.03 vs. 29.89±4.03, $P < 0.001$), and serum hCG level 14 days after transfer (861.75±568.97 vs. 619.49 ±470.08, $P < 0.001$), lower the total Gn dose in cycle (1728.88±788.45 vs. 1833.67±613.50, $P < 0.001$). The mean of total Gn dose in cycle and serum HCG level 14 days after transfer were 1808.01 IU and 695.30 IU/L respectively, thereby setting as the cutoff values. Besides, there were statistically highly significant distribution differences of six COH protocols, fertilization methods, cycle type, no. of embryos transferred and cleavage-stage embryo or blastocyst among pregnancies between Nanjing and Changzhou (all $P < 0.001$), whereas no difference of infertility type , maternal BMI and paternal BMI were found.

Factors influencing live birth probability throughout gestational weeks

As shown in Table 2, the overall rate of pregnancy loss in IVF/ICSI clinical pregnancies was 12.5% (685/5485). Maternal age, maternal BMI, COH protocol, cycle type, no. of embryos transferred and cleavage-stage embryo or blastocyst were significantly associated with the survival time during pregnancy by log-rank test after adjusted by maternal age (all log-rank $P < 0.05$, data not shown).

We found couples in ART pregnancies demonstrated a significantly increased risk of PL as maternal age

Table 1 Demographics and clinical characteristics of clinical pregnancies conceived through ART

Variables	Total	Nanjing	Changzhou	P
Total number	5485	4165	1320	
Maternal age	30.01 ± 4.03	29.89 ± 4.03	30.42 ± 4.03	<0.001*
Maternal BMI	22.08 ± 3.03	22.04 ± 2.99	22.21 ± 3.16	0.227
Paternal BMI	24.23 ± 3.09	24.18 ± 2.98	24.37 ± 3.39	0.131
Infertility type				0.593
Primary	2781(53.0%)	2165(52.8%)	616(53.7%)	
Secondary	2466(47.0%)	1935(47.2%)	531(46.3%)	
COH protocol				<0.001*
GnRH-a long protocol	3406(63.1%)	2311(56.7%)	1095(83.0%)	
GnRH-a short protocol	1573(29.2%)	1448(35.5%)	125(9.5%)	
GnRH antagonist protocol	95(1.8%)	95(2.3%)	0(0.0%)	
Minimal stimulation protocol	186(3.4%)	111(2.7%)	75(5.7%)	
GnRH-a rolonged protocol	123(2.3%)	108(2.6%)	15(1.1%)	
Other protocol	13(0.2%)	4(0.1%)	9(0.7%)	
Total Gn dose	1808.01 ± 662.11	1833.67 ± 613.50	1728.88 ± 788.45	<0.001*
Groups of total Gn dose				<0.001*
< 1808.01	3181(59.0%)	2344(57.6%)	837(63.4%)	
≥ 1808.01	2208(41.0%)	1725(42.4%)	483(36.6%)	
Fertilization methods				<0.001*
IVF	4543(83.9%)	3641(88.8%)	902(68.3%)	
ICSI	875(16.1%)	457(11.2%)	418(31.7%)	
Cycle type				<0.001*
Fresh	2675(51.9%)	2202(57.5%)	473(35.8%)	
Frozen	2477(48.1%)	1630(42.5%)	847(64.2%)	
No. of embryos transferred				<0.001*
1	474(8.7%)	442(10.7%)	32(2.4%)	
2	4324(79.6%)	3088(75.0%)	1236(93.6%)	
3	655(11.5%)	585(14.2%)	52(3.9%)	
Cleavage-stage embryo or blastocyst				
Cleavage-stage embryo	3860(73.3%)	2540(64.4%)	1320(100.0%)	
Blastocyst	1405(26.7%)	1405(35.6%)	0(0.0%)	
Serum hCG levels 14 days after transfer	695.30 ± 515.44	619.49 ± 470.08	861.75 ± 568.97	<0.001*
Groups of serum hCG levels 14 days after transfer				<0.001*
< 695.30	2205(52.2%)	1598(55.5%)	607(46.3%)	
≥ 695.30	1988(47.8%)	1283(44.5%)	705(53.7%)	

(HR=1.31, 95% CI=1.17-1.45, P_{trend}<0.001) grows when age was divided into four subgroups. Moreover, compared with women <30 years old, those aged 36-40 years (HR=1.63, 95% CI=1.28-2.08, P < 0.001) and older than 40 years (HR=4.14, 95% CI=2.63-6.52, P < 0.001) had significantly shorter survival pregnancy weeks. Besides, obese women (BMI≥28, HR=1.52, 95% CI=1.11-2.10, P = 0.010) tended to have higher risk of PL compared with the normal BMI group (BMI=18.5-25), yet there was significant heterogeneity for maternal BMI (BMI≥28) in two reproductive medicine centers (Nanjing and Changzhou) based on heterogeneity test (P for heterogeneity test was 0.02) (Additional file 1: Table S1). What's more, pregnancies received COH protocol like GnRH antagonist protocol (HR=3.49, 95% CI=2.46-4.94, P < 0.001) and minimal stimulation protocol (HR=1.83, 95% CI=1.31-2.54, P < 0.001) had higher risk of PL than GnRH-a long protocol.

Cycle type was significantly associated with the survival time during pregnancy by Cox analysis adjusted for maternal age as well (Log-rank P < 0.001). Notable, the

Table 2 Cox analysis of risk of pregnancy loss throughout pregnancy in ART clinical pregnancies

Variables	No. of PL/total (685/ 5485)	PL rate	HR (95% CI)[a]	p^a
Maternal age				
< 30	292/2556	11.4%	1.00[Reference]	
30–35	283/2361	12.0%	1.06(0.90–1.25)	0.508
36–40	84/472	17.8%	1.63(1.28–2.08)	<0.001*
> 40	20/53	37.7%	4.14(2.63–6.52)	<0.001*
P_{trend}			1.31(1.17–1.45)	<0.001*
Maternal BMI				
< 18.5	50/509	9.8%	0.85(0.63–1.13)	0.260
18.5–25	487/4009	12.1%	1.00[Reference]	
25–28	97/641	15.1%	1.24(1.00–1.55)	0.051
≥ 28	42/235	17.9%	1.52(1.11–2.10)	0.010*
Paternal BMI				
< 18.5	9/103	8.7%	0.67(0.33–1.35)	0.264
18.5–25	405/3309	12.2%	1.00[Reference]	
25–28	189/1344	14.1%	1.15(0.96–1.37)	0.120
≥ 28	69/603	12.3%	0.95(0.74–1.23)	0.691
Infertility type				
Primary	337/2781	12.1%	1.00[Reference]	
Secondary	319/2466	12.9%	0.99(0.85–1.16)	0.908
COH protocol[d]				
GnRH-a long protocol	391/3406	11.5%	1.00[Reference]	
GnRH-a short protocol	186/1573	11.8%	0.93(0.77–1.11)	0.373
GnRH antagonist protocol	35/95	36.8%	3.49(2.46–4.94)	<0.001*
Minimal stimulation protocol	44/186	23.7%	1.83(1.31–2.54)	<0.001*
GnRH-a rolonged protocol	12/123	9.8%	0.84(0.48–1.50)	0.689
Other protocol	5/13	38.5%	3.70(1.53–8.95)	0.004*
The total Gn dose[b]				
< 1808.01	373/3181	11.7%	1.00[Reference]	
≥ 1808.01	301/2208	13.6%	1.12(0.96–1.30)	0.161
Fertilization methods				
IVF	579/4543	12.7%	1.00[Reference]	
ICSI	98/875	11.2%	0.87(0.70–1.08)	0.205
Cycle type				
Fresh	282/2675	10.5%	1.00[Reference]	
Frozen	337/2477	13.6%	1.30(1.11–1.53)	0.001*
No. of embryos transferred				
1	82/474	17.3%	1.00[Reference]	
2	516/4324	11.9%	0.71(0.56–0.90)	0.005*
3	84/637	13.2%	0.67(0.49–0.91)	0.010*
P_{trend}			0.81(0.69–0.96)	0.012*
Cleavage-stage embryo or blastocyst[d]				
Cleavage-stage embryo	466/3860	12.1%	1.00[Reference]	

Table 2 Cox analysis of risk of pregnancy loss throughout pregnancy in ART clinical pregnancies *(Continued)*

Variables	No. of PL/total (685/ 5485)	PL rate	HR (95% CI)[a]	P[a]
Blastocyst	198/1405	14.1%	1.10(1.01–1.19)	*0.030*[*]
Serum hCG levels 14 days after transfer[c]				
< 695.30	334/2205	15.1%	1.00[Reference]	
≥ 695.30	115/1988	5.8%	0.36(0.29–0.45)	*<0.001*[*]

[a]Adjusted for maternal age
[b]The cutoff value was the mean of total Gn dose in cycle
[c]The cutoff value was the mean of serum hCG levels 14 days after transfer
[d]GnRH antagonist protocol was not utilized in Changzhou, and they only transferred cleavage-stage embryos

risk of loss increased after frozen cycles (HR=1.30, 95% CI=1.11-1.53, P = 0.001). However, heterogeneity was also significant for cycle type (P = 0.011) between two reproductive medicine centers (Nanjing and Changzhou). After two and three embryos transfer, couples demonstrated 29% (HR=0.71, 95% CI=056-0.90, P = 0.005) and 33% (HR=0.67, 95% CI=0.49-0.91, P = 0.010) decreased risk of PL than those after one embryos transfer. And, a significant locus-dosage effect was detected between three groups and risk of PL (adjusted HR=0.81, 95% CI=0.69-0.96, P_{trend}=0.012). In addition, pregnancies after blastocyst transfer had higher risk than those after cleavage-stage embryo transfer after accounting for maternal age (HR=1.10, 95% CI=1.01-1.19, P = 0.030). However, after stratification analysis, we found only cleavage-stage embryos were transferred in Changzhou and the difference was no more significant. Moreover, on day 14 after transfer, women with hCG≥695.30 IU/L had an HR of 0.36 (95% CI=0.29-0.45, P < 0.001) compared to those with hCG lower than 695.30 IU/L.

To get insight into the independent effects of characteristics and clinical features of pregnancies on survival time during ART pregnancy, we performed stepwise backward Cox proportional hazard analysis. As shown in Table 3, four independent factors were determined, including maternal age (compared with maternal age<30, P = 0.027 for maternal age between 36 and 40 years, P < 0.001 for maternal age>40 years), COH protocol (compared with GnRH-a long protocol, P value<0.001 for both GnRH antagonist protocol and mini-stimulation protocol), cycle type (P = 0.030) and serum hCG level 14 days after transfer (P < 0.001). Kaplan-Meier plots of live birth by maternal age, COH protocol, cycle type and serum hCG level 14 days after transfer were shown in Fig. 1.

Risk factors for early miscarriage and late miscarriage

In Table 4, among the 685 pregnancy loss cycles, a total of 460 ended as early SA, 191 as late SA. The rate of early miscarriage in ART clinical pregnancies was 8.4% (460/ 5485) while the rate of late miscarriage in ART clinical pregnancies after 12 weeks of gestational age was 3.8% (191/5025). Of those clinical pregnancies, women aged

36-40 years (HR=2.14, 95% CI=1.62-2.83, P < 0.001) and over 40 years (HR=6.04, 95% CI=3.76-9.69, P < 0.001) were more likely to encounter early pregnancy loss in contrast to those younger than 30 years old. Besides, treated by GnRH antagonist and minimal stimulation COH protocol (both P < 0.001), blastocyst transferred (P = 0.006), and frozen embryo transferred (P < 0.001) were more likely to encounter early pregnancy loss. What's more, there was a significant decrease of risk of early SA in pregnancies after two embryos transferred compared with those following one embryo transfer (P < 0.001). Serum hCG level at higher level on day 14 after transfer was linked with a significant 78% and 32% decreased risk of early SA and late SA (P < 0.001). Moreover, maternal BMI≥28 had a positive impact on late PL rather than early PL. Notably, in contrast to fresh cycle, women who received frozen cycle embryo had a significant decrease of risk of late SA (P = 0.045), while frozen cycle was linked with higher risk of early PL. After stepwise backward Cox proportional hazard analysis, we found that maternal age, COH protocol, cycle type and hCG level 14 days after transfer had independent effects on live birth probability of ART clinical pregnancies before 12 weeks of gestational age (In Table 5). However, none of factors for PL investigated in this study had independent effects on late miscarriage (data not shown).

Discussion

This retrospective cohort study on the risk of PL throughout ART pregnancy included 5485 ART clinical pregnancies with data of gestational weeks, 685 of which suffered pregnancy loss. The main findings of this study were that maternal age, COH protocol, cycle type and hCG level 14 days after transfer significantly affected the reproductive pregnancy loss of ART population. Besides, the incidence of PL decreased as pregnancy progresses, early SA therefore occurred more frequently than the late one. To our knowledge, this is the first retrospective cohort study to extensively explore the different risk factors of early miscarriage and late miscarriage after IVF/ICSI.

The negative effect of maternal reproductive age on the risk of PL has been consistently reported and studied

Table 3 Stepwise Cox regression analysis on live birth probability of ART clinical pregnancies

Variables	β^a	SE^b	HR	95% CI	P
Maternal age (reference: <30)					
30–35	0.0733	0.1102	1.08	0.87–1.34	0.506
36–40	0.3758	0.1697	1.46	1.04–2.03	*0.027*[*]
> 40	1.1000	0.3222	3.00	1.60–5.65	*<0.001*[*]
COH protocol (reference: GnRH-a long protocol)					
GnRH-a short protocol	0.0326	0.1191	1.03	0.82–1.30	0.784
GnRH antagonist protocol	0.8914	0.2698	2.44	1.44–4.14	*<0.001*[*]
Minimal stimulation protocol	0.7869	0.2152	2.20	1.44–3.35	*<0.001*[*]
GnRH-a rolonged protocol	−0.1192	0.4160	0.89	0.39–2.01	0.774
Other protocol	1.3692	0.5070	3.93	1.46–10.62	*0.007*[*]
Cycle Type (reference: Fresh)					
Frozen	0.2296	0.1057	1.26	1.02–1.55	*0.030*[*]
Serum hCG levels 14 days after transfer (reference: < 695.30)					
≥ 695.30	−1.0848	0.1180	0.34	0.27–0.43	*<0.001*[*]

HR hazard ratio, *CI* confidence interval
[a]β is the estimated parameter of the regression model
[b]SE is the standard error of the regression model

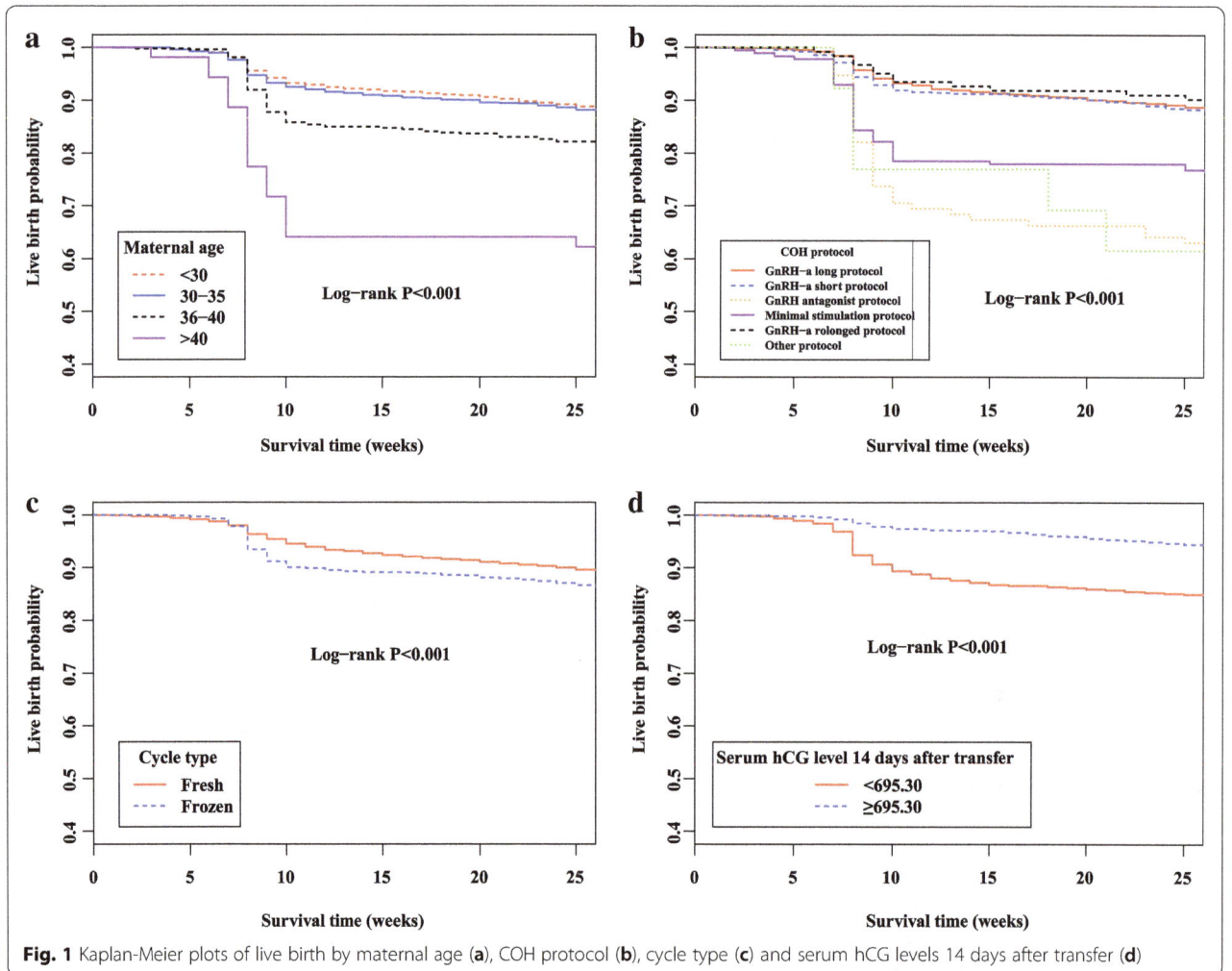

Fig. 1 Kaplan-Meier plots of live birth by maternal age (**a**), COH protocol (**b**), cycle type (**c**) and serum hCG levels 14 days after transfer (**d**)

Table 4 Comparison of early miscarriage and late miscarriage in ART clinical pregnancies

Variables	Early miscarriage				Late miscarriage			
	N[c] (%)	n (%)	HR (95%CI)[a]	P[a]	N[d] (%)	n (%)	HR (95%CI)[a]	P[a]
Maternal age								
< 30	2556(47.0)	180(39.5)	1.00		2376(47.7)	94(49.7)	1.00	
30–35	2361(43.4)	188(41.2)	1.14(0.93–1.40)	0.215	2173(43.6)	80(42.3)	0.93(0.69–1.25)	0.630
36–40	472(8.7)	69(15.1)	2.14(1.62–2.83)	<0.001*	403(8.1)	15(7.9)	0.94(0.54–1.62)	0.823
> 40	53(1.0)	19(4.2)	6.04(3.76–9.69)	<0.001*	34(0.7)	0(0.0)	0	0.992
Maternal BMI								
< 18.5	509(9.4)	32(7.0)	0.82(0.57–1.18)	0.282	477(9.7)	15(8.1)	0.82(0.52–1.51)	0.647
18.5–25	4009(74.3)	335(73.3)	1.00		3674(74.4)	130(70.3)	1.00	
25–28	641(11.9)	65(14.2)	1.19(0.91–1.55)	0.205	576(11.7)	24(13.0)	1.20(0.78–1.86)	0.407
≥28	235(4.4)	25(5.5)	1.35(0.90–2.03)	0.145	210(4.3)	16(8.6)	2.09(1.22–3.57)	0.007*
Paternal BMI								
< 18.5	103(1.9)	8(1.8)	1.07(0.53–2.16)	0.859	95(1.9)	1(0.5)	0.00(0.00 – +∞)	0.992
18.5–25	3309(61.7)	266(58.6)	1.00		3043(62.0)	120(64.9)	1.00	
25–28	1344(25.1)	129(28.4)	1.17(0.95–1.45)	0.137	1215(24.8)	50(27.0)	1.06(0.76–1.48)	0.728
≥ 28	603(11.3)	51(11.2)	1.08(0.80–1.46)	0.616	552(11.3)	14(7.6)	0.64(0.37–1.12)	0.118
Infertility type								
Primary	2781(53.0)	227(51.1)	1.00		2554(53.2)	92(51.7)	1.00	
Secondary	2466(47.0)	217(48.9)	0.94(0.78–1.14)	0.544	2249(46.8)	86(48.3)	1.10(0.81–1.49)	0.538
COH protocol[b]								
GnRH-a long protocol	3406(63.1)	243(53.4)	1.00		3163(64.0)	125(67.9)	1.00	
GnRH-a short protocol	1573(29.2)	132(29.0)	1.00(0.80–1.26)	0.974	1441(29.2)	48(26.1)	0.85(0.60–1.21)	0.370
GnRH antagonist protocol	95(1.8)	29(6.4)	4.11(2.78–6.08)	<0.001*	66(1.3)	5(2.7)	1.95(0.80–4.78)	0.144
Minimal stimulation protocol	186(3.4)	40(8.8)	2.39(1.67–3.43)	<0.001*	146(3.0)	1(0.5)	0.18(0.02–1.29)	0.088
GnRH-a rolonged protocol	123(2.3)	8(1.8)	0.90(0.44–1.82)	0.765	115(2.3)	3(1.6)	0.67(0.21–2.11)	0.492
Other protocol	13(0.2)	3(0.7)	3.27(1.04–10.23)	0.042*	10(0.2)	2(1.1)	5.52(1.36–22.40)	0.017*
The total Gn dose								
< 1808.01	3181(59.0)	252(55.4)	1.00		2929(59.4)	104(56.2)	1.00	
≥ 1808.01	2208(41.0)	203(44.6)	1.08(0.89–1.30)	0.440	2005(40.6)	81(43.8)	1.15(0.86–1.54)	0.355
Fertilization methods								
IVF	4543(83.9)	386(84.6)	1.00		4157(83.8)	162(86.6)	1.00	
ICSI	875(16.1)	70(15.4)	0.93(0.72–1.20)	0.562	805(16.2)	25(13.4)	0.81(0.53–1.23)	0.320
Cycle type								
Fresh	2675(51.9)	161(39.1)	1.00		2514(53.0)	106(60.6)	1.00	
Frozen	2477(48.1)	251(60.9)	1.67(1.37–2.04)	<0.001*	2226(47.0)	69(39.4)	0.73(0.54–0.99)	0.045*
No. of embryos transferred								
1	474(8.7)	64(14.0)	1.00		410(8.2)	16(8.4)	1.00	
2	4324(79.6)	330(72.1)	0.61(0.47–0.80)	<0.001*	3994(80.2)	157(82.6)	0.99(0.59–1.65)	0.961
3	637(11.7)	64(14.0)	0.63(0.44–0.89)	0.010*	573(11.5)	17(8.9)	0.75(0.38–1.51)	0.425
Cleavage-stage embryo or blastocyst[b]								
Cleavage-stage embryo	3860(73.3)	305(68.2)	1.00		3555(73.8)	135(73.8)	1.00	
Blastocyst	1405(26.7)	142(31.8)	1.15(1.04–1.27)	0.006*	1263(26.2)	48(26.2)	1.00(0.85–1.18)	0.994

Table 4 Comparison of early miscarriage and late miscarriage in ART clinical pregnancies *(Continued)*

Variables	Early miscarriage				Late miscarriage			
	N[c] (%)	n (%)	HR (95%CI)[a]	P[a]	N[d] (%)	n (%)	HR (95%CI)[a]	P[a]
Serum hCG levels 14 days after transfer								
< 695.30	2187(52.2)	248(82.7)	1.00		1939(49.8)	79(59.8)	1.00	
≥ 695.30	2006(47.8)	52(17.3)	0.22(0.16–0.30)	<0.001*	1954(50.2)	53(40.2)	0.68(0.48–0.96)	0.030*

[a]Adjusted for maternal age
[b]GnRH antagonist protocol was not utilized in Changzhou, and they only transferred cleavage-stage embryos
[c]the number of clinical pregnancies
[d]the number of clinical pregnancies after 12 weeks of gestational age

in previous studies [19, 20]. Age of the female is the most important risk factor in determining pregnancy success rates both in natural conception and after ART [4]. It is partly because of obvious decline in ovarian germ cells supply, decrease in oocyte quality and ultimately leading to ovarian reproductive failure [21]. In this study, women>40 years old had approximately 37.7% PL rate, and they showed significant decline in survival probability of ART clinical pregnancies progressed to a live birth compared with those <30 years old. Some studies suggested that the decreased fecundity and fertility rate occurred due in part to decreased follicle reserves [22] and increased aneuploidy [23] in the older female. In addition, chromosome abnormality decreases as pregnancy progresses and occurs mostly before 12 weeks of pregnancy [14], which makes the association of older parental age with early SA credible. Now, pre-implantation genetic screening of embryos prior to transfer may reduce early pregnancy wastage resulting from aneuploidy, but safety and risks of the technology need further investigation.

Controlled ovarian hyperstimulation is a fundamental step of IVF/ICSI and over time IVF techniques have developed to satisfy the needs of fertility patients and the improvement of ART success rate. The present results suggest that for the purpose of increasing survival probabilities of ART pregnancies, the GnRH-a long protocol is a better option for IVF/ICSI stimulation compared to GnRH antagonist and minimal stimulation protocol. Using Gn and CC in ART cycles is associated with chromosomal abnormalities in an IVF embryo and subsequent early miscarriage after transfer [24]. Moreover, patients with poor ovarian reserve prefer considering minimal stimulation protocol, and GnRH antagonist protocols are applied to "poor responders" and women at high-risk of developing OHSS, thus oocyte/embryo quality and development was inferior to that of the agonist group. However, data from earlier studies don't support the finding and indicate that the usage of GnRH antagonist is not associated with reduction of the likelihood of achieving live birth, compared with GnRH-a protocols [25]. Therefore, further investigation is needed

Table 5 Stepwise Cox regression analysis on live birth probability of ART clinical pregnancies before 12 weeks of gestational age

Variables	β[a]	SE[b]	HR	95% CI	P
Maternal age (reference: <30)					
30–35	0.1196	0.1392	1.13	0.86–1.48	0.390
36–40	0.5253	0.1956	1.69	1.15–2.48	0.007*
> 40	1.3087	0.3324	3.70	1.93–7.10	<0.001*
COH protocol (reference: GnRH-a long protocol)					
GnRH-a short protocol	0.2526	0.1460	1.29	0.97–1.71	0.084
GnRH antagonist protocol	1.2436	0.2953	3.47	1.94–6.19	<0.001*
Minimal stimulation protocol	1.1429	0.2310	3.14	2.00–4.93	<0.001*
GnRH-a rolonged protocol	0.0747	0.5109	1.08	0.40–2.93	0.884
Other protocol	1.4356	0.5868	4.20	1.33–13.27	0.014*
Cycle Type (reference: Fresh)					
Frozen	0.5059	0.1287	1.66	1.29–2.13	<0.001*
Serum hCG levels 14 days after transfer (reference: < 695.30)					
≥ 695.30	−1.6353	0.1687	0.19	0.14–0.27	<0.001*

HR hazard ratio, *CI* confidence interval, *P<0.05
[a]β is the estimated parameter of the regression model
[b]SE is the standard error of the regression model

to clarify the matter and future developments have to be focused on the optimization of COH protocols.

As for the association of cycle type and the occurrence of PL, we found the rate of loss, especially early miscarriage, increased after frozen IVF/ICSI cycles. We considered that embryo may inevitably be damaged by cryopreservation technology, which may damage the ability of embryo development and thus result in abortion. However, a meta-analysis showed that this difference did not reach statistical significance [26], and even in a multicenter randomized trial, the opposite result showed in infertile women with PCOS [27]. Thus, it is necessary to examine the effect of hormone level. To our surprise, frozen embryos after implantation showed significant lower late SA probability compared to fresh ones in our findings, which was consistent with the two multicenter randomized trials involving infertile women with the PCOS and ovulatory women [27, 28]. However, after stepwise backward Cox proportional hazard analysis, this different was no more significant, which could be due to difference in cryopreservation protocols, freezing day (cleavage-stage or blastocyst), number or quality of frozen embryos transferred.

Serum hCG has been used to be the main endocrine determinant of ongoing pregnancy, and then whether serum hCG level measured on the 14th day after transfer is sufficient in predicting final live birth outcomes needs to be confirmed. It was a significant observation in our findings that the hCG level of live birth was markedly higher than that of PL especially early abortion, which was agreement with another study that estimates the cutoff value of 50 IU/L (75% sensitivity, 81% specificity, $P < 0.001$) to predict ongoing pregnancy [29] as well. However, no hCG cutoff level had a sensitivity or specificity of 100% for pregnancies, making it essential to continue routine monitoring of ART pregnancy outcomes.

In addition to the above, we found BMI, freezing day (cleavage-stage or blastocyst) and no. of embryos transferred affected PL, but the three factors were not significant any more after stepwise COX regression. The incidence of PL progressively ascended as maternal BMI categories increased, which is consistent with a recent study [30]. And the association of female obesity (BMI>28 kg/m^2) with a significant decreased possibility of ART baby's survival after 12 weeks of gestational age was another interesting observation. It is suggested that maternal obesity can impair embryo development and the mechanism that Stella insufficiency in oocytes mediates developmental defects in early embryos has been elucidated in a recent study [31]. Besides, it is explained that the higher risk in subjects with high BMI may be due to the action of a hormone named leptin, which is produced predominantly in the adipose tissue [32].

In our finding, more than one embryo transfer was a protective factor of fetal loss in ART pregnancies after accounting for maternal age and the association of two embryos transfer with a significant decreased risk of early loss is an interesting observation. Although the results of a previous study also suggested that live birth and pregnancy rates following single embryo transfer were lower than those following double embryo transfer, so are the chances of multiple pregnancy including twins [33]. Multiple gestations lead to an increased risk of complications in both the fetuses and the mothers, so the optimal and recommended choice is the limit to the number of embryos to transfer [34].

This study was limited by some data availability as there is no routine ART surveillance system. We could not have data of other PL risk factors like microbial infections to resolve existing data gap. Secondly, the data covered in the article derived from two centers in Nanjing and Changzhou, so we would not obtain sufficient and identical characteristics and clinical features of pregnancies for lack data of some variables in either of centers. Lastly, in this retrospective cohort study, we could not investigate the mechanism of miscarriage during pregnancy weeks and the sample size is not enough, so the large-scale prospective cohort study should be carried out to in China.

Conclusions

In conclusion, the ultimate aim of assisted reproductive medicine practitioners would still be the improvement of IVF/ICSI efficacy in terms of take-home-baby rates. Therefore, with these findings in this study, clinicians may make it better to evaluate an infertile couple's risk of PL based on the maternal age at the time of treatment, COH protocol, cycle type and serum hCG level 14 days after transfer and the gestational week of the fetus. Additionally, these factors had significant impact on miscarriage mainly before 12 weeks of gestational age. Hopefully, these findings may offer some suggestions of population risks of pregnancy loss for reproductive health epidemiologists and contribute to future study on its etiology.

Abbreviations
ART: Assisted reproductive technology; BMI: Body mass index; CC: Clomiphene citrate; CDC: Centers for Disease Control; CI: Confidence interval; COH: Controlled ovarian hyperstimulation; ET: Embryo transfer; Gn: Gonadotropin; GnRH-a: Gonadotropin-releasing hormone agonist; hCG: Human chorionic gonadotropin; HR: Hazard ratio; ICSI: Intracytoplasmic sperm injection; IVF: In vitro fertilization; PCOS: Polycystic ovarian syndrome; PGD: Preimplantation genetic diagnosis; PGS: Preimplantation genetic screening; PL: Pregnancy loss; SA: Spontaneous abortion

Acknowledgements

The authors thank all of medics in Reproductive Medicine Center of the Affiliated Nanjing Maternity and Child Health Hospital of Nanjing Medical University and Reproductive Medicine Center of the Affiliated Changzhou Maternity and Child Health Care Hospital of Nanjing Medical University for recording all the data in this study through the years.

Funding

Supported by National Key Research & Development Program (2016YFC1000200, 2016YFC1000204), the State Key Program of National Natural Science of China (31530047), Science Foundation for Distinguished Young Scholars in Jiangsu (BK20160046), National Natural Science Foundation of China (81602927), Cheung Kong Scholars Programme of China, the QingLan Project of the Jiangsu Province, Jiangsu Specially-Appointed Professor project, Priority Academic Program Development of Jiangsu Higher Education Institutions (PAPD), Clinical medicine research fund of the Chinese medical association (17020420711), Innovation fund of state key laboratory of reproductive medicine (SKLRM-GC201802), Top-notch Academic Programs Project of Jiangsu Higher Education Institutions (PPZY2015A067), Jiangsu Provincial Medical Youth Talent (QNRC2016304), and Natural Science Foundation of Jiangsu Province (BK20161031).

Authors' contributions

LH and JD contributed to conception and design. HL contributed to analysis and interpretation of data, drafting and revising the article. JZ, MC, YW, FW, FL and XC contributed to acquisition of data. JZ, HM, GJ, HS, LC, XL and ZH contributed to revising the article critically for important intellectual content. All authors read and approved the final manuscript.

Competing interests

The authors declare that they have no competing interests.

Author details

[1]Department of Reproduction, the Affiliated Changzhou Maternity and Child Health Care, Hospital of Nanjing Medical University, Changzhou 213003, Jiangsu, China. [2]Department of Epidemiology, School of Public Health, Nanjing Medical University, Nanjing 211166, China. [3]State Key Laboratory of Reproductive Medicine, Nanjing Medical University, Nanjing 211166, China. [4]Department of Reproduction, the Affiliated Nanjing Maternity and Child Health, Hospital of Nanjing Medical University, Nanjing 210004, China.

References

1. Boivin J, Bunting L, Collins JA, Nygren KG. International estimates of infertility prevalence and treatment-seeking: potential need and demand for infertility medical care. Hum Reprod. 2007;22:1506–12.
2. Sunderam S, Kissin DM, Crawford SB, Folger SG, Jamieson DJ, Warner L, Barfield WD. Centers for Disease C, Prevention. Assisted Reproductive Technology Surveillance - United States, 2012. MMWR Surveill Summ. 2015; 64:1–29.
3. Robinson GE. Pregnancy loss. Best Pract Res Clin Obstet Gynaecol. 2014;28: 169–78.
4. Nybo Andersen AM, Wohlfahrt J, Christens P, Olsen J, Melbye M. Maternal age and fetal loss: population based register linkage study. BMJ. 2000;320: 1708–12.
5. Wang JX, Norman RJ, Wilcox AJ. Incidence of spontaneous abortion among pregnancies produced by assisted reproductive technology. Hum Reprod. 2004;19:272–7.
6. Assefa N, Berhane Y, Worku A. Pregnancy rates and pregnancy loss in eastern Ethiopia. Acta Obstet Gynecol Scand. 2013;92:642–7.
7. Farr SL, Schieve LA, Jamieson DJ. Pregnancy loss among pregnancies conceived through assisted reproductive technology, United States, 1999-2002. Am J Epidemiol. 2007;165:1380–8.
8. Buck Louis GM, Sapra KJ, Schisterman EF, Lynch CD, Maisog JM, Grantz KL, Sundaram R. Lifestyle and pregnancy loss in a contemporary cohort of women recruited before conception: the LIFE study. Fertil Steril. 2016;106:180–8.
9. Delabaere A, Huchon C, Deffieux X, Beucher G, Gallot V, Nedellec S, Vialard F, Carcopino X, Quibel T, Subtil D, et al. Epidemiology of loss pregnancy. J Gynecol Obstet Biol Reprod (Paris). 2014;43:764–75.
10. Giakoumelou S, Wheelhouse N, Cuschieri K, Entrican G, Howie SE, Horne AW. The role of infection in miscarriage. Hum Reprod Update. 2016;22:116–33.
11. Negro R, Schwartz A, Gismondi R, Tinelli A, Mangieri T, Stagnaro-Green A. Increased pregnancy loss rate in thyroid antibody negative women with TSH levels between 2.5 and 5.0 in the first trimester of pregnancy. J Clin Endocrinol Metab. 2010;95:E44–8.
12. Hipp H, Crawford S, Kawwass JF, Chang J, Kissin DM, Jamieson DJ. First trimester pregnancy loss after fresh and frozen in vitro fertilization cycles. Fertil Steril. 2016;105:722–8.
13. Wang JX, Davies MJ, Norman RJ. Polycystic ovarian syndrome and the risk of spontaneous abortion following assisted reproductive technology treatment. Hum Reprod. 2001;16:2606–9.
14. Jia CW, Wang L, Lan YL, Song R, Zhou LY, Yu L, Yang Y, Liang Y, Li Y, Ma YM, Wang SY. Aneuploidy in Early Miscarriage and its Related Factors. Chin Med J (Engl). 2015;]:2772–2776.
15. McNamee KM, Dawood F, Farquharson RG. Mid-trimester pregnancy loss. Obstet Gynecol Clin N Am. 2014;41:87–102.
16. Winter E, Wang J, Davies MJ, Norman R. Early pregnancy loss following assisted reproductive technology treatment. Hum Reprod. 2002;17:3220–3.
17. Chen CD, Chiang YT, Yang PK, Chen MJ, Chang CH, Yang YS, Chen SU. Frequency of low serum LH is associated with increased early pregnancy loss in IVF/ICSI cycles. Reprod BioMed Online. 2016;33:449–57.
18. Abd ElHafeez S, Torino C, D'Arrigo G, Bolignano D, Provenzano F, Mattace-Raso F, Zoccali C, Tripepi G. An overview on standard statistical methods for assessing exposure-outcome link in survival analysis (part II): the Kaplan-Meier analysis and the cox regression method. Aging Clin Exp Res. 2012;24:203–6.
19. Spandorfer SD, Davis OK, Barmat LI, Chung PH, Rosenwaks Z. Relationship between maternal age and aneuploidy in in vitro fertilization pregnancy loss. Fertil Steril. 2004;81:1265–9.
20. Khalil A, Syngelaki A, Maiz N, Zinevich Y, Nicolaides KH. Maternal age and adverse pregnancy outcome: a cohort study. Ultrasound Obstet Gynecol. 2013;42:634–43.
21. Baird DT, Collins J, Egozcue J, Evers LH, Gianaroli L, Leridon H, Sunde A, Templeton A, Van Steirteghem A, Cohen J, et al. Fertility and ageing. Hum Reprod Update. 2005;11:261–76.
22. Ziebe S, Loft A, Petersen JH, Andersen AG, Lindenberg S, Petersen K, Andersen AN. Embryo quality and developmental potential is compromised by age. Acta Obstet Gynecol Scand. 2001;80:169–74.
23. Franasiak JM, Forman EJ, Hong KH, Werner MD, Upham KM, Treff NR, Scott RT Jr. The nature of aneuploidy with increasing age of the female partner: a review of 15,169 consecutive trophectoderm biopsies evaluated with comprehensive chromosomal screening. Fertil Steril. 2014;101:656–63. e651
24. Shoham Z, Zosmer A, Insler V. Early miscarriage and fetal malformations after induction of ovulation (by clomiphene citrate and/or human menotropins), in vitro fertilization, and gamete intrafallopian transfer. Fertil Steril. 1991;55:1–11.
25. Lambalk CB, Banga FR, Huirne JA, Toftager M, Pinborg A, Homburg R, van der Veen F, van Wely M. GnRH antagonist versus long agonist protocols in IVF: a systematic review and meta-analysis accounting for patient type. Hum Reprod Update. 2017;23:560–79.

26. Roque M, Lattes K, Serra S, Sola I, Geber S, Carreras R, Checa MA. Fresh embryo transfer versus frozen embryo transfer in in vitro fertilization cycles: a systematic review and meta-analysis. Fertil Steril. 2013;99:156–62.

27. Chen ZJ, Shi Y, Sun Y, Zhang B, Liang X, Cao Y, Yang J, Liu J, Wei D, Weng N, et al. Fresh versus frozen embryos for infertility in the polycystic ovary syndrome. N Engl J Med. 2016;375:523–33.

28. Shi Y, Sun Y, Hao C, Zhang H, Wei D, Zhang Y, Zhu Y, Deng X, Qi X, Li H, et al. Transfer of fresh versus frozen embryos in ovulatory women. N Engl J Med. 2018;378:126–36.

29. Urbancsek J, Hauzman E, Fedorcsak P, Halmos A, Devenyi N, Papp Z. Serum human chorionic gonadotropin measurements may predict pregnancy outcome and multiple gestation after in vitro fertilization. Fertil Steril. 2002; 78:540–2.

30. Provost MP, Acharya KS, Acharya CR, Yeh JS, Steward RG, Eaton JL, Goldfarb JM, Muasher SJ. Pregnancy outcomes decline with increasing body mass index: analysis of 239,127 fresh autologous in vitro fertilization cycles from the 2008-2010 Society for Assisted Reproductive Technology registry. Fertil Steril. 2016;105:663–9.

31. Han L, Ren C, Li L, Li X, Ge J, Wang H, Miao YL, Guo X, Moley KH, Shu W, Wang Q. Embryonic defects induced by maternal obesity in mice derive from Stella insufficiency in oocytes. Nat Genet. 2018;50:432–42.

32. Mitchell M, Armstrong DT, Robker RL, Norman RJ. Adipokines: implications for female fertility and obesity. Reproduction. 2005;130:583–97.

33. McLernon DJ, Harrild K, Bergh C, Davies MJ, de Neubourg D, Dumoulin JC, Gerris J, Kremer JA, Martikainen H, Mol BW, et al. Clinical effectiveness of elective single versus double embryo transfer: meta-analysis of individual patient data from randomised trials. BMJ. 2010;341:c6945.

34. Practice Committee of the American Society for Reproductive Medicine. Electronic address Aao, Practice Committee of the Society for Assisted Reproductive T. Guidance on the limits to the number of embryos to transfer: a committee opinion. Fertil Steril. 2017;107:901–3.

3

Endometrium metabolomic profiling reveals potential biomarkers for diagnosis of endometriosis at minimal-mild stages

Jingjie Li[1†], Lihuan Guan[2†], Huizhen Zhang[2], Yue Gao[2], Jiahong Sun[2], Xiao Gong[4], Dongshun Li[2], Pan Chen[3], Xiaoyan Liang[1], Min Huang[2] and Huichang Bi[2*]

Abstract

Background: The sensitivity and specificity of non-invasive diagnostic methods for endometriosis, especially at early stages, are not optimal. The clinical diagnostic indicator cancer antigen 125 (CA125) performs poorly in the diagnosis of minimal endometriosis, with a sensitivity of 24%. Therefore, it is urgent to explore novel diagnostic biomarkers. We evaluated the metabolomic profile variation of the eutopic endometrium between minimal-mild endometriosis patients and healthy women by ultra-high-performance liquid chromatography coupled with electrospray ionization high-resolution mass spectrometry (UHPLC-ESI-HRMS).

Methods: Our study comprised 29 patients with laparoscopically confirmed endometriosis at stages I-II and 37 infertile women who underwent diagnostic laparoscopy combined with hysteroscopy from January 2014 to January 2015. Eutopic endometrium samples were collected by pipelle endometrial biopsy. The metabolites were quantified by UHPLC-ESI-HRMS. The best combination of biomarkers was then selected by performing step-wise logistic regression analysis with backward elimination.

Results: Twelve metabolites were identified as endometriosis-associated biomarkers. The eutopic endometrium metabolomic profile of the endometriosis patients was characterized by a significant increase in the concentration of hypoxanthine, L-arginine, L-tyrosine, leucine, lysine, inosine, omega-3 arachidonic acid, guanosine, xanthosine, lysophosphatidylethanolamine and asparagine. In contrast, the concentration of uric acid was decreased. Metabolites were filtered by step-wise logistic regression with backward elimination, and a model containing uric acid, hypoxanthine, and lysophosphatidylethanolamine was constructed. Receiver-operating characteristic (ROC) analysis confirmed the prognostic value of these parameters for the diagnosis of minimal/mild endometriosis with a sensitivity of 66.7% and a specificity of 90.0%.

Conclusions: Metabolomics analysis of the eutopic endometrium in endometriosis was effectively characterized by UHPLC-ESI-HRMS-based metabolomics. Our study supports the importance of purine and amino acid metabolites in the pathophysiology of endometriosis and provides potential biomarkers for semi-invasive diagnosis of early-stage endometriosis.

Keywords: Endometriosis, Metabolomics, UHPLC-ESI-HRMS, Eutopic endometrium

* Correspondence: bihchang@mail.sysu.edu.cn
†Equal contributors
2School of Pharmaceutical Sciences in Sun Yat-sen University, 132# Waihuandong Road, Guangzhou, University City, Guangzhou 510006, People's Republic of China
Full list of author information is available at the end of the article

Background

Endometriosis is a chronic, benign gynaecological disorder characterized by the presence of endometrial cells at extrauterine sites and associated with chronic pain and infertility. This disease is a highly prevalent disease, presenting in 10–15% of reproductive age women and approximately 25 to 50% of infertile women [1, 2]. Endometriosis has a severe impact on socioeconomics and the quality of life of patients [3]. Endometriosis is classified into minimal (I), mild (II), moderate (III) and severe (IV) stages [4]. The incidence of minimal or mild endometriosis is more frequent than advanced endometriosis. Minimal or mild endometriosis is peritoneal or ovarian endometriotic implants and filmy adhesions on the fallopian tubes or ovaries. The presence of early-stage endometriosis is associated with poor oocyte quality, lower fertilization rate and embryonic developmental competence [5, 6]. However, no substantial pelvic anatomical changes have been identified. In addition, atypical symptoms or even no symptoms increase the difficulty of diagnosis in minimal or mild endometriosis, which can be delayed on average by 8 to 11 years [7]. Currently, the sensitivity and specificity of non-invasive diagnostic methods for endometriosis, especially early-stage, are not optimal. The clinical diagnostic indicator cancer antigen 125 (CA125) performs poorly in diagnosing minimal endometriosis, with a sensitivity of 24% [8]. Therefore, it is urgent to explore novel diagnostic biomarkers.

Metabolomics has emerged as a powerful and reliable tool to identify metabolites and biomarkers present in the biological system under a given physiological condition. Metabolites not only represent the final products of biological regulatory processes but also act as communicators between the information-rich genome and the functional phenotype. In the past few years, several studies identified a list of potential diagnostic candidates in peritoneal fluid, blood and urine from endometriosis patients at different stages of disease and menstrual cycle [9, 10]. However, potential biomarkers from the eutopic endometrium remain unknown. Therefore, in the current study, ultra-high-performance liquid chromatography coupled with electrospray ionization high-resolution mass spectrometry (UHPLC-ESI-HRMS) was used to investigate the metabolomic profile of the eutopic endometrium between minimal/mild endometriosis patients and controls. Twelve metabolites were identified as endometriosis-associated biomarkers. The eutopic endometrium metabolomic profile of endometriosis patients was characterized by a significant increase in the concentration of hypoxanthine, L-arginine, L-tyrosine, leucine, lysine, inosine, omega-3 arachidonic acid, guanosine, xanthosine, lysophosphatidylethanolamine and asparagine. In contrast, the concentration of uric acid was decreased. Our study provides potential biomarkers for the semi-invasive diagnose of endometriosis at minimal-mild stages.

Methods

Subject selection

Patient recruitment was carried out at the Sixth Hospital of Sun Yat-sen University, and analysis of the endometrium metabolomic profiles was performed at the School of Pharmaceutical Sciences at Sun Yat-sen University. Eutopic endometrium was collected from 68 volunteers (21–38 years old, body mass index less than 30 kg/m^2) from January 2014 to January 2015 who underwent diagnostic laparoscopy combined with hysteroscopy because of infertility. Clinical diagnosis and classification of subjects were performed through laparoscopic surgery to visually confirm the presence of endometriotic lesions. Surgery was carried out on the third to fifth day after menstrual cessation. All participants had regular menstrual cycles (between 21 and 35 days) without hormonal treatment or use of an intrauterine device in the 3 months before sample collection. Endometrial tissues were obtained via Pipelle biopsy during surgery on the 3rd-5th day after the end of their menstrual bleeding. The severity of endometriosis was determined according to the American Society of Reproductive Medicine revised system [4]. Patients diagnosed with endometrial polyp, endometritis, submucous myoma or hydrosalpinx should be excluded after confirmation with hysteroscopy combined with laparoscopy and further confirmation by histology. Two volunteers diagnosed by hysteroscopy with endometrial polyps were excluded. No other pathologies were detected in the 68 volunteers. Three volunteers were highly suspicious for endometrioma on 2 ultrasounds with more than 3 months interval. The mean sizes of the cysts were 8 mm, 7 mm and 8 mm, which were confirmed during surgery. Clinical information associated with each sample group is summarized in Table 1. After collection, specimens were immediately placed into microtubes and preserved in liquid nitrogen until analysis. This study received the approval of the institutional review board, and all patients gave their written informed consent (approval number: G2012021).

Sample preparation for metabolomics

Endometrial tissues were obtained from 37 healthy women (Control) and 29 women with endometriosis. Sample preparation was performed according to a previous report with slight modifications [11]. Briefly, 400 μL of 50% chilled methanol was added to 20 mg of tissue sections in tubes containing ceramic beads for homogenization by using a Precellys 24 homogenizer (Bertin, France). The supernatant was transferred into a fresh tube, and 800 μL of chilled 100% acetonitrile was added to precipitate the protein.

Table 1 Characteristics of participants for endometriosis patients and controls

	Endometriosis patients ($n = 29$)	Control group ($n = 37$)	P
Age (years)	29.69 ± 3.19	29.74 ± 3.43	0.9543
BMI (kg/m^2)	21.04 ± 2.08	21.89 ± 3.22	0.2916
AMH (ng/ml)	4.35 ± 2.74	6.4 ± 4.68	0.0661
Uric acid(μmol/l)	271.2 ± 67.38	289.1 ± 63.15	0.3018
The day of sampling	8.667 ± 0.2108	8.45 ± 0.3033	0.5576
The length of menstruation	5.19 ± 0.3209	5 ± 0.3839	0.7044
Endometriosis stage			
I stage	19	N/A	
II stage	10	N/A	
Ovarian endometriomas	3	N/A	

Samples were centrifuged at 18000×g at 4 °C for 15 min. A total of 500 μL of supernatant was transferred to a fresh tube and dried under vacuum. Samples were re-suspended in 200 μL of 70% acetonitrile for hydrophobic interaction liquid chromatography (HILIC) mode or in 35% acetonitrile for reversed-phase liquid chromatography (RPLC) mode and then centrifuged at 18000×g at 4 °C for 5 min. Finally, 5 μL of supernatant was transferred to a UPLC vial and injected for UHPLC-ESI-HRMS analysis. The quality control (QC) samples comprised 5 μL of each sample, representing a universal set of metabolites for this study. In addition, blank samples were 70% acetonitrile or 35% acetonitrile.

UHPLC-ESI-HRMS measurements of endometrial tissues

According to our previously reported method [12], chromatography was performed using an Ultimate 3000 HPLC system (Dionex Corporation, Sunnyvale, CA) coupled to a Q Exactive™ benchtop Orbitrap high-resolution mass spectrometer (Thermo Fisher Scientific, San Jose, CA). For the HILIC mode, an Atlantis Silica HILIC 3 μm column (100 mm × 2.1 mm, Waters, Milford, MA, USA), total run time 30 min, was employed. Solvent A was 95% acetonitrile containing 10 mM ammonium formate and 0.1% formic acid, and solvent B was 10 mM ammonium formate and 0.1% formic acid in 50% acetonitrile. The linear gradient used was as follows: holding in 100% A for 0–1 min, increasing to 100% B linearly for 20 min and washing the column for the next 4.9 min, then returning to 100% A until 30 min for column equilibration with a flow rate of 0.3 mL/min. For the RPLC mode, samples were injected onto an Xterra MS C18 5 μm column (100 mm × 2.1 mm, Waters, Milford, MA, USA). The mobile phase consisted of 0.1% formic acid in water (A) and 100% acetonitrile (B).

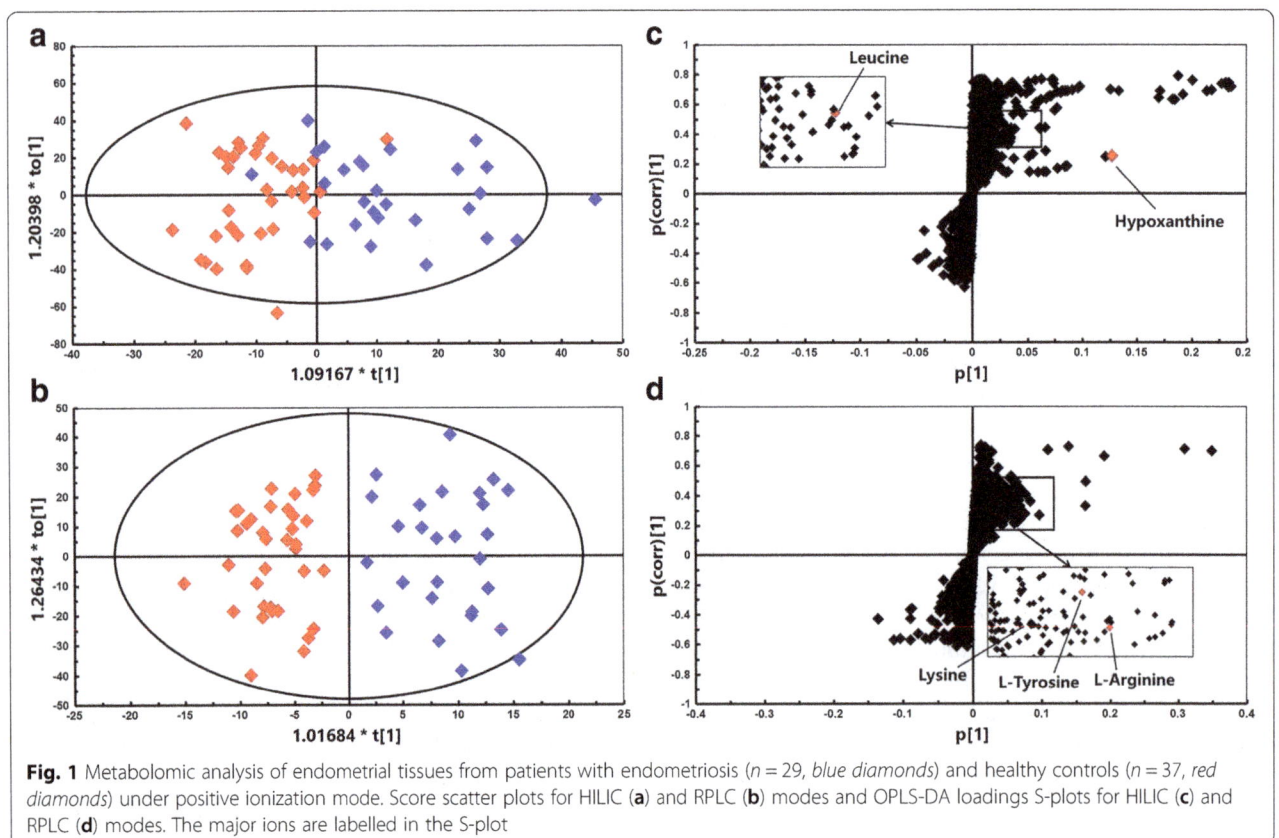

Fig. 1 Metabolomic analysis of endometrial tissues from patients with endometriosis ($n = 29$, *blue diamonds*) and healthy controls ($n = 37$, *red diamonds*) under positive ionization mode. Score scatter plots for HILIC (**a**) and RPLC (**b**) modes and OPLS-DA loadings S-plots for HILIC (**c**) and RPLC (**d**) modes. The major ions are labelled in the S-plot

The flow rate was kept at 0.3 mL/min during a 22-min run with the following gradient: 100% A for 2 min to 52% A at 4 min to 30% A at 11 min to 25% A at 14 min and kept at 100% B from 16 min to 17 min and 100% A from 18 min to 22 min. The column temperature was kept at 40 °C. Mass spectrometry was performed with an electrospray ionization source both in positive and negative ionization modes under the following conditions: the spray voltage was 3.5 kV. The capillary and aux gas heater temperature were 300 °C and 350 °C, respectively. Nitrogen was used as sheath gas (40 arbitrary) and auxiliary gas (10 arbitrary). Data were acquired from 80 to 900 mass-to-charge (m/z) for mass scanning, and the step collision energy 15, 30, 45 eV was used for MS/MS fragmentation of ions. QC samples were injected intermittently to account for the reproducibility and stability of the UHPLC-ESI-HRMS data [13].

Data analysis

The mass spectra data were pre-processed by SIEVE 2.2 (Thermo Fisher Scientific, San Jose, CA) to remove the background and generate a multivariate data matrix containing aligned peak areas with matched m/z and retention times. Then, SIMCA 13.0 software (Umetrics, Kinnelon, NJ) was applied to find the features that were responsible for the discrimination of the groups. An orthogonal partial least squares discriminant analysis (OPLS-DA) was used to maximize the group discrimination. The candidate markers were selected by examining the S-plot based on the variable importance (VIP) value, which was more than 1.0. The identification of the metabolites was confirmed by comparisons of fragmentation spectra and m/z through three main online databases: Metlin (http://metlin.scripps.edu), HMDB (http://www.hmdb.ca/), and mzcloud (https://www.mzcloud.org/) [14, 15]. To assess the strength of association between individual metabolites and minimal/mild endometriosis, a step-wise logistic regression analysis with backward elimination was used to establish a model and filter crucial metabolites. The receiver operating characteristic (ROC) curve was plotted, and the area under the curve (AUC) was calculated. The optimal point on the ROC curve provided the best trade-off between sensitivity and specificity. Statistical testing was carried out by SPSS 19.0 software (IBM Analytics, USA). Data were assessed for normality of distribution using the Shapiro–Wilk test first. Unpaired Student's t-test or the non-parametric Mann–Whitney U-test was evaluated with a 95% confidence level for statistical analysis between the two groups. False discovery rate (FDR) control was performed by the SAS PROC MULTITEST with the FDR option

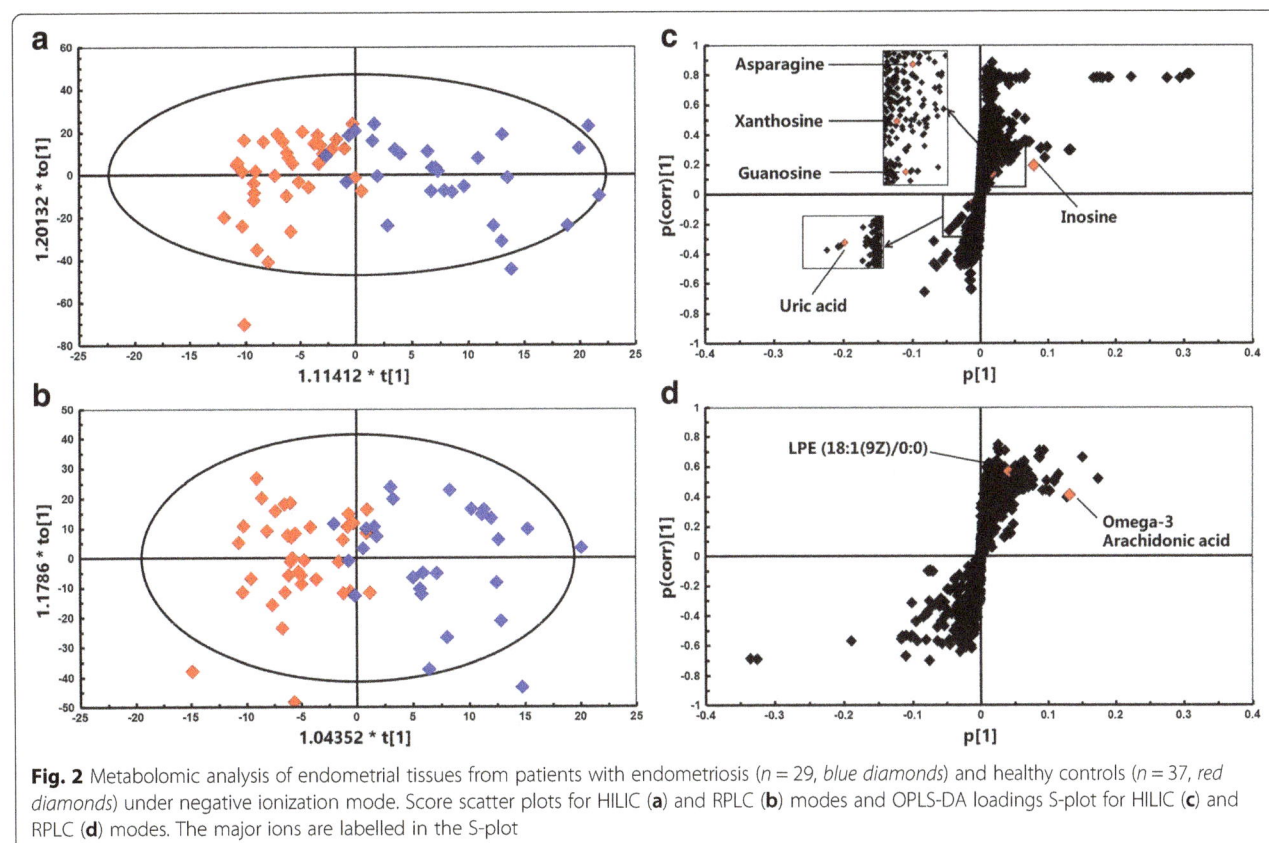

Fig. 2 Metabolomic analysis of endometrial tissues from patients with endometriosis (n = 29, *blue diamonds*) and healthy controls (n = 37, *red diamonds*) under negative ionization mode. Score scatter plots for HILIC (a) and RPLC (b) modes and OPLS-DA loadings S-plot for HILIC (c) and RPLC (d) modes. The major ions are labelled in the S-plot

Current Progress in Reproductive Biology and Endocrinology

(SAS Inst, Cary, North Carolina, USA). *P*-values less than 0.05 were considered statistically significant while controlling FDR at 0.05.

Results
Characteristics of participants with endometriosis and controls
Clinical information associated with each sample group is summarized in Table 1. A total of 66 volunteers were recruited in this study. Twenty-nine patients had laparoscopically confirmed endometriosis, staged as minimal ($n = 19$) and mild ($n = 10$). Three patients had a laparoscopically documented presence of ovarian endometrioma. All of the endometriomas were histologically confirmed. The mean sizes of all the cysts were less than 1 cm. Age, BMI, menstrual cycle, AMH and uric acid in serum were comparable between the two groups ($P > 0.05$). Both the mean day of sampling and the length of menstruation were not significantly different between the endometriosis patients and the control group. No volunteer had a history of smoking in this study.

Multivariate statistical analysis of difference between the endometriosis and control groups
The alignment of all the features in all samples generated a data matrix by SIEVE 2.2 software with an abundance of 5388 features under HILIC mode and 3424 features under RPLC mode. To compare the overall variation of metabolic profiles between the endometriosis patients and healthy controls, a classification model was built by the supervised OPLS-DA, which revealed a clear separation between the two groups (Figs. 1a, b and 2a, b). The model also showed that samples from humans had great individual differences. An OPLS-DA loadings S-plot was performed to highlight significantly different variables in the two groups (Figs. 1c, d and 2c, d). Each point represented a detected ion (variables). The further away from the plot origin an ion point lies, the more the ion contributes to the difference between the two study groups. Therefore, variables plotted at the top or bottom were changed most significantly. Metabolite features of interest were selected by a VIP value > 1.0. With such a strategy, 450 variables from the HILIC mode results and 469

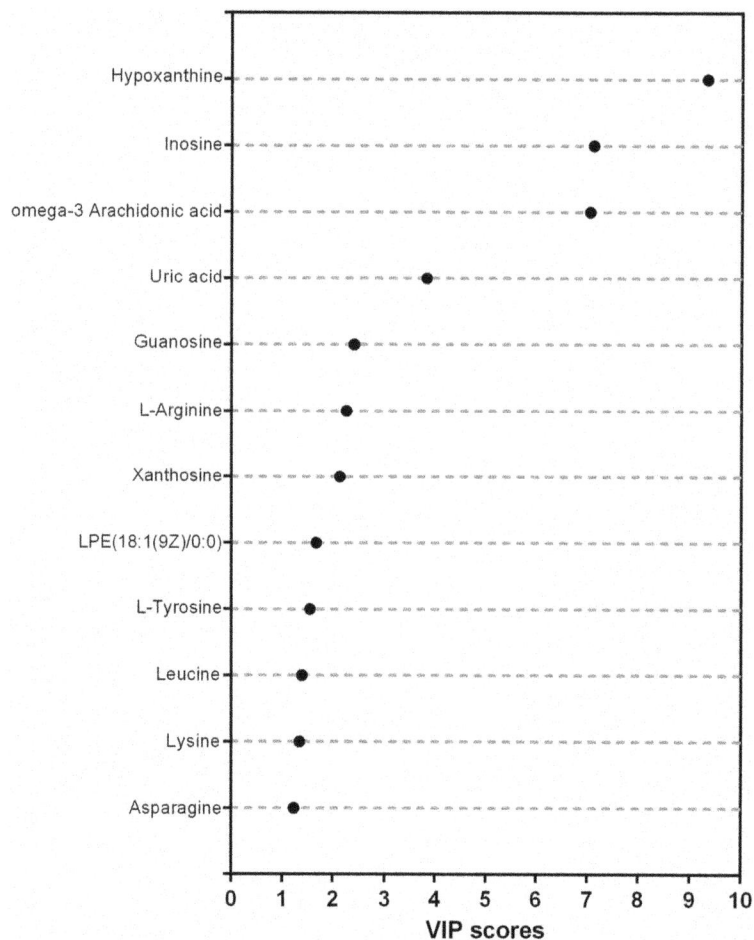

Fig. 3 Identified metabolites with increasing contributions to the difference in metabolomic profiles between the two groups based on VIP scores

variables from the RPLC mode results were considered to have impact on the model.

Identification of detected metabolites

The m/z of the selected variables and their MS/MS fragmentation spectra were used for comparison with compounds annotated in the online databases. Finally, 27 metabolites from positive and negative ionization modes were uniquely identified on the basis of exact mass and retention time. Among them, levels of 12 metabolites corresponding to high variable importance (VIP > 1) (Fig. 3) were different between the endometriosis and control groups ($P < 0.05$). In addition, their detailed information is summarized in Table 2 and labelled in the S-plot (Figs. 1c, d and 2c, d). Obviously, levels of hypoxanthine, L-arginine, L-tyrosine, leucine, lysine, inosine, omega-3 arachidonic acid, guanosine, xanthosine, lysophosphatidylethanolamine and asparagine were higher in the endometriosis group than in the control group, whereas the level of uric acid was higher in the control group (Fig. 4). It is noteworthy that the xanthosine level in the endometriosis group was 2.53-fold higher than that of the control group, while the amount of uric acid was decreased by half, indicating that purine metabolism was disturbed in endometriosis patients. After using step-wise multivariate logistic regression analysis with backward elimination, a model with three predictors was established, including uric acid, hypoxanthine

and lysophosphatidylethanolamine, with a sensitivity of 66.7% (95% CI: 0.417–0.875) and a specificity of 90.0% (95% CI: 0.600–1.000). The receiver operating characteristic (ROC) curve shows improved effects of adding separate variables to the model. The apparent AUC of the ROC curve for the model predicting endometriosis at the minimal/mild stages was 0.868 (95% CI: 0.774–0.963) (Fig. 5). The combination of three variables led to a curve with significantly better performance and allows very good discrimination between endometriosis patients at early stages and controls.

Discussion

In the current study, we applied a UHPLC-ESI-HRMS-based metabolome profiling approach to investigate metabolic changes in the eutopic endometrium samples from endometriosis patients and identified metabolites for early-diagnosed endometriosis. In this regard, 11 metabolites including hypoxanthine, L-arginine, L-tyrosine, leucine, lysine, inosine, omega-3 arachidonic acid, guanosine, xanthosine, lysophosphatidylethanolamine and asparagine were significantly increased in the endometriosis group, whereas the uric acid level was decreased. The global metabolomics and subsequent multivariate analysis clearly distinguished metabolic changes in the endometriosis patients from those in the matched controls. A combination of three predictors (uric acid, hypoxanthine and lysophosphatidylethanolamine) shows a very good potential for use in diagnosing endometriosis at early stages.

Table 2 Summary of the data from the 12 features found in positive and negative ionization modes contributing to the discrimination of endometrial tissues between endometriosis patients and healthy controls

m/z[a]	t_R (min)[b]	Metabolite	Molecular formula	Adduct	Fold change[c]	P value[d]	Adj P value[e]
HILIC mode							
131.0462	10.793	Asparagine	$C_4H_8N_2O_3$	M-H	1.44	0.013	0.0173
132.1019	8.833	Leucine	$C_6H_{13}NO_2$	M + H	1.68	0.002	0.0120
137.0455	4.431	Hypoxanthine	$C_5H_4N_4O$	M + H	1.64	0.033	0.0360
167.0209	5.283	Uric acid	$C_5H_4N_4O_3$	M-H	0.54	0.000	0.0053
267.0737	4.539	Inosine	$C_{10}H_{12}N_4O_5$	M-H	1.58	0.037	0.0370
282.0844	6.017	Guanosine	$C_{10}H_{13}N_5O_5$	M-H	1.55	0.023	0.0276
283.0685	4.771	Xanthosine	$C_{10}H_{12}N_4O_6$	M-H	2.53	0.008	0.0137
RPLC mode							
147.1125	0.696	Lysine	$C_6H_{14}N_2O_2$	M + H	1.54	0.008	0.0137
175.1186	0.703	L-Arginine	$C_6H_{14}N_4O_2$	M + H	1.41	0.004	0.0137
182.0808	1.091	L-Tyrosine	$C_9H_{11}NO_3$	M + H	1.47	0.006	0.0137
303.2329	15.245	Omega-3 Arachidonic acid	$C_{20}H_{32}O_2$	M-H	1.57	0.005	0.0137
478.2935	10.770	LPE (18:1(9Z)/0:0)	$C_{23}H_{46}NO_7P$	M-H	1.20	0.013	0.0173

[a]m/z is the detected mass to charge ratio from LC-MS/MS runs
[b]Retention time in minutes
[c]The fold change of the endometriosis group vs the control group (a higher ratio indicates a higher level of expression of a compound in the EMS group)
[d]P value is the significance level of the difference between the two groups
[e]P values were adjusted for false discovery rate correction at the significance level of 5%
LPE lysophosphatidylethanolamine, PC phosphatidylcholine

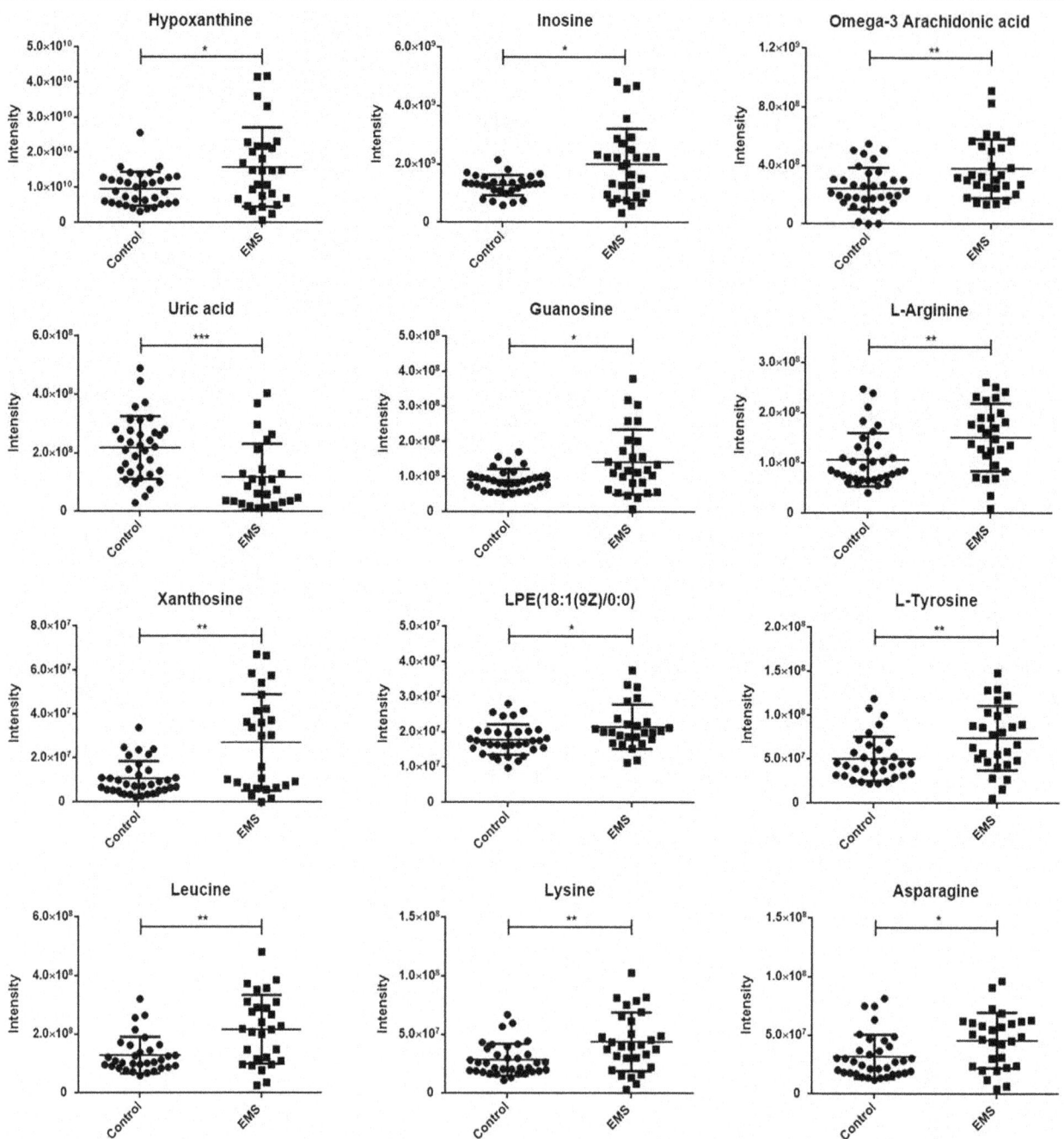

Fig. 4 Scatter diagram of 12 selected metabolites. Data are expressed as the mean ± SD. *P < 0.05, **P < 0.01, ***P < 0.001, endometriosis patients (EMS, n = 29) vs healthy controls (Control, n = 37)

However, a study with a larger sample size is needed to obtain stronger evidence and avoid wide confidence intervals in the future.

Endometriosis is a disease characterized by the presence of endometrial glands and stroma at ectopic sites. This gynaecological disease occurs in approximately 10% of women of reproductive age, who present symptoms including dyspareunia, dysmenorrhoea, chronic pelvic pain and subfertility [16]. Laparoscopy is the gold standard

for the diagnosis of endometriosis. However, laparoscopy is an invasive operation with several limitations, such as surgery-associated risks and financial burden [17]. So far, it has not been able to accurately predict the presence of endometriosis based on non-invasive way. Ultrasound could efficiently detect the presence of ovarian endometriomas, but it is inadequate for the diagnosis of peritoneal endometriosis, deep endometriosis and endometriosis-associated adhesions. CA125 is the most frequently

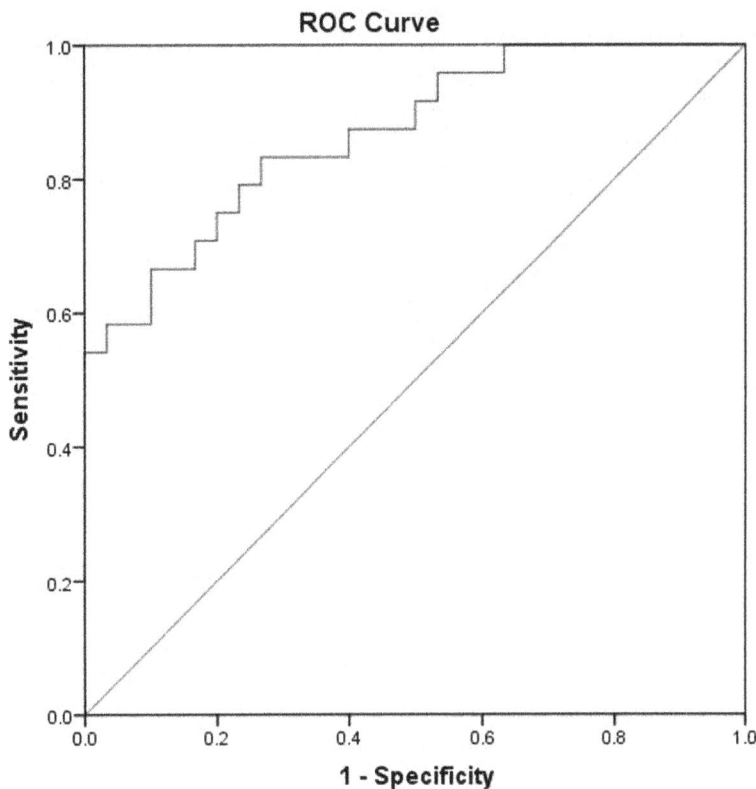

Fig. 5 Receiver operating characteristic curves for the model of endometriosis at minimal/mild stages

studied biomarker for endometriosis [18]. However, it may be more beneficial for diagnosing advanced stages (III–IV) compared to early stages (I - II) [19]. Hirsch et al. showed that CA 125 performs poorly in diagnosing minimal endometriosis, with a sensitivity of 24% [8]. At present, over 100 potential biomarkers of endometriosis have been reported; however, few markers were useful for the detection of minimal–mild endometriosis [20]. The diagnosis of endometriosis can be delayed, on average, by 8 to 11 years, which leads to significant symptoms [7]. Thus, the cost-effectiveness of endometriosis diagnosis and therapy should be urgently improved.

Increasing evidence shows that metabolomics using easily accessible human biosamples has become an effective tool to explore diagnostic biomarkers and investigate disease progression [21–24]. Metabolomics analysis in endometriosis has been performed in peripheral blood, peritoneal fluid, follicular fluid and urine [25–28]. According to the widely accepted theory of retrograde menstruation, the endometrium is the source of ectopic endometriotic foci. Previous studies showed that the eutopic endometrium contributed to the pathogenesis of endometriosis due to the increase of proliferation, migration and invasion of ectopic endometrium [29–33]. In this study, we did not detect a significant difference in patients' uric acid level in serum. However, uric acid level was

reduced by about half in the eutopic endometrium of patients. The differential expression of uric acid in the serum and endometrium indicated that the eutopic endometrium was more representative, stable and similar to ectopic lesions compared to other samples. In addition, we utilized a semi-invasive way of sampling. The pipelle endometrial biopsy can be used without cervical dilatation in the outpatient department and causes minimal discomfort. Thus, metabolomics analysis via pipelle endometrial biopsy is a viable method to explore molecular markers of endometriosis. All the samples were obtained strictly on the third to fifth day after menstrual cessation because we tried to examine samples in the early follicle phase. Although theoretically we should sample on the same day of the menstrual cycle, each patient's menstrual period and speed of follicle growth varies. We chose this time to collect samples based on hysteroscopic surgical requirements and patient compliance. Unfortunately, we did not collect enough data on patients with advanced endometriosis to analyse because few patients in stages III-IV in our centre had not been exposed to hormonal drugs within 3 months.

Purine metabolites, including inosine, xanthosine, guanosine and hypoxanthine, were significantly upregulated in the eutopic endometrium, whereas uric acid, as the end product of purine metabolism, was remarkably downregulated. This observation indicates that local purine salvage is potentially impaired. Multiple enzymes participate in the purine metabolism process. Among them, purine nucleoside phosphorylase (PNP) is one of the essential enzymes mediating the generation of uric acid from purines. High levels of expression of this enzyme are postulated to reflect extensive programmed cell death during the implantation process [34, 35]. In addition, pharmacological inhibition of PNP has been demonstrated to be embryo-lethal or teratogenic [34]. Our data indicated that the accumulation of these purine metabolites and decrease in uric acid level in the eutopic endometrium may be due to suppressed PNP expression. A previous study applied parallel gene expression profiling using high-density oligonucleotide microarrays to investigate the regulation of gene expression in the endometrium [36], and reduction of PNP expression was found in endometriosis patients, which supports our hypothesis.

Endometriosis has been known to exhibit similar features of malignancy [37, 38]. Clinical and microscopic examination proved that endometriosis exhibited cancer-like characteristics, demonstrated by uncontrolled growth, cell invasion, neovascularization and apoptosis [39]. Almost all of the amino acids have been reported to be upregulated in carcinoma tissues in previous studies [40]. In cancer cells, a high energy demand leads to the alteration of biochemistry including citric acid cycle dysfunction [41]. Therefore, alternative routes of carbon backbone delivery are required. The increased ectopic endometrium levels of L-arginine, L-tyrosine, leucine, lysine and asparagine observed in the present study might be caused by the alteration of energy metabolism and high turnover of structural protein. These observations are in agreement with a study carried out on serum samples of endometriosis [42] and metabolic alterations observed in oesophageal cancer patients [43, 44].

Conclusion

Metabolomics provides a powerful approach to explore diagnostic biomarkers by analysing changes in metabolic profiles. Overall, this study is the first to demonstrate a comprehensive analysis of metabolic changes in the eutopic endometrium in endometriosis at early stages. Metabolites involved in purine, amino acid and arachidonic acid metabolic pathways could be potential biomarkers for early diagnosis of endometriosis. These findings provide potential biomarkers for semi-invasive diagnosis of endometriosis at minimal-mild stages in clinical practice. The implications of these individual metabolites in the pathophysiology and analysis of metabolites in all stages of endometriosis have now to be further studied.

Funding

The authors would like to acknowledge the support from the National Natural Science Foundation of China (No. 81601347, 81503156, 81320108027), Natural Science Foundation of Guangdong Province (No. 2014A030310096) and Public Welfare Research and Capacity Building Fund of Guangdong (No. 2016A020218006).

Authors' contributions

JJL conceived of the study, wrote the manuscript and supervised patient recruitment. LHG, HZZ, YG and DSL contributed to the study execution and analysis and interpretation of the data. XG performed data analysis and interpretation. JHS and PC reviewed the manuscript. HCB, MH and XYL supervised patient recruitment, collected and evaluated data, and drafted, edited and approved the final version of this paper for submission. All authors read and approved the final manuscript.

Competing interests

The authors declare that they have no competing interests.

Author details

[1]Center of Reproductive Medicine, the Sixth Affiliated Hospital, Sun Yat-sen University, Guangzhou, China. [2]School of Pharmaceutical Sciences in Sun Yat-sen University, 132# Waihuandong Road, Guangzhou, University City, Guangzhou 510006, People's Republic of China. [3]Pharmacy Department, the First Affiliated Hospital, Sun Yat-sen University, Guangzhou, China. [4]School of Public Health, Guangdong Pharmaceutical University, Guangzhou, China.

References

1. Olive DL, Pritts EA. Treatment of endometriosis. N Engl J Med. 2001;345: 266–75.
2. Counseller VS, Crenshaw JL Jr. A clinical and surgical review of endometriosis. Am J Obstet Gynecol. 1951;62:930–42.
3. Simoens S, Dunselman G, Dirksen C, Hummelshoj L, Bokor A, Brandes I, Brodszky V, Canis M, Colombo GL, DeLeire T, et al. The burden of endometriosis: costs and quality of life of women with endometriosis and treated in referral centres. Hum Reprod. 2012;27:1292–9.
4. Revised American Society for Reproductive Medicine classification of endometriosis. Fertil Steril. 1996;1997(67):817–21.
5. Barnhart K, Dunsmoor-Su R, Coutifaris C. Effect of endometriosis on in vitro fertilization. Fertil Steril. 2002;77:1148–55.
6. Bergendal A, Naffah S, Nagy C, Bergqvist A, Sjoblom P, Hillensjo T. Outcome of IVF in patients with endometriosis in comparison with tubal-factor infertility. J Assist Reprod Genet. 1998;15:530–4.
7. Hadfield R, Mardon H, Barlow D, Kennedy S. Delay in the diagnosis of endometriosis: a survey of women from the USA and the UK. Hum Reprod. 1996;11:878–80.
8. Hirsch M, Duffy J, Davis CJ, Nieves Plana M, Khan KS. International collaboration to harmonise O, measures for E: diagnostic accuracy of cancer antigen 125 for endometriosis: a systematic review and meta-analysis. BJOG. 2016;123:1761–8.
9. Ahn SH, Singh V, Tayade C. Biomarkers in endometriosis: challenges and opportunities. Fertil Steril. 2017;107:523–32.
10. Marianna S, Alessia P, Susan C, Francesca C, Angela S, Francesca C, Antonella N, Patrizia I, Nicola C, Emilio C. Metabolomic profiling and biochemical evaluation of the follicular fluid of endometriosis patients. Mol BioSyst. 2017;13:1213–22.
11. Cheema AK, Pathak R, Zandkarimi F, Kaur P, Alkhalil L, Singh R, Zhong X, Ghosh S, Aykin-Burns N, Hauer-Jensen M. Liver metabolomics reveals increased oxidative stress and fibrogenic potential in gfrp transgenic mice in response to ionizing radiation. J Proteome Res. 2014;13:3065–74.
12. Bi H, Krausz KW, Manna SK, Li F, Johnson CH, Gonzalez FJ. Optimization of harvesting, extraction, and analytical protocols for UPLC-ESI-MS-based metabolomic analysis of adherent mammalian cancer cells. Anal Bioanal Chem. 2013;405:5279–89.

13. Want EJ, Masson P, Michopoulos F, Wilson ID, Theodoridis G, Plumb RS, Shockcor J, Loftus N, Holmes E, Nicholson JK. Global metabolic profiling of animal and human tissues via UPLC-MS. Nat Protoc. 2013;8:17–32.

14. Yu T, Wang Y, Zhang H, Johnson CH, Jiang Y, Li X, Wu Z, Liu T, Krausz KW, Yu A, et al. Metabolomics reveals mycoplasma contamination interferes with the metabolism of PANC-1 cells. Anal Bioanal Chem. 2016;408:4267–73.

15. Zhang H, Jiang Y, Wu J, Zheng C, Ran X, Li D, Huang M, Bi H. Metabolic mapping of Schisandra sphenanthera extract and its active lignans using a metabolomic approach based on ultra high performance liquid chromatography with high-resolution mass spectrometry. J Sep Sci. 2017;40:574–86.

16. Dunselman GA, Vermeulen N, Becker C, Calhaz-Jorge C, D'Hooghe T, De Bie B, Heikinheimo O, Horne AW, Kiesel L, Nap A, et al. ESHRE guideline: management of women with endometriosis. Hum Reprod. 2014;29:400–12.

17. Slack A, Child T, Lindsey I, Kennedy S, Cunningham C, Mortensen N, Koninckx P, McVeigh E. Urological and colorectal complications following surgery for rectovaginal endometriosis. BJOG. 2007;114:1278–82.

18. Check JH. CA-125 as a biomarker for malignant transformation of endometriosis. Fertil Steril. 2009;91:e35. author reply e36

19. Mol BW, Bayram N, Lijmer JG, Wiegerinck MA, Bongers MY, van der Veen F, Bossuyt PM. The performance of CA-125 measurement in the detection of endometriosis: a meta-analysis. Fertil Steril. 1998;70:1101–8.

20. May KE, Conduit-Hulbert SA, Villar J, Kirtley S, Kennedy SH, Becker CM. Peripheral biomarkers of endometriosis: a systematic review. Hum Reprod Update. 2010;16:651–74.

21. Zhang A, Sun H, Wang X. Serum metabolomics as a novel diagnostic approach for disease: a systematic review. Anal Bioanal Chem. 2012;404:1239–45.

22. Patel NR, McPhail MJ, Shariff MI, Keun HC, Taylor-Robinson SD. Biofluid metabonomics using (1)H NMR spectroscopy: the road to biomarker discovery in gastroenterology and hepatology. Expert Rev Gastroenterol Hepatol. 2012;6:239–51.

23. Weiss RH, Kim K. Metabolomics in the study of kidney diseases. Nat Rev Nephrol. 2011;8:22–33.

24. Rhee EP, Gerszten RE. Metabolomics and cardiovascular biomarker discovery. Clin Chem. 2012;58:139–47.

25. Vicente-Munoz S, Morcillo I, Puchades-Carrasco L, Paya V, Pellicer A, Pineda-Lucena A. Pathophysiologic processes have an impact on the plasma metabolomic signature of endometriosis patients. Fertil Steril. 2016;106:1733–41. e1731

26. Vicente-Munoz S, Morcillo I, Puchades-Carrasco L, Paya V, Pellicer A, Pineda-Lucena A. Nuclear magnetic resonance metabolomic profiling of urine provides a noninvasive alternative to the identification of biomarkers associated with endometriosis. Fertil Steril. 2015;104:1202–9.

27. Cordeiro FB, Cataldi TR, Perkel KJ, Do Vale Teixeira da Costa L, Rochetti RC, Stevanato J, Eberlin MN, Zylbersztejn DS, Cedenho AP, Turco EG. Lipidomics analysis of follicular fluid by ESI-MS reveals potential biomarkers for ovarian endometriosis. J Assist Reprod Genet. 2015;32:1817–25.

28. Rizner TL. Diagnostic potential of peritoneal fluid biomarkers of endometriosis. Expert Rev Mol Diagn. 2015;15:557–80.

29. Joshi NR, Su RW, Chandramouli GV, Khoo SK, Jeong JW, Young SL, Lessey BA, Fazleabas AT. Altered expression of microRNA-451 in eutopic endometrium of baboons (Papio anubis) with endometriosis. Hum Reprod. 2015;30:2881–91.

30. Laudanski P, Charkiewicz R, Tolwinska A, Szamatowicz J, Charkiewicz A, Niklinski J. Profiling of selected MicroRNAs in proliferative Eutopic endometrium of women with ovarian endometriosis. Biomed Res Int. 2015;2015:760698.

31. Goteri G, Altobelli E, Tossetta G, Zizzi A, Avellini C, Licini C, Lorenzi T, Castellucci M, Ciavattini A, Marzioni D. High temperature requirement A1, transforming growth factor beta1, phosphoSmad2 and Ki67 in eutopic and ectopic endometrium of women with endometriosis. Eur J Histochem. 2015;59:2570.

32. Chelariu-Raicu A, Wilke C, Brand M, Starzinski-Powitz A, Kiesel L, Schuring AN, Gotte M. Syndecan-4 expression is upregulated in endometriosis and contributes to an invasive phenotype. Fertil Steril. 2016;106:378–85.

33. Li Y, An D, Guan YX, Kang S. Aberrant methylation of the E-cadherin gene promoter region in endometrium and ovarian Endometriotic cysts of patients with ovarian endometriosis. Gynecol Obstet Investig. 2017;82:78–85.

34. Witte DP, Wiginton DA, Hutton JJ, Aronow BJ. Coordinate developmental regulation of purine catabolic enzyme expression in gastrointestinal and postimplantation reproductive tracts. J Cell Biol. 1991;115:179–90.

35. Hong L, Mulholland J, Chinsky JM, Knudsen TB, Kellems RE, Glasser SR. Developmental expression of adenosine deaminase during decidualization in the rat uterus. Biol Reprod. 1991;44:83–93.

36. Kao LC, Germeyer A, Tulac S, Lobo S, Yang JP, Taylor RN, Osteen K, Lessey BA, Giudice LC. Expression profiling of endometrium from women with endometriosis reveals candidate genes for disease-based implantation failure and infertility. Endocrinology. 2003;144:2870–81.

37. Karanjgaokar VC, Murphy DJ, Samra JS, Mann CH. Malignant transformation of residual endometriosis after hysterectomy: a case series. Fertil Steril. 2009;2037(92):e2019–21.

38. Lin J, Zhang X, Chen Y. Mutagen sensitivity as a susceptibility marker for endometriosis. Hum Reprod. 2003;18:2052–7.

39. Munksgaard PS, Blaakaer J. The association between endometriosis and gynecological cancers and breast cancer: a review of epidemiological data. Gynecol Oncol. 2011;123:157–63.

40. Denkert C, Budczies J, Weichert W, Wohlgemuth G, Scholz M, Kind T, Niesporek S, Noske A, Buckendahl A, Dietel M, Fiehn O. Metabolite profiling of human colon carcinoma–deregulation of TCA cycle and amino acid turnover. Mol Cancer. 2008;7:72.

41. Chen JQ, Russo J. Dysregulation of glucose transport, glycolysis, TCA cycle and glutaminolysis by oncogenes and tumor suppressors in cancer cells. Biochim Biophys Acta. 2012;1826:370–84.

42. Dutta M, Joshi M, Srivastava S, Lodh I, Chakravarty B, Chaudhury K. A metabonomics approach as a means for identification of potential biomarkers for early diagnosis of endometriosis. Mol BioSyst. 2012;8:3281–7.

43. Zhang J, Liu L, Wei S, Nagana Gowda GA, Hammoud Z, Kesler KA, Raftery D. Metabolomics study of esophageal adenocarcinoma. J Thorac Cardiovasc Surg. 2011;141:469–75. 475 e461–464

44. Zhang J, Bowers J, Liu L, Wei S, Gowda GA, Hammoud Z, Raftery D. Esophageal cancer metabolite biomarkers detected by LC-MS and NMR methods. PLoS One. 2012;7:e30181.

4

Reproductive outcomes in women with unicornuate uterus undergoing in vitro fertilization: a nested case-control retrospective study

Yanrong Chen[1,2,3†], Victoria Nisenblat[1,3†], Puyu Yang[1,2,3], Xinyu Zhang[1,2,3] and Caihong Ma[1,2,3,4*]

Abstract

Background: Unicornuate uterus, a congenital uterine malformation resulting from unilateral maldevelopment of Mullerian duct, is more prevalent in women with infertility. Owing to relative rarity of the condition, the evidence on the associated reproductive outcomes is derived from small heterogeneous studies that report different clinical endpoints and often do not account for the anatomical variations of unicornuate uterus. The aim of this study was to evaluate the embryological and clinical outcomes following IVF-ICSI treatment in women with unicornuate uterus without rudimentary functional cavity (ESHRE-ESGE class IVb).

Methods: Retrospective nested case-control study comprised 342 women with unicornuate uterus and 1026 matched controls who underwent IVF-ICSI cycles between October 2012 and October 2016. Cumulative live birth rate upon one complete IVF cycle, including transfers of all resulting embryos was considered as a primary outcome measure.

Results: Baseline characteristics were comparable between the unicornuate uterus and control groups except for higher rate of primary infertility in unicornuate uterus. Ovarian response to stimulation did not differ between the groups. Transfer of day-3 embryos in fresh cycle resulted in lower clinical pregnancy rate (35.9% vs. 43.9%, $p = 0.028$) and live-birth rate (26.9% vs. 35.2%, $p = 0.017$) per transfer, but the difference was not observed when either cleavage frozen-thaw embryos or blastocysts were transferred. Implantation rate was lower and miscarriage rate was higher in women with unicornuate uterus but the difference between the groups did not reach statistical significance. Transfer of cleavage embryos resulted in significantly higher miscarriage rate and lower live-birth rate in fresh versus frozen-thaw cycles in each group, whereas fresh and frozen-thaw blastocyst embryos had comparable outcomes. Upon completion of one IVF-ICSI cycle, the cumulative pregnancy rate (53.1% vs. 65.7, $p < 0.001$) and cumulative live birth rate (42.4% vs. 54.6%, $p < 0.001$) were significantly lower in women with unicornuate uterus compared to those in women with normal uterus. Cumulative outcomes were superior when embryos were cultured to blastocyst stage.

Conclusions: Women with unicornuate uterus have lower clinical pregnancy and live birth rate after IVF-ICSI treatment compared to women with normal uterus. The treatment outcomes are improved with blastocyst culture, which warrants evaluation in prospective setting.

Keywords: Unicornuate uterus, ART, IVF-ICSI, Reproductive outcomes, Cumulative live birth rate

* Correspondence: macaihong@263.net; bysy@bjmu.edu.cn
†Yanrong Chen and Victoria Nisenblat contributed equally to this work.
[1]Center for Reproductive Medicine, Department of Obstetrics and Gynecology, Peking University Third Hospital, Beijing 100191, China
[2]National Clinical Research Center for Obstetrics and Gynecology, Beijing 100191, China
Full list of author information is available at the end of the article

Background

Congenital uterine defects represent a wide range of abnormalities of uterine anatomy that result from elongation, fusion and absorption disorders of the bilateral Müllerian ducts during embryogenesis between 6 and 20 weeks of gestation [1]. The prevalence of uterine malformations is estimated at 5.5% in general population and at approximately 8% in women with infertility [2]. Unicornuate uterus is caused by maldevelopment of one Müllerian duct and is relatively uncommon, representing 2.5–13.2% of all uterine malformations [2]. It occurs in 0.1% of unselected population and is more prevalent in women with infertility (0.5%), miscarriage (0.5%) or both (3.1%) [2]. The European Society of Human Reproduction and Embryology–European Society for Gynecological Endoscopy (ESHRE–ESGE) recognizes two types of unicornuate uterus: 1) hemi-uterus with a rudimentary functional contralateral cavity, communicating or non-communicating, due to a partial Mullerian duct development (class IVa) and 2) isolated hemi-uterus caused by a unilateral agenesis of Mullerian duct (class IVb) [3, 4]. Ovarian development usually is not compromised, although ovary on the affected side may be misplaced higher in the abdomen or even absent in rare cases [5]. Coincidental renal anomalies are common and there is an increased risk of developing endometriosis or chronic pain due to hematometra in women with rudimentary horn [5, 6].

It has been widely recognized that unicornuate uterus is associated with increased risk of miscarriage, ectopic pregnancy in rudimentary horn and adverse obstetrics outcomes [5–7]. The relationship between unicornuate uterus and infertility is less clear. A retrospective observational study in 3181 women reported that 23.7% of women with unicornuate uterus were diagnosed with subfertility [8]. A meta-analysis of 25 studies on women with different Mullerian anomalies revealed that a probability of spontaneous conception was not different in women with unicornuate uterus compared with the controls, although these conclusions were based on two small retrospective studies [7]. Several investigators demonstrated poorer outcomes of assisted reproductive technology (ART) treatments in women with unicornuate uterus compared to those with normal anatomy [9–13]. Most of these studies, however, included low number of patients, focused on varying treatment endpoints and presented reproductive outcomes in different ways, all of which challenge the evaluation and synthesis of the reported data. Moreover, none of these studies stratified the outcomes by the type of unicornuate uterus, which may influence reproductive outcomes owing to variations in uterine vascularity, degree of uterine muscle development and presence of other concurrent pelvic pathology [14].

The aim of this study was to evaluate the embryological and clinical outcomes in women with unicornuate uterus without rudimentary horn (ESHRE-ESGE class IVb) following one complete ART cycle including the transfer of all the resulting fresh and frozen-thaw embryos, with a focus on the cumulative birth rate as a primary outcome measure.

Methods

Study design and participants

Retrospective nested case control study was conducted at the Reproductive Centre of the Peking University Third Hospital, a tertiary university hospital and a center of excellence in Reproductive Medicine in China. We assessed the medical records of all women who underwent in vitro fertilization (IVF) or intracytoplasmic sperm injection (ICSI) cycles between October 1st, 2012 and October 31st, 2016. Patients were identified through the hospital electronic database.

In addition to the routine pre-treatment work-up, which included history, gynecological examination, baseline reproductive hormones, thyroid function, tubal patency test, pelvic ultrasound and male partner semen analysis, women with any suspected uterine pathology underwent hysteroscopy with or without laparoscopy to confirm the diagnosis and karyotype as deemed appropriate within the clinical context. The inclusion criteria in the study group (unicornuate uterus group) were as follows: 1) unicornuate uterus class IVb (isolated hemi-uterus without functional rudimentary cavity) diagnosed by 3D transvaginal sonography (3D-TVS) and by hysteroscopy, with or without laparoscopy and MRI (Magnetic Resonance Imaging); 2) first IVF/ICSI cycle in our center. The exclusion criteria were: 1) other uterine malformations (septum, unicornuate uterus class IVa, bicornuate uterus); 2) endometrial lesions (polyps, endometrial hyperplasia, intrauterine adhesions); 3) uterine fibroids distorting uterine cavity diagnosed by TVS or hysteroscopy; 4) sonographic features of adenomyosis; 5) chromosomal abnormality of male or female partner; 6) patients who undertook a donor oocyte program or had preimplantation genetic diagnosis (PGD)/preimplantation genetic screening (PGS); 7) patients who had cancelled IVF cycle that did not result in embryo transfer (ET). The control group included women with normal uterus who otherwise met the similar selection criteria and underwent IVF treatment during the study period. Controls were randomly selected from the same database, matched in a ratio of 1:3 by age, BMI, cause of infertility, and number of embryos transferred.

ART treatment protocols

All participants underwent ovarian stimulation by using either long GnRH agonist downregulation or antagonist protocol, using either recombinant or human menopausal gonadotrophins. Human chorionic gonadotrophin (hCG) trigger was administered when there were at least one to three follicles above 18 mm. Stimulation protocol, type of gonadotrophins and starting dose were at discretion of the treating clinician in discussion with the patient. Ultrasound-guided transvaginal oocyte retrieval was performed 36–38 h after the trigger injection according to the department protocol. Oocytes were inseminated either by conventional IVF or by ICSI depending on sperm quality. Fertilization was assessed 17–19 h after insemination and was defined by the presence of two pronuclears (2PN) and two polar bodies (PBs). An embryo quality was assessed 68–72 h (day 3) after insemination according to the Istanbul Consensus Workshop on Embryo Assessment criteria [15]. Day-3 cleavage embryos were either transferred or cultured for the additional 48 h to the blastocyst stage. The blastocysts were evaluated on day 5 by using Gardner morphological grading system [16]. All spare embryos were cryopreserved for future use. Two cryopreservation methods including vitrification and slow freezing were used.

Day-3 or day-5 embryos were transferred in a fresh cycle with luteal support by vaginal and/or intramuscular progesterone, unless there were medical indications for freezing all the embryos. When the cryopreserved embryos generated from the index stimulation cycle were available, frozen-thaw embryo transfer (FET) was performed in a natural or artificial estradiol and progesterone endometrium priming as described previously [17]. The best morphological grade embryos were selected for transfer and if were not available, the decision to transfer lower quality embryo was based on clinical circumstances and patient wishes after appropriate counselling. ETs were performed by using a soft catheter (K-Soft 5100; Cook, Queensland, Australia). Serum hCG was measured 14 days after ET and was considered positive for hCG level ≥ 10 IU. Transvaginal ultrasonography at 30 days after transfer confirmed clinical pregnancy if intrauterine gestational sac was demonstrated.

Outcome measures

Cumulative live birth rate was a primary outcome measure and was calculated by the number of first live births generated from a single IVF/ICSI cycle including all the fresh or frozen-thaw ETs generated from the index cycle divided by all women who received treatment. Live birth was defined as a pregnancy that led to delivery of at least one living child, irrespective of the duration of gestation.

Secondary outcomes included the following: 1) implantation rate (the number of gestational sacs divided by the number of transferred embryos); 2) miscarriage rate (loss of clinical pregnancy before 24 weeks of gestation divided by the number of clinical pregnancies); 3) cumulative clinical pregnancy rate (number of first clinical pregnancies from a single IVF/ICSI cycle including all the fresh or frozen-thaw ETs generated from the index cycle divided by all women who received treatment); 4) clinical pregnancy per transfer cycle (number of clinical pregnancies divided by the number of women who had transfer); and 5) live birth rate per transfer cycle (number of live births divided by the number of women who had transfer). The 'per cycle' parameters were calculated separately for fresh and frozen-thaw ET cycles.

Statistical analysis

The Student's t-test was used for comparison of continuous variables between the groups. The chi-squared test or Fisher's exact test, where appropriate, were used for comparisons of categorical variables. Results are presented as mean ± standard deviation (SD) or as percentages. The multivariable logistic regression analyses were employed to delineate the independent prognostic risk factors for cumulative live birth rate. Statistical significance was set at a probability (p) value < 0.05 (two--sided). All statistical analyses were performed using SPSS 23.0 software (SPSS, Inc., Chicago, IL, USA).

Results

Overall 1368 women were included in the study. Of them, 342 patients with unicornuate ESHRE-ESGE class IVb uterus comprised the study group and 1026 women served as controls. There was no significant difference between the groups with respect to age, BMI, baseline FSH, duration and cause of infertility (Table 1). Majority of women in both groups were nulliparous. Primary infertility was significantly more common in women with unicornuate uterus ($p = 0.005$). The characteristics of the ART cycles and the embryology outcomes are summarized in Table 2. There was no difference in number of women assigned to a specific stimulation protocol or in number of ICSI cycles. Both groups did not differ in ovarian response to simulation, had comparable yield of oocytes and of cleavage stage embryos, and had similar fertilization rate. The endometrium on hCG trigger day was significantly thinner in women with unicornuate uterus compared to that in controls, but this difference was of marginal clinical value (10.08 ± 1.57 vs. 10.78 ± 1.55, $p<0.001$).

Each woman completed one IVF-ICSI treatment including all fresh and frozen-thaw ETs of the embryos generated from this cycle. There was a total of 1939 ET cycles, which included 500 ET cycles in the study group and 1439 ET cycles in controls. The number of embryos transferred per fresh or frozen-thaw cycle, either at cleavage or blastocyst stage was similar between the study and control groups. The clinical outcomes of fresh ETs are presented in Table 3. Cleavage day-3 stage embryos were transferred in majority of fresh ET cycles:

Table 1 Baseline characteristics of the study population

	Unicornuate uterus n = 342 women	Controls n = 1026 women	p-value
Age (years), mean ± SD	30.53 ± 4.20	30.61 ± 4.28	p = 0.784
BMI (kg/m^2), mean ± SD	22.95 ± 3.36	22.63 ± 2.93	p = 0.120
Basal FSH (mIU/ml), mean ± SD	6.21 ± 2.40	5.95 ± 2.59	p = 0.089
Primary infertility, n (%)	215/342 (62.9%)	556/1026 (54.2%)	p = 0.005
Infertility duration (years), mean ± SD	4.17 ± 3.24	4.26 ± 3.11	p = 0.640
Nulliparity, n (%)	328/342 (95.9%)	961/1026 (93.7%)	p = 0.124
Cause of infertility			p = 0.891
Tubal factor, n (%)	216/342 (63.2%)	684/1026 (66.7%)	
Male factor, n (%)	63/342 (18.4%)	176/1026 (17.2%)	
Endometriosis, n (%)	5/342 (1.5%)	12/1026 (1.2%)	
PCOS, n (%)	11/342 (3.2%)	26/1026 (2.5%)	
POR, n (%)	13/342 (3.8%)	37/1026 (3.6%)	
Unexplained, n (%)	34/342 (9.9%)	91/1026 (8.9%)	

BMI body mass index, FSH follicle stimulating hormone, PCOS polycystic ovary syndrome, POR poor ovarian response

1216 transfers of cleavage stage embryos and 84 transfers of blastocysts. In women with unicornuate uterus transfer of day-3 embryos in fresh cycle was associated with lower rates of clinical pregnancy (35.9% vs. 43.9%, $p = 0.028$), live birth (26.9% vs. 35.2%, $p = 0.017$) and multiple live birth (4.9% vs. 9.7%, $p = 0.024$) compared to those in controls. Implantation rate was also lower (23.7% vs. 28.0%, $p = 0.073$) and miscarriage rate was higher (25.0% vs. 19.7%, $p = 0.283$) in unicornuate uterus but the difference did not reach statistical significance. For fresh cycle blastocyst transfers the comparison between the two groups failed to demonstrate significant difference for any of the outcome parameters. The results of frozen-thaw ET (FET) are illustrated in Table 4. There were 307 cycles of cleavage stage ET and 332 cycles of blastocyst transfer. No significant difference was observed between the study and control groups with respect to any of the clinical endpoints when either cleavage stage or blastocyst embryos were transferred, although there was a similar trend towards lower clinical pregnancy and live birth rate in unicornuate uterus group.

The results of the comparisons between fresh and frozen-thaw ETs stratified by the type of embryos transferred in each group is summarized in Additional file 1: Table S1. Transfer of day-3 embryos in fresh cycle resulted in significantly higher implantation and clinical pregnancy rate, but significantly lower miscarriage rate than in frozen-thaw cycle in both the unicornuate uterus or control

Table 2 Characteristics of IVF-ICSI stimulation cycles

	Unicornuate uterus n = 342 women	Control n = 1026 women	p-value
Number of IVF/ICSI cycles, n	342	1026	
ICSI, n (%)	26.3% (90/342)	30.5% (310/1026)	p = 0.146
GnRH agonist protocol, % (n)	55.8% (191/342)	61.0% (626/1026)	p = 0.092
Total gonadotrophin dose (IU), mean ± SD	2778.29 ± 866.62	2730.50 ± 1214.06	p = 0.501
EM thickness on HCG-day (mm), mean ± SD	10.08 ± 1.57	10.78 ± 1.55	p < 0.001
E2 on hCG-day (pmol/L), mean ± SD	9661.81 ± 6011.21	9442.79 ± 5834.27	p = 0.580
LH on hCG-day (mIU/ml), mean ± SD	2.76 ± 1.42	2.81 ± 1.47	p = 0.651
P on hCG-day (nmol/L), mean ± SD	1.73 ± 1.79	1.62 ± 2.91	p = 0.526
Oocytes collected, mean ± SD	13.11 ± 7.77	12.28 ± 6.02	p = 0.073
2PN embryos, mean ± SD	7.63 ± 5.88	7.10 ± 4.60	p = 0.113
Day-3 embryos, mean ± SD	5.24 ± 5.30	4.95 ± 4.21	p = 0.363

E2 estradiol, EM endometrial, hCG human chorionic gonadotrophin, ICSI intracytoplasmic sperm injection, IVF in vitro fertilization, 2PN two pronuclear zygote, P progesterone

Table 3 Reproductive outcomes calculated per fresh ET cycle

	Unicornuate uterus $n = 342$ women	Control $n = 1026$ women	OR (95% CI)	p-value
Cleavage day-3 ET cycles, n	223	993		
Embryos per transfer, mean ± SD	1.87 ± 0.49	1.93 ± 0.46		$p = 0.123$
Implantation rate, % (n)	23.7% (99/418)	28.0% (535/1914)	0.847 (0.703–1.021)	$p = 0.073$
Clinical pregnancy rate, % (n)	35.9% (80/223)	43.9% (436/993)	0.817 (0.676–0.987)	$p = 0.028$
Miscarriage rate, % (n)	25.0% (20/80)	19.7% (86/436)	1.267 (0.829–1.937)	$p = 0.283$
Live birth rate, % (n)	26.9% (60/223)	35.2% (350/993)	0.763 (0.605–0.963)	$p = 0.017$
Multiple live birth rate, % (n)	4.9% (11/223)	9.7% (96/993)	0.510 (0.278–0.936)	$p = 0.024$
Blastocyst ET cycles, n	59	25		
Embryos per transfer, mean ± SD	1.07 ± 0.25	1.16 ± 0.37		$p = 0.192$
Implantation rate, % (n)	34.9% (22/63)	34.5% (10/29)	1.013 (0.553–1.853)	$p = 0.967$
Clinical pregnancy, % (n)	37.3% (22/59)	40.0% (10/25)	0.932 (0.520–1.670)	$p = 0.815$
Miscarriage rate, % (n)	18.2% (4/22)	20.0% (2/10)	0.909 (0.198–4.173)	$p = 0.903$
Live birth rate, % (n)	30.5% (18/59)	32.0% (8/25)	0.953 (0.479–1.899)	$p = 0.892$
Multiple live birth rate, % (n)	3.4% (2/59)	0	0.966 (0.921–1.013)	$p = 0.351$

ET embryo transfer, CI confidence interval, OR odds ratio

groups. The outcomes of the blastocyst transfers were not different between the fresh and frozen-thaw cycles in either group.

The cumulative outcomes of one complete ART treatment with all the ETs generated from a single stimulation-oocyte retrieval cycle are presented in Table 5. The cumulative clinical pregnancy rate was significantly lower in women with unicornuate uterus than that in controls (53.1% vs. 65.7%, $p < 0.001$). Likewise, the unicornuate uterus group had significantly lower cumulative live birth rate compared to the women with normal uterine anatomy (42.4% vs. 54.6%, $p < 0.001$) (Table 5A). Among women with unicornuate uterus, transfer of cleavage embryos resulted in significantly lower clinical pregnancy and live birth than transfer of blastocyst embryos (47.5% vs. 65.1%, $p = 0.006$ and 38.2% vs. 53.0%, $p = 0.021$), respectively (Table 5B).

Table 4 Reproductive outcomes per FET cycle

	Unicornuate uterus $n = 342$ women	Control $n = 1026$ women	OR (95% CI)	p-value
Cleavage day-3 FET cycles, n	93	214		
Embryos survival rate, % (n)	90.2% (203/225)	91.9% (475/517)		$p = 0.478$
Embryos per transfer, mean ± SD	2.18 ± 0.59	2.21 ± 0.68		$p = 0.743$
Implantation rate, % (n)	16.7% (34/203)	20.4% (97/475)	0.820 (0.575–1.169)	$p = 0.267$
Clinical pregnancy, % (n)	32.3% (30/93)	35.5% (76/214)	0.908 (0.643–1.283)	$p = 0.581$
Miscarriage rate, % (n)	6.7% (2/30)	9.2% (7/76)	0.724 (0.159–3.288)	$p = 0.672$
Live birth rate, % (n)	30.1% (28/93)	32.2% (69/214)	0.934 (0.648–1.346)	$p = 0.712$
Multiple live birth rate, % (n)	4.3% (4/93)	9.8% (21/214)	0.438 (0.155–1.241)	$p = 0.105$
Blastocyst FET cycles, n	125	207		
Embryos survival rate, % (n)	97.9% (141/144)	98.7% (234/237)		$p = 0.677$
Embryos per transfer, mean ± SD	1.13 ± 0.34	1.13 ± 0.34		$p = 0.949$
Implantation rate, % (n)	34.0% (48/141)	36.8% (86/234)	0.926 (0.697–1.231)	$p = 0.596$
Clinical pregnancy, % (n)	36.8% (46/125)	40.1% (83/207)	0.918 (0.619–1.219)	$p = 0.550$
Miscarriage rate, % (n)	21.7% (10/46)	10.8% (9/83)	2.005 (0.878–4.576)	$p = 0.094$
Live birth rate, % (n)	28.8% (36/125)	35.7% (74/207)	0.806 (0.579–1.121)	$p = 0.192$
Multiple live birth rate, % (n)	1.6% (2/125)	1.4% (3/207)	1.104 (0.187–6.516)	$p = 0.913$

FET frozen embryo transfer, CI confidence interval, OR odds ratio, SD standard deviation

Table 5 Cumulative reproductive outcomes from one complete ART cycle including fresh and frozen-thaw ETs

A. Cumulative outcomes in women with unicornuate uterus and in controls[a]

	Unicornuate	Control	OR (95% CI)	p-value
	n = 335 women	n = 920 women		
Number of IVF/ICSI cycles, n	335	920		
Number of ET cycles, n	486	1206		
Fresh ET cycles, n	277	916		
FET cycles, n	209	290		
Cumulative pregnancy rate, % (n)	53.1% (178/335)	65.7% (604/920)	0.809 (0.724–0.904)	p<0.001
Cumulative live birth rate, % (n)	42.4% (142/335)	54.6% (502/920)	0.777 (0.677–0.892)	p<0.001

B. Cumulative outcomes in women with unicornuate uterus group stratified by the type of embryos transferred[b]

	Cleavage day-3 ET	Blastocyst ET	OR (95% CI)	p-value
	n = 217 women	n = 83 women		
Number of IVF-ICSI cycles, n	217	83		
Number of ET cycles, n	251	148		
Fresh ET cycles, n	185	64		
FET cycles, n	66	84		
Cumulative pregnancy rate, % (n)	47.5% (103/217)	65.1% (54/83)	0.730 (0.591–0.901)	p = 0.006
Cumulative live birth rate, % (n)	38.2% (83/217)	53.0% (44/83)	0.722 (0.554–0.939)	p = 0.021

ART assisted reproductive technologies, CI confidence interval, ET embryo transfer, FET frozen-thaw ET, ICSI intracytoplasmic sperm injection, IVF in vitro fertilization, OR odds ratio

[a]only women who either achieved pregnancy or utilized all the embryos resulting from the index stimulation cycle were included in this analysis

[b] only women who had one type of embryos transferred in both fresh and FET cycles, either only cleavage or only blastocysts, were included in this analysis

Our study used the cumulative live birth as a dependent variable, unicornuate uterus, infertility type, protocol type, basal FSH and oocytes collected as independent variables, analyzed by the method of multivariable logistic regression. The unicirnuate uterus (OR 0.756, 95%CI 0.586–0.974, $p = 0.030$) and infertility type (OR 0.487, 95%CI 0.391–0.607, $p < 0.001$) were the independent factors of the cumulative live birth.

Discussion

This study aimed to evaluate the IVF-ICSI treatment outcomes in infertile women with unicornuate uterus without functional rudimentary cavity. We considered cumulative live birth rate after one cycle of ovarian stimulation - oocyte retrieval with all the resulting fresh and frozen-thaw ET cycles as a primary outcome measure and reported the data from 342 women with unicornuate uterus and 1026 randomly selected matched controls from the same cohort. To the best of our knowledge, this is the largest report that includes well-characterized women with specific phenotype of unicornuate uterus and accounts for multiple confounding factors that may impact the treatment outcomes.

Our results demonstrate that unicornuate uterus did not affect ovarian response to stimulation and embryology outcomes. Overall the IVF-ICSI endpoints in women unicornuate uterus without functional rudimentary cavity are reassuring but are inferior to those in women with normal uterus. In women with unicornuate uterus, the odds of achieving clinical pregnancy following one complete IVF-ICSI cycle were 24% lower (OR 0.809, 95%CI 0.724–0.904) and the odds of live birth were 28% lower (OR 0.777, 95% CI 0.677–0.892) than in women with normal uterine anatomy after control for important demographic and clinical confounders.

This is in line with the results of previous observational studies that demonstrated lower pregnancy rate and/or live-birth in women with unicornuate uterus than in controls with normal uterine morphology [6, 10, 11, 18]. In contrast, Jayaprakasan et al., did not observe difference in ART outcomes between women with uterine malformations and normal uterus, but the study included only 6 women with bicornuate uterus, while arcuate uterus represented majority of the evaluated uterine malformations [13]. When we stratified the outcomes by the type of embryos transferred, statistically significant difference between the groups with respect to clinical pregnancy and live birth were observed only for fresh cleavage stage embryos, while transfer of frozen-thaw cleavage or of blastocyst embryos resulted in only non-significantly lower outcomes in unicornuate uterus group.

In contrast with previously demonstrated lower implantation rate in unicornuate uterus [18], in this study implantation rate was only non-significantly reduced in women with unicornuate uterus, which is in agreement with the findings reported by Ozgur et al. [10]. The association between unicornuate uterus and miscarriage following either natural or assisted conception were previously reported by several investigators [6, 10, 11, 13, 18, 19]. In this study, there was only non-significant increase in miscarriage rate in the overall group of women with unicornuate uterus. However, women who had a transfer of fresh cleavage stage embryos had significantly higher miscarriage rate and lower live-birth rate compared to those who had frozen-thaw cycles, which held true for women with either unicornuate or normal uterus. This observation is consistent with the results of recent randomized controlled trial (RCT) that demonstrated that frozen ET cycles were associated with higher rate of live birth and lower rate of miscarriage in women with PCOS [20]. Transfer of blastocyst stage embryos did not appear to be associated with different outcomes in either group. Importantly, however, the cumulative reproductive outcomes in women with unicornuate uterus were significantly higher when embryos were cultured to the blastocyst stage with 37% higher odds to achieve clinical pregnancy (OR 0.730, 95%CI 0.591–0.901) and 39% higher odds to achieve live-birth (OR 0.722, 95%CI 0.554–0.939) compared to the transfer of cleavage stage embryos. Improved implantation and pregnancy rates have been increasingly reported for transferred blastocysts compared to cleavage embryos in IVF cycles. This finding should be interpreted with caution in view of relative paucity of blastocyst ET cycles in this study. The most recent Cochrane library systematic review concluded that in general IVF population, the live birth rate per fresh transfer was significantly higher with blastocyst culture compared to cleavage stage embryos, whereas there was no difference between the groups in cumulative live birth rates following both fresh and frozen-thaw cycles resulting from one egg collection [21]. Higher likelihood of failure to make embryo transfer along with lower availability for surplus embryos with blastocyst culture are possible explanation. This meta-analysis, however, included earlier studies employing slow freezing and overall reported low quality evidence for the cumulative outcomes, hence the effect of the day of transfer on cumulative pregnancy and live birth rate remains unclear. In this study women with unicornuate uterus had higher rate of primary infertility, similarly to the observed in previous studies [6]. Unicornuate uterus has been recognized in association with adverse obstetrics and neonatal outcomes, including preterm labor, fetal malpresentation, fetal growth restriction and perinatal death [5–7]. The possible causative factors include reduced uterine muscle mass, aberrant uterine vasculature and smaller size of uterine cavity [5, 14]. The underlying mechanism by which unicornuate uterus affects fertility and ART treatment outcomes is unclear. It has been proposed that derangements in endometrial vascularization with deleterious effect on endometrial receptivity and implantation could play a role [14]. It is also possible that mechanical factor is more likely to be present in unicornuate uterus due to presence of a single tube. Unicornuate uterus has been also associated with increased risk of ectopic pregnancy and endometriosis, particularly in women with functional rudimentary uterine cavity. In our cohort, tubal factor accounted for majority of causes of infertility, 63.2%, which is higher than the estimated ~ 18% in general population of women who undergo ART [22].

The strengths of this study are in its relatively large sample size of well-characterized cohort and the utilized strategies to control for confounding, including carefully 1:3 matched controls and multiple subgroup analyses. In addition, the study reports the cumulative success rate after one complete stimulation cycle, which is a more appropriate way to estimate the ART treatment outcomes than presenting a data per an individual transfer cycle. The information presented this study helps to refine patient counselling and directs the clinicians towards more effective tailored interventions.

The main limitations of this study are its retrospective nature and no information on the obstetrics and neonatal outcomes. Furthermore, not all women that commenced ART treatment in 2016 utilized their available embryos from the index stimulation cycle and were not included in estimation of cumulative live birth rate. Finally, culture to blastocyst was performed in relatively small number of treatment cycles as the shift towards blastocyst embryo transfer has occurred in our center in the last several years.

Conclusion

In summary, women with unicornuate uterus have lower clinical pregnancy and live-birth rate after IVF-ICSI treatment compared to women with normal uterine morphology with similar baseline characteristics. Culture to blastocyst is associated with the improved treatment cycle outcomes. The findings of this study require further validation in large well-defined cohort of women with unicornuate uterus in different population. It is unrealistic to expect a single-center interventional RCT that focuses on management of unicornuate uterus as the condition is infrequent. Multi-center initiatives or non-randomized prospective studies would help to evaluate the contribution of blastocyst transfer, especially single blastocyst transfer approach to improvement of ART treatment outcomes in women with unicornuate uterus.

Acknowledgements
We thank the medical and administrative staff of the Reproductive Medical Center of Peking University Third Hospital for their assistance with maintaining the electronic database and assistance with data collection.

Funding

This study was supported by the 'Capital's Funds for Health Improvement and Research (2014-1-4091)' and 'Key Clinical Program of Peking University Third Hospital (BYSY2015002)'.

Authors' contributions

YC: performed the data collection, analysis and produced the first draft of the manuscript; VN: contributed to the concept, study design, data analysis and preparation of the manuscript; PY and XZ were involved in critical discussions; CM: initiated and coordinated the research, contributed to study design, critical discussions and preparation of the manuscript. All authors read and approved the final manuscript.

Competing interests

The authors declare that they have no competing interests.

Author details

[1]Center for Reproductive Medicine, Department of Obstetrics and Gynecology, Peking University Third Hospital, Beijing 100191, China. [2]National Clinical Research Center for Obstetrics and Gynecology, Beijing 100191, China. [3]Key Laboratory of Assisted Reproductive, Ministry of Education, Beijing 100191, China. [4]Beijing, China.

References

1. Engmann L, Schmidt D, Nulsen J, Maier D, Benadiva C. An unusual anatomic variation of a unicornuate uterus with normal external uterine morphology. Fertil Steril. 2004;82(4):950–3.
2. Chan YY, Jayaprakasan K, Zamora J, Thornton JG, Raine-Fenning N, Coomarasamy A. The prevalence of congenital uterine anomalies in unselected and high-risk populations: a systematic review. Hum Reprod Update. 2011;17(6):761–71.
3. Grimbizis GF, Gordts S, Di Spiezio SA, Brucker S, De Angelis C, Gergolet M, et al. The ESHRE-ESGE consensus on the classification of female genital tract congenital anomalies. Gynecol Surg. 2013;10(3):199–212.
4. Grimbizis GF, Di Spiezio SA, Saravelos SH, Gordts S, Exacoustos C, Van Schoubroeck D, et al. The Thessaloniki ESHRE/ESGE consensus on diagnosis of female genital anomalies. Gynecol Surg. 2016;13:1–16.
5. Reichman D, Laufer MR, Robinson BK. Pregnancy outcomes in unicornuate uteri: a review. Fertil Steril. 2009;91(5):1886–94.
6. Fedele L, Zamberletti D, Vercellini P, Dorta M, Candiani GB. Reproductive performance of women with unicornuate uterus. Fertil Steril. 1987;47(3): 416–9.
7. Venetis CA, Papadopoulos SP, Campo R, Gordts S, Tarlatzis BC, Grimbizis GF. Clinical implications of congenital uterine anomalies: a meta-analysis of comparative studies. Reprod BioMed Online. 2014;29(6):665–83.
8. Raga F, Bauset C, Remohi J, Bonilla-Musoles F, Simón C, Pellicer A. Reproductive impact of congenital mü¨ llerian anomalies. Fertil Steril. 1997; 12(10):2277–81.
9. Lavergne N, Aristizabal J, Zarka V, Erny R, Hedon B. Uterine anomalies and in vitro fertilization: what are the results? Eur J Obstet Gynecol Reprod Biol. 1996;68(1–2):29–34.
10. Ozgur K, Bulut H, Berkkanoglu M, Coetzee K. Reproductive outcomes of IVF patients with unicornuate uteri. Reprod BioMed Online. 2017;34(3):312–8.
11. Li X, Ouyang Y, Yi Y, Lin G, Lu G, Gong F. Pregnancy outcomes of women with a congenital unicornuate uterus after IVF-embryo transfer. Reprod BioMed Online. 2017;35(5):583–91.
12. Liu J, Wu Y, Xu S, Su D, Han Y, Wu X. Retrospective evaluation of pregnancy outcomes and clinical implications of 34 Han Chinese women with unicornuate uterus who received IVF-ET or ICSI-ET treatment. J Obstet Gynaecol. 2017;37(8):1020–4.
13. Jayaprakasan K, Chan YY, Sur S, Deb S, Clewes JS, Raine-Fenning NJ. Prevalence of uterine anomalies and their impact on early pregnancy in women conceiving after assisted reproduction treatment. Ultrasound Obstet Gynecol. 2011;37(6):727–32.
14. Taylor E, Gomel V. The uterus and fertility. Fertil Steril. 2008;89(1):1–16.
15. Alpha Scientists in Reproductive M, Embryology ESIGo. The Istanbul consensus workshop on embryo assessment: proceedings of an expert meeting. Hum Reprod. 2011;26(6):1270–83.
16. Schoolcraft WB, Gardner DK, Lane M, Schlenker T, Hamilton F, Meldrum DR. Blastocyst culture and transfer: analysis of results and parameters affecting outcome in two in vitro fertilization programs. Fertil Steril. 1999;72(4):604–9.
17. Xu YYNV, Lu C, Li R, Qiao J, Zhen X, Wang S. Pretreatment with coenzyme Q10 improves ovarian response and embryo quality in low-prognosis young women with decreased ovarian reserve: a randomized controlled trial. Reprod Biol Endocrinol. 2018; in press
18. Heinonen PK, Kuismanen K, Ashorn R. Assisted reproduction in women with uterine anomalies. Eur J Obstet Gynecol Reprod Biol. 2000;89(2):181–4.
19. Akar ME, Bayar D, Yildiz S, Ozel M, Yilmaz Z. Reproductive outcome of women with unicornuate uterus. ANZJOG. 2005;45(2):148–50.
20. Chen ZJ, Shi Y, Sun Y, Zhang B, Liang X, Cao Y, et al. Fresh versus frozen embryos for infertility in the polycystic ovary syndrome. NEJM. 2016;375(6): 523–33.
21. Glujovsky D, Farquhar C, Quinteiro Retamar AM, Alvarez Sedo CR, Blake D. Cleavage stage versus blastocyst stage embryo transfer in assisted reproductive technology. Cochrane Database Syst Rev. 2016;6:CD002118. https://doi.org/10.1002/14651858.CD002118.pub5.25.
22. Centers for Disease Control and Prevention, Society for Assisted Reproductive Technology. 2004 Assisted Reproductive Technology Success Rates: National Summary and Fertility Clinic Reports, Department of Health and Human Services, Centers for Disease Control and Prevention, 2006.

5

The dynamic changes in the number of uterine natural killer cells are specific to the eutopic but not to the ectopic endometrium in women and in a baboon model of endometriosis

Josephine A. Drury[1], Kirstin L. Parkin[2,3], Lucy Coyne[4,5], Emma Giuliani[2,6], Asgerally T. Fazleabas[2] and Dharani K. Hapangama[1,4*] [iD]

Abstract

Background: Endometriosis is a common condition associated with growth of endometrial-like tissue beyond the uterine cavity. Previous reports have suggested a role for uNK cells in the pathogenesis of endometriosis postulating that survival and accumulation of menstrual endometrial tissue in the peritoneal cavity may relate to a reduction in the cytotoxic activity of peripheral blood NK cells. We aimed to assess the differences in percentage of uNK cells and their phenotypical characterization in eutopic and ectopic endometrial samples from women with and without endometriosis and baboons with induced endometriosis.

Methods: Eutopic and ectopic endometrial samples from 82 women across the menstrual cycle with/without endometriosis and from 8 baboons before and after induction of endometriosis were examined for CD56 and NKp30 expression with immunohistochemistry, quantified using computer assisted image analysis. Curated secretory phase endometrial microarray datasets were interrogated for NK cell receptors and their ligands. In silico data was validated by examining the secretory phase eutopic endometrium of women with and without endometriosis ($n = 8$/group) for the immuno-expression of BAG6 protein.

Results: The percentage of uNK cells increased progressively from the proliferative phase with the highest levels in the late secretory phase in the eutopic endometrium of women with and without endometriosis. The percentage of uNK cells in ectopic lesions remained significantly low throughout the cycle. In baboons, induction of endometriosis increased the percentage of uNK in the ectopic lesions but not NKp30. Published eutopic endometrial microarray datasets demonstrated significant upregulation of NKp30 and its ligand BAG6 in women with endometriosis compared with controls. Immunohistochemical staining scores for BAG6 was also significantly higher in secretory phase eutopic endometrium from women with endometriosis compared with the endometrium of healthy women ($n = 8$/group).

Conclusions: The dynamic increase in the percentage of uNK cells in the secretory phase is preserved in the endometrium of women with endometriosis. The low number of uNK cells in human and baboon ectopic lesions may be due to their exaggerated reduction in hormonal responsiveness (progesterone resistance).

Keywords: Uterine natural killer cells, Endometriosis, Humans, Primate, Baboon

* Correspondence: dharani@liv.ac.uk
[1]Department of Women's and Children's Health, Institute of Translational Medicine, University of Liverpool, Liverpool, UK
[4]Department of Gynecology, Liverpool Women's Hospital, Liverpool, UK
Full list of author information is available at the end of the article

Background

[1, 2] Endometrial leucocytes are postulated to play an important role in normal endometrial functions [3] and CD56^{bright} CD16$^-$ uterine Natural killer (uNK) cells are the predominant leucocyte subset in the secretory phase endometrium [4]. They are likely to have functions in inflammatory modulation, angiogenesis, apoptosis, and extracellular matrix remodelling and these activities may continue into the decidual tissue of the very early stages of pregnancy [5, 6]. NK cells are terminally activated by specific receptors such as NK cell p30 related protein (NKp30) receptor, through their corresponding ligands which are up-regulated on the surface of cells that are deemed to be a threat to the body, such as cancer cells [7]. Intriguingly, decidual uNK cells, which have attenuated cytotoxicity [8] express NKp30, and most available data on uNK cells focus on pregnant decidua while the evidence regarding NKp30 expression in non-pregnant uNK cells is limited.

The purported importance of uNK cells, and in particular their numbers, is well documented in the pathogenesis of a variety of female reproductive disorders such as recurrent miscarriage [9], sporadic miscarriage [10], recurrent implantation failure [11], fibroids [12], fetal growth restriction and pre-eclampsia [13].

Endometriosis is a common, benign, chronic inflammatory gynaecological disease often associated with subfertility [14], characterized by the presence of endometrial glands and stroma-like tissue outside the uterine cavity [14]. The eutopic endometrium of women with endometriosis has been shown to be different to that of women without endometriosis [14–17] while persistent proliferation and progesterone resistance is known to exist in ectopic lesions [14, 16, 18, 19]. The pathogenesis of endometriosis is not fully understood, although the theory of retrograde menstruation, where subsequent deposition of shed endometrium in the pelvic cavity gives rise to endometriotic deposits, is the most widely accepted [14]. Previous reports have suggested a role for uNK cells in the pathogenesis of endometriosis [20–22] postulating that survival and accumulation of menstrual endometrial tissue in the peritoneal cavity may relate to a reduction in the cytotoxic activity of peripheral blood NK cells [23]. Jones et al. investigated various leukocyte subpopulations in endometriosis and adenomyosis, however, the data is expressed relative to the number of leukocyte antigen positive cells [21]. There are no comprehensive studies that describe the uNK cell numbers relative to the endometrial stromal niche cells in eutopic and ectopic endometrium of women with endometriosis published to date that utilise a validated analytic method to ensure reproducibility or generalisability of data. Furthermore, cycle phase specific changes in uNK cell numbers including proliferative phase, mid-secretory and late-secretory phase in relation to endometriosis have not yet been described. Studying the establishment of the disease in humans is challenging since it is impossible to know how long the disease has been present at the point of surgical diagnosis and the correlation between symptoms and disease severity is poor. The baboon model of induction of endometriosis thus provides a unique opportunity to study the natural course of endometriosis following the initial establishment of the disease [24].

Since uNK cells are of great interest to reproductive biologists and immunologists as a target for therapies, we aimed to assess the uNK cell numbers and their NKp30 activation status in a well characterised patient population with or without endometriosis across different phases of the menstrual cycle and to examine the early stages of disease establishment in the baboon model of induction of endometriosis. Ectopic lesions excised from women and baboons were also examined and compared to the eutopic endometrium. To overcome the deficiencies in previous publications on the subject we employed a validated and reproducible computer assisted tool [25] in our analysis and further examined curated micro-array data, which was validated by examining the differential expression of one of the identified gene products (BAG6) in the eutopic endometrium of women with and without endometriosis.

Methods

Endometrial biopsies were taken from 30 patients with surgically diagnosed peritoneal endometriosis at American Fertility Society stages I–IV and 30 healthy fertile controls (at least one live birth without a history of subfertility, recurrent miscarriage or endometriosis, confirmed by laparoscopy) undergoing laparoscopic sterilization [16] at Liverpool Women's Hospital, Liverpool, UK (tertiary referral centre). All women included had regular menstrual cycles (26–30 days), were not on any hormonal therapy and were not using an intrauterine device. Endometrial biopsies were grouped by cycle stage: 10 proliferative, 10 mid-secretory and 10 late-secretory phase per group, with cycle stage confirmed by histological dating according to modifications of Noyes criteria [26]. Samples were fixed in 10% buffered formalin for 24 h prior to embedding in paraffin blocks for immunohistochemistry.

Ectopic lesions: Human

Peritoneal red/blue ectopic lesions (no ovarian or deep infiltrating endometriosis lesions were included) histologically confirmed to contain endometrium-like cells (glandular and or stromal components) were excised from 22 patients (day 2 to day 30 of menstrual cycle; 2 menstrual, 6 proliferative, 10 mid-secretory, 4 late secretory). Seven of these also had matched eutopic endometrial biopsies.

Baboon samples

Tissues obtained from previously well-described baboon model of endometriosis induction was utilised for this study [24, 27–29]. As previously described [24], animals were housed in the animal care facility at the University of Illinois, Chicago, USA, and all studies were approved by the University of Illinois IACUC. Laparoscopy confirmed the absence of spontaneous endometriosis and endometrium was harvested from each animal at day 9 to 12 post-ovulation, prior to the induction of endometriosis (control, $n = 5$). Endometriosis was then induced in ten female baboons (*Papio anubis*) by intra-peritoneal inoculation of autologous menstrual endometrial tissue on the first or second day of menstruation on two consecutive menstrual cycles, as previously reported [24]. Disease progression was monitored by consecutive laparoscopies and video recording at 3 ($n = 8$), and 15 months (n = 8) after induction of endometriosis. Following each laparoscopy, a laparotomy was performed and eutopic/ectopic endometrial tissue was harvested at day 9–12 post-ovulation. The animals were euthanized at 15 months post-induction as required by the IACUC approval.

Ectopic lesions: Baboon

Blue ectopic lesions were harvested at day 9–12 post-ovulation at 3 months ($n = 4$) and 15 months ($n = 5$) post-inoculation. Each lesion was taken from a different animal.

Immunohistochemistry

Expression of CD56, NKp30 and BAG6 was determined by immunohistochemistry. 3 μm (human) or 5 μm (baboon)-thick paraffin sections were incubated with either monoclonal mouse anti-human CD56 (NCAM, clone 1B6 Novocastra Leica Biosystem, Newcastle, UK) antibody at 1:50, polyclonal goat anti-human NKp30 antibody (sc-20,477, Santa Cruz Biotechnology, Inc) at 1:100 dilution or polyclonal rabbit anti-human BAG6 antibody (HPA053291, ATLAS antibodies, Cambridge Biosciences UK) at 1:500 for 1 h at room temperature in a humidified chamber. Detection was with ImmPRESS anti-mouse, anti-goat or anti-rabbit polymer (Vector Laboratories, Peterborough, UK) respectively and visualisation was with ImmPACT DAB (Vector Laboratories, Peterborough, UK). The sections were counterstained in Gill 2 Haematoxylin, dehydrated, cleared and mounted in Consul Mount (Thermo Scientific, Runcorn, UK). Mouse, goat or rabbit negative control IgG (0.5 μg/ml Vector Laboratories, Peterborough, UK) replaced the respective primary antibody as a negative control.

Image analysis

Ten high-resolution images were captured using a Nikon Eclipse 50i Microscope, Nikon Corporation, Surrey, UK and Nikon DS Fi1 digital camera (Nikon) at 400× magnification for each sample and edited to leave only stromal cells. The ratio of the area occupied between positive CD56 or NKp30 cells (brown stain) and total endometrial stromal cells (blue stain) was assessed using computer assisted image analysis with color deconvolution (Image J software, NIH) for each image (10 images for each sample) [25]. The average percent of positive staining as a total of the stromal cells present was then calculated for each sample (previously shown to be equivalent to counting uNK cells) [25]. The investigators were blinded to the identification of the endometrial tissue sections during the analysis.

Semi-quantitative quickscore for BAG6

The immunostaining was first broadly evaluated to identify the location of the positively stained areas. Subsequently, the *functionalis* glands from each section were analysed semi-quantitatively using a modified Quickscore method incorporating both staining intensity and abundance [30–32].

Bioinformatics analysis

The role of key receptors on human NK cells was examined by collating a list of inhibitory and activating receptors, adhesion molecules or co-stimulatory molecules [33]. Curated datasets containing microarray data from secretory phase patients with endometriosis ($n = 60$; 24 early-secretory and 36 mid-secretory phase) compared with normal endometrium ($n = 25$; 9 early-secretory and 16 mid-secretory phase) [34, 35] were examined using the meta-analysis function in the Illumina BaseSpace Correlation Engine for the gene list described above and tabulated.

Statistical analysis

Graphpad prism was used for all analyses. Cell densities of related and non-related groups were compared by non-parametric tests as appropriate (Kruskall Wallis and Mann–Whitney U-test). Parametric and non-parametric tests were used to compare differences between groups as appropriate. Data are presented as median (range). Statistical significance was set at $P < 0.05$.

Results

Demographic characteristics

There were no statistically significant differences in age, BMI or smoking status between the two groups of women although the control group tended to be older (Table 1).

Parity was significantly higher in the control group ($P < 0.0001$). However, this was expected since proven fertility was part of the inclusion criteria for this cohort of women.

In the baboons, the average number of endometriotic lesions after the inoculation of endometrial tissue was

Table 1 Clinical characteristics of study women

Demographic data	Control group $N = 30$	Endometriosis group $N = 30$	Ectopic group $N = 22$	P value (control v endometriosis)
Age, median (range)	40 (25–47)	36 (18–45)	40 (24–51)	$P = 0.056$
BMI, median (range)	27 (20–42)	26 (20–38)	27.1 (18–32)	$P = 0.37$
Parity, median (range)	2 (1–4)	1 (0–3)	1 (0–2)	$P < 0.0001$
Smoker	9/30 (30%)	5/30 (17%)	1/22 (5%)	$P = 0.36$
Endometriosis stage, median (range)	–	2 (1–4)	4 (1–4)	N/A

Control group consists of 10 patients with proliferative phase endometrium, 10 patients with mid-secretory phase endometrium and 10 patients with late-secretory phase endometrium. Endometriosis group consists of 10 patients with proliferative phase endometrium, 10 patients with mid-secretory phase endometrium and 10 patients with late-secretory phase endometrium. The ectopic group consists of ectopic lesions excised from women with endometriosis, 2 menstrual, 6 proliferative, 10 mid-secretory and 4 late secretory phase. Mann-Whitney U test for age, BMI and parity; Fisher's Exact test for smoking status

20.2 ± 11.5 at 3 months and 20.3 ± 8.1 at 15 months. No lesions were visualized before the induction of the disease in any animal.

The dynamic CD56 and NKp30 expression pattern observed in human eutopic endometrium across the cycle is preserved in women with endometriosis

In fertile control women, the percentage of uNK cells in the stromal compartment rose significantly in the eutopic endometrium across the menstrual cycle (Kruskal-Wallis test $P = 0.0038$), with the highest levels seen in the late secretory phase (7.35% (2.6–10.6)). Mann Whitney U test showed significantly higher CD56 in eutopic endometrial biopsies taken from fertile control women in the late secretory phase compared with proliferative phase ($P = 0.002$, Fig. 1c). Although the same trend was seen across the menstrual cycle in the eutopic endometria of women with endometriosis, the increase bordered on statistical significance (Kruskal-Wallis test $P = 0.05$). However it was noted that there appeared to be an earlier rise in the percentage of uNK cells in the endometriosis group - in the mid-secretory phase of the cycle (7.1% (1.7–36.8)) compared to the fertile control group (3.6% (2.3–26.6)). Eutopic endometrial CD56 co-localised with NKp30 on serial sections of late secretory endometrium (Fig. 2). There was a statistically significant increase in %NKp30 across the cycle from proliferative to late-secretory phase eutopic endometrium in both the fertile control group and endometriosis group (Kruskal-Wallis test $P < 0.0001$ and $P = 0.03$ respectively, Fig. 1d). NKp30 was significantly higher in the late-secretory phase eutopic endometrium compared with proliferative phase in both fertile control (Mann Whitney U test $P = 0.0002$) and endometriosis patients (Mann Whitney U test $P = 0.01$). In fertile control patients, there was also a significant increase in NKp30 from mid-late secretory phase endometrium (Mann Whitney U test $P = 0.0004$). There was a strong correlation between CD56 and NKp30 in control patients ($r = 0.63$, $P = 0.0002$), whilst the correlation in the eutopic endometrium of endometriosis patients was not statistically significant ($r = 0.35$, $P = 0.06$) (Additional file 1: Figure S1). The ratio of eutopic endometrium NKp30:

CD56 was calculated across the cycle to give an indication of relative uNK cell activation and had a small decrease across the menstrual cycle in the endometriosis group (Fig. 1e, Kruskal-Wallis test $P = 0.05$).

CD56 expression in human ectopic endometriotic lesions

Ectopic lesions excised from women showed a low %CD56+ cells throughout the menstrual cycle (KW test $P = 0.3$), similar to the levels seen in proliferative phase eutopic endometrium (Fig. 1f). In the mid-secretory phase, %CD56+ was significantly lower in ectopic lesions than in eutopic endometrium (Mann Whitney U test $P = 0.004$, $n = 10$ per group). In paired eutopic and ectopic endometrium the percentage of uNK cells was significantly lower in the matched ectopic endometrium ($P = 0.03$, $n = 7$, Wilcoxon matched pairs signed rank test, Fig. 1g).

CD56 and NKp30 expression in baboon eutopic endometrium with induction of endometriosis

Compared to pre-induction controls the median (range) %CD56+ cells (1.1% (0.8–3.0) $n = 5$; KW test, $P = 0.17$, Fig. 3) was not statistically significantly different at 3 months (2.0% (1.3–2.5) $n = 8$) and 15 months (1.8% (0.8–3.4) n = 8) in the eutopic endometrium post-induction of endometriosis although the median levels were slightly higher. The median %NKp30+ cells also remained similar after induction of endometriosis in the eutopic tissue. Interestingly, induction of endometriosis resulted in a trend to slightly lower ratio of NKp30:CD56 in the eutopic endometrium at 3 and 15 months compared to pre-induction controls (KW test $P = 0.19$, Fig. 3).

CD56 and NKp30 expression in baboon ectopic endometriotic lesions

In baboons at 3 months post-induction of endometriosis, %CD56+ were similar in both eutopic endometrium and ectopic lesions (Fig. 3b). Yet, 15 months after the induction of endometriosis, the ectopic lesions from half of the animals (2/4) demonstrated three fold greater %CD56+ cells when compared with their eutopic endometrium (Fig. 3b). Furthermore, the %NKp30+ uNK cells at 3 months and 15 months post-induction

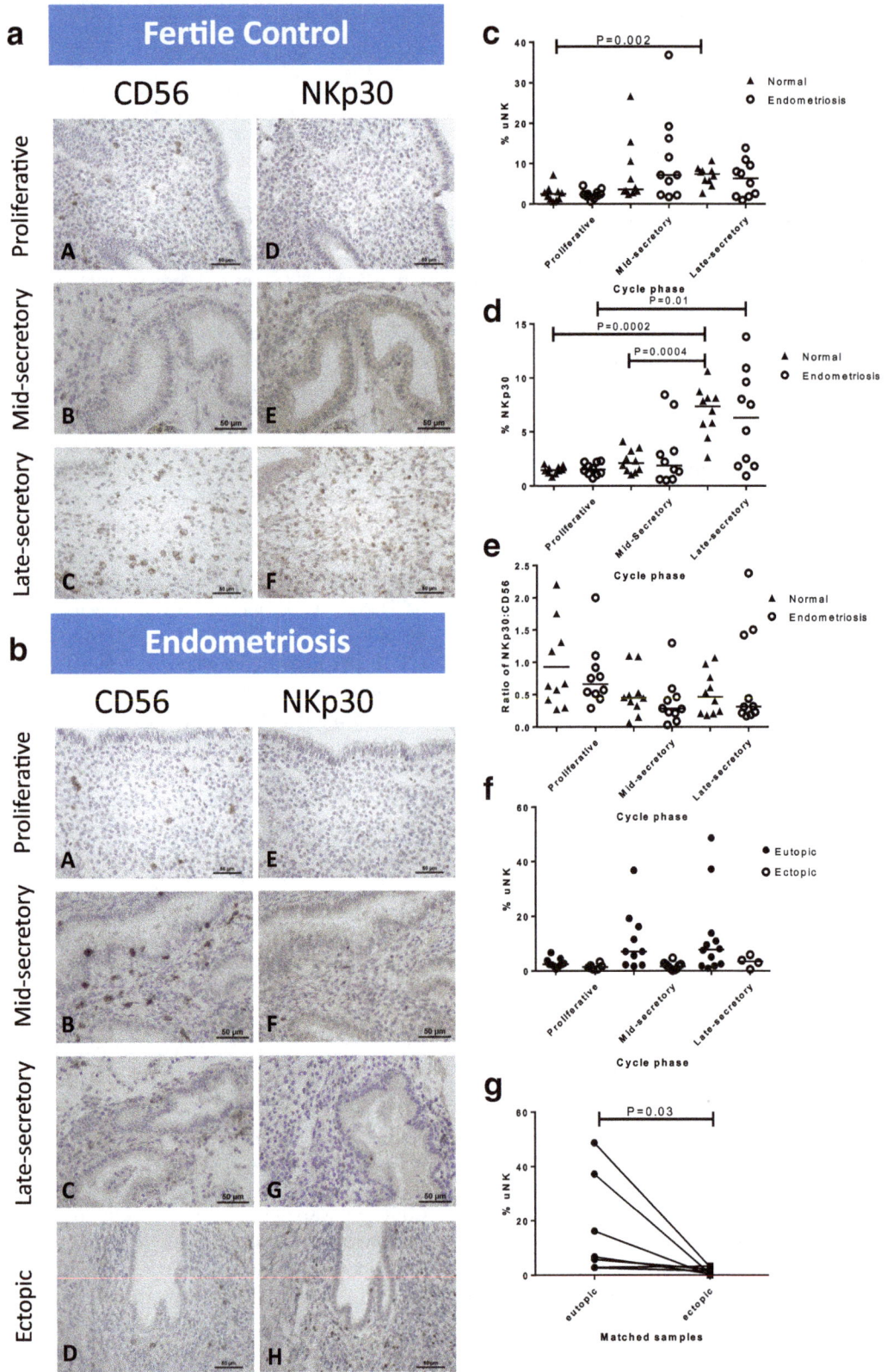

Fig. 1 (See legend on next page.)

(See figure on previous page.)
Fig. 1 Expression of CD56 and NKp30 in human endometrium. Representative micrographs showing CD56 expression by immunohistochemistry (brown DAB staining) in eutopic endometrial stromal cells of fertile control women (**a**, A-C) and in women with endometriosis (**b**, A-C) (400× magnification). NKp30 expression in eutopic endometrial stromal cells from fertile control women (**a**, D-F) and women with endometriosis (**b**, E-G). Staining in ectopic lesions are shown in (**b** D) (uNK cells) and (**b** H) (NKp30). Graphs comparing %CD56 (1c), %NKp30 (**d**) and ratio of NKp30:CD56 (**e**) in ectopic lesions (n = 6–9) and at different time points in the menstrual cycle (PP = proliferative phase; MSP = mid-secretory phase; LSP = late-secretory phase; n = 10 for each group in human samples (in both fertile controls 'normal' and patients with endometriosis). (**f**) Graph showing percentage of CD56 + uNK cells in eutopic endometrium and ectopic lesions across the menstrual cycle (n = 9 ectopic lesions with matched eutopic endometrium in 7/36 cases) demonstrating that levels remain low in ectopic lesions. (**g**) Graph showing percentage of CD56+ uNK cells in matched eutopic and ectopic endometrium (n = 7). P = 0.03, Wilcoxon matched pairs signed rank test

of endometriosis appeared raised in the ectopic lesions from 1 or 2 animals when compared with eutopic endometrium (Fig. 3c).

Bioinformatics analysis of differential expression of genes encoding NK cell receptors and ligands in secretory phase endometrium

Of the 92 genes examined, 60 were significantly up- or down- regulated (Additional file 2: Table S1) in endometrial samples of women with endometriosis relative to control women. The 10 most significantly up/down-regulated genes are shown below in Table 2.

NKp30 (NCR3) and its ligand BAT3 (BAG6) were significantly upregulated in 6/6 and 4/6 secretory phase datasets from endometriosis patients respectively compared with control patients (1.2–1.7 fold change and 1.4–2.3 fold change respectively, Additional file 2: Table S1).

In accordance with the immunohistochemistry data, NCAM1 (CD56) was not differentially regulated in 5/6 datasets.

Considering the other NK cell regulatory genes that were significantly altered in the majority of the

endometriosis datasets (4–6/6), either a particular receptor (e.g. KIR3DL2) or the ligand (e.g. NECL2) was differentially expressed, but paired alteration of both the receptor and its ligand was not observed (Additional file 2: Table S1).

In vivo validation of in silico data

We subsequently chose one of the gene products identified in our bioinformatics analysis, BAG6 for further study. BAG6 expression was not previously reported in the human endometrium, and we confirmed the expression of BAG6 protein in the endometrium. The strongest immuno-staining for BAG6 was in the endometrial epithelial compartment (highest quickscores in the luminal epithelium) but staining was also observed in stromal and vascular cells. Eutopic endometrium from women with endometriosis in the secretory phase showed significantly higher immunoexpression scores for BAG6 (Fig. 4) supporting our in silico data.

Discussion

We have shown that the cyclical percentage change of uNK cells that occurs in healthy fertile endometrium,

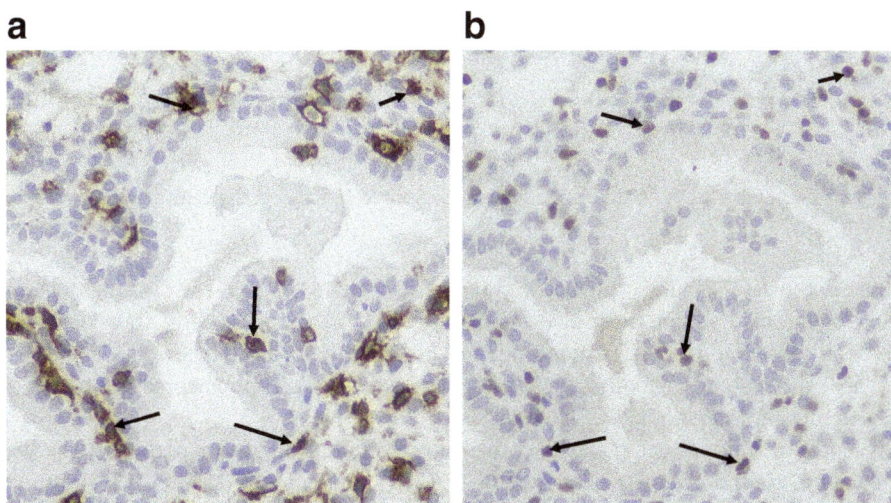

Fig. 2 Co-localisation of CD56 (**a**) and NKp30 (**b**) positive cells on serial sections from late secretory endometrium. Examples of cells stained with both markers are shown by black arrows

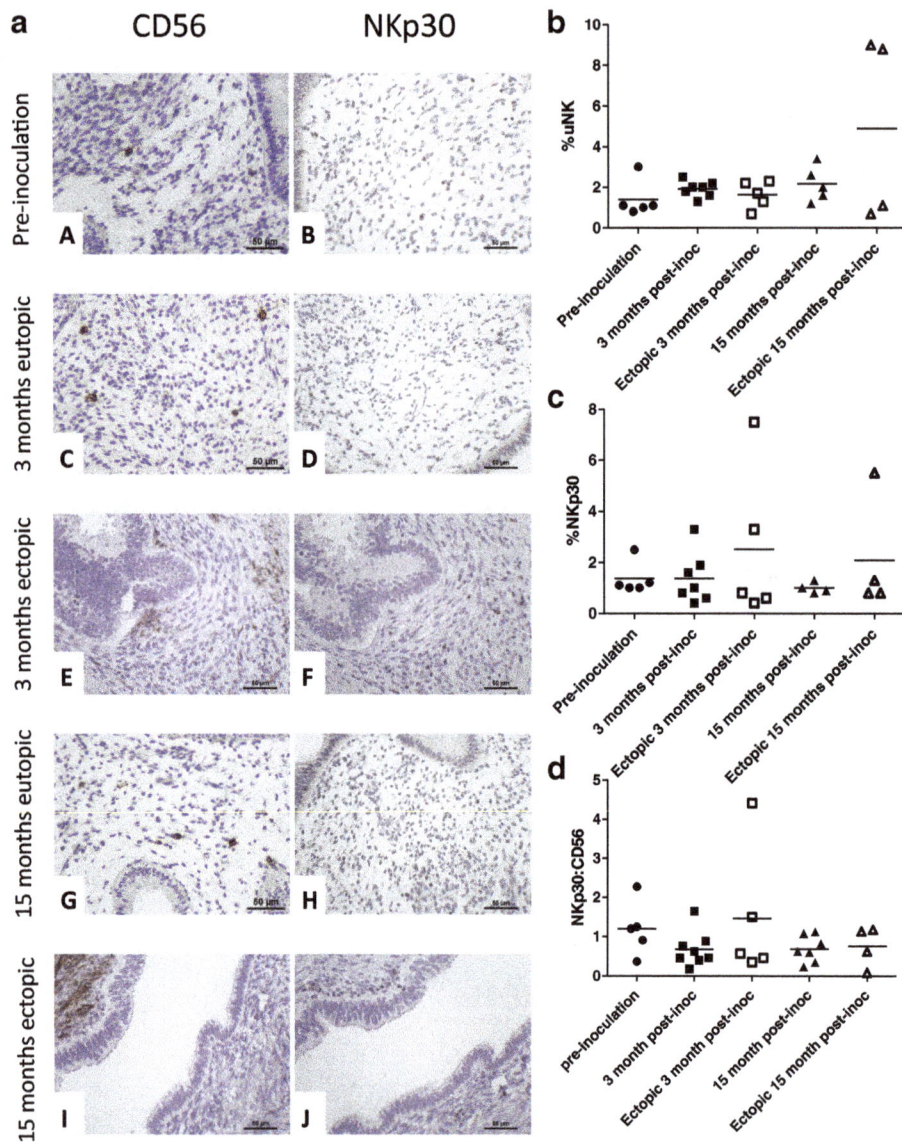

Fig. 3 Expression of CD56 and NKp30 in a baboon model of induced endometriosis. **a** Representative micrographs depicting CD56 (*A, C, E, G, I*), or NKp30 (*B, D, F, H, J*) expression in eutopic endometrial stroma cells of baboon samples during the three time-points: pre-inoculation (*A, B*), 3 (*C, D*) and 15 months (*G, H*) post-inoculation of the disease and expression in ectopic endometrial lesions 3 months (*E, F*) and 15 months (*I, J*) post-inoculation (400× magnification). Graphs comparing percentage of stromal CD56$^+$ (**b**), NKp30$^+$ (**c**) and ratio of NKp30$^+$ to CD56 (**d**) cells prior to inoculation ($n = 5$), at 3 ($n = 7$) and 15 months ($n = 5$) in eutopic endometrium after the induction of endometriosis and in ectopic lesions at 3 ($n = 5$) and 15 months ($n = 4$) after induction of endometriosis

with a clear increase in the late-secretory phase of the cycle, is preserved in the eutopic endometrium of women with endometriosis. This observation was supported in the baboon model where induction of endometriosis was not associated with a significant increase in %CD56+ cells in the mid-secretory eutopic endometrial samples compared with pre-inoculation control samples. The use of the primate model of endometriosis (proposed to be the gold standard animal model of endometriosis) allowed us to document the precisely timed changes in eutopic uNK

cells induced by the establishment of endometriosis, particularly at the very early stages of the disease, which is not feasible to attain in women due to the significant delay in diagnosis and poor correlation between symptoms and disease severity.

It is tempting to speculate that the animals with higher %uNK in ectopic lesions 15 months post-inoculation may be less likely to have lesions that persist as active endometriotic deposits and that those with low %uNK are able to evade the body's immune surveillance

Table 2 Top differentially regulated NK cell related genes in endometriosis

Gene	Gene Description	Specificity	Overall Gene score	Up/down-regulated
NCR3	natural cytotoxicity triggering receptor 3	6 out of 6	135.1	Up
SIGLEC7	sialic acid binding Ig-like lectin 7	5 out of 6	99.5	Up
CADM1	cell adhesion molecule 1	4 out of 6	234.7	Down
SELPLG	selectin P ligand	4 out of 6	158. 6	Up
COL1A1	collagen, type I, alpha 1	4 out of 6	158.1	Up
KIR3DL2	killer cell immunoglobulin-like receptor, three domains, long cytoplasmic tail, 2	4 out of 6	138.48	Up
BAG6	BCL2-associated athanogene 6	4 out of 6	136.0	Up
COL6A1	collagen, type VI, alpha 1	3 out of 6	162.0	Up
HCST	hematopoietic cell signal transducer	3 out of 6	154.9	Up
KIR2DS2	killer cell immunoglobulin-like receptor, two domains, short cytoplasmic tail, 2	3 out of 6	147.4	Up

Table showing the most significantly differentially regulated NK cell related genes examined. Specificity refers to the number of biological datasets in which the gene was found to be differentially regulated. Overall gene score is a measure of the fold change in the individual datasets combined with the number of datasets in which the particular gene was differentially regulated

mechanisms thus contributing to disease establishment. However, at present, there is insufficient evidence to suggest that uNK cells play a role in the establishment of ectopic endometriotic lesions despite the increasing evidence for a role in infertility [20, 36].

We have also demonstrated, that NKp30, an activating receptor of uNK cells, is expressed in endometrial uNK cells in the non-pregnant endometrium of humans and in baboons and that the NKp30 expression increases in the late secretory phase in humans. Furthermore, this

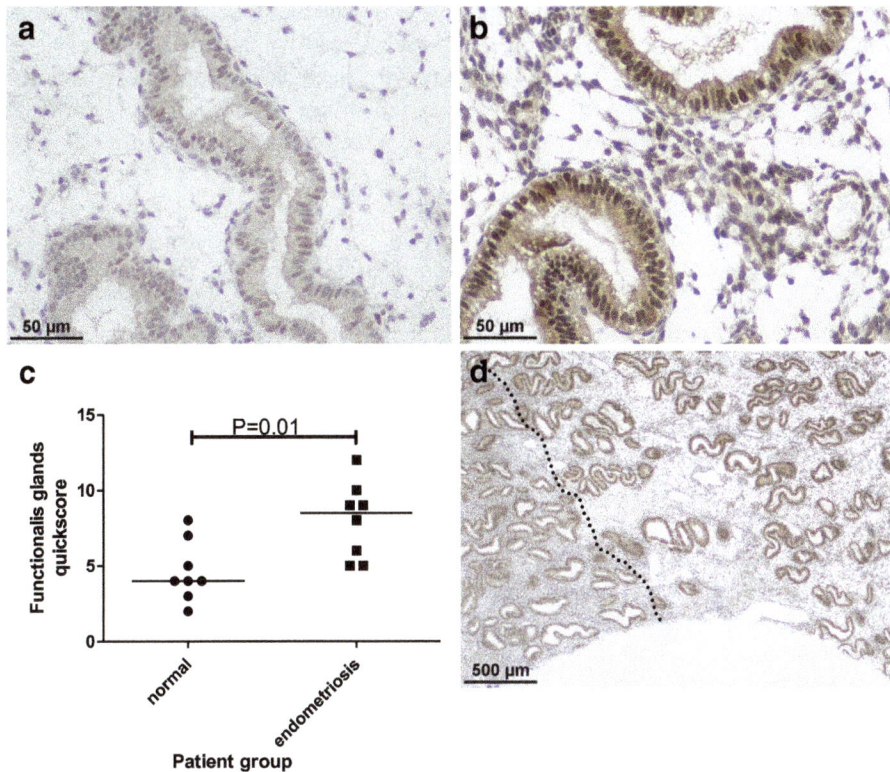

Fig. 4 BAG6 expression in mid-secretory phase human endometrium. Representative micrographs depicting BAG6 expression in the functional layer of the endometrium from **a** fertile control women (400× magnification) and **b** women with endometriosis (400× magnification). **c** Quickscore data comparing BAG6 immuno staining in the endometrium of normal control women compared with women with endometriosis during the mid-secretory phase and demonstrating significantly increased BAG6 immunoexpression scores in the endometriosis group (n = 8/group, P = 0.01, Mann Whitney U test). In full thickness endometrium, a gradient in staining intensity was observed from the *functionalis* to the *basalis* layer (D, 40× magnification). The *basalis/functionalis* demarcation is indicated by the dotted line with the *basalis* to the left of the line and the *functionalis* to the right

increase of eutopic endometrial NKp30 expression and the highest level of NKp30 were observed in the late secretory phase of the cycle in women with/without endometriosis in agreement with some of the previous work [37]. Previous reports on NKp30 expression in uNK cells from non-pregnant endometrium are contradictory. FACS analysis of uNK cells isolated from mid-secretory phase did not show significant NKp30 expression [38] yet menstrual blood NK cells (with uNK phenotype, CD56^{bright}, CD16^{dim}) showed NKp30 expression [39]. Our data suggest a possible explanation to these seemingly contradictory reports. We propose that the menstrual blood NK cells studied by van der Molen et al. are likely to originate from the late-secretory endometrium. It seems that, in the late secretory phase, there is also an influx of other NKp30 expressing cells such as T cells [40–42]. Interestingly there was a strong, significant correlation between CD56+ cells and NKp30 in the normal eutopic endometrium which was lost in the endometriosis samples, further suggesting the NKp30+ expressing cells in women with endometriosis may be related to a T cell subpopulation.

In agreement with previous reports [21, 43] ectopic lesions had significantly low uNK cell numbers. Previous authors have also suggested that the ectopic lesions may have an increased number of CD3 and CD8 expressing T cells [21], which may express Nkp30 [42]. We also observed low Nkp30 expression in ectopic lesions, similar to the eutopic endometrium at the proliferative phase of the cycle. NKp30 is a natural cytotoxicity receptor (NCR) [38, 44], and ligand induced down-regulation of the receptor expression has been proposed as an immune surveillance evading mechanism in some tumors [45]. If low NKp30 expression is associated with reduced uNK cell cytotoxic activity, this may allow established human ectopic endometriotic cells to persist and evade immuno-clearance. Additional studies using the baboon model may help to determine whether NKp30 in uNK cells plays a role in propagation of ectopic lesions. Ectopic endometriotic lesions are postulated to have a progesterone resistant phenotype [46], which may further explain the observed low percentage of uNK cells in the human lesions.

The immune cell composition in the endometrium at the time of implantation is considered pivotal for successful conception; whereas at the end of the implantation window, during the late secretory phase, the main function of the endometrium is effective shedding and regeneration when no pregnancy ensues. Therefore, it is possible that as part of the innate immune system, uNK cells could play a role in both these contrasting functions of the eutopic endometrium as the most abundant leukocyte subpopulation in the human endometrium at both the mid and late secretory phase [47]. Endometriosis is a clinically challenging condition, associated with subfertility, with reported aberrations in mid-secretory phase endometrial function; whereas abnormal shedding of an aberrant late secretory phase endometrium [15, 19, 48] is postulated to explain its pathogenesis. Our data suggest that possible higher amounts of activated (NKp30 expressing) uNK cells in the eutopic endometrium of a subset of women with endometriosis may indicate possible functional aberrations in these cells in the late secretory endometrium. Further studies are warranted in the future to examine the functional differences in the production of cytokines and other immune modulators to determine how that may change the endometrial phenotype of the shedding endometrium of women with endometriosis.

Through systems biology and reviewing published literature, we have highlighted the complex nature of uNK cell activation and function. The final activation status or function of uNK cells will depend on the homeostasis of all the uNK cell activation/inhibitory receptors or the availability of the corresponding ligands, the vast majority of which were differentially regulated in the endometria of women with endometriosis. BAG6 is one of the ligands for NKp30, and was one of the genes identified in our in silico study (Table 2 and Additional file 1: Figure S1). BAG6 has multiple functions including apoptosis, gene regulation, protein synthesis, protein quality control, and protein degradation. We have demonstrated that human endometrium expresses BAG6 protein for the first time, and revealed an increased immuno-expression for BAG6 in secretory endometrium of women with endometriosis validating our in silico study. BAG6 has also been shown to be expressed on dendritic cells and cells after malignant transformation, where it serves as the ligand for NKp30 triggering NK cell cytotoxicity [49]. Further studies are warranted to elucidate the exact functional relevance of the presence of this protein in the endometrium.

Furthermore, we have previously published evidence for eutopic endometrial gene expression alterations subsequent to the induction of ectopic endometriotic lesions in baboons [29]. These published changes in eutopic endometrial gene expression included many of the endometriosis specific eutopic endometrial gene alterations reported in the human [29]. Interestingly, 40 of the 92 genes encoding NK cell receptors and ligands in our list were also amongst the differentially regulated gene list in the baboon eutopic endometrium at 6 months after induction of endometriosis (reported in Additional file 3: Table S2 in Afshar et al. [29], and in Additional file 3: Table S2), suggesting a close homology between the baboon model of endometriosis induction with the human disease.

Conclusions

Our results suggest that the dynamic increase in the percentage of uNK cells in the secretory phase is preserved in the eutopic endometrium of women with endometriosis. Further work is indicated to assess if the observed uNK cell dynamics are perturbed in the subset of women with endometriosis who are also sub-fertile. We hypothesize that lower uNK cells associated with ectopic endometrial cells may permit the early establishment of these lesions and that NKp30 expressing uNK cells (and possibly T cells) may have a role in endometrial shedding/regeneration. However, our knowledge on the putative role of uNK cells in endometriosis is far from complete and further studies are required to explore the intricate function of these cells and explain their involvement in the pathogenic mechanisms of endometriosis.

Additional files

Additional file 1: Figure S1. A. Graph showing correlation between CD56 and NKp30 in control human patients ($n = 30$). Spearman rank correlation $r = 0.63$, $P = 0.0002$. **B.** Graph showing correlation between CD56 and NKp30 in patients with endometriosis ($n = 30$). Spearman rank correlation $r = 0.35$, $P = 0.058$ (PDF 131 kb)

Additional file 2: Table S1. Output from bioinformatics analysis showing differential expression of genes encoding NK cell receptors and ligands in secretory phase endometrium from endometriosis patients when compared with the endometrium of control women without endometriosis ordered by specificity and overall gene score. Full gene list examined is shown in the second tab. (XLSX 26 kb)

Additional file 3: Table S2. The differentially expressed genes in post ovulatory eutopic endometrium of baboons 6 months after induction of endometriosis ($n = 4$) compared with the same of control animals (n = 4) published in Additional file 3: Table S2, in Afshar et al. [29] (bioset 2) was interrogated to identify 40 out of 92 genes encoding for uNK cell receptor/ligand described in 2nd tab of the Additional file 2: Table S1 (bioset 1) amongst these altered genes. *NCR3*, *CADM1* and *HCST* genes which were amongst the top 10 up-regulated genes in the human eutopic endometriosis (in Table 1) were amongst these, suggesting a close homology of the baboon model with the human disease (XLSX 12 kb)

Acknowledgements
Authors are grateful to Dr. Areege Kamal and Dr. Judith Bulmer for their insightful advice on the study.

Funding
This research was supported by The RCOG Endometriosis Millennium Fund (LC, DH), Wellbeing of Women's Project grants RG1073 and RG1487 (DH), and Liverpool Women's Hospital (LC, JAD) and NIH RO1 HD 083273 to ATF.

Authors' contributions
DKH and AF obtained the Ethical approval, and DKH conceived the study design. The human samples and clinical data were collected by DKH, and baboon samples by AF. Experiments were carried out, and data collected, by LC, JD, KP and EG. Data analyzed and interpreted by JD, KP, LC, EG and DKH; in silico analysis was by JD and DKH, JD produced final table and figures and JD, KP, LC, EG and DKH produced the initial drafts. All authors had final approval of the submitted version.

Competing interests
The authors declare that they have no competing interests.

Author details
[1]Department of Women's and Children's Health, Institute of Translational Medicine, University of Liverpool, Liverpool, UK. [2]Department of Obstetrics, Gynecology and Reproductive Biology, College of Human Medicine, Michigan State University, Grand Rapids, MI, USA. [3]Department of Microbiology and Molecular Genetics, Michigan State University, East Lansing, MI, USA. [4]Department of Gynecology, Liverpool Women's Hospital, Liverpool, UK. [5]Hewitt Fertility Centre; Liverpool Women's Hospital, Liverpool, UK. [6]Department of Obstetrics and Gynecology, Grand Rapids Medical Education Partners/Michigan State University, Grand Rapids, MI, USA.

References
1. Hapangama DK, Kamal AM, Bulmer JN. Estrogen receptor beta: the guardian of the endometrium. Hum Reprod Update. 2015;21:174–93.
2. Dunk C, Smith S, Hazan A, Whittle W, Jones RL. Promotion of angiogenesis by human endometrial lymphocytes. Immunol Investig. 2008;37:583–610.
3. Berbic M, Fraser IS. Regulatory T cells and other leukocytes in the pathogenesis of endometriosis. J Reprod Immunol. 2011;88:149–55.
4. King A. Uterine leukocytes and decidualization. Hum Reprod Update. 2000;6:28–36.
5. Quenby S, Nik H, Innes B, Lash G, Turner M, Drury J, Bulmer J. Uterine natural killer cells and angiogenesis in recurrent reproductive failure. Hum Reprod. 2009;24:45–54.
6. Vacca P, Moretta L, Moretta A, Mingari MC. Origin, phenotype and function of human natural killer cells in pregnancy. Trends Immunol. 2011;32:517–23.
7. Vacca P, Cantoni C, Prato C, Fulcheri E, Moretta A, Moretta L, Mingari MC. Regulatory role of NKp44, NKp46, DNAM-1 and NKG2D receptors in the interaction between NK cells and trophoblast cells. Evidence for divergent functional profiles of decidual versus peripheral NK cells. Int Immunol. 2008;20:1395–405.
8. Kopcow HD, Allan DSJ, Chen X, Rybalov B, Andzelm MM, Ge BX, Strominger JL. Human decidual NK cells form immature activating synapses and are not cytotoxic. Proc Natl Acad Sci U S A. 2005;102:15563–8.
9. Tang AW, Alfirevic Z, Quenby S. Natural killer cells and pregnancy outcomes in women with recurrent miscarriage and infertility: a systematic review. Hum Reprod. 2011;26:1971–80.
10. Zenclussen AC, Fest S, Sehmsdorf US, Hagen E, Klapp BF, Arck PC. Upregulation of decidual P-selectin expression is associated with an increased number of Th1 cell populations in patients suffering from spontaneous abortions. Cell Immunol. 2001;213:94–103.
11. Tuckerman E, Mariee N, Prakash A, Li TC, Laird S. Uterine natural killer cells in peri-implantation endometrium from women with repeated implantation failure after IVF. J Reprod Immunol. 2010;87:60–6.
12. Kitaya K, Yasuo T. Leukocyte density and composition in human cycling endometrium with uterine fibroids. Hum Immunol. 2010;71:158–63.
13. Williams PJ, Bulmer JN, Searle RF, Innes BA, Robson SC. Altered decidual leucocyte populations in the placental bed in pre-eclampsia and foetal growth restriction: a comparison with late normal pregnancy. Reproduction. 2009;138:177–84.
14. Sourial S, Tempest N, Hapangama DK. Theories on the pathogenesis of endometriosis. International Journal of Reproductive Medicine. 2014;2014:9.

15. Hapangama DK, Raju RS, Valentijn AJ, Barraclough D, Hart A, Turner MA, Platt-Higgins A, Barraclough R, Rudland PS. Aberrant expression of metastasis-inducing proteins in ectopic and matched eutopic endometrium of women with endometriosis: implications for the pathogenesis of endometriosis. Hum Reprod. 2012;27:394–407.

16. Hapangama DK, Turner MA, Drury JA, Quenby S, Hart A, Maddick M, Martin-Ruiz C, von Zglinicki T. Sustained replication in endometrium of women with endometriosis occurs without evoking a DNA damage response. Hum Reprod. 2009;24:687–96.

17. Hapangama DK, Turner MA, Drury JA, Quenby S, Saretzki G, Martin-Ruiz C, Von Zglinicki T. Endometriosis is associated with aberrant endometrial expression of telomerase and increased telomere length. Obstetrical & Gynecological Survey. 2008;63:711–3.

18. Bulun SE. Mechanisms of disease endometriosis. N Engl J Med. 2009;360:268–79.

19. Hapangama DK, Turner MA, Drury J, Heathcote L, Afshar Y, Mavrogianis PA, Fazleabas AT. Aberrant expression of regulators of cell-fate found in eutopic endometrium is found in matched ectopic endometrium among women and in a baboon model of endometriosis. Hum Reprod. 2010;25:2840–50.

20. Giuliani E, Parkin KL, Lessey BA, Young SL, Fazleabas AT. Characterization of uterine NK cells in women with infertility or recurrent pregnancy loss and associated endometriosis. Am J Reprod Immunol. 2014;72:262–9.

21. Jones RK, Bulmer JN, Searle RF. Phenotypic and functional studies of leukocytes in human endometrium and endometriosis. Hum Reprod Update. 1998;4:702–9.

22. Izumi G, Koga K, Takamura M, Makabe T, Satake E, Takeuchi A, Taguchi A, Urata Y, Fujii T, Osuga Y. Involvement of immune cells in the pathogenesis of endometriosis. J Obstet Gynaecol Res. 2018;44:191–8.

23. Oosterlynck DJ, Cornillie FJ, Waer M, Vandeputte M, Koninckx PR. Women with endometriosis show a defect in natural-killer activity resulting in a decreased cytotoxicity to autologous endometrium. Fertil Steril. 1991;56:45–51.

24. Fazleabas AT. A baboon model for inducing endometriosis. Methods Mol Med. 2006;121:95–9.

25. Drury JA, Tang AW, Turner MA, Quenby S. A rapid, reliable method for uNK cell density estimation. J Reprod Immunol. 2013;97:183–5.

26. Murray MJ, Meyer WR, Zaino RJ, Lessey BA, Novotny DB, Ireland K, Zeng DL, Fritz MA. A critical analysis of the accuracy, reproducibility, and clinical utility of histologic endometrial dating in fertile women. Fertil Steril. 2004;81:1333–43.

27. Braundmeier AG, Fazleabas AT. The non-human primate model of endometriosis: research and implications for fecundity. Mol Hum Reprod. 2009;15:577–86.

28. Hastings JM, Fazleabas AT. A baboon model for endometriosis: implications for fertility. Reprod Biol Endocrinol. 2006;4(Suppl 1):S7.

29. Afshar Y, Hastings J, Roqueiro D, Jeong JW, Giudice LC, Fazleabas AT. Changes in eutopic endometrial gene expression during the progression of experimental endometriosis in the baboon. Papio anubis Biol Reprod. 2013;88:44.

30. Schiessl B, Innes BA, Bulmer JN, Otun HA, Chadwick TJ, Robson SC, Lash GE. Localization of angiogenic growth factors and their receptors in the human placental bed throughout normal human pregnancy. Placenta. 2009;30:79–87.

31. Valentijn AJ, Palial K, Al-Lamee H, Tempest N, Drury J, Von Zglinicki T, Saretzki G, Murray P, Gargett CE, Hapangama DK. SSEA-1 isolates human endometrial basal glandular epithelial cells: phenotypic and functional characterization and implications in the pathogenesis of endometriosis. Hum Reprod. 2013;28:2695–708.

32. Mathew D, Drury JA, Valentijn AJ, Vasieva O, Hapangama DK. In silico, in vitro and in vivo analysis identifies a potential role for steroid hormone regulation of FOXD3 in endometriosis-associated genes. Hum Reprod. 2016;31:345–54.

33. Nk cells: receptors and functions [http://www.nature.com/nri/posters/nkcells/index.html].

34. Tamaresis JS, Irwin JC, Goldfien GA, Rabban JT, Burney RO, Nezhat C, DePaolo LV, Giudice LC. Molecular classification of endometriosis and disease stage using high-dimensional genomic data. Endocrinology. 2014;155:4986–99.

35. Burney RO, Talbi S, Hamilton AE, Vo KC, Nyegaard M, Nezhat CR, Lessey BA, Giudice LC. Gene expression analysis of endometrium reveals progesterone resistance and candidate susceptibility genes in women with endometriosis. Endocrinology. 2007;148:3814–26.

36. Glover LE, Crosby D, Thiruchelvam U, Harmon C, Ni Chorcora C, Wingfield MB, O'Farrelly C. Uterine natural killer cell progenitor populations predict successful implantation in women with endometriosis-associated infertility. Am J Reprod Immunol. 2018;79

37. Ponnampalam AP, Weston GC, Trajstman AC, Susil B, Rogers PAW. Molecular classification of human endometrial cycle stages by transcriptional profiling. Mol Hum Reprod. 2004;10:879–93.

38. Manaster I, Mizrahi S, Goldman-Wohl D, Sela HY, Stern-Ginossar N, Lankry D, Gruda R, Hurwitz A, Bdolah Y, Haimov-Kochman R, et al. Endometrial NK cells are special immature cells that await pregnancy. J Immunol. 2008;181:1869–76.

39. van der Molen RG, Schutten JHF, van Cranenbroek B, ter Meer M, Donckers J, Scholten RR, van der Heijden OWH, Spaanderman MEA, Joosten I. Menstrual blood closely resembles the uterine immune micro-environment and is clearly distinct from peripheral blood. Hum Reprod. 2014;29:303–14.

40. Shivhare SB, Bulmer JN, Innes BA, Hapangama DK, Lash GE. Menstrual cycle distribution of uterine natural killer cells is altered in heavy menstrual bleeding. J Reprod Immunol. 2015;112:88–94.

41. Tang Q, Grzywacz B, Wang HB, Kataria N, Cao Q, Wagner JE, Blazar BR, Miller JS, Verneris MR. Umbilical cord blood T cells express multiple natural cytotoxicity receptors after IL-15 stimulation, but only NKp30 is functional. J Immunol. 2008;181:4507–15.

42. Golden-Mason L, Cox AL, Randall JA, Cheng LL, Rosen HR. Increased natural killer cell cytotoxicity and NKp30 expression protects against hepatitis C virus infection in high-risk individuals and inhibits replication in vitro. Hepatology. 2010;52:1581–9.

43. Bulmer JN, Jones RK, Searle RF. Intraepithelial leukocytes in endometriosis and adenomyosis: comparison of eutopic and ectopic endometrium with normal endometrium. Hum Reprod. 1998;13:2910–5.

44. Hanna J, Goldman-Wohl D, Hamani Y, Avraham I, Greenfield C, Natanson-Yaron S, Prus D, Cohen-Daniel L, Arnon TI, Manaster I, et al. Decidual NK cells regulate key developmental processes at the human fetal-maternal interface. Nat Med. 2006;12:1065–74.

45. Pietra G, Manzini C, Rivara S, Vitale M, Cantoni C, Petretto A, Balsamo M, Conte R, Benelli R, Minghelli S, et al. Melanoma cells inhibit natural killer cell function by modulating the expression of activating receptors and Cytolytic activity. Cancer Res. 2012;72:1407–15.

46. Bulun SE, Cheng YH, Yin P, Imir G, Utsunomiya H, Attar E, Innes J, Julie Kim J. Progesterone resistance in endometriosis: link to failure to metabolize estradiol. Mol Cell Endocrinol. 2006;248:94–103.

47. Osuga Y, Koga K, Hirota Y, Hirata T, Yoshino O, Taketani Y. Lymphocytes in endometriosis. Am J Reprod Immunol. 2011;65:1–10.

48. Leyendecker G, Herbertz M, Kunz G, Mall G. Endometriosis results from the dislocation of basal endometrium. Hum Reprod. 2002;17:2725–36.

49. Binici J, Koch J. BAG-6, a jack of all trades in health and disease. Cell Mol Life Sci. 2014;71:1829–37.

6

Pretreatment with coenzyme Q10 improves ovarian response and embryo quality in low-prognosis young women with decreased ovarian reserve: a randomized controlled trial

Yangying Xu[1,2,3], Victoria Nisenblat[2,3], Cuiling Lu[2,3], Rong Li[2,3], Jie Qiao[2,3], Xiumei Zhen[2,3*] and Shuyu Wang[1*]

Abstract

Background: Management of women with reduced ovarian reserve or poor ovarian response (POR) to stimulation is one of the major challenges in reproductive medicine. The primary causes of POR remain elusive and oxidative stress was proposed as one of the important contributors. It has been suggested that focus on the specific subpopulations within heterogeneous group of poor responders could assist in evaluating optimal management strategies for these patients. This study investigated the effect of anti-oxidant treatment with coenzyme Q10 (CoQ10) on ovarian response and embryo quality in young low-prognosis patients with POR.

Methods: This prospective, randomized controlled study included 186 consecutive patients with POR stratified according to the POSEIDON classification group 3 (age < 35, poor ovarian reserve parameters). The participants were randomized to the CoQ10 pre-treatment for 60 days preceding IVF-ICSI cycle or no pre-treatment. The number of high quality embryos was a primary outcome measure.

Results: A total of 169 participants were evaluated (76 treated with CoQ10 and 93 controls); 17 women were excluded due to low compliance with CoQ10 administration. The baseline demographic and clinical characteristics were comparable between the groups. CoQ10 pretreatment resulted in significantly lower gonadotrophin requirements and higher peak E2 levels. Women in CoQ10 group had increased number of retrieved oocytes (4, IQR 2–5), higher fertilization rate (67.49%) and more high-quality embryos (1, IQR 0–2); $p < 0.05$. Significantly less women treated with CoQ10 had cancelled embryo transfer because of poor embryo development than controls (8.33% vs. 22.89%, $p = 0.04$) and more women from treatment group had available cryopreserved embryos (18.42% vs. 4.3%, $p = 0.012$). The clinical pregnancy and live birth rates per embryo transfer and per one complete stimulation cycle tended to be higher in CoQ10 group but did not achieve statistical significance.

Conclusion: Pretreatment with CoQ10 improves ovarian response to stimulation and embryological parameters in young women with poor ovarian reserve in IVF-ICSI cycles. Further work is required to determine whether there is an effect on clinical treatment endpoints.

Keywords: Poor ovarian response, POSEIDON stratification, Oxidative stress, Coenzyme Q10, In vitro fertilization, High-quality embryos, Clinical outcomes

---

* Correspondence: janez2012@sina.com; yushu57200@126.com
[2]Reproductive Medical Center, Department of Obstetrics and Gynecology, Peking University Third Hospital, Beijing 100123, China
[1]Department of Reproduction, Beijing Obstetrics and Gynecology Hospital, Capital Medical University, Beijing 100026, China
Full list of author information is available at the end of the article

Background

Poor response to controlled ovarian hyperstimulation (COH) remains one of the main challenges of the assisted reproductive technology (ART) treatments. Despite impressive advances in the field, many women exhibit inadequate response to gonadotrophins, referred to as 'poor or low responders' and have higher odds of cycle cancellation, fewer oocytes at retrieval, lower oocyte quality and reduced number of embryos for transfer. Collectively, this results in serial failure of the ART cycles and is frustrating for both patients and their caregivers. The exact incidence of the condition is hard to establish owing to variable definitions in literature with the estimates ranging from 5.6 to 35.1% of ART cycles [1]. Multiple interventions have been proposed to improve reproductive outcomes in women with poor ovarian response (POR), but the randomized intervention studies and meta-analyses of these studies reveal conflicting results [2, 3]. Currently, the evidence-based therapeutic strategies to improve ovarian response and reproductive outcomes in women with POR are lacking, and treating clinicians often offer empirical treatments with little clinical evidence to support their use [4]. Furthermore, it has been increasingly acknowledged that the available ovarian reserve tests are not reliable to predict pregnancy after assisted conception [5]. We do not have universally accepted tests to predict response to treatment, which is of important value for counseling couples regarding their treatment pathways and for setting patients' expectations.

It has been proposed that a heterogeneity of the included population is the main barrier in evaluating the interventions and the factors that guide prognosis for POR [6]. An internationally-agreed consensus on the definition of POR reached by an ESHRE Campus Workshop held in Bologna in 2010 suggests that at least 2 out of 3 features must be present: (1) advanced maternal age or any other risk factor for POR; (2) previous POR; (3) abnormal ovarian reserve test [7]. This uniform definition, however, implies that POR constitutes heterogeneous group of women with respect to age, previous reproductive experience and ovarian reserve tests that may have different response to the interventions [6]. While age-dependent decline in ovarian reserve and oocyte quality accounts for poor response in older women, an underlying etiology for its occurrence earlier in life is less clear. It is possible that younger women with compromised ovarian reserve represent a distinct subpopulation within POR group, and their fertility prognosis may differ from that of older women with low ovarian reserve markers or from similar age women with adequate ovarian reserve parameters but suboptimal response to ovarian stimulation [8].

Taking the above considerations into account, the recently established POSEIDON group (Patient-Oriented Strategies Encompassing Individualize Oocyte Number) proposed a new stratification of women with POR undergoing ART treatments, which includes 4 subgroups based on women's age, ovarian reserve parameters and previous response to ovarian stimulation [9]. The POSEIDON concept introduces personalized medicine approach to the POR population and is expected to be more effective in identifying the subsets of patients who could benefit from specific interventions [10].

The physiology of poor ovarian response is not fully understood and the molecular events underlying POR remain unknown. Oxidative stress and mitochondrial dysfunction are among the most investigated possible mechanisms [11]. Mitochondria are the most abundant organelles in oocytes and early embryos that generate approximately 90% of reactive oxygen species (ROS), the end products of oxygen metabolism, and convert ROS into an inactive state via antioxidant defense mechanisms [12]. Higher levels of ROS accumulating in mitochondria during multiple physiological conditions contribute to mitochondrial dysfunction and increase in oxidative stress. This, in turn, leads to oxidative damage to DNA and other intra-cellular aberrations, which are similar to the age-related changes [12, 13]. Thus, improving mitochondrial function by supplementing antioxidants has been proposed as one of the important strategies to enhance reproductive performance [11, 14].

Coenzyme Q10 (CoQ10) is a lipid-soluble coenzyme and is an essential component of the inner mitochondrial membrane. CoQ10 is primarily involved in electron transport in the mitochondrial respiratory chain and oxidative phosphorylation to produce adenosine triphosphate (ATP). CoQ10 acts as an antioxidant by inhibiting lipid peroxidation and DNA oxidation, thus is capable of strengthening endogenous antioxidant system within a cell [15]. CoQ10 supplementation has been shown to improve cardiovascular function and male fertility [16–18]. Reduced concentrations of CoQ10 in plasma have been associated with hypogonadism and altered levels of other steroid hormones [19]. Decrease in CoQ10 level is commonly observed in individuals in late 30th and appears to co-occur with the age-related decline in fertility and increased rate of embryo aneuploidy, suggesting a contribution of the reduced expression of CoQ10 to ovarian ageing [20]. Several animal studies have demonstrated that CoQ10 protects ovarian reserve, counteracts physiological ovarian ageing by restoring mitochondrial function and increases the rate of embryo cleavage and blastocyst formation [21–23]. In the clinical setting, CoQ10 supplementation led to better response to ovulation induction and decreased odds of fetal aneuploidy in 35–43-year-old women [24, 25]. To date, however, no study has investigated whether CoQ10 pretreatment could improve the ART treatment outcomes in young subpopulation of poor responders in a randomized setting.

On the above evidence, this study focused on investigating the effect of CoQ10 supplementation on response to ovarian stimulation in the group of young women with diminished ovarian reserve, corresponding to the Poseidon's stratification group 3 [9]. We hypothesized that increased oxidative stress has a prominent effect on premature decline of ovarian function in these women, which could be amenable to anti-oxidant therapy.

Methods

Study design and randomization

This was a prospective randomized controlled study, conducted at the Reproductive Medical Center of the Peking University Third Hospital, a tertiary university hospital and a center of excellence in Reproductive Medicine in China. The study is reported according to the CONSORT guidelines. The flow of the patients in this study is presented in Fig. 1.

All the participants were randomized 1:1 to either CoQ10 treatment (study group) or no treatment (control group) followed by an ART cycle. The randomization was performed over the period of 14 months (between June 2, 2015 and July 31, 2016) by using the computer-generated randomization codes, which were then placed in the sealed, opaque sequentially numbered envelopes by a third party (nurse practitioner) who was not directly involved in the patient management or in the randomization process. The envelopes were handed out to the participants upon completing the informed consent. The study participants and the investigators were not blinded to the patient grouping. The participants were followed through one completed ART cycle until all frozen embryos generated from the index cycle were used or until delivery in those who achieved pregnancy.

Study population

All consecutive women who were found to have POR and were referred to IVF-ET cycle in our institution were approached. POR was defined according to the ESHRE Bologna criteria [7]. The study inclusion criteria were: age < 35 years, anti-Mullerian hormone (AMH) < 1.2 ng/ml, and antral follicle count (AFC) < 5, the parameters that corresponded to a low prognosis group 3 as per the POSEIDON stratification [9]. Exclusion criteria were: age ≥ 35 years, history of ovarian surgery, endocrine or autoimmune disease (e.g. diabetes, thyroid disease or presence of anti-thyroid antibodies or PCOS), chromosomal abnormality, uterine malformations, more than 3 previous IVF cycles, treatment with cholesterol-lowering drugs, previous treatment with anti-oxidants (last 5 years) or known allergy to CoQ10 or ubiquinol (the water-soluble isoform of CoQ10). All the participants completed the questionnaire with demographic, medical and reproductive information and underwent clinical examination, pelvic ultrasound, chromosome analysis, AMH test, reproductive endocrine profile and thyroid studies. All the included women were specifically asked about any previous treatment with anti-oxidants such as CoQ10, ubiquinol, vitamin A, vitamin E, vitamin C, beta-carotene or selenium, including the duration and time of treatment.

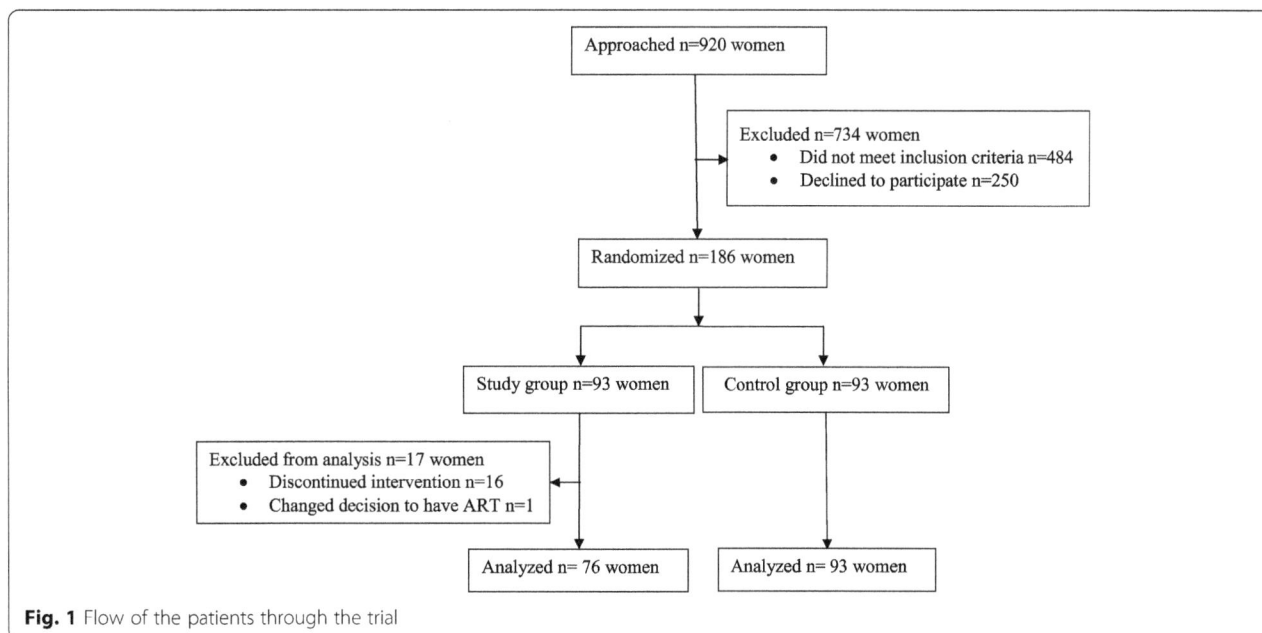

Fig. 1 Flow of the patients through the trial

Treatment protocols

The intervention in the study group included oral administration of CoQ10 (GNC Holdings Inc., Pittsburg, PA, USA) 200 mg three times a day, for a period of 60 days in an open label fashion. The ART treatment (in vitro fertilization (IVF) or intracytoplasmic sperm injection (ICSI)) was commenced in the first menstrual cycle upon completion of CoQ10 treatment. The control group commenced ART (IVF or ICSI) after enrollment without any additional treatment.

Ovarian stimulation and oocyte retrieval

All participants underwent ovarian stimulation with the short GnRH-antagonist protocol. A combination of recombinant follicle stimulating hormone (FSH) (Gonal-F, 225 IU/day, Merck Serono SA Aubonne Branch) and human menopausal gonadotrophin (Menotropins for injection FSH 75 IU: LH 75 IU, 225 IU/day, Livzon Pharmaceutical Group Inc.) in a fixed-dose was started on Day 2 of the menstrual cycle with the option to adjust dose according to response after 4 days of stimulation (Day 6 of menstrual cycle). GnRH antagonist (Cetrorelix 250 µg/day, Merck Serono, Darmstadt, Germany) was started when a leading follicle of 12 mm was achieved. Recombinant human chorionic gonadotrophin (hCG) trigger (Ovidrele 250 µg; Merck Serono S.p.A, Rome, Italy) was administered when at least one follicle was above 18 mm. The cycle was cancelled when there were no follicles with diameter ≥ 14 mm after 8–9 days of gonadotrophin therapy or when peak E2 level was below 250 pmol/l.

Ultrasound-guided transvaginal oocyte retrieval was performed 36–38 h after the trigger injection by using a 17-gauge double-lumen needle (Cook Medical) and a vacuum pump (Cook Medical) under pressure at 125 mmHg. Each follicle sized above 12–14 mm was drained, and follicle flushing was not performed. The cumulus-oocyte complexes (COCs) were removed from the collection fluid using a sterile glass pipette and washed in G-IVF Plus media (Vitrolife, Sweden) and transported to the laboratory.

Oocyte insemination and embryo culture

Oocytes were inseminated either by conventional IVF or by ICSI depending on sperm quality. Oocytes undergoing IVF insemination were placed into a dish with G-IVF (Vitrolife) covered in mineral oil. Oocytes undergoing ICSI were denuded and injected if maturation status was confirmed by the presence of the first polar body (PB). Fertilization was assessed 17–19 h after insemination and was defined by the presence of two pronuclears (2PN) and two PBs. All embryos were transferred to GM medium (G-M, Life Global, CT, USA) for a further 48 h of culture.

Embryo development and quality were assessed 68–72 h (day 3) after insemination, based on the number of blastomeres, blastomere symmetry, percentage of fragmentation, and quality of cytoplasm according to the criteria established by the Istanbul Consensus Workshop on Embryo Assessment [26]. All supernumerary day-3 embryos were cryopreserved by vitrification (JIEYING laboratory Inc., Canada) for future use.

Endometrial preparation and embryo transfer

All patients underwent transfer of day-3 embryos in a fresh cycle and subsequent frozen embryo transfer (FET) when the cryopreserved embryos generated from the index stimulation cycle were available. The embryos with the best morphological grade were selected for transfer. In absence of high-quality embryos, transfer of any embryo quality was considered after careful patient counselling.

In a fresh cycle, the luteal phase was supported with progesterone intravaginal gel (Crinone 8% 90 mg/day, Merck-Serono) commenced on the day of oocyte retrieval until 14 days after embryo transfer. In women with positive pregnancy test, luteal support was continued until 8 weeks gestation. The protocols used for FET utilized either natural cycle or artificial estradiol and progesterone endometrium priming in normo-ovulatory and oligo-ovulatory women, respectively. In natural cycle, ovulation was tracked with transvaginal ultrasound and urine LH kit. Oral dydrogesterone (Duphaston, 20 mg daily for 7 days; Abbott Biologicals B.V.) was commenced for luteal phase support 3 days after LH surge on the day of embryo transfer until 8 weeks gestation. In artificial FET protocol, oral estradiol valerate (Progynova 6 mg/day, Schering, Berlin, Germany) was initiated on the third day of the menstrual cycle and endometrial thickness was monitored with transvaginal ultrasonography. When the endometrial thickness exceeded 8 mm, luteal support with progesterone intravaginal gel (Crinone 8% 90 mg, daily; Merck-Serono), combined with oral dydrogesterone (Duphaston, 20 mg daily for 7 days; Abbott Biologicals B.V.) was added and embryo transfer was performed after 5 days. Hormonal treatment was stopped if pregnancy test was negative or continued until 11 weeks gestation with tapering off after 10 weeks. Single or double cleavage-stage embryo transfer were performed by using a soft catheter (K-Soft 5100; Cook, Queensland, Australia) without ultrasound guidance. Serum hCG was measured 14 days after embryo transfer and was considered positive for hCG level ≥ 10 IU. Transvaginal ultrasonography at 30 days after transfer was used to confirm clinical pregnancy.

Hormone assay procedures

All the hormonal assays were performed at the endocrine laboratory of the Peking University Third Hospital

Reproductive Centre by using commercially available kits. Serum concentrations of hCG were determined by using the commercially available ELISA kit (Beckman DXI800, Beckman, USA) according to the manufacturer's instructions. Serum levels of anti-Mullerian hormone (AMH) were measured by automated assays using commercially available kit (Ashlab, USA). Serum luteinizing hormone (LH), FSH, estradiol (E2), and Progesterone (P) were tested using the Immulite 1000 assay based on chemiluminescence (DPC, Poway, CA).

The lower detection limit of the hCG and the AMH assays was 0.5 IU/L and 0.06 ng/ml respectively. The intra- and inter-assay coefficient of variation (CV) for hCG activity was 5% and for AMH was 8%. The lower detection limit of LH, FSH, E2 and P was 0.05 IU/L, 0.12 IU/L, 73.4 pmol/L, 0.64 nmol/L, respectively. The CV of LH and FSH was 6% and of E_2 and P was 10%.

Outcome measures

The primary outcome measure was the number of high quality day-3 embryos generated from one stimulation cycle. High quality embryos were defined as embryos that reached 6 to 8-cell stage with cytoplasmic fragmentation occupying less than 10% of the embryo surface and had equal size blastomeres.

The secondary outcomes included ovarian response parameters (duration of stimulation, total dose of gonadotrophins, peak E2 level and endometrial thickness on the day of hCG trigger), embryological parameters (number of oocytes retrieved, fertilization rate, number of patients with frozen embryos and number of patients who did not achieve embryo transfer) and clinical parameters (miscarriage, clinical pregnancy and live birth rate). Fertilization rate was defined as the number of 2PN embryos divided by the number of inseminated oocytes. Clinical pregnancy was defined as a presence of intrauterine gestational sac observed on ultrasound after 30 days of embryo transfer. Miscarriage was defined as a loss of clinical pregnancy before 24 weeks of gestation. Live birth was defined as the birth of at least one living child, irrespective of the duration of gestation. Clinical pregnancy and live birth rate were calculated per embryo transfer cycle as number of pregnancies/live births divided per number of women who had transfer. Cumulative pregnancy and live birth rate were defined as the number of clinical pregnancies/live births generated from the index ART cycle following fresh or frozen embryo transfer divided by all women who received treatment. In addition, markers of ovarian reserve, including AMH, day 3 FSH and AFC were evaluated before and after CoQ10 treatment in the participants from the intervention (study) group.

Sample size calculation

The sample size calculation for this study was based on the number of high quality embryos as primary outcome. In our center women with poor response have an average 0.6–0.8 high quality embryos per woman. To detect a difference of 50% in primary outcome measure (from 0.6–0.8 to 1.0–1.2 embryos per woman) with alpha 0.05 and power 0.80, the required sample size was estimated at 76 women in each arm. When accounted for a drop out rate of 20%, each arm required 92 women.

Statistical analysis

The Student's t-test or Mann-Whitney U test were used for comparisons of continuous variables between the groups depending on the distribution of the data. The chi-squared test or Fisher's exact test, where appropriate, were used for comparisons of categorical variables. Results are presented as mean ± standard deviation (SD), median and interquartile range (IQR) or as percentages. Statistical significance was set at a probability (p) value < 0.05. All statistical analyses were performed using SPSS 22.0 software (IBM Corp., Armonk, NY, USA).

Results

A total of 436 women met inclusion criteria. Of them, 186 women agreed to participate and were enrolled in the study, 93 women in each arm. Among the participants who were randomized to the intervention (CoQ10 treatment) group, 17 women were excluded from the analysis for the following reasons: one woman changed her mind to undergo ART and 16 women discontinued CoQ10 treatment due to the compliance issues. Overall, 76 women were retained in the study group and 93 women comprised the control group. All the participants shared the features of POSEIDON group 3, i.e. low prognosis patients younger than 35 years old with poor ovarian reserve pre-stimulation parameters. Baseline characteristics were comparable between the two groups with respect to age, BMI, duration of infertility, parity, ovarian reserve tests and causes of infertility (Table 1). Most participants were diagnosed with primary infertility and were ART treatment-naïve.

In the treatment group, no local or systemic side effects related to the use of oral CoQ10 were reported. Sequential measurements of ovarian reserve markers before and after CoQ10 treatment are presented in Table 2. The levels of basal day-3 FSH were significantly lower after 60 days supplementation of CoQ10 compared to the pre-treatment levels in the same group of women. In contrast, the levels of AMH and AFC were almost identical before and after CoQ10 treatment (Table 2).

Table 1 Baseline characteristics of the study population

Variables	Study group ($n = 76$)	Control group ($n = 93$)	p-value
Demographic characteristics			
Age (years), mean ± SD	32.50 ± 3.30	31.92 ± 3.68	0.29
BMI (kg/m^2), mean ± SD	21.85 ± 2.51	22.24 ± 3.07	0.37
Infertility duration (years), median (IQR)	3 (2, 4)	3 (2, 3)	0.32
Primary infertility, n (%)	48/76 (63.15)	65/93 (69.89)	0.71
Nulliparity, n (%)	72/76 (94.74)	86/93 (92.47)	0.76
Previous ART treatments, n (%)	11/76 (14.47)	20/93 (21.51)	0.43
Ovarian reserve markers			
AMH (ng/ml), median (IQR)	0.57 (0.35, 0.80)	0.56 (0.35, 0.80)	0.46
AFC, median (IQR)	5 (3, 6)	4 (3, 6)	0.17
Day 3 FSH (IU/ml), median (IQR)	12.25 (9.39, 15.50)	12.6 (9.95, 15.60)	0.58
Diagnosis of infertility in addition to POR			
Tubal factor, n (%)	13/76 (17.11)	22/93 (23.66)	0.61
Male factor, n (%)	22/76 (28.95)	25/93 (26.88)	0.82
Unexplained, n (%)	22/76 (28.95)	25/93 (26.88)	0.82

AMH - anti-Mullerian hormone; AFC - antral follicle count; BMI – body mass index; IQR – interquartile range; POR – poor ovarian reserve; SD – standard deviation

The parameters of ovarian response to stimulation and the embryology outcomes of ART cycles in the study population are summarized in Table 3. The amount of gonadotrophin used was significantly lower in CoQ10 treatment group than in controls ($p = 0.03$). The duration of gonadotrophin therapy tended to be shorter in the participants treated with CoQ10, but the difference did not reach statistical significance ($p = 0.08$). Peak E2 serum concentrations were significantly higher in the CoQ10 group, but there was no difference in the mean endometrial thickness on the day of hCG trigger between the two groups. In the CoQ10 treatment group there were fewer cancelled cases due to suboptimal ovarian response (5.23%, 4/76) compared to the control group (10.75%, 10/93) although this difference failed to achieve statistical significance, $p = 0.27$. Overall, 94.74% (72/76) women from the CoQ10 group and 89.25% (83/93) women from the control group received hCG and underwent oocyte retrieval. The median number of retrieved oocytes was significantly higher after CoQ10 pretreatment (4, IQR 2–5), than in controls (2, IQR 1–2), $p = 0.002$. Most women had conventional IVF and the number of ICSI cycles was comparable between the groups. The median number of fertilized oocytes and

fertilization rate were significantly higher in women treated with CoQ10 than in controls, $p < 0.05$. The median number of high quality day-3 embryos available per patient in the CoQ10 group was 1 (IQR 0–2) and in control group was 0 (IQR 0–1.75), with significant difference in favor of CoQ10 treatment, $p = 0.03$.

Among the patients in CoQ10 group who underwent oocyte retrieval, there was significantly lower number of women who did not achieve embryo transfer because of failure to retrieve oocytes or due to the absence of useable embryos (8.33%, 6/72) compared to women from the control group (22.89%, 19/83), $p = 0.04$ (Table 4). Collectively, embryos were available for 66 women in the CoQ10 group and 64 women in the control group, all of whom underwent fresh embryo transfer. The number of fresh embryo transfer cycles in the CoQ10 groups was comparable to that in controls. More patients in the CoQ10 group had cryopreserved embryos (18.42%, 14/76 vs. 4.3%, 4/93, respectively, $p = 0.02$) and the number of frozen-thaw embryo transfers from the index stimulation cycle was significantly higher, $p = 0.01$ (Table 4). In 14.29%, 2/14 women from the CoQ10 group with available cryopreserved embryos and in 25%, 1/4 controls, embryos did not recover after thawing. One to two

Table 2 Ovarian reserve markers before and after CoQ10 treatment in the study group

Variables	Before CoQ10 ($n = 76$)	After CoQ10 ($n = 76$)	p-value
AMH (ng/ml), median (IQR)	0.57 (0.35, 0.80)	0.59 (0.38, 0.80)	0.91
AFC(n), median (IQR)	5 (3, 6)	5 (3, 7)	0.94
Day 3 FSH (IU/ml), median (IQR)	12.25 (9.39, 15.50)	10.50 (9.23, 12.60)	0.006

AMH - anti-Mullerian hormone; AFC - antral follicle count; FSH - follicle stimulating hormone; IQR - interquartile range

Table 3 ART cycle stimulation parameters and embryology outcomes

Variable	Study group (n = 76)	Control group (n = 93)	p- value
Cycle stimulation			
Total dose of Gn (IU), median (IQR)	2000 (1200, 4275)	3075 (1900, 4275)	0.03
Duration of stimulation (days), median (IQR)	10 (9, 11)	11 (9, 12)	0.08
Peak E2 concentration (pmol/l), median (IQR)	2349 (892, 4784)	1685 (1125, 3042)	0.02
Endometrial thickness on the day of hCG trigger (mm), mean ± SD	10.12 ± 1.93	10.34 ± 1.50	0.13
Patients who had oocyte retrieval	72/76 (94.74)	83/93 (89.25)	0.82
Cancelled cycles [a], n (%)	4/76 (5.23)	10/93 (10.75)	0.27
Embryology outcomes			
Retrieved oocytes, median (IQR)	4 (2, 5)	2 (1, 4)	0.002
ICSI cycles, n (%)	24/76 (31.58)	19/93 (20.43)	0.20
Fertilized oocytes (2PN), median (IQR)	0.80 (0.50, 0.93)	0.50 (0.33, 1.0)	0.01
Fertilization rate [b], n (%)	191/253 (67.49)	191/283 (45.06)	0.001
Number of high quality embryos, median (IQR)	1 (0, 2)	0 (0, 1.75)	0.03

[a]Included women in who did not respond to stimulation and did not have oocyte retrieval
[b]Calculated as following: the number of total 2PN embryos divided by the number of total inseminated oocytes
E2 – estradiol; Gn – gonadotrophin; hCG – human chorionic gonadotrophin; IQR – interquartile range; LH - luteinizing hormone; P - progesterone, 2PN – two pronuclear, SD - standard deviation

embryos were replaced into the uterus in each transfer cycle with higher median number in the CoQ10 group (2, IQR 1–2) than in controls (1, IQR 1–2), $p = 0.04$.

In the CoQ10 group there were 23 clinical pregnancies following fresh embryo transfer and one additional pregnancy following frozen-thaw embryo transfer. In the control group there were 16 clinical pregnancies after fresh embryo transfer and no pregnancies after frozen-thaw transfer. The were no spontaneously conceived pregnancies in either group. Successful live birth was achieved in 22 women from the CoQ10 (21 after fresh and 1 after frozen-thaw transfer) and in 14 women from the control group. Clinical pregnancy rate and live birth rate per fresh embryo transfer cycle were 34.85% and 31.82% in women treated with CoQ10, and 25% and 21.88% in controls, respectively. The clinical estimates for frozen-thaw embryo transfer were not calculated due to the paucity of the available data. When the transfers of all embryos originating from the complete ART cycle were considered, in women treated with CoQ10 the

Table 4 Clinical reproductive outcomes

Variable	Study group (n = 76)	Control group (n = 93)	p-value
Number of fresh ET cycles[a], n (%)	66/76 (86.84)	64/93 (68.82)	0.35
Patients who had oocyte retrieval but no ET [b], n (%)	6/72 (8.33)	19/83 (22.89)	0.04
Number of FET cycles, n (%)	12/76 (15.79)	3/93 (3.23)	0.01
Patients with cryopreserved embryos, n (%)	14/76 (18.42)[c]	4/93 (4.30)[d]	0.012
Number of embryos per ET[e], median (IQR)	2 (1,2)	1 (1,2)	0.04
Clinical pregnancy rate per fresh ET[f], n (%)	23/66 (34.85)	16/64 (25.00)	0.24
Cumulative clinical pregnancy rate[g], n (%)	24/76 (31.58)	16/93 (17.20)	0.11
Multiple pregnancy, n (%)	4/76 (5.26)	3/93 (3.23)	0.70
Spontaneous miscarriage, n (%)	2/23 (8.67)	2/16 (12.50)	0.73
Live birth rate per fresh ET[f], n (%)	21/66 (31.82)	14/64 (21.88)	0.33
Cumulative live birth rate[g], n (%)	22/76 (28.95)	14/93 (15.54)	0.08

[a]All patients with available embryos had fresh ET
[b]Included women who had hCG andoocyte retrieval but did not have oocytes or useable embryos
[c]Embryos for 2women from this group did not survive the thawing (2/14, 14.29%)
[d]Embryos for 1 woman from this group did not survive the thawing (1/4, 25%)
[e]All the transferred embryos were day-3 cleavage stage embryos
[f]Calculated as follows: the number of clinical pregnancies/ live births originated from fresh ET divided by the number of women with transferred embryos
[g]Calculated as follows: the number of clinical pregnancies/ live births originated from one completed ART cycle including fresh and frozen-thaw ETs divided by the number of women treated
ET – embryo transfer; FET – frozen-thaw embryo transfer; IQR – interquartile range

cumulative clinical pregnancy rate after one complete cycle was 31.58%, 24/76 and the cumulative live birth rate was 28.95%, 22/76. In the control group, the cumulative clinical pregnancy rate was 17.20%, 16/93 and the cumulative live birth rate was 15.54%, 14/93, respectively. Miscarriage rate was 8.67% in women from the CoQ10 group and 12.5% in controls. Although women from the CoQ10 group had higher clinical pregnancy and live birth rates with lower occurrence of pregnancy loss, the difference between the treatment and control groups failed to achieve statistical significance for each of these outcomes.

Discussion

In this study we demonstrated potential benefit of CoQ10 treatment in improving ovarian response to gonadotrophin stimulation in young women with low ovarian reserve. To the best of our knowledge, this is the first study that evaluated an effect of anti-oxidant treatment in specific phenotypic subgroup of women with POR.

Our results demonstrate that pre-treatment with CoQ10 resulted in significant decrease in the total amount of gonadotrophin needed to achieve ovarian response, shorter duration of stimulation, higher peak E2 levels and the number of oocytes retrieved. CoQ10 treatment led to significant increase in fertilization rate and in the number of high quality embryos. There was significantly lower rate of cancelled cycles because of no response to stimulation, less cancelled embryo transfers because of failed embryo development and larger number of cycles with cryopreserved embryos in the CoQ10 treated group than in controls. The clinical pregnancy and live birth rates were higher after CoQ10 treatment then in controls, but these differences failed to achieve significance, presumably due to insufficient sample size. Taken together, our data suggest that CoQ10 administration enhances ovarian response to stimulation and improves oocyte and embryo quality.

The findings of this study are approximately in line with previous reports that linked CoQ10 with improved reproductive outcomes. Small randomized placebo-controlled study in 24 participants (10 women in CoQ10 and 14 in placebo group) have demonstrated higher peak concentration of E2, increased number of high quality cleavage embryos, and a trend towards decreased aneuploidy and higher clinical pregnancy rate after 60 days treatment with 600 mg CoQ10 [25]. However, the study was underpowered and failed to demonstrate significant difference in clinical outcomes between the groups [25]. Another randomized controlled study in 101 young women with PCOS demonstrated that addition of CoQ10 in a dose of 180 mg during ovulation induction with clomiphene citrate improved ovarian response in clomiphene-resistant women and resulted in higher clinical pregnancy rate [24]. Retrospective analysis in 797 IUI and 253 IVF cycles in women older than 36–37 years revealed that addition of 600 mg CoQ10 to dehydroepiandrosterone (DHEA) over the period longer than 1 month resulted in lower dose of gonadotrophins and higher number of mature follicles than in women treated with DHEA alone [27]. The authors did not demonstrate significant difference in the embryological or clinical outcomes, and the comparisons with untreated controls were not available [27].

The plausible effect of CoQ10 on reproductive function is attributed to its effect on the antioxidative capacity and energy production in the oocyte [10, 28, 29]. CoQ10, the only synthesized lipid soluble antioxidant in humans, is an essential component of the mitochondrial respiratory chain, serving an important antioxidant function both in mitochondria and in lipid membranes [15]. ROS-induced DNA damage in ovary leads to genomic instability, mutations and apoptosis of oocytes, and is thought to be ameliorated by an antioxidant activity of CoQ10 [22]. CoQ10 has been also shown to improve mitochondrial function and restore energy production by mitochondria [23]. Mitochondrial dysfunction in oocytes results in decreased oxidative phosphorylation and suboptimal levels of mitochondria-generated ATP, which has been strongly associated with poor reproductive performance, including diminished ovarian reserve, poor oocyte quality, abnormal fertilization and deranged preimplantation embryo development [29, 30]. Energy production by mitochondria is important for steroid hormone biosynthesis, oocyte maturation, fertilization, and early embryonic development [31, 32]. It has been demonstrated that CoQ10 supplemented in aged animal model has improved mitochondrial membrane potential, mitochondrial ATP production and mitotic spindle orientation [21]. Treatment with CoQ10 increased the number of ovulated oocytes and reduced ROS in oocytes to the levels observed in young animals, indicating this is an effective strategy to reverse the effect of reproductive ageing [33]. In humans, levels of CoQ10 in the follicular fluid positively correlated with oocyte maturation, embryo grade and pregnancy rate in women undergoing ART [34, 35]. While oocyte appears to be the main target of CoQ10, it remains unclear whether anti-oxidant treatment also improves uterine environment. We did not demonstrate any differences in endometrial thickness, but there were no data to confidently comment on the effect of CoQ10 in intra-uterine milieu.

CoQ10 has been also associated with improved ovarian reserve. In rodents, CoQ10 administration reversed ovarian toxicity of cisplatin, leading to increase in the serum AMH concentrations, improved AMH-positive follicle count and lower number of atretic follicles [22]. Exposure to CoQ10 restored ovarian reserve in mice with induced accelerated oocyte loss [21]. Currently, however, there is relative paucity of information concerning the exact mechanism by which CoQ10 influences ovarian reserve in humans and it is difficult to conclude whether CoQ10 rescues follicles from apoptosis or enhances primordial follicle activation. In this study there was significant decrease in baseline FSH levels after 60 days of CoQ10 administration. It is possible that a change in FSH levels could also have occurred without CoQ10 treatment over a period of two-three months, but this seems unlikely considering that previous study in 287 infertile men showed 14% decline in FSH levels after 3 months of CoQ10 supplementation with continuing decrease throughout 12 months therapy [18]. In contrast, we did not observe improvement in other ovarian reserve markers, namely AMH and AFC and such discrepancy between our and animal studies could be explained by different treatment protocols and variation in physiological parameters between species. In rodents, 8–12 weeks of CoQ10 exposure corresponds to about ¼ of the life span, which is considerably longer interval in relation to a reproductive cycle when compared to analogous treatment period in humans. It has been supposed that two months exposure to CoQ10 could improve energy production in the ovary but might not be long enough to restore prolonged effect of oxidative damage [25]. It should be noted that it takes about three months for a primordial follicle to reach the preovulatory stage [36]. AMH is predominantly produced upon transition from the primordial to primary follicles when they are recruited from the dormant pool and represents early stages of growth [37]. Thus, short duration of CoQ10 administration is likely to influence late events of follicle maturation but may not be sufficient to improve follicle recruitment evidenced by AMH levels. Indeed, the study that reported significant increase in antral follicles in CoQ10, included women who were treated with CoQ10 for an average of 8.8 ± 6.2 months [27].

The optimal timing, duration and dose of CoQ10 supplementation remain unclear. In this study, the duration of treatment was selected arbitrary based on previous study in IVF population [25]. It could be argued that CoQ10 treatment implies a delay in initiation of ART cycle and thus longer pretreatment period may be less acceptable to the patients. It has been demonstrated that CoQ10 is well tolerated and safe for healthy adults at intake of up to 900 mg/day [38]. We were guided by previous experience in selecting the dose of CoQ10, although this was rather intuitive choice [18, 24, 25, 27].

The main strength of this study is that it focused on a specific phenotype within a broad heterogeneous group of women with POR. All the participants shared similar demographic and clinical characteristics and had comparable pre-treatment markers of ovarian activity. In addition, we utilized an unbiased randomization process and applied the similar laboratory and clinical protocols to all the participants.

The important limitation of our study was its small sample size and we were unable to detect significant differences in clinical outcomes. Live birth is an ultimate outcome of infertility treatment and is more appropriate estimate for patient counseling. The POSEIDON group has recently suggested that the number of oocytes needed to obtain at least one euploid embryo per patient is a more practical treatment endpoint for the studies in women with POR and helps to define the short-term goals for management [10]. In adopting this approach, we chose the number of high quality embryos as a primary outcome measure and calculated the sample size accordingly. High drop-out rate in the study group due to CoQ10 discontinuation was additional limiting factor that should be considered in future studies. In line with the reported by others, CoQ10 administration did not cause any adverse reactions or side effects in this study [39], but all women who discontinued treatment reported difficulty to comply with the CoQ10 regime requiring three times a day administration. Finally, in this study we did not evaluate the levels of oxidative stress markers before or after treatment and did not assess the influence of other lifestyle factors that may pose women at higher risk. A threshold effect of CoQ10 may vary on individual level due to interference with other environmental exposures leading to oxidative stress and this should be considered in the design of future studies.

Conclusions

In summary, pretreatment with CoQ10 increases ovarian response to stimulation and improves oocyte and embryo quality in young low prognosis patients with diminished ovarian reserve. There is a possible beneficial effect on clinical pregnancy and live birth rates, but this needs to be confirmed in larger randomized controlled studies. Further work is required to establish the optimal length, timing and dosage of treatment and to evaluate the therapeutic effect of CoQ10 supplementation in other subgroups of low prognosis women with POR.

Acknowledgements
We sincerely thank the women who participated in the study. We also thank the medical and nursing staff of the Reproductive Medical Center of Peking University Third Hospital for their assistance in patient recruitment and management.

Funding
This study was supported by National key research and development project (2016YFC1000302) and the scientific research foundation for the returned overseas Ministry of Education (A70538–3).

Authors' contributions

YYX took part in the patient enrolment, management and follow-up, performed data analysis and prepared the first draft of the manuscript; VN contributed to study design, data analysis and preparation of the manuscript; CL was involved in embryological experiments and contributed to study design; RL and JQ contributed to study design and were involved in critical discussions; XZ contributed to the concept, design and preparation of the manuscript and was involved in patient enrolment and management; SW coordinated the research and contributed to study design and critical discussions. All authors read and approved the final manuscript.

Competing interests

The authors declare that they have no competing interests.

Author details

[1]Department of Reproduction, Beijing Obstetrics and Gynecology Hospital, Capital Medical University, Beijing 100026, China. [2]Reproductive Medical Center, Department of Obstetrics and Gynecology, Peking University Third Hospital, Beijing 100123, China. [3]Key Laboratory of Assisted Reproduction, Ministry of Education, Beijing, China.

References

1. Oudendijk JF, Yarde F, Eijkemans MJ, Broekmans FJ, Broer SL. The poor responder in IVF: is the prognosis always poor? A systematic review. Hum Reprod Update. 2012;18:1–11.
2. Pandian Z, McTavish AR, Aucott L, Hamilton MP, Bhattacharya S. Interventions for 'poor responders' to controlled ovarian hyper stimulation (COH) in in-vitro fertilisation (IVF). Cochrane Database Syst Rev. 2010;20: CD004379.
3. Szymusik I, Marianowski P, Zygula A, Wielgos M. Poor responders in IVF, is there any evidence based treatment for them? Neuro Endocrinol Lett. 2015; 36:209–13.
4. Patrizio P, Vaiarelli A, Setti L, Tobler KJ, Shoham G, Leong M, et al. How to define, diagnose and treat poor responders? Responses from a worldwide survey of IVF clinics. Reprod BioMed Online. 2015;30:581–92.
5. Domingues TS, Rocha AM, Serafini PC. Tests for ovarian reserve: reliability and utility. Curr Opin Obstet Gynecol. 2010;22:271–6.
6. Papathanasiou A, Searle BJ, King NM. Trends in 'poor responder' research: lessons learned from RCTs in assisted conception. Hum Reprod Update. 2016;22
7. Ferraretti AP, La Marca A, Fauser BC, Tarlatzis B, Nargund G, Gianaroli L. ESHRE consensus on the definition of 'poor response' to ovarian stimulation for in vitro fertilization: the bologna criteria. Hum Reprod. 2011;26:1616–24.
8. Szymusik I, Marianowski P, Zygula A, Wielgos M. Management of poor responders in IVF: is there anything new? Biomed Res Int. 2014;2014:352098.
9. Poseidon Group (Patient-Oriented Strategies Encompassing IndividualizeD Oocyte Number), Alviggi C, Andersen CY, Buehler K, Conforti A, De Placido G, et al. A new more detailed stratification of low responders to ovarian stimulation: from a poor ovarian response to a low prognosis concept. Fertil Steril. 2016;105(6):1452–3.
10. Humaidan P, Alviggi C, Fischer R, Esteves SC. The novel POSEIDON stratification of 'low prognosis women in assisted reproductive technology' and its proposed marker of successful outcome[J]. F1000research. 2016;5:2911.
11. Blerkom JV. Mitochondrial function in the human oocyte and embryo and their role in developmental competence. Mitochondrion. 2011;11:797–813.
12. Nickel A, Kohlhaas M, Maack C. Mitochondrial reactive oxygen species production and elimination. J Mol Cell Cardiol. 2014;73:26–33.
13. Wilson DM 3rd, Sofinowski TM, McNeill DR. Repair mechanisms for oxidative DNA damage. Front Biosci. 2003;8:d963–81.
14. Bentov Y, Casper RF. The aging oocyte—can mitochondrial function be improved? Fertil Steril. 2013;99:18–22.
15. Bentinger M, Brismar K, Dallner G. The antioxidant role of coenzyme Q. Mitochondrion. 2007;7:S41.
16. Rosenfeldt F, Hilton D, Pepe S, Krum H. Systematic review of effect of coenzyme Q10 in physical exercise, hypertension and heart failure. Biofactors. 2003;18:91–100.
17. Balercia G, Mosca F, Mantero F, Boscaro M, Mancini A, Ricciardo-Lamonica G, et al. Coenzyme Q(10) supplementation in infertile men with idiopathic asthenozoospermia: an open, uncontrolled pilot study. Fertil Steril. 2004;81:93–8.
18. Reza Safarinejad M. The effect of coenzyme Q10 supplementation on partner pregnancy rate in infertile men with idiopathic oligo astheno teratozoospermia: an open-label prospective study. Int Urol Nephrol. 2012; 44:689–700.
19. Mancini A, Festa R, Raimondo S, Pontecorvi A, Littarru GP. Hormonal influence on coenzyme Q10 levels in blood plasma. Int J Mol Sci. 2011; 12:9216–25.
20. Miles MV, Horn PS, Tang PH, Morrison JA, Miles L, DeGrauw T, Pesce AJ. Age-related changes in plasma coenzyme Q10 concentrations and redox state in apparently healthy children and adults. Clin Chim Acta. 2004;347:139–44.
21. Ben-Meir A, Burstein E, Borrego-Alvarez A, Chong J, Wong E, Yavorska T, et al. Coenzyme Q10 restores oocyte mitochondrial function and fertility during reproductive aging. Aging Cell. 2015;14:887–95.
22. Ozcan P, Ficicioglu C, Kizilkale O, Yesiladali M, Tok OE, Ozkan F, et al. Can coenzyme Q10 supplementation protect the ovarian reserve against oxidative damage? J Assist Reprod Genet. 2016;33:1223–30.
23. Marriage BJ, Clandinin MT, Macdonald IM, Glerum DM. Cofactor treatment improves ATP synthetic capacity in women with oxidative phosphorylation disorders. Mol Genet Metab. 2004;81:263–72.
24. El Refaeey A, Selem A, Badawy A. Combined coenzyme Q10 and clomiphene citrate for ovulation induction in clomiphene-citrate-resistant polycystic ovary syndrome. Reprod BioMed Online. 2014;29:119–24.
25. Bentov Y, Hannam T, Jurisicova A, Esfandiari N, Casper RF. Coenzyme Q10 supplementation and oocyte aneuploidy in women undergoing IVF-ICSI treatment. Clin Med Insights Reprod Health. 2014;8:31–6.
26. Alpha Scientists in Reproductive Medicine and ESHRE Special Interest Group of Embryology. The Istanbul consensus workshop on embryo assessment: proceedings of an expert meeting. Hum Reprod. 2011;26(6):1270–83. https://doi.org/10.1093/humrep/der037.
27. Gat I, Blanco Mejia S, Balakier H, Librach CL, Claessens A, Ryan EA. The use of coenzyme Q10 and DHEA during IUI and IVF cycles in patients with decreased ovarian reserve. Gynecol Endocrinol. 2016; https://doi.org/10.3109/09513590.2015.1137095.
28. Torner H, Brüssow KP, Alm H, Ratky J, Pöhland R, Tuchscherer A, Kanitz W. Mitochondrial aggregation patterns and activity in porcine oocytes and apoptosis in surrounding cumulus cells depends on the stage of pre-ovulatory maturation. Theriogenology. 2004;61:1675–89.
29. Fragouli E, Wells D. Mitochondrial DNA assessment to determine oocyte and embryo viability. Semin Reprod Med. 2015;33:401–9.
30. Meldrum DR. Aging gonads, glands, and gametes: immutable or partially reversible changes? Fertil Steril. 2013;99(1):1–4.
31. Bentov Y, Yavorska T, Esfandiari N, Jurisicova A, Casper RF. The contribution of mitochondrial function to reproductive aging. J Assist Reprod Genet. 2011;28:773–83.
32. Crane FL. The evolution of coenzyme Q. Biofactors. 2008;32:5–11.
33. Burstein E, Perumalsamy A, Bentov Y, Esfandiari N, Jurisicova A, Casper RF. Co-enzyme Q10 supplementation improves ovarian response and mitochondrial function in aged mice. Fertil Steril. 2009;92:S31.
34. Turi A, Giannubilo SR, Brugè F, Principi F, Battistoni S, Santoni F, et al. Coenzyme Q10 content in follicular fluid and its relationship with oocyte fertilization and embryo grading. Arch Gynecol Obstet. 2012;285:1173–6.
35. Akarsu S, Gode F, IsikA Z, Günnur Dikmen Z, Agah Tekindal M. The association between coenzyme Q10 concentrations in follicular fluid with

embryo morphokinetics and pregnancy rate in assisted reproductive techniques. J Assist Reprod Genet. 2017;34:599–605.

36. Gougeon A. Regulation of ovarian follicular development in primates: facts and hypotheses. Endocr Rev. 1996;17:121–55.

37. Visser JA, Schipper I, Laven JSE, Themmen APN. Anti-Müllerian hormone: an ovarian reserve marker in primary ovarian insufficiency. Nat Rev Endocrinol. 2012;8:331–41.

38. Ikematsu H, Nakamura K, Harashima S, Fujii K, Fukutomi N. Safety assessment of coenzyme Q10 (Kaneka Q10) in healthy subjects: a double-blind, randomized, placebo-controlled trial. Regul Toxicol Pharmacol. 2006; 44:212–8.

39. Pfeffer G, Majamaa K, Turnbull DM, Thorburn D, Chinnery PF. Treatment for mitochondrial disorders. Cochrane Database Syst Rev. 2012;4(4):CD004426.

7

Spermatogenesis improved by suppressing the high level of endogenous gonadotropins in idiopathic non-obstructive azoospermia: a case control pilot study

Xuechun Hu[1†], Zheng Ding[2†], Zhiwei Hong[1,3†], Zhichuan Zou[1], Yuming Feng[1], Ruilou Zhu[4], Jinzhao Ma[1], Xie Ge[1], Chaojun Li[4*] and Bing Yao[1*]

Abstract

Background: Elevated plasma gonadotropins were associated with desensitization of Sertoli and Leydig cells in the male testis. Testis spermatogenesis ability would be improved via inhibiting high endogenous gonadotropin in patients with severe oligozoospermia. Whether it would be beneficial for non-obstructive azoospermia (NOA) patients was still unclear.

Methods: Goserelin, a gonadotropin releasing hormone agonist (GnRHα) was used to suppress endogenous gonadotropin levels (gonadotropin reset) in the NOA patients, improving the sensitization of the Sertoli and Leydig cells. Then human menopausal gonadotropin (hMG) and human chorionic gonadotropin (hCG) were injected to stimulate them to ameliorate the ability of testicular spermatogenesis. The main outcome measure was the existence of spermatozoa in the semen or by testicular sperm extraction (TESE). Elevation of inhibin B and/or ameliorative expression pattern of ZO-1 was the secondary objective.

Results: A total of 35 NOA men who failed to retrieve sperm via TESE were enrolled. Among these, 10 patients without treatment were selected as control group and secondary TESE was performed 6 months later. Of the 25 treated men, inhibin B was elevated in 11 patients in the first 4 weeks (Response group), while only 5 patients had constant increase in the following 20 weeks (Response group 2). Of the 5 men, 2 men acquired sperm (Response group 2B), while 3 failed (Response group 2A). Immunofluorescence of mouse vasa homologue (MVH) and ZO-1 showed that both positive MVH signals and ZO-1 expression were significantly increased in the Response group 2, but only Response group 2B showed ameliorative ZO-1 distribution.

Conclusions: Gonadotropin reset, a new therapeutic protocol with GnRHα, was able to improve the ability of testicular spermatogenesis in the NOA patients through restoring the sensitivity of Sertoli and Leydig cells, which were reflected by elevated inhibin B and ameliorative ZO-1 expression and distribution.

Keywords: Gonadotropin reset, NOA, GnRHα

* Correspondence: licj@nju.edu.cn; 2424572228@qq.com
†Xuechun Hu, Zheng Ding and Zhiwei Hong contributed equally to this work.
4MOE Key Laboratory of Model Animals for Disease Study, Model Animal Research Center and the Medical School of Nanjing University, National Resource Center for Mutant Mice, Nanjing 210061, China
1Center of Reproductive Medicine, Nanjing Jinling Hospital, the Medical School of Nanjing University, Nanjing 210002, China
Full list of author information is available at the end of the article

Background

Non-obstructive azoospermia (NOA) affects approximately 1% of the general population and 10–20% of infertile men worldwide [1, 2]. A series of factors were associated with NOA, for example, hypogonadotropic hypogonadism (HH), Y microdeletion, chromosomal abnormalities etc. [3]. The causes and the underlying mechanism of idiopathic NOA still remain unclear. Testicular sperm extraction (TESE) or microdissection testicular sperm extraction (micro-TESE) combined with intracytoplasmic sperm injection (ICSI) was the approach recommended for idiopathic NOA [4]. However, the total rate of sperm retrieval was only about 50% [5]. Thus, efficient medical treatment strategies are required.

Hormone replacement therapy would improve the ability of the testis to produce spermatozoa in idiopathic NOA patients [6, 7]. For example, the improvement of spermatogonial DNA synthesis was demonstrated by Shinjo and coworkers [8], the elevation of intra-testicular testosterone levels was demonstrated by Kato and coworkers and the hypertrophic change of leydig cells was demonstrated by Oka and coworkers, respectively [9, 10]. Recently, a multi-institutional prospective study conducted by Shiraishi and coworkers provided a stronger evidence of the efficiency of hormone therapy [6]. However, the total rate of acquiring sperm was only about 10–20%. A possible explanation of the low success rate was that high plasma gonadotropins in the patients led to dysregulated function of FSH and LH receptors (FSHR, LHR) in Sertoli and leydig cells [7, 11, 12]. As demonstrated by in vivo and in vitro studies, desensitization and downregulation of FSH signaling in Sertoli cells was induced by the chronic stimulation of FSH [13–15]. Considering the risk of high plasma gonadotropins, a 'gonadotropin reset' with leuprolide acetate, a gonadotropin releasing hormone agonist (GnRHα), was proposed to induce a hypogonadotrophic state by Foresta and coworkers [11]. Thus, the FSHR and LHR in the testis would be 'released' and subsequent exogenous hormone stimulation would be beneficial for testis spermatogenesis, as great success has been achieved in the treatment of hypogonadotropic hypogonadism via hormone replacement therapy. Moreover, gonadotropin reset with GnRHα had been demonstrated to improve the function of Sertoli cells and subsequently enhance the sperm concentration in patients with severe oligozoospermia [11, 16]. However, to our knowledge, there is no data of gonadotropin reset with GnRHα in the NOA patients.

Inhibin B is secreted by Sertoli cells and is involved in the negative feedback of plasma FSH [17]. The expression of inhibin B was regulated by FSH and plasma inhibin B level was considered as a marker of Sertoli cell function [18]. Plasma inhibin B level was also closely related with spermatogenesis. Low levels of inhibin B was demonstrated in patients with bad semen quality which may be related with the dysfunction of Sertoli cells [11, 18]. Moreover, elevated inhibin B levels may indicate improved function of Sertoli cells, reflecting better spermatogenesis environment [11] .

Cell-cell junction in the seminiferous epithelium played an important role in spermatogenesis including self-renewability and differentiation of spermatogonial stem cells into mature spermatozoa [19]. Blood testis barrier (BTB) mainly includes tight junctions (TJ) that are present between adjacent Sertoli cells [19]. Redistribution of the TJs to the cytoplasmic compartment or decreased expression was associated with abnormal spermatogenesis [20, 21]. NOA patients were also accompanied with dysfunction of TJ proteins, such as occludin 11 etc. [21]. Zonula occludens-1 (ZO-1) is a membrane protein that distributed peripherally, and interacted together and anchored membrane proteins to the actin cytoskeleton [22]. However, the expression pattern of ZO-1 has never been reported in the NOA patients.

Hence, in the present study, we tried to suppress the high endogenous gonadotropin levels in the NOA patients with goserelin, another GnRHα to release and restore the receptors' function and then stimulate them using human menopausal gonadotropin (hMG) and human chorionic gonadotropin (hCG) to improve the ability of testicular spermatogenesis. Inhibin B, ZO-1 and mouse vasa homologue (MVH, a marker of germ cells) were detected to evaluate the response to the intervention.

Methods

Subjects

The study protocol was approved by the Research Ethics Committee of Nanjing Jinling Hospital and informed consent was obtained from all the participants. Semen samples from the patients with azoospermia were analyzed at least twice at an interval of 3 weeks according to the WHO Laboratory Manual for the Examination and Processing of Human Semen (5th edition) [23]. Totally, 175 patients aged between 18 and 45 with FSH plasma level > 5.5 IU/L were included. Patients with history of cryptorchidism (0), varicocele (15) or testicular trauma (0), medical treatment before (33), genital infections (8), Y Microdeletion (6), chromosomal abnormalities (7), both sides of the testes were less than 8 ml (37) and men who acquired sperm with TESE (8) were excluded (Fig. 1). Patients with Sertoli cell only syndrome (SCOS, 18) and maturation arrest (MA, 8) were also excluded. Finally, 35 patients diagnosed with hypospermatogenesis (HP) as shown by histological analysis in Fig. 2 were enrolled.

Study design

The overall experimental design was presented in Fig. 3. 3.6 mg goserelin (AstraZeneca, UK Limited) was given

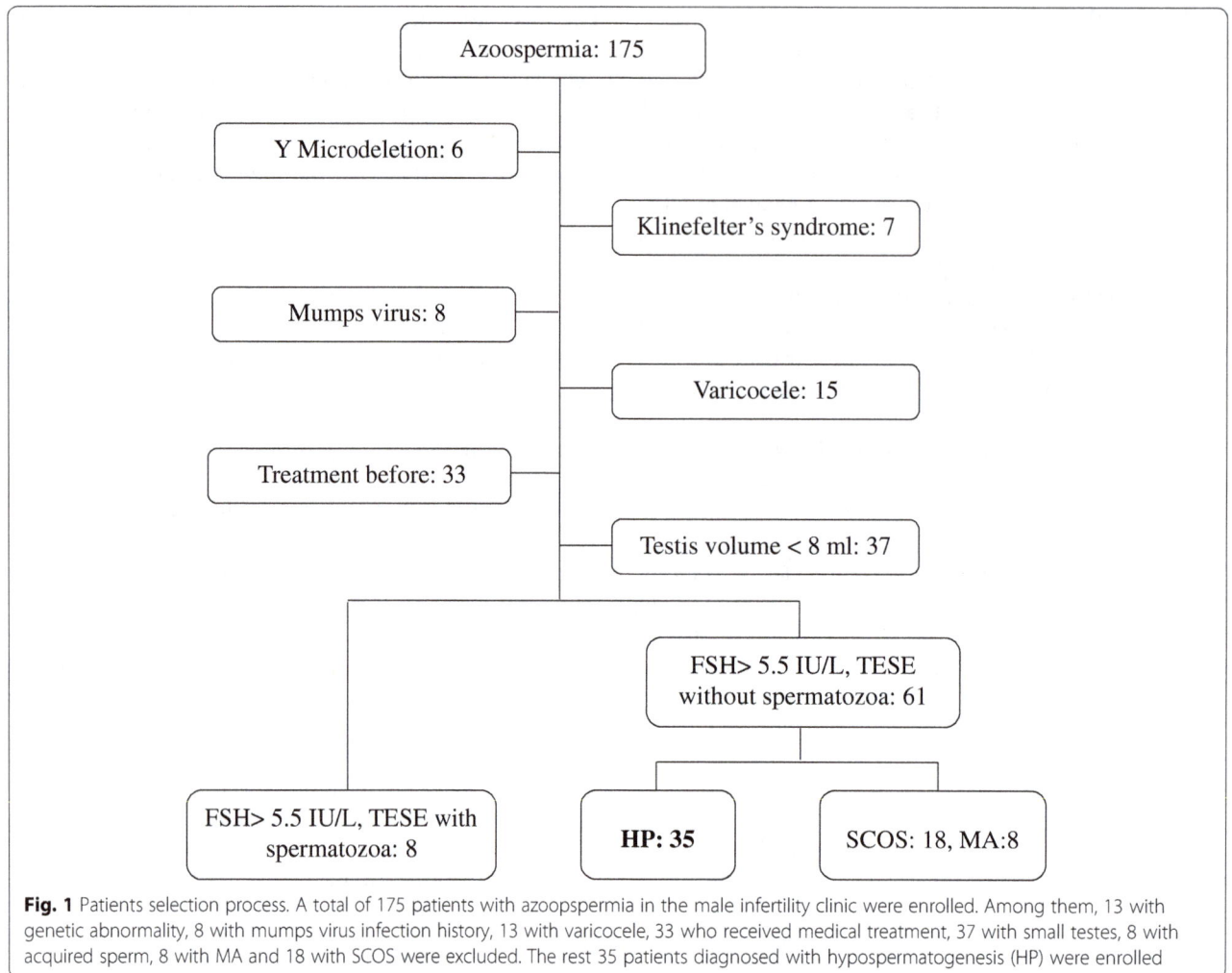

Fig. 1 Patients selection process. A total of 175 patients with azoopspermia in the male infertility clinic were enrolled. Among them, 13 with genetic abnormality, 8 with mumps virus infection history, 13 with varicocele, 33 who received medical treatment, 37 with small testes, 8 with acquired sperm, 8 with MA and 18 with SCOS were excluded. The rest 35 patients diagnosed with hypospermatogenesis (HP) were enrolled

to patients once every 4 weeks through subcutaneous injection for 24 weeks. hCG (Pregnyl, N.V. Organon Oss, Holland) was administered via intramuscular injection with a dose of 2000 IU, once a week for 20 weeks. hMG (Urofollitropin for Injection, Livzon Pharm Group Inc., China) was also administered through intramuscular injection at a dose of 150 IU, twice a week for 16 weeks. Ten patients who did not agree with the treatment were selected as the control group. All patients received the secondary TESE 24 weeks later.

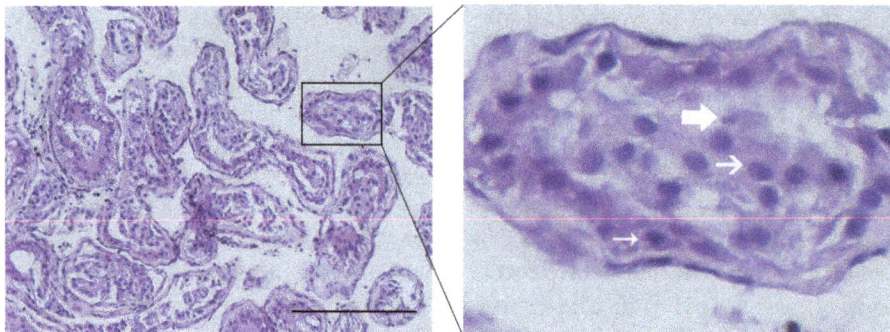

Fig. 2 Histological analysis. The typical hematoxylin and eosin (H&E) staining of the testis specimens of the enrolled patients showed hypospermatogenesis (HP). The narrow arrow indicated the spermatocyte, the broad arrow indicated the elongated spermatid, and the medium arrow indicated the round spermatid. Scale bar, 200 μm

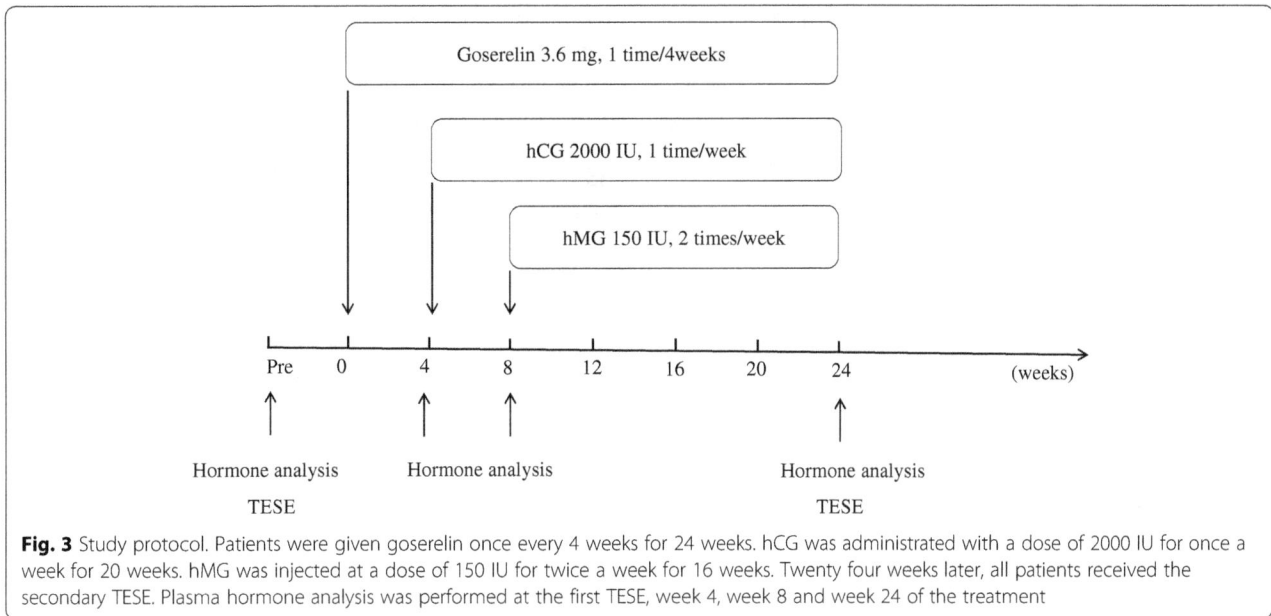

Fig. 3 Study protocol. Patients were given goserelin once every 4 weeks for 24 weeks. hCG was administrated with a dose of 2000 IU for once a week for 20 weeks. hMG was injected at a dose of 150 IU for twice a week for 16 weeks. Twenty four weeks later, all patients received the secondary TESE. Plasma hormone analysis was performed at the first TESE, week 4, week 8 and week 24 of the treatment

Clinical monitoring

All enrolled patients were informed of the possible side effects during the period of treatment. Informed consents were acquired from all the men. Semen parameters were analyzed by the computer aided semen analysis (CASA) system (WLJY-9000). Body mass index and testicular volume measurement were carried out. Testicular volume uses an ellipsoid approximation (volume = length * width * depth * 0.523) by ultrasound (nemio-XG580, Toshiba, Tokyo, Japan). Blood samples were obtained at 8–11 a.m. and centrifuged at 1800 g for 10 min. Plasma inhibin B was detected by electrochemical luminescence method (Roche, Mannheim, Germany). The levels of FSH, luteinizing hormone (LH), total testosterone, estrogen (E2) and prolactin (PRL) were determined by radio-immunoassay (Beckman Coulter, Brea, USA). The normal range of FSH is 1–5.5 U/L, 1–6.3 U/L for LH, 9.4–37 nmol/L for testosterone and 18.22–311.27 pg/mL for inhibin B. Apart from these, blood pressure, hematological parameters including blood corpuscle, biochemical and lipid parameters were detected to evaluate the safety of therapeutic protocol.

H& E and immunofluorescence staining

Testes specimens were collected by testicular fine needle aspiration cytology (FNAC) for histopathological and immunofluorescent analysis as described previously [24]. Briefly, the testes were fixed in 4% paraformaldehyde. Following routine pathological procedure, the section slides were prepared. Subsequently, the slides were stained with hematoxylene-eosin (H&E). The steps required for staining of the testicular sections with ZO-1 (ab96587, Abcam, USA) and MVH (ab13840, Abcam, USA) antibodies were the same as described previously [25]. Briefly, the sections were hydrated with gradient alcohol followed by dewaxing with xylene, blocked with 5% bovine serum albumin (BSA, Sigma) for 1 h at room temperature and finally incubated with ZO-1 and MVH antibodies at 4 °C overnight. The following day, the samples were washed with PBS for three times, and incubated with anti-rabbit IgG H&L secondary antibody for 1 h in the dark. Finally, the sections were visualized using a fluorescence microscope. Quantification of MVH-positive signals and mean fluorescence intensity of ZO-1 per tubule area were calculated referring to the study of bai and coworkers [26] and then the data in NOA groups were normalized by OA group, 30 tubules from each group were calculated.

Statistical analysis

All data were evaluated for normal distribution by the Kolmogorov–Smirnov test. The variables conformed to normal distribution was summarized as mean ± standard deviation, and those departed from normal distribution were summarized as medians and interquartile intervals. Differences between the groups at baseline and differences at different time points for each group were calculated by Student's t-test. $p < 0.05$ was considered as statistically significant.

Results
Characteristics of studied men

The baseline data of all the participants were presented in Table 1. The plasma FSH and LH levels were significantly higher than normal range while the inhibin B was lower than normal range. The plasma total testosterone level and body mass index (BMI) were in the normal

Table 1 Patients' characteristics of all the enrolled patients

Variables	Treatment	Control	P
Age	25.8 ± 3.4	26.6 ± 3.3	0.53
BMI (kg/m^2)	22.2 ± 1.9	22.5 ± 1.1	0.70
FSH (IU/L)	18.8 ± 7.2	20.8 ± 5.6	0.43
LH (IU/L)	9.1 ± 3.6	10.2 ± 3.3	0.52
Total testosterone (nmol/L)	13.2 ± 4.3	12.6 ± 4.0	0.46
Estradiol (pmol/L)	127.9 ± 69.6	122.9 ± 47.2	0.84
PRL (mIU/L)	220.9 ± 81.1	203.7 ± 61.9	0.55
Inhibin B (pg/mL)	13.6 ± 13.1	14.1 ± 14.1	0.95
Testicular volume (mL)	10.7 ± 1.8	11.2 ± 1.9	0.46

range. No parameters showed difference between the control group and the treatment group at the baseline.

Therapeutic response of the plasma hormones

The dynamic change of plasma hormones were shown in Fig. 4. The levels of plasma FSH, LH, and total testosterone were significantly suppressed by goserelin in the first 4 weeks (Fig. 4a-c). Later, hCG and hMG demonstrated little influence on the plasma FSH and LH levels, but total testosterone showed significant increase (Fig. 4c). Interestingly, 11 of the 25 treated patients showed elevated inhibin B levels with goserelin alone in the first 4 weeks and were considered as Response group (Fig. 4d), while the other 14 showed no change were seen as No response group. The baseline levels of plasma inhibin B were significantly higher in the Response group by further analysis (Fig. 4f). Among the 11 patients, 5 showed constant increase of inhibin B in the following 20 weeks (Response group 2, Fig. 4e), while the other 6 were hewed back to the baseline (Response group 1). Finally, 2 men in the Response group 2 acquired spermatozoa (Response group 2B), while the other 3 failed to acquire (Response group 2A). One man in the Response group 2B acquired sperm in the semen. Sperm concentration was 1.42 * 10^6/ml and the total sperm count was 3.98*10^6. No significant difference of PRL or E2 was observed during the whole process (data not shown). No sperm was found in the secondary TESE in the control group and no significant change of plasma inhibin B, FSH, LH or total testosterone was observed between two TESEs in the control group (Additional file 1: Figure S1).

Therapeutic response in the testes

H&E staining of the testis specimens were performed. No significant difference was found in the No response group (Fig. 5c) or Response group 1 (Fig. 5d) between the two TESEs. Germ cells in the Response group 2A were increased significantly but no mature spermatozoa were found (Fig. 5e). Excitingly, mature spermatozoa were observed in the Response group 2B (Fig. 5f). No

obvious morphological change was found in Sertoli cells. Furthermore, MVH and ZO-1, markers of germ cells and BTB, were stained in the testis specimens. As shown in Fig. 6b, positive MVH signals were rarely observed in the seminiferous tubules and the expression and distribution of ZO-1 was abnormal (punctuate and discrete) in the NOA patients compared with OA patients whose ZO-1 distribution was consecutive (Fig. 6a). During the secondary TESE, the expression of MVH and ZO-1 were slightly affected in both No response group (Fig. 6c) and Response group 1 (Fig. 6d). However, the positive MVH signals and expression of ZO-1 were significantly increased in the Response group 2A (Fig. 6e), but the distribution of ZO-1 was not changed. Interestingly, not only mature spermatozoa were observed but also the expression and distribution of ZO-1 were recovered in a degree in the Response group 2B (Fig. 6f). Moreover, the MVH-positive cells and mean fluorescence intensity of ZO-1 per tubule area were then quantified as shown in Fig. 6g and h.

Side effects

The treatment was well tolerated by all the enrolled patients and no cases offended with side effects. During GnRHα treatment alone in the first 4 weeks, 40% of the patients exhibited symptoms of androgenic deprivation such as mild loss of libido, erectile dysfunction, asthenia etc. hCG therapy in the follow-up treatment restored the concentration of testosterone and abolished these side effects. During the whole period, no significant difference of BMI, blood pressure or testicular volume was observed. Gynecomastia was not seen in any of the subjects. Hematological parameters including blood corpuscle, biochemical and lipid parameters remained stable during the whole treatment period (data not shown). No other side effects were discovered in the enrolled patients.

Discussion

As mentioned previously, TESE or micro-TESE combined with ICSI was the only recommended treatment for NOA patients till date [1, 2]. However, the patients who failed to acquire sperm in the TESE remained a problem in the whole world. A series of studies have been reported regarding the treatment strategies for NOA patients including empirical medical therapies like testolactone [27, 28], hormone replacement therapy etc. [8, 9]. However, the results were not ideal. In 2012, Shiraishi and coworkers tried to trigger 'gonadotropin reset' with high-dose hCG stimulation. As a result, the high gonadotropins in NOA patients were decreased and the ability of testicular spermatogenesis was improved [7]. This indicated that gonadotropin reset is an efficient approach in the NOA patients. However, the dose of hCG was too high in clinical practice. Therefore, we enrolled

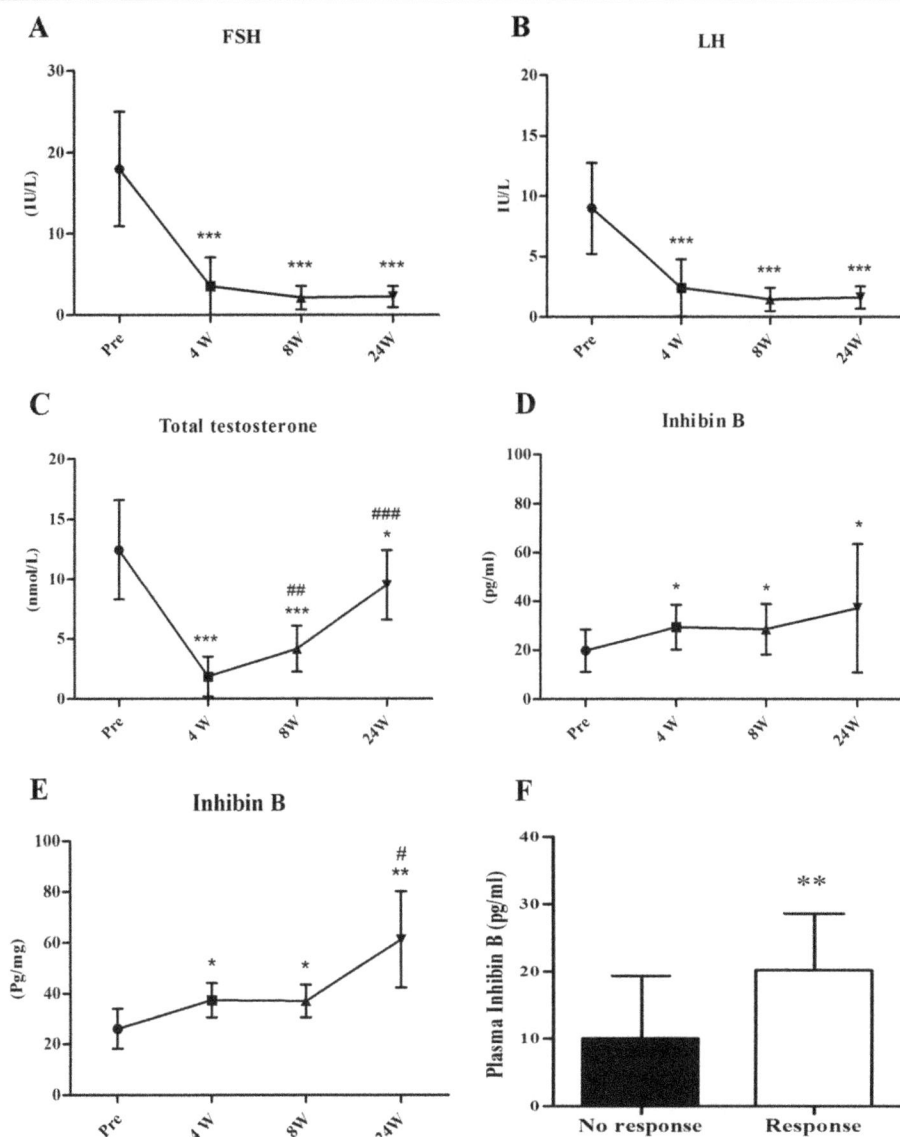

Fig. 4 Dynamic changes in plasma hormone levels. **a-c** The dynamic changes of FSH, LH, T levels through the whole treatment period were shown. **d** The dynamic change of inhibin B in the Response group (Response group 1 + 2). **e** The dynamic change of inhibin B in the Response group 2. **f** The level of inhibin B at baseline in the No response group and the Response group (Response group 1 + 2). Results were shown as mean ± SD. **a-d** *$P < 0.05$ compared with the value before the treatment (Pre); **$P < 0.01$ compared to the value before the treatment; ***$P < 0.001$ compared with the value before the treatment; ##$P < 0.01$ compared with value at week 4. ###$P < 0.001$ compared with value at week 4; **e** *$P < 0.05$ compared with the value before the treatment, **$P < 0.01$ compared to the value before the treatment, #$P < 0.015$ compared with value at week 8; **f** *$P < 0.05$ compared with No response group

patients with NOA and explored another way to fulfill gonadotropin reset with GnRHα in the present study.

As we all know, spermatogenesis is regulated via a complex array of paracrine, endocrine and juxtacrine regulatory cross-talk involving Leydig, Sertoli, peritubular, germ cells etc. [29]. FSH and testosterone were believed to play vital roles in spermatogenesis by stimulating Sertoli cells [30]. However, the precise mechanism still remain unclear. Studies in animals demonstrated that FSH was involved in the proliferation of early stage germ cells, and testosterone is one of the most important factors for initiating and

maintaining spermatogenesis [31, 32]. As we all know, plasma FSH levels were often elevated in patients with NOA [7]. Significantly elevated FSH levels had been demonstrated to decrease FSH-FSHR signaling pathway in the testes of NOA patients. The possible explanation may be: (i) the uncoupling reaction of the FSHR from the effector system led to the constant phosphorylation of the C-terminal, intracellular domain of FSHR [33, 34]; (ii) decreased number of FSHRs was mediated by extensive clustering and internalization of the FSH–FSHR complex and by reduced expression of the receptor as a result

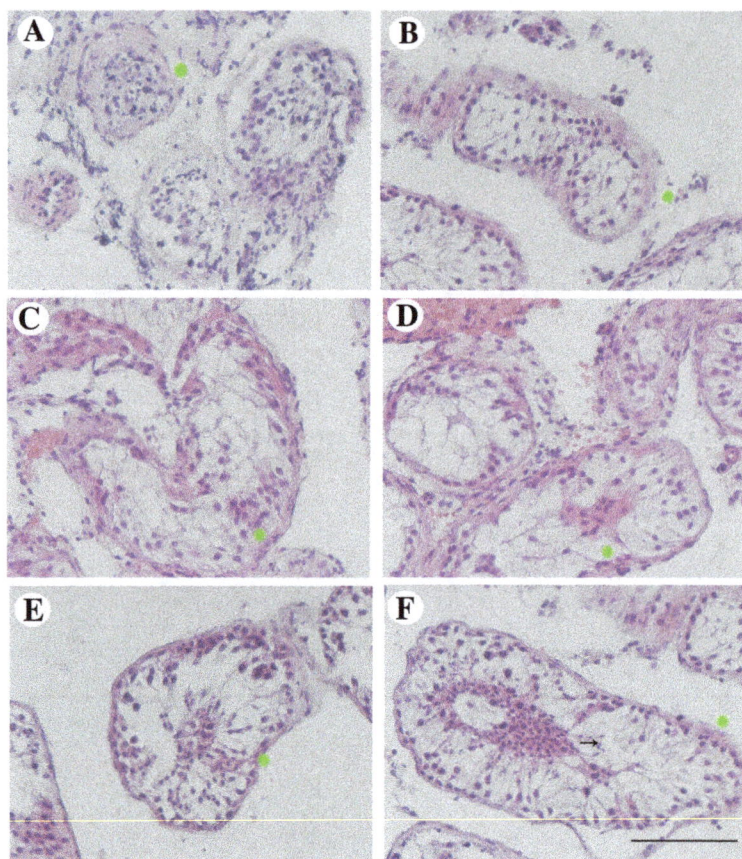

Fig. 5 H&E staining of the testes before and after treatment. **a** The typical image of the testes specimens from OA patients. **b** The typical image in the first TESE. **c-f** The typical image of No response group, Response group 1, Response group 2A, Response 2B during the secondary TESE. Scale bar, 100 μm. Green color represented the Sertoli cells. The arrow indicated the mature sperm

of both decreased transcription levels and reduced half-life of mRNA [15, 35]. In view of the effects of high endogenous FSH, Foresta and coworkers have demonstrated that, leuprolide acetate treatment decreased the high endogenous gonadotropin levels, thus activating the FSH receptors. Followed by stimulation with exogenous FSH, the semen quality of the patients were significantly improved [11]. Based on these results, we tried to regulate endogenous gonadotropin levels with goserelin in the NOA patients in the present study. As a result, inhibin B was significantly lower than normal range in the NOA patients (Table 1), indicating injuried function of Sertoli cells. Interestingly, inhibin B levels were elevated in 11 of the 25 patients, indicating Sertoli cell function was improved after inhibition of endogenous gonadotropins in the first 4 weeks. The other 14 showed no response. This may be due to the excessive damage of Sertoli cells in the testis as the basic plasma inhibin B levels were significantly lower than the Response group ($p = 0.009$, Fig. 4f) which is consistent with the result of Foresta and coworkers who had demonstrated that the function of Sertoli cells was severely injuried and remained

irresponsive to hormone treatment while the basic plasma inhibin B was low [11]. During the following 20 weeks, only 5 patients of the Response group (Response group 2) showed a constant increase of inhibin B, while the other 6 (Response group 1) did not. There was no difference observed in the basic plasma inhibin B levels between Response group 1 and 2, but an increased tendency was shown in Response group 2 (*P = 0.06*). This might possibly be due to that the function of Sertoli cells were incomplete in the Response group 1, i.e., the cells were not enough to initiate and maintain spermatogenesis as there was no significant change of the MVH signals after treatment (Fig. 5d and 6d). The inhibin B levels would be higher in presence of germ cells as they are also considered to be the source and involved in the secretion of inhibin B [36, 37]. Correspondingly, significant increase of positive signals of MVH in Response group 2 indicated the proliferation and meiosis of the germ cells after the treatment (Fig. 6e-h), therefore, the inhibin B levels were elevated. All of these indicated that plasma inhibin B level may act as a good marker to predict spermatogenesis in the testis and to evaluate the response of the therapies in the NOA patients.

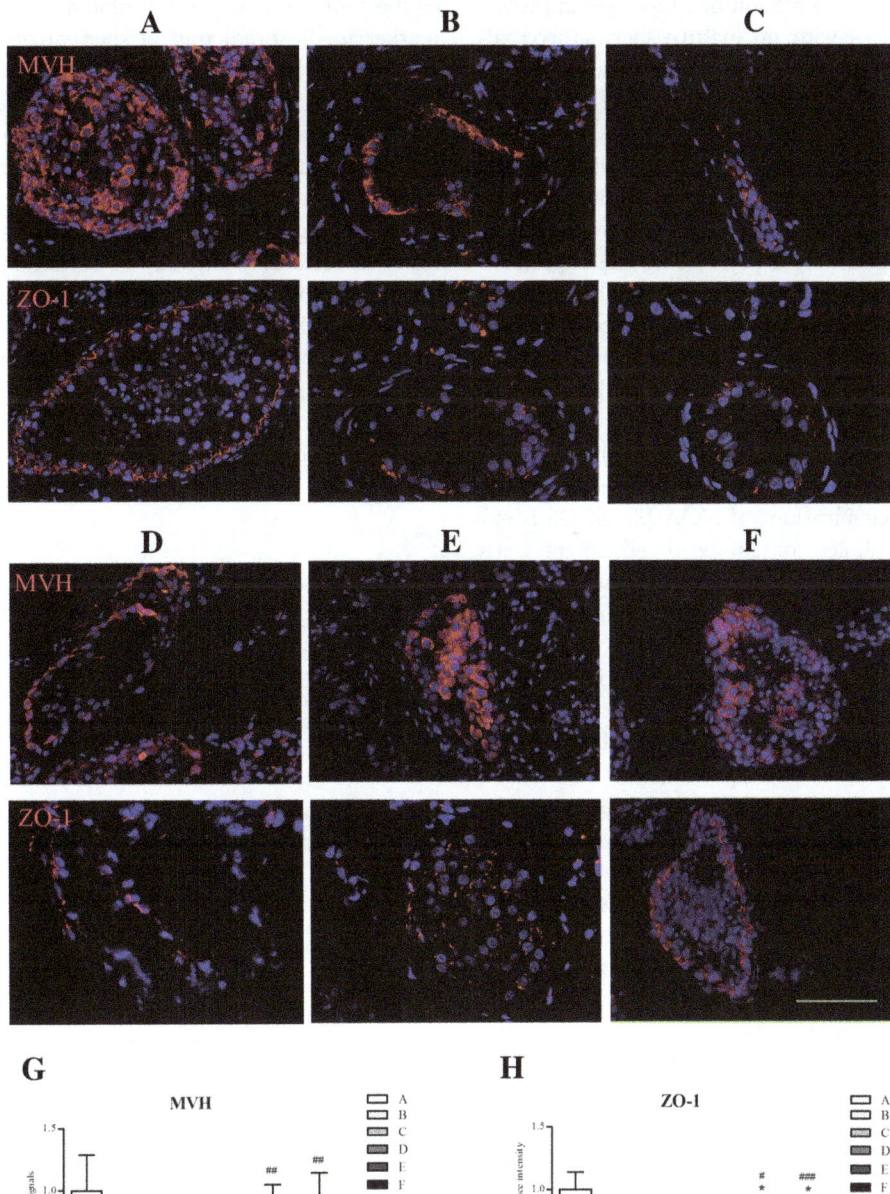

Fig. 6 Immunofluorescence staining MVH and ZO-1 in the testis specimens. **a** The OA specimen were selected as positive control. **b** The typical images in the first TESE. **c-f** The typical images of patients in No response group, Response group 1, Response group 2A, Response group 2B during the secondary TESE. Scale bar, 100 μm. **g** Quantification of MVH-positive cells per tubule area in each group was then counted, 30 tubules from each group were calculated. **h** Relative mean fluorescence intensity of ZO-1 was calculated as total fluorescence intensity per tubule area, 30 tubules from each group were calculated. Results were shown as mean + SD. $*P < 0.05$, $**P < 0.01$, $***P < 0.001$ compared with OA group; $^{\#}P < 0.05$, $^{\#\#}P < 0.01$, $^{\#\#\#}P < 0.001$ compared with NOA patients during the first TESE.

As mentioned previously, BTB played an important role in the spermatogenesis [19]. Aberrant expressions of TJs were associated with abnormal spermatogenesis [38]. ZO-1, occludin, and claudin are the TJ proteins identified in the testis [39]. In the present study, the distribution of ZO-1 was punctuate and discrete in NOA patients as shown in Fig. 6b compared with patients of OA whose ZO-1 distribution were normal and consecutive. The expression and distribution of ZO-1 were improved in Response group 2B with mature spermatozoa were observed in the testis while only expression of ZO-1 was improved in Response group 2A with no mature spermatozoa, although the number of germ cells was increased significantly (Fig. 6e, f). This indicated that well-distributed ZO-1 played an important role in the sperm maturation changes, which was consistent with other studies [39, 40]. Under the physiological conditions, the main factor affecting the TJ formation is the endogenous testosterone [29]. Besides, FSH may also play a key role in the expression and localization of TJ proteins [29]. The ameliorative expression and distribution of ZO-1 in the Response group 2B also indicated the effectiveness of the protocol in restoring the function of FSHRs and LHRs and the elevation of intra-testicular testosterone levels by subsequent hCG treatment that has been demonstrated by others [9, 10].

As known previously, HP, MA and SCOS were the three main histological classifications of NOA [3]. SCOS is excluded here as no tubules contain germ cells in the testis specimens of the patients [41], hence the possibility of acquiring sperm was very low [6]. Spermatogenesis of MA was often arrested at the spermatogonial or primary spermatocyte stage. It was mainly related to the presence of a genetic lesion or toxicant exposure [41]. The process of spermatogenesis in HP was almost intact, but reduced to a certain extent. Hence, we supposed that it was related with terrible testis microenvironment and improve the microenvironment via hormone may be beneficial for spermatogenesis [7]. HP were also believed to be the ideal objects for medical treatment in the previous studies [6, 7]. Moreover, the cost of the treatment was high. Therefore, the clinical trial was performed in patients who are more likely to succeed. Besides, there is a deficiency in the present study. The effectiveness of the protocol in the study was lack of strict "control group" who should be given only hCG combined with hMG in the process, that is to say, the role of goserelin in the study was lack of evidence. However, the elevation of inhibin B in the first 4 weeks during which goserelin was given alone indicated the positive effect of it. Moreover, Foresta and coworkers had demonstrated that FSH alone would not enhance plasma inhibin B in patients with high endogenous gonadotropins as the Sertoli cells were irresponsive [11]. Therefore, the reactivity to FSH was restored via the use of goserelin in the present study as reflected by constant increased inhibin B following hMG treatment was another proof for the role of goserelin, which is also consistent with the result of Foresta and coworkers [11].

Conclusions

This was a preliminary prospective study, and we initially explored the therapeutic protocol in patients with NOA. Although only 2 of the 25 treated patients succeeded to acquire sperm, the plasma inhibin B levels were significantly elevated in 5 patients (25%). This indicated the effectiveness

of the protocol and plasma inhibin B may be a good biomarker in the prediction of spermatogenesis. Destruction of BTB may be related with the arrest of spermatogenesis in the NOA patients, while ameliorative BTB would be beneficial for spermatogenesis, indicating that BTB might be a therapeutic target in the NOA patients. In a word, 'gonadotropin reset' was able to improve the ability of testicular spermatogenesis in the NOA patients which may be a result of restored sensitivity of Sertoli and Leydig cells to gonadotropins. More rigorous randomized controlled trial studies should be carried out to explore the effect of the therapeutic protocol in NOA patients. The limited success rate of the present study indicated us that the etiology or mechanism of NOA should be further studied and more efficient therapeutic protocols should be explored.

Abbreviations

BTB: Blood tesis barrier; FNAC: Fine needle aspiration cytology; GnRHα: Gonadotropin releasing hormone agonist; hCG: Human chorionic gonadotropin; hMG: Human menopausal gonadotropin; HP: Hypospermatogenesis; ICSI: Intracytoplasmic sperm injection; MA: Maturation arrest; NOA: Non-obstructive azoospermia; SCOS: Sertoli cell only syndrome; TESE: Testicular sperm extraction; ZO-1: Zonula occludens-1

Acknowledgements

The authors would like to sincerely thank Yifeng Ge, Yong Shao, Rong Zeng and Cencen Wang for their excellent technical supports and other helps during the experiments.

Funding

This work was supported by the Research Funds for Jiangsu province key research and development plan (BE2016750), the Research Funds for Military family planning (16JS012), the Jiangsu Province Natural Science Foundation (BK20170620) and China Postdoctoral Science Foundation (2017M613434).

Authors' contributions

All authors had made important roles in the design and viewing of the study. XH wrote the manuscript, took part in the enrollment of the patients, performing the experiments and elucidation of the data. ZD and ZH participated in the design of the study and assisted to modify the manuscript. ZZ and YF assisted to enroll patients. RZ, JM, XG assisted to perform the experiments and elucidate the data. BY and CL designed the protocol and provided support in the whole process. All the authors have read, and agreed with the final manuscript.

Competing interests

The authors declare that they have no competing interests.

Author details

[1]Center of Reproductive Medicine, Nanjing Jinling Hospital, the Medical School of Nanjing University, Nanjing 210002, China. [2]Nanjing Jiangning Hospital, the Affiliated Jiangning Hospital of Nanjing Medical University,

Nanjing 210000, China. ³Department of Urology, Fujian Provincial Hospital, Fuzhou 350000, China. ⁴MOE Key Laboratory of Model Animals for Disease Study, Model Animal Research Center and the Medical School of Nanjing University, National Resource Center for Mutant Mice, Nanjing 210061, China.

References

1. Aziz N. The importance of semen analysis in the context of azoospermia. Clinics (Sao Paulo). 2013;68(Suppl 1):35–8.

2. Esteves SC, Miyaoka R, Agarwal A. An update on the clinical assessment of the infertile male. [corrected]. Clinics (Sao Paulo). 2011;66:691–700.

3. Esteves SC. Clinical management of infertile men with nonobstructive azoospermia. Asian J Androl. 2015;17:459–70.

4. Belva F, De Schrijver F, Tournaye H, Liebaers I, Devroey P, Haentjens P, Bonduelle M. Neonatal outcome of 724 children born after ICSI using non-ejaculated sperm. Hum Reprod. 2011;26:1752–8.

5. Tsujimura A, Matsumiya K, Miyagawa Y, Tohda A, Miura H, Nishimura K, Koga M, Takeyama M, Fujioka H, Okuyama A. Conventional multiple or microdissection testicular sperm extraction: a comparative study. Hum Reprod. 2002;17:2924–9.

6. Shiraishi K, Ishikawa T, Watanabe N, Iwamoto T, Matsuyama H. Salvage hormonal therapy after failed microdissection testicular sperm extraction: a multi-institutional prospective study. Int J Urol. 2016;23:496–500.

7. Shiraishi K, Ohmi C, Shimabukuro T, Matsuyama H. Human chorionic gonadotrophin treatment prior to microdissection testicular sperm extraction in non-obstructive azoospermia. Hum Reprod. 2012;27:331–9.

8. Shinjo E, Shiraishi K, Matsuyama H. The effect of human chorionic gonadotropin-based hormonal therapy on intratesticular testosterone levels and spermatogonial DNA synthesis in men with non-obstructive azoospermia. Andrology. 2013;1:929–35.

9. Kato Y, Shiraishi K, Matsuyama H. Expression of testicular androgen receptor in non-obstructive azoospermia and its change after hormonal therapy. Andrology. 2014;2:734–40.

10. Oka S, Shiraishi K, Matsuyama H. Effects of human chorionic gonadotropin on testicular interstitial tissues in men with non-obstructive azoospermia. Andrology. 2017;5:232–9.

11. Foresta C, Bettella A, Spolaore D, Merico M, Rossato M, Ferlin A. Suppression of the high endogenous levels of plasma FSH in infertile men are associated with improved Sertoli cell function as reflected by elevated levels of plasma inhibin B. Hum Reprod. 2004;19:1431–7.

12. Heidargholizadeh S, Aydos SE, Yukselten Y, Ozkavukcu S, Sunguroglu A, Aydos K. A differential cytokine expression profile before and after rFSH treatment in Sertoli cell cultures of men with nonobstructive azoospermia. Andrologia. 2017;49:e12647.

13. Gnanaprakasam MS, Chen CJ, Sutherland JG, Bhalla VK. Receptor depletion and replenishment processes: in vivo regulation of gonadotropin receptors by luteinizing hormone, follicle stimulating hormone and ethanol in rat testis. Biol Reprod. 1979;20:991–1000.

14. O'Shaughnessy PJ, Brown PS. Reduction in FSH receptors in the rat testis by injection of homologous hormone. Mol Cell Endocrinol. 1978;12:9–15.

15. Themmen AP, Blok LJ, Post M, Baarends WM, Hoogerbrugge JW, Parmentier M, Vassart G, Grootegoed JA. Follitropin receptor down-regulation involves a cAMP-dependent post-transcriptional decrease of receptor mRNA expression. Mol Cell Endocrinol. 1991;78:R7–13.

16. Foresta C, Selice R, Moretti A, Pati MA, Carraro M, Engl B, Garolla A. Gonadotropin administration after gonadotropin-releasing-hormone agonist: a therapeutic option in severe testiculopathies. Fertil Steril. 2009;92:1326–32.

17. Hayes FJ, Pitteloud N, DeCruz S, Crowley WF Jr, Boepple PA. Importance of inhibin B in the regulation of FSH secretion in the human male. J Clin Endocrinol Metab. 2001;86:5541–6.

18. Iliadou PK, Tsametis C, Kaprara A, Papadimas I, Goulis DG. The Sertoli cell: Novel clinical potentiality. Hormones (Athens). 2015;14:504–14.

19. Weinbauer GF, Wessels J. 'Paracrine' control of spermatogenesis. Andrologia. 1999;31:249–62.

20. Fink C, Weigel R, Fink L, Wilhelm J, Kliesch S, Zeiler M, Bergmann M, Brehm R. Claudin-11 is over-expressed and dislocated from the blood-testis barrier in Sertoli cells associated with testicular intraepithelial neoplasia in men. Histochem Cell Biol. 2009;131:755–64.

21. Haverfield JT, Meachem SJ, O'Bryan MK, McLachlan RI, Stanton PG. Claudin-11 and connexin-43 display altered spatial patterns of organization in men with primary seminiferous tubule failure compared with controls. Fertil Steril. 2013;100:658–66.

22. Pummi K, Malminen M, Aho H, Karvonen SL, Peltonen J, Peltonen S. Epidermal tight junctions: ZO-1 and occludin are expressed in mature, developing, and affected skin and in vitro differentiating keratinocytes. J Invest Dermatol. 2001;117:1050–8.

23. World Health Organization. Laboratory manual for the examination and processing of human semen. 5th ed. Geneva: World Health Organization; 2010. p. 10–56.

24. Foresta C, Varotto A, Scandellari C. Assessment of testicular cytology by fine needle aspiration as a diagnostic parameter in the evaluation of the azoospermic subject. Fertil Steril. 1992;57:858–65.

25. Hu X, Ge X, Liang W, Shao Y, Jing J, Wang C, Zeng R, Yao B. Effects of saturated palmitic acid and omega-3 polyunsaturated fatty acids on Sertoli cell apoptosis. Syst Biol Reprod Med. 2018;64:1–13.

26. Bai S, Cheng L, Zhang Y, Zhu C, Zhu Z, Zhu R, Cheng CY, Ye L, Zheng K. A germline-specific role for the mTORC2 component Rictor in maintaining Spermatogonial differentiation and intercellular adhesion in mouse testis. Mol Hum Reprod. 2018;24:244–59.

27. Pavlovich CP, King P, Goldstein M, Schlegel PN. Evidence of a treatable endocrinopathy in infertile men. J Urol. 2001;165:837–41.

28. Reifsnyder JE, Ramasamy R, Husseini J, Schlegel PN. Role of optimizing testosterone before microdissection testicular sperm extraction in men with nonobstructive azoospermia. J Urol. 2012;188:532–6.

29. Shiraishi K, Matsuyama H. Gonadotropin actions on spermatogenesis and hormonal therapies for spermatogenic disorders [review]. Endocr J. 2017;64:123–31.

30. Regueira M, Artagaveytia SL, Galardo MN, Pellizzari EH, Cigorraga SB, Meroni SB, Riera MF. Novel molecular mechanisms involved in hormonal regulation of lactate production in Sertoli cells. Reproduction. 2015;150:311–21.

31. de Kretser DM, Loveland KL, Meinhardt A, Simorangkir D, Wreford N. Spermatogenesis. Hum Reprod. 1998;13(Suppl 1):1–8.

32. Pakarainen T, Zhang FP, Makela S, Poutanen M, Huhtaniemi I. Testosterone replacement therapy induces spermatogenesis and partially restores fertility in luteinizing hormone receptor knockout mice. Endocrinology. 2005;146:596–606.

33. Conti M, Toscano MV, Petrelli L, Geremia R, Stefanini M. Involvement of phosphodiesterase in the refractoriness of the Sertoli cell. Endocrinology. 1983;113:1845–53.

34. Sanchez-Yague J, Hipkin RW, Ascoli M. Biochemical properties of the agonist-induced desensitization of the follicle-stimulating hormone and luteinizing hormone/chorionic gonadotropin-responsive adenylyl cyclase in cells expressing the recombinant gonadotropin receptors. Endocrinology. 1993;132:1007–16.

35. Fletcher PW, Reichert LE Jr. Cellular processing of follicle-stimulating hormone by Sertoli cells in serum-free culture. Mol Cell Endocrinol. 1984;34:39–49.

36. Allenby G, Foster PM, Sharpe RM. Evidence that secretion of immunoactive inhibin by seminiferous tubules from the adult rat testis is regulated by specific germ cell types: correlation between in vivo and in vitro studies. Endocrinology. 1991;128:467–76.

37. Levi M, Hasky N, Stemmer SM, Shalgi R, Ben-Aharon I. Anti-Mullerian hormone is a marker for chemotherapy-induced testicular toxicity. Endocrinology. 2015;156:3818–27.

38. Liu Z, Mao J, Wu X, Xu H, Wang X, Huang B, Zheng J, Nie M, Zhang H. Efficacy and outcome predictors of gonadotropin treatment for male congenital hypogonadotropic hypogonadism: a retrospective study of 223 patients. Medicine (Baltimore). 2016;95:e2867.

39. Furuse M, Fujita K, Hiiragi T, Fujimoto K, Tsukita S. Claudin-1 and -2: novel integral membrane proteins localizing at tight junctions with no sequence similarity to occludin. J Cell Biol. 1998;141:1539–50.

40. Byers S, Graham R, Dai HN, Hoxter B. Development of Sertoli cell junctional specializations and the distribution of the tight-junction-associated protein ZO-1 in the mouse testis. Am J Anat. 1991;191:35–47.

41. McLachlan RI, Rajpert-De Meyts E, Hoei-Hansen CE, de Kretser DM, Skakkebaek NE. Histological evaluation of the human testis–approaches to optimizing the clinical value of the assessment: mini review. Hum Reprod. 2007;22:2–16.

8

FMR1 expression in human granulosa cells increases with exon 1 CGG repeat length depending on ovarian reserve

Julia Rehnitz[1,3]*, Diego D. Alcoba[1,2], Ilma S. Brum[2], Jens E. Dietrich[3], Berthe Youness[1], Katrin Hinderhofer[4], Birgitta Messmer[1], Alexander Freis[3], Thomas Strowitzki[3] and Ariane Germeyer[3]

Abstract

Background: *Fragile-X-Mental-Retardation-1- (FMR1)-gene* is supposed to be a key gene for ovarian reserve and folliculogenesis. It contains in its 5′-UTR a triplet-base-repeat (CGG), that varies between 26 and 34 in general population. CGG-repeat-lengths with 55–200 repeats (pre-mutation = PM) show instable heredity with a tendency to increase and are associated with premature-ovarian-insufficiency or failure (POI/POF) in about 20%. *FMR1*-mRNA-expression in leucocytes and granulosa cells (GCs) increases with CGG-repeat-length in PM-carriers, but variable *FMR1*-expression profiles were also described in women with POI without PM-*FMR1* repeat-length. Additionally, associations between low numbers of retrieved oocytes and elevated *FMR1*-expression levels have been shown in GCs of females with mid-range PM-CGG-repeats without POI. Effects of *FMR1*-repeat-lengths-deviations ($n < 26$ or $n > 34$) below the PM range ($n < 55$) on ovarian reserve and response to ovarian stimulation remain controversial.

Methods: We enrolled 229 women undergoing controlled ovarian hyperstimulation for IVF/ICSI-treatment and devided them in three ovarian-response-subgroups: Poor responder (POR) after Bologna Criteria, polycystic ovary syndrome (PCO) after Rotterdam Criteria, or normal responder (NOR, control group). Subjects were subdivided into six genotypes according to their be-allelic CGG-repeat length. *FMR1*-CGG-repeat-length was determined using ALF-express-DNA-sequencer or ABI 3100/3130 × 1-sequencer. mRNA was extracted from GCs after follicular aspiration and quantitative *FMR1*-expression was determined using specific TaqMan-Assay and applying the $\Delta\Delta CT$ method. Kruskall-Wallis-Test or ANOVA were used for simple comparison between ovarian reserve (NOR, POR or PCO) and CGG-subgroups or cohort demographic data. All statistical analysis were performed with SPSS and statistical significance was set at $p \leq 0.05$.

Results: A statistically significant increase in *FMR1*-mRNA-expression-levels was detected in GCs of PORs with heterozygous normal/low-CGG-repeat-length compared with other genotypes ($p = 0.044$).

Conclusion: Female ovarian response may be negatively affected by low CGG-alleles during stimulation. In addition, due to a low-allele-effect, folliculogenesis may be impaired already prior to stimulation leading to diminished ovarian reserve and poor ovarian response. A better understanding of *FMR1* expression-regulation in GCs may help to elucidate pathomechanisms of folliculogenesis disorders and to develop risk-adjusted treatments for IVF/ICSI-therapy. Herewith *FMR1*-genotyping potentially provides a better estimatation of treatment outcome and allows the optimal adaptation of stimulation protocols in future.

Keywords: *FMR1* expression, Granulosa cells, *FMR1* CGG repeat length, *FMR1* genotype

* Correspondence: julia.rehnitz@med.uni-heidelberg.de
[1]Reproduction Genetics Unit, Department of Gynecological Endocrinology and Fertility Disorders, University Women's Hospital, Heidelberg, Germany
[3]Department of Gynecological Endocrinology and Fertility Disorders, University Women's Hospital, Heidelberg, Germany
Full list of author information is available at the end of the article

Background

A sufficient ovarian reserve is crucial for female fertility and, consequently, a successful pregnancy. Diminished ovarian reserve can considerably affect the success rates of assisted reproductive techniques (ARTs) [1]. The response to controlled ovarian hyperstimulation, in addition to oocyte quality, reflects female reproductive potential. Therefore, understanding the mechanisms underlying ovarian response patterns are necessary for improving ART approaches.

FMR1 (fragile X mental retardation 1) gene is one of the major genes of interest in this field, as it is associated with premature ovarian insufficiency (POI) and its endpoint premature ovarian failure (POF; OMIM accession number: 615723) and, as its protein FMRP is mainly localized in granulosa cells within the ovary [2, 3]. The *FMR1* gene contains a CGG repeat of variable size (generally, approximately 30 repeats long) in its 5′-untranslated region (UTR) of exon 1 [4]. If the repeat length extends over 200 (full mutation: FM), individuals can develop the fragile X syndrome (OMIM accession number: 300624), which is linked with a mental retardation caused by *FMR1* gene silencing and loss of fragile X mental retardation 1 protein (FMRP) [5]. While FM-carriers do not show an increased risk for the development of POI/POF, premutation (PM) carriers frequently (~ 20%) suffer from this disorder [2], known as fragile X-associated POI (FXPOI) as well. They have > 54 and < 200 CGG repeats in their *FMR1* gene and demonstrate a repeat length instability with a tendency of increasing repeat lengths from one generation to the next.

In leukocytes and lymphoblastoid cells of male and female *FMR1* PM carriers, *FMR1* mRNA was shown to be overexpressed, while its protein level was decreased [6, 7]. This inverse correlation can be explained by the presence of a regulatory feedback mechanism, where high levels of *FMR1* mRNA may be toxic and lead to the development of pathologies in PM carriers [8]. For the PM-associated neurological disorder FXTAS (fragile X-associated tremor/ataxia syndrome) symptoms are explained by the formation of intranuclear inclusions by the extended CGG triplet block, that result from aberrant protein binding to specific hairpin structures within the nucleus. Sequestration of the *FMR1*-PM mRNA thereby leads to elevated transcription rates [9, 10]. Although similar results and mechanisms are expected in women with POI as well, extensive studies on women and on female germline cells have not been conducted. Previously, we detected alterations in *FMR1* expression levels in leukocytes of women with POI, which were shown to be independent of the PM status [3]. Chen et al. demonstrated that CGG repeat length, regardless of the PM status, in human neuronal and kidney cells may act as positive or negative modulators of *FMR1* translation [11]. Additionally, several studies demonstrated that CGG repeats below 26 or above

34 may affect ovarian reserve and fertility as well [12–16]. According to the repeat lengths at both alleles (low < 26 repeats; normal 26–34 repeats; high 35–55 repeats) women can be divided into six different *FMR1*-CGG-genotypes: high/high, high/low, normal/high, normal/normal, normal/low, and low/low [17]. A pathological effect of CGG repeats outside the range of 26–34 repeats remains controversial, since it was not observed in studies with different experimental settings [18–22].

FMR1 expression levels in leukocytes and other cell types may not be equivalent to the levels in germline cells. During folliculogenesis, oocytes are surrounded by granulosa cells (GCs), forming a functional entity. These cells are necessary for the proper development of oocytes before ovulation. In the human ovaries, GCs represent the main source of FMRP [3], which led us to analyze *FMR1* mRNA expression directly in human GCs, thereby avoiding potential bias originating from the usage of animal models or different human cell types or lines. This study aimed to evaluate the effects of different *FMR1* genotypes, according to the allele specific CGG repeat length, on the expression of this gene in GCs in an ovarian response-dependent manner.

Elizur et al. demonstrated a significant non-linear association between CGG repeat length and *FMR1* expression levels in GCs of female PM carriers, with the highest *FMR1* expression level in women with mid-range CGG repeat length (80–120 triplets), which was shown to be associated with a low number of oocytes retrieved during in vitro fertilization (IVF) [23]. Mid-range PM carrier status is also supposed to demonstrate the highest risk for developing POI/POF in women [24].

To the best of our knowledge, association studies analyzing *FMR1* mRNA expression profiles in GCs with aberrant *FMR1* CGG repeat numbers below the PM threshold have not been performed to date. Therefore, we evaluated the effects of the six *FMR1* genotypes (i.e. low, normal and high repeat numbers for each allele) on the *FMR1* mRNA expression profile in GCs, using GCs obtained from women with different ovarian response patterns: women with poor ovarian response (POR), women with normal ovarian function (NOR), and women with polycystic ovary syndrome (PCOS).

Methods

We aimed to evaluate if *FMR1*-CGG-repeat-lengths aberrations from normal range (n: 26–34) influence the mRNA-expression in GCs of women in an ovarian response depending manner.

Study population

A total of 229 women that underwent controlled ovarian hyperstimulation for either IVF or IVF with intracytoplasmic sperm injection (ICSI) treatment at the Department of

Gynecological Endocrinology and Reproductive Medicine, University Women's Hospital, Heidelberg, from February 2013 to August 2016 were prospectively recruited for our study. We collected GCs and blood samples from all patients. Additionally, their medical records and questionnaires were assessed in order to obtain demographic information (age at presentation and body mass index [BMI]), baseline hormone levels (serum follicle stimulating hormone [FSH], luteinizing hormone [LH], estradiol [E₂], and anti-Müllerian hormone [AMH]), and reproductive parameters (antral follicle count [AFC], total number of oocytes recovered, and mature [MII] oocytes retrieved). Patients were divided into three response groups. According to the Bologna Criteria [25], patients were included into the POR group ($n = 70$); in case of clinically documented PCOS, according to the Rotterdam Criteria [26], patients were included in the PCO group ($n = 8$). Those who did not fulfill criteria for POR or PCO groups were included in the NOR group, which served as a control ($n = 151$).

Ethical approval
All patients signed an informed consent form and completed a clinical questionnaire. This study was approved by the local ethical committee of the University of Heidelberg, Germany (number S-602/2013), and conducted according to the principles expressed in the Declaration of Helsinki.

CGG repeat length analysis
DNA samples were prepared as described previously [27] from 10 ml of blood samples with EDTA. To analyze CGG repeat length in the 5′-UTR of FMR1 exon 1, polymerase chain reaction (PCR) analysis and subsequent analysis of this region with the ALFexpress DNA sequencer (Amersham 1050; Pharmacia Biotech, Freiburg, Germany) or ABI 3100/3130xl sequencer (Life Technologies/Applied Biosystems, Foster City, CA, USA) were performed. PCR mixture (total volume, 30 ml) contained 0.25 μM of each primer (for forward and reverse primer sequences see Fu et al., 1991), 0.2 mM of dATP, dCTP, and dTTP each, 50 μM dGTP, 150 μM deaza-dGTP, 0.12 U KAPA Hot Start Taq polymerase, 1× PCR buffer, 1.5 mM MgCl₂, 1× Enhancer (Qiagen GmbH, Hilden, Germany), and 50 ng of genomic DNA. PCR conditions were as follows: 3 min at 94 °C for the first denaturation step; 35 cycles of amplification with a time-temperature profile of 15 s at 94 °C, 15 s at 66 °C, 15 s at 72 °C; and the additional incubation for 8 min at 72 °C in the last cycle. The forward primer was labeled with the fluorescent Cy5 or FAM dye (Eurofins Genomics, Ebersberg, Germany). For the analysis using ALFexpress sequencer, a 5 μl aliquot of PCR mix was mixed with 5 μl of 6× loading solution (5 mg/ml Blue Dextran (Carl Roth GmbH + Co. KG, Karlsruhe, Germany) in formamide (Merck KGaA, Darmstadt, Germany)) and

1 μl of 250-bp internal marker. All samples following the denaturation at 95 °C for 5 min were analyzed on 6% denaturing polyacrylamide gel with 7 M urea. A 70–397 nucleotide size marker labeled with Cy5 dye was used for the determination of CGG repeat numbers. Allele sizes and peak areas of fluorescent products were analyzed with the Fragment Manager software (Pharmacia Biotech, Freiburg, Germany). To analyze the samples on the ABI 3100/3130xl sequencer, 1 μl of PCR product was mixed with 10.5 μl of Hi-Di-formamide and 0.5 μl of GeneScan ROX standard (Applied Biosystems, Foster City, CA, USA) and loaded. The obtained data were analyzed with the GeneMapper software (Applied Biosystems, Foster City, CA, USA). When the presence of PM was suspected, Southern blot was performed using a-^{32}P-dCTP radioactively-labeled p2 probe containing FMR1 exon 1 with CGG repeat as described previously [28].

Non-PM allele length classification
A CGG repeat length of 26–34 was considered a normal repeat length range according to prior studies [4, 14–16, 20]. We classified the patients according to the repeat lengths at both alleles (low < 26 repeats; normal 26–34 repeats; high 35–55 repeats) into six different genotypes: high/high, high/low, normal/high, normal/normal, normal/low, and low/low, as previously described [17]. PM carriers were not included in the study.

Ovarian stimulation
Ovarian stimulation was performed using either the long protocol of gonadotropin-releasing hormone (GnRH) agonist administration (long GnRH agonist protocol) or GnRH antagonist protocol. The appropriate protocol was selected by the physicians in charge. In the long GnRH agonist protocol an initial down-regulation using a GnRH-agonist at day 20+ 1 of the menstrual cycle was used. On day two of following cycle, gonadotropins (mainly recFSH or HMG) were injected daily to induce proper follicle maturation. When follicles reached 18 mm diameter, ovulation was induced by HCG injection and the oocytes were retrieved via ultrasound-guided follicular puncture after 36 h in 14 ml round bottom tubes containing PBS (1× Phosphate-buffered saline) and heparin (250 μl Heparin / 500 ml PBS). In the GnRH-antagonist protocol, gonadotropins (mainly recFSH or HMG) were injected daily to induce proper follicle maturation beginning at day 2 of menstrual cycle. When the leading follicle reached 14 mm average diameter, a GnRH-antagonist was used to prevent preterm spontaneous ovulation. At stage of 18 mm diameter follicle size, oocytes were retrieved after ovulation induction as described above. The cumulative dose of gonadotropins was determined based on the patients' response and the decisions made by the physicians in charge.

Retrieval of GCs

GCs were retrieved from the follicular fluid after the transvaginal ultrasound-guided follicle puncture for IVF treatment that was performed with an ovum aspiration needle (Premium Fas Single Lumen, #4551 NS-AS1; Gynétics Medical Products N.V., Lommel, Belgium) connected to a vacuum pump (Cook Medical, K-MAR-5200, Bloomington, IN, USA). The aspirated follicular fluid was collected in 14 mL round-bottom tubes (Falcon, 352,001, NY, USA), and kept at 37 °C in a test-tube heater (Cook Medical, K-FTH-1012, Bloomington, IN, USA) or in a Thermo-Cell-Transporter (Labotect, Thermo-Cell-Transporter 3018, Rosdorf, Germany). Follicular fluid was transferred to a 100-mm cell culture dish (Thermo Fisher Scientific, Nunc, Waltham, MA, USA) on a table heated to 37 °C (Workstation L126 Dual, K-Systems, Birkerød, Denmark). GCs were identified morphologically as epithelial cell aggregates within the follicular fluid using a Nikon SMZ1500 zoom-stereomicroscope (Nikon Instruments Europe B.V., Amsterdam, Netherlands). In most cases granulosa cells (GCs) were picked up directly from the follicular fluid without additional washing. A brief washing step in either Multipurpose Handling Medium (MHM) or Sydney IVF Fertilization medium (Cook, K-SIFM-20, Bloomington, IN, USA) was considered necessary, if the follicular fluid was bloody. In some cases, i.e. bloody follicular fluid and a lot of Cumulus-Oocyte-Complexes (COCs), the MHM used for keeping COCs during the search also became bloody. In those cases GCs were briefly washed in Sydney IVF Fertilization medium that was also used to wash COCs before in vitro culture. We did not check for pH variations in Sydney IVF Fertilization medium after washing GCs and therefore cannot exclude a possible impact. However, only equilibrated Sydney IVF Fertilization medium was used for washing of COCs. The Sydney IVF Fertilization medium was then used immediately to wash GCs. Thus, the time during which Sydney IVF Fertilization medium was used outside the CO^2-incubator was kept to a minimum.

Mural GCs were aspirated in a 2.5 µl volume with a sterile tip (ep Dualfilter T.I.P.S. 10 µl S, Eppendorf, Wesseling-Berzdorf, Germany), transferred to 1.5-ml tubes (Sarstedt, Nümbrecht, Germany) pre-filled with 12–13 µl of RNAlater stabilization solution (Ambion, AM7020, Life Technologies, Carlsbad, CA, USA), and stored at 4 °C.

RNA extraction

GCs in the stabilizing solution were centrifuged at $5000 \times g$ for 5 min, and the supernatants were removed. mRNA was directly isolated from the GCs using TRIzol (Life Technologies, Carlsbad, CA, USA) according to the manufacturer's instructions [29, 30] with PEQGOLD PHASETRAP A 1.5 ml tubes (VWR International GmbH, Darmstadt, Germany). mRNA was dissolved in RNAse-free water and the concentration and purity were detected using NanoDrop 2000c UV-spectrometer (NanoDrop Products, Wilmington, DE, USA). cDNA samples were synthesized after oligo-dT priming with SuperScript III First-Strand Synthesis System (Invitrogen by Life Technologies, Carlsbad, CA, USA) and the M-MLV Reverse Transcriptase, RNase H Minus, Point Mutant (Promega, Madison, WI, USA).

Gene expression analysis

TaqMan predesigned gene expression assays for *FMR1* (Hs00924544_m1) and two housekeeping genes, *HPRT* and *TBP* (Hs99999909_m1; Hs00427620_m1, respectively), as well as the TaqMan universal PCR master mix were purchased from Applied Biosystems (Life Technologies, Carlsbad, CA, USA) and the experiments were performed according to the manufacturer's instructions. The samples were analyzed in triplicates, and standard PCR conditions were used, with Fast Forward 7500 real-time PCR-system (Applied Biosystems, Life Technologies, Carlsbad, CA, USA). Relative gene expression was analyzed using $\Delta\Delta Ct$ method [31]. cDNA obtained from the COV 434 granulosa cells [32] was used as a calibrator in each run.

Statistical analysis

Data distribution was first determined by Shapiro-Wilk-Test. For simple comparison between ovarian reserve- (NOR, POR, or PCO) or CGG-subgroups, and the analysis of cohort demographic data, Kruskall-Wallis test or analysis of variance (ANOVA) were used. When statistically significant differences were obtained between groups, a post hoc test [Tukey's honestly significant difference (HSD) or Dunn's tests] was performed to identify which of the analyzed subgroups differed. In order to adjust the significance level, the Bonferroni correction was applied. Additionally, the χ2-test, supplemented by the adjusted residuals, was used for between- group comparisons (clinical ovarian reserve classification and genotype). Results are presented as mean ± standard deviation (SD), or median and interquartile range (percentile 25-percentile 75; respectively 1rst-3rd quartile). For $n < 3$, the data are presented as median and minimum and maximum value (minimum–maximum). Statistical analyses were performed with SPSS (Statistical Package for the Social Sciences V. 22.0; IBM Corporation, NY, USA), and statistical significance was set at $p \leq 0.05$.

Results

General study population

Cohort demographics

Of 229 patients participating in our study, 151 were classified as NORs, 70 belonged to the POR group, while eight patients were included in the PCO group (Table 1). No differences in BMI and estradiol (E_2) levels, diagnosed at early follicular phase, were determined between

Table 1 Cohort demographics

Demographic	NOR		POR		PCO		p value
	n	Median (P25-P75)	n	Median (P25-P75)	n	Median (P25-P75)	
Age*	151	35.1 ± 4.2^A	70	37.4 ± 4.6^B	8	31.3 ± 3.8^C	0.001
BMI	149	23.6 (20.5–27.3)	65	22.3 (20.7–25.4)	8	26.3 (20.9–32.1)	0.352
AFC	84	$6 (4.5–9)^A$	35	$2.5 (1.5–3.5)^B$	6	$16.25 (12.1–20)^C$	< 0.001
FSH (U/L)	137	$7.2 (6–8.8)^A$	59	$8.6 (6.1–11.1)^B$	7	$6.1 (5.8–7.2)^{AB}$	0.013
LH (U/L)	139	$5.3 (3.7–6.8)^A$	62	$5.5 (3.5–6.5)^A$	8	$12.9 (9.6–17.5)^B$	< 0.001
Estradiol	133	43 (34.5–58.2)	59	49.2 (31.1–76.0)	8	41.7 (31.1–46.4)	0.810
AMH	142	$2.47 (1.4–3.8)^A$	69	$0.88 (0.5–1.1)^B$	8	$9.37 (4.5–14.6)^C$	< 0.001
Total oocytes	149	$9 (6–13)^A$	64	$3 (2–5.7)^B$	8	$22 (4.2–36)^A$	< 0.001
MII oocytes	117	$7 (5–11)^A$	43	$3 (2–5)^B$	6	$16 (8–27.2)^A$	< 0.001
FMR1	138	0.75 (0.5–1.2)	57	0.8 (0.5–1.2)	8	0.9 (0.46–1.43)	0.947

BMI body mass index, *AFC* antral follicle count, *FSH* follicle stimulating hormone, *LH* luteinizing hormone, *AMH* anti-Müllerian-hormone, *MII* oocytes, mature oocytes, *FMR1* fragile X mental retardation 1 gene relative gene expression in granulosa cells of the patients normalized by two house-keeping genes and a granulosa cell calibrator (see MM-part for details)
All other values represent median values, with 1st and 3rd quartile parenthesized
Different letters in one row signify statistical difference
p values represent significance levels between normal responders (NOR), poor responders (POR), and polycystic ovarian syndrome group (PCO)
*Mean ± standard deviation

the ovarian response groups. The age of patients of the 3 response groups differed whereby PCO patients were the youngest (Table 1).

As expected, FSH ($p = 0.013$), LH, AMH, AFC, the number of total oocytes retrieved, and the number of MII oocytes differed significantly ($p < 0.001$ for all; Table 1) between these three groups, which demonstrated the appropriate patient selection.

In the three groups treatment distribution between IVF, ICSI and IVF/ICSI-splitting was comparable between NOR and PCO with 69.3%, respectively 62.5% for ICSI-treatments and with 26.7%, respectively 25% for IVF-treatments. However, in the POR group the percentage of IVF was higher (45.2%) and no splitting was performed in our population.

FMR1 mRNA expression

Relative mRNA *FMR1* expression in GCs did not differ between the three response groups ($p = $ n.s.; Table 1).

FMR1 genotype groups
Cohort demographics

To evaluate the potential effects of CGG repeat number aberrations on ovarian response and/or mRNA *FMR1* expression in human GCs of IVF/ICSI patients, we divided the patients according to their allele CGG repeat lengths into six genotype groups: high/high, high/low, normal/high, normal/normal, normal/low, and low/low groups.

As age distribution in all genotype groups was similar, we did not perform any further age-dependent analyses. FSH, LH, AMH, AFC, the number of total oocytes retrieved, and the number of MII oocytes did not differ between different genotype groups ($p = $ n.s. for all; Table 2).

Ovarian response

The correlation analysis of the CGG genotypes and three ovarian response groups showed no significant differences in genotype distribution ($p = $ n.s.; Table 3), demonstrating that different genotypes in general are not associated with the ovarian response in our study population.

FMR1 mRNA expression

Different genotypes in general were not shown to be related with *FMR1* expression levels ($p = $ n.s.; Table 4). However, analysis of *FMR1* expression related to ovarian response showed that the normal/low genotype in PORs is significantly associated with an increase in *FMR1* expression in GCs ($p = 0.044$; Table 4).

Further analysis of the different genotypes in POR group demonstrated that the *FMR1* expression in normal/low genotype group is significantly different compared with that in both normal/high or normal/normal genotype groups ($p = 0.008$ and $p = 0.027$, respectively; Fig. 1).

Discussion

Poor ovarian response is one of the major factors limiting the success rate of infertility treatments. *FMR1* is involved in folliculogenesis and the CGG repeat length in PM range was shown to be associated with the development of POI. An association between high *FMR1* mRNA expression levels in GCs in mid-range *FMR1* PM-carriers and the lowest total number of retrieved oocytes during IVF, compared with the other analyzed groups, was demonstrated already earlier [23] suggesting that via the exact level of *FMR1* expression ovarian response may be judged.

Table 2 Cohort demographic analysis of groups formed according to *FMR1* genotypes

Demographics	All patients												p value
	high/high		high/low		high/normal		normal/normal		normal/low		low/low		
	n	(P25-P75)	n	(P25-P75)	n	(P25-P75)	n	(P25-P75)	n	(P25-P75)	n	(P25-P75)	
Age[a]	2	34 ± 5.6	3	28.6 ± 1.1	25	35.4 ± 4.4	123	35.7 ± 4.5	65	35.9 ± 4.7	8	36.3 ± 3.2	0.163
AFC	2	6 (6–6)	0	–	18	3 (1.8–7.1)	62	5.75 (3–9.12)	38	5 (3–6.1)	3	5.5 (3.5–10)	0.239
FSH	2	9.5 (6.6–12.4)	2	7.3 (6.9–7.7)	23	8.3 (6.1–10.9)	110	7.1 (5.7–8.7)	56	7.8 (6.2–9.3)	7	7.9 (5.2–10.3)	0.323
LH	2	9.2 (6.7–11.7)	3	4.8 (4.7–6.1)	24	5.7 (3.7–10.1)	113	5.4 (3.5–7.1)	56	5.3 (3.7–6.4)	8	4.9 (3.6–6)	0.338
Estradiol	2	55.8 (51.5–68.2)	3	47.3 (31.2–63.1)	23	45.6 (38.2–76)	108	40.6 (32.4–58.2)	54	43.6 (34.3–57.9)	7	55.7 (41.5–76)	0.372
AMH	2	1.24 (0.94–1.55)	2	2.49 (2.48–2.5)	25	0.88 (0.55–3.35)	120	1.86 (1.06–3.68)	59	1.87 (1.14–3.16)	8	1.37 (1.03–1.64)	0.426
Total oocyte number	2	2.5 (2–3)	3	9 (7–14)	23	6 (2–14)	120	7 (4–12)	63	7 (5–12)	8	4.5 (3.2–6)	0.210
MII oocyte number	2	2 (2–2)	2	6.5 (6–7)	16	6 (2–15)	92	6 (3–9)	49	6 (4.5–9)	5	5 (3–8.5)	0.739

BMI body mass index, *AFC* antral follicle count, *FSH* follicle stimulating hormone, *LH* luteinizing hormone, *AMH* anti-Müllerian-hormone, *MII* oocytes mature oocytes.

[a]Age, mean ± standard deviation is presented

All other values are presented as median and 1st and 3rd quartile parenthesized

p values represent significance levels between the six evaluated *FMR1* genotypes

Here, we aimed to analyze the effects of CGG repeat length aberrations outside the PM stage on the *FMR1* expression in human GCs, and its potential correlation with different ovarian response patterns. We detected a significant effect of normal/low CGG repeat length in the POR group on gene expression with significantly elevated *FMR1* mRNA expression levels in this group.

The impact of different *FMR1* CGG repeat lengths below the PM range as a potentially important marker of female fertility and ovarian response remains controversial. Different results obtained by analyzing the non-PM *FMR1* GCC repeat lengths may be partially explained by the difference in study endpoints. While some groups focused on ovarian reserve or response to ovarian stimulation depending on different *FMR1* CGG haplo- and genotypes, others considered the age of menopause or AMH-level as CGG-dependent factors [12–22]. Also, in the pathogenesis of other folliculogenesis disorders the CGG repeat length is supposed to be involved. In PCO patients with normal/low *FMR1* genotype statistically, for

example, higher rates of autoimmunity and lower pregnancy rates were detected [33].

In our study the number of PCO patients included was quite low and low alleles were not detected in our PCO group. The low number of PCO in our study can be explained by our clinical procedures, where in vitro maturation (IVM) is the protocol of choice offered to patients with PCO due to an increased risk of developing ovarian hyperstimulation syndrome instead of the classical IVF/ICSI treatment. Patients undergoing IVM treatment were not included in this study. The exclusion of PCO patients from our analysis does not affect the demonstrated results, leading to the same conclusions. Nevertheless, for future studies consideration of *FMR1*-genotype dependent *FMR1*-expression variations in GCs of PCO-patients, especially those with low alleles, may be promising, too.

Furthermore, one of the limitations of our study is, that we did not specifically check for CGG mosaics. Therefore, we cannot exclude existing mosaics in our patients, unless it is described, that only 1% of cases are affected by this [34].

Additionally, we opine that the discrepancies in distribution of ART-treatments between NOR and PCO with POR are of minor importance, since our study evaluated the gene expression in GCs after follicular aspiration prior to fertilization in dependence of ovarian response and *FMR1*-genotype and not the reproductive outcome.

We here evaluated for the first time the putative effects of aberrant non-PM *FMR1* CGG repeat numbers on female fertility based on the individual *FMR1* mRNA gene expression levels in GCs, the *FMR1* target cells in the ovary, that are highly relevant for proper folliculogenesis and oocyte maturation. We thereby aimed to help elucidate the controversially discussed impact of

Table 3 *FMR1* genotype distribution in patients with different ovarian response patterns

Frequencies	NOR - n (%)	POR - n (%)	PCO - n (%)
high/high	1 (0.7)	1 (1.4)	0 (0.0)
high/low	3 (2.0)	0 (0.0)	0 (0.0)
high/normal	13 (8.7)	10 (14.5)	2 (25.0)
normal/normal	79 (53.0)	38 (55.1)	6 (75.0)
normal/low	47 (31.5)	18 (26.1)	0 (0.0)
low/low	6 (4.0)	2 (2.9)	0 (0.0)

NOR normal responders, *POR* poor responders, *PCO* polycystic ovary syndrome patients

Ovarian response distribution among the six *FMR1* genotypes (*p* = 0.54)

Table 4 *FMR1* mRNA gene expression levels in different *FMR1* genotype and ovarian response groups (age-independent)

FMR1 Expression	high/high		high/low		high/normal		normal/normal		normal/low		low/low		*p* value
	n	(P25-P75)	n	(P25-P75)	n	(P25-P75)	n	(P25-P75)	n	(P25-P75)	n	(P25-P75)	
All patients	1[a]	0.309	3	0.32 (0.26–1.54)	21	0.67 (0.51–1.21)	109	0.73 (0.47–1.25)	59	0.84 (0.55–1.27)	8	0.68 (0.19–1.69)	0.475
NOR	1[a]	0.309	3	0.32 (0.26–1.54)	10	0.95 (0.53–1.47)	71	0.71 (0.48–1.25)	45	0.77 (0.52–1.09)	6	0.68 (0.16–1.9)	0.630
POR	0	–	0	–	9	0.56 (0.47–0.69)	32	0.78 (0.43–1.2)	14	1.1 (0.95–1.5)	2	0.77 (0.2–1.3)	0.044
PCO	0	–	0	–	2	1.05 (0.92–1.19)	6	0.83 (0.35–1.53)	0	–	0	–	0.505

Distribution of *FMR1*-expression in GCs among the six genotypes related to different ovarian response groups. Normal/low genotypes demonstrated elevated *FMR1* expression in case of poor response (*p* = 0.044)
[a]Descriptive analysis only, due to the number of patients
p values represent significance-levels between the six genotypes and are calculated as described in the Material and Method part

CGG repeat length aberrations on female fertility and ovarian reserve [12–22]. We believe that our findings can contribute to resolve this contentious issue as it combines *FMR1*-gene-expression analysis in GCs with the ovarian response of patients. Our obtained results herein are in line with our previously obtained data, showing different PM-independent *FMR1* expression levels in POI patients [3].

As POR may be considered as a clinical stage putatively leading to the development of POI, we used female GCs and focused on women showing different response to controlled ovarian stimulation, to evaluate the potential association between their *FMR1* mRNA expression and different *FMR1* genotypes, together with different ovarian response patterns directly in female germline.

We demonstrated that patients belonging to the POR group, with a normal/low CGG genotype, show a significantly increased *FMR1* expression levels in GCs, compared with those in the other genotype groups (normal/normal

and normal/high). Combined with NOR and PCO such an effect was not detected. This can be due to the limited sample size. So we appreciate further studies to clarify this issue. If such a low allele effect only in POR with larger sample sizes persists, it can be hypothesized, that women with a normal/low CGG repeat length *FMR1* genotype suffer from POR due to their elevated *FMR1* mRNA expression levels that negatively affect the response to controlled ovarian hyperstimulation. Alternatively, poor response of these patients could be the visible endpoint of an already impaired folliculogenesis whose proper process is depending on a sound *FMR1*/FMRP expression regulation. The low-CGG-allele thereby putatively influences this expression regulation. This would be in line with the results of a previous study, that showed in patients carrying heterozygous low CGG repeat length alleles a significantly increased percentage of poor-quality embryo morphology and a lower potential of conceiving after ART [35]. One possible mechanism explaining such a

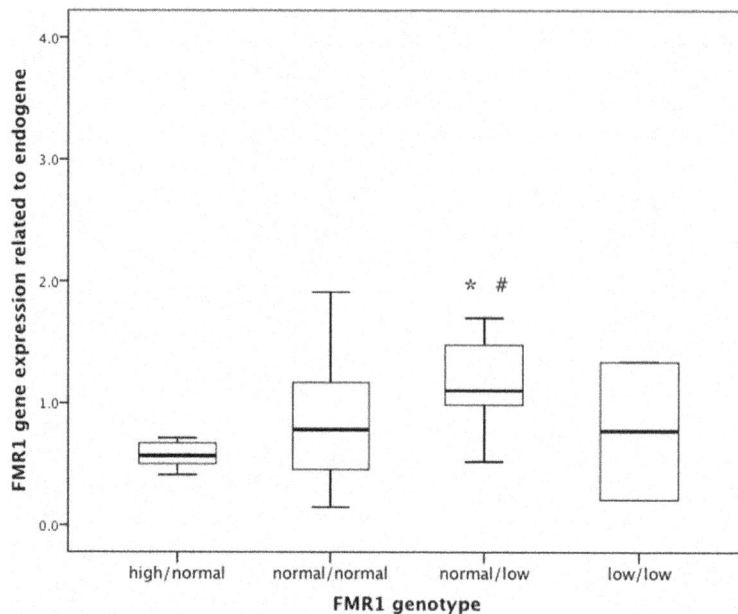

Fig. 1 *FMR1* gene expression in poor responder group (POR) depending on *FMR1* genotype. * Statistically different from high/normal group (*p* = 0.008); # statistically different from normal/normal group (*p* = 0.027)

low-allele effect only in POR may be a skewed X Inactivation, as it is described in PM carrier women suffering from FXTAS (Fragile-X-Associated Tremor/Ataxia Syndrome) 1 [36].

Due to the limited low/low genotype numbers in POR ($n = 2$) and NOR ($n = 6$) we could not detect an effect on the FMR1 mRNA expression in POR, neither in NOR with two low alleles. So, if this effect is even more pronounced when two low alleles are present, stays speculative. To elucidate this further studies with larger sample sizes are needed, that especially include more patients with homozygous and heterozygous low alleles.

If the CGG repeat length acts as a positive or negative modulator of the FMR1 translation, as previously hypothesized [11], low CGG repeat numbers may induce gene transcription in POR patients putatively via altered binding capacity of transcriptional factors and/or other regulatory elements such as non coding RNAs (microRNAs, long non coding RNAs), variable CpG methylation and histone modifications. Evaluating these factors in a CGG repeat length depending setting with regards to altered FMR1 expression levels would therefore be of major interest in future studies.

The elevated FMR1 mRNA levels of POR with normal/low genotype, similar to the situation in female PM-carriers, may also have a toxic effect and lead to altered FMRP levels. Therefore, in future studies the level of FMRP in dependence of FMR1 genotype, the level of RNA and the ovarian response should be evaluated. In such a study, altered FMRP-level as potential cause of the poor response and negative effects on proper oocyte and embryo development after fertilization might be identified. So further experiments aiming at the reproductive outcome depending on different genotypes, FMR1/FMRP expression level and ovarian response are advisable.

In conclusion, analysis of FMR1 expression in GCs obtained from women with different ovarian reserves can help to obtain a better insight into the FMR1/FMRP expression regulatory mechanism and its putative effects on female fertility and folliculogenesis disorders. To the best of our knowledge, we are the first group analyzing the impact of the CGG genotype on the ovarian response and FMR1 expression directly at the locus of interest in GCs, although larger samples are needed to substantiate the results of this pilot project. Also, functional studies are needed that evaluate involved regulatory elements in order to clarify if and how high mRNA-expression-level of FMR1 and the CGG repeat length impact follicular maturation and ovarian response.

Conclusions

Heterozygous low CGG repeat numbers are associated with significantly elevated FMR1-expressions profiles in granulosa cells of women with poor ovarian response. If the genotype directly affects female ovarian response or, if this low response is caused by impaired folliculogenesis prior to stimulation due to a low-allele-effect stays speculative. Our results may contribute to a better understanding of FMR1 expression-regulation in GCs in order to elucidate underlying pathomechanisms of different folliculogenesis disorders and are potentially of value to develop risk-adjusted treatments during IVF/ICSI therapy, in which FMR1 genotyping provides the better estimate of treatment outcome and allows the optimal adaptation of stimulation protocols in future.

Abbreviations
AFC: Antral Follicle Count; AMH: Anti-Müllerian Hormone; ART: Assisted Reproductive Techniques; BMI: Body Mass Index; COC: Cumulus Oocyte Complex; E_2: Estradiol; FMR1: Fragile X Mental Retardation I gene; FMRP: Fragile X Mental Retardation I protein; FSH: Follicle Stimulating Hormone; FXPOI: Fragile X-associated POI; FXTAS: Fragile X-associated tremor/ataxia syndrome; GC: Granulosa Cells; GnRH: Gonadotropin-releasing Hormone; ICSI: Intracytoplasmic Sperm Injection; IVF: In vitro fertilization; IVM: In vitro maturation; LH: Luteinizing Hormone; MII: Mature Oocytes; NOR: Normal responders; PCOS: Polycystic Ovarian Syndrome; PM: Pre-mutation; POF/POI: Premature Ovarian Failure/Insufficiency; POR: Poor responders

Acknowledgements
We acknowledge financial support by DFG within the funding programme Open Access Publishing, by the Baden-Württemberg Ministry of Science, Research and the Arts and by Ruprecht-Karls-Universität Heidelberg.

Funding
This study was supported by DFG (German Research Foundation): RE 3647/1-1 to JR.

Authors' contributions
Each author contributed substantially to the drafting or critical revision of the manuscript, and approved the final version. JR, AG, TS and DDA conceived and designed the study. Data acquisition, data analysis and interpretation, and statistical analyses were performed by JR, DDA, ISB, JED, KH, BY, BM, AG, AF, TS.

Competing interests
The authors declare that they have no competing interests.

Author details
[1]Reproduction Genetics Unit, Department of Gynecological Endocrinology and Fertility Disorders, University Women's Hospital, Heidelberg, Germany. [2]Department of Physiology, Institute of Health Sciences, Federal University of Rio Grande do Sul, Porto Alegre, Brazil. [3]Department of Gynecological Endocrinology and Fertility Disorders, University Women's Hospital, Heidelberg, Germany. [4]Laboratory of Molecular Genetics, Institute of Human Genetics, Heidelberg University, Heidelberg, Germany.

References

1. Barad DH, Weghofer A, Gleicher N. Age-specific levels for basal follicle-stimulating hormone assessment of ovarian function. Obstet Gynecol. 2007;109:1404–10.
2. Sullivan AK, Marcus M, Epstein MP, Allen EG, Anido AE, Paquin JJ, Yadav-Shah M, Sherman SL. Association of FMR1 repeat size with ovarian dysfunction. Hum Reprod. 2005;20:402–12.
3. Schuettler J, Peng Z, Zimmer J, Sinn P, von Hagens C, Strowitzki T, Vogt PH. Variable expression of the fragile X mental retardation 1 (FMR1) gene in patients with premature ovarian failure syndrome is not dependent on number of (CGG)n triplets in exon 1. Hum Reprod. 2011;26:1241–51.
4. Fu YH, Kuhl DP, Pizzuti A, Pieretti M, Sutcliffe JS, Richards S, Verkerk AJ, Holden JJ, Fenwick RG Jr, Warren ST, et al. Variation of the CGG repeat at the fragile X site results in genetic instability: resolution of the Sherman paradox. Cell. 1991;67:1047–58.
5. Devys D, Lutz Y, Rouyer N, Bellocq JP, Mandel JL. The FMR-1 protein is cytoplasmic, most abundant in neurons and appears normal in carriers of a fragile X premutation. Nat Genet. 1993;4:335–40.
6. Kenneson A, Zhang F, Hagedorn CH, Warren ST. Reduced FMRP and increased FMR1 transcription is proportionally associated with CGG repeat number in intermediate-length and premutation carriers. Hum Mol Genet. 2001;10:1449–54.
7. Primerano B, Tassone F, Hagerman RJ, Hagerman P, Amaldi F, Bagni C. Reduced FMR1 mRNA translation efficiency in fragile X patients with premutations. RNA. 2002;8:1482–8.
8. Hagerman PJ, Hagerman RJ. The fragile-X premutation: a maturing perspective. Am J Hum Genet. 2004;74:805–16.
9. Greco CM, Berman RF, Martin RM, Tassone F, Schwartz PH, Chang A, Trapp BD, Iwahashi C, Brunberg J, Grigsby J, et al. Neuropathology of fragile X-associated tremor/ataxia syndrome (FXTAS). Brain J Neurol. 2006;129:243–55.
10. Greco CM, Hagerman RJ, Tassone F, Chudley AE, Del Bigio MR, Jacquemont S, Leehey M, Hagerman PJ. Neuronal intranuclear inclusions in a new cerebellar tremor/ataxia syndrome among fragile X carriers. Brain J Neurol. 2002;125:1760–71.
11. Chen LS, Tassone F, Sahota P, Hagerman PJ. The (CGG)n repeat element within the 5′ untranslated region of the FMR1 message provides both positive and negative cis effects on in vivo translation of a downstream reporter. Hum Mol Genet. 2003;12:3067–74.
12. Gleicher N, Weghofer A, Oktay K, Barad D. Relevance of triple CGG repeats in the FMR1 gene to ovarian reserve. Reprod BioMed Online. 2009;19:385–90.
13. Gustin SL, Ding VY, Desai M, Leader B, Baker VL. Evidence of an age-related correlation of ovarian reserve and FMR1 repeat number among women with "normal" CGG repeat status. J Assist Reprod Genet. 2015;32:1669–76.
14. Gleicher N, Weghofer A, Barad DH. Ovarian reserve determinations suggest new function of FMR1 (fragile X gene) in regulating ovarian ageing. Reprod BioMed Online. 2010;20:768–75.
15. Pastore LM, Young SL, Baker VM, Karns LB, Williams CD, Silverman LM. Elevated prevalence of 35–44 FMR1 trinucleotide repeats in women with diminished ovarian reserve. Reprod Sci. 2012;19:1226–31.
16. Pastore LM, Young SL, Manichaikul A, Baker VL, Wang XQ, Finkelstein JS. Distribution of the FMR1 gene in females by race-ethnicity: women with diminished ovarian reserve versus women with normal fertility (SWAN study). Fertil Steril. 2017;107:205–211.e1.
17. Gleicher N, Weghofer A, Lee IH, Barad DH. Association of FMR1 genotypes with in vitro fertilization (IVF) outcomes based on ethnicity/race. PLoS One. 2011;6:e18781.
18. Voorhuis M, Onland-Moret NC, Fauser BC, Ploos van Amstel HK, van der Schouw YT, Broekmans FJ. The association of CGG repeats in the FMR1 gene and timing of natural menopause. Hum Reprod. 2013;28:496–501.
19. Banks N, Patounakis G, Devine K, DeCherney AH, Widra E, Levens ED, Whitcomb BW, Hill MJ. Is FMR1 CGG repeat length a predictor of in vitro fertilization stimulation response or outcome? Fertil Steril. 2016;105:1537–46. e1538
20. Maslow BS, Davis S, Engmann L, Nulsen JC, Benadiva CA. Correlation of normal-range FMR1 repeat length or genotypes and reproductive parameters. J Assist Reprod Genet. 2016;33:1149–55.
21. Morin SJ, Tiegs AW, Franasiak JM, Juneau CR, Hong KH, Werner MD, Zhan Y, Landis J, Scott RT Jr. FMR1 gene CGG repeat variation within the normal range is not predictive of ovarian response in IVF cycles. Reprod BioMed Online. 2016;32:496–502.
22. Ruth KS, Bennett CE, Schoemaker MJ, Weedon MN, Swerdlow AJ, Murray A. Length of FMR1 repeat alleles within the normal range does not substantially affect the risk of early menopause. Hum Reprod. 2016;31:2396–403.
23. Elizur SE, Lebovitz O, Derech-Haim S, Dratviman-Storobinsky O, Feldman B, Dor J, Orvieto R, Cohen Y. Elevated levels of FMR1 mRNA in granulosa cells are associated with low ovarian reserve in FMR1 premutation carriers. PLoS One. 2014;9:e105121.
24. Mailick MR, Hong J, Greenberg J, Smith L, Sherman S. Curvilinear association of CGG repeats and age at menopause in women with FMR1 premutation expansions. Am J Med Genet B Neuropsychiatr Genet. 2014;165B(8):705–11.
25. Ferraretti AP, La Marca A, Fauser BC, Tarlatzis B, Nargund G, Gianaroli L, Definition Ewgo POR. ESHRE consensus on the definition of 'poor response' to ovarian stimulation for in vitro fertilization: the bologna criteria. Hum Reprod. 2011;26:1616–24.
26. Rotterdam EA-SPcwg. Revised 2003 consensus on diagnostic criteria and long-term health risks related to polycystic ovary syndrome (PCOS). Hum Reprod. 2004;19:41–7.
27. Fassnacht W, Mempel A, Strowitzki T, Vogt PH. Premature ovarian failure (POF) syndrome: towards the molecular clinical analysis of its genetic complexity. Curr Med Chem. 2006;13:1397–410.
28. Stoyanova V, Oostra BA. The CGG repeat and the FMR1 gene. Methods Mol Biol. 2004;277:173–84.
29. Chomczynski P, Sacchi N. Single-step method of RNA isolation by acid guanidinium thiocyanate-phenol-chloroform extraction. Anal Biochem. 1987;162:156–9.
30. Chomczynski P. A reagent for the single-step simultaneous isolation of RNA, DNA and proteins from cell and tissue samples. BioTechniques. 1993;15:532–4. 536-537
31. Winer J, Jung CK, Shackel I, Williams PM. Development and validation of real-time quantitative reverse transcriptase-polymerase chain reaction for monitoring gene expression in cardiac myocytes in vitro. Anal Biochem. 1999;270:41–9.
32. van den Berg-Bakker CA, Hagemeijer A, Franken-Postma EM, Smit VT, Kuppen PJ, van Ravenswaay Claasen HH, Cornelisse CJ, Schrier PI. Establishment and characterization of 7 ovarian carcinoma cell lines and one granulosa tumor cell line: growth features and cytogenetics. Int J Cancer. 1993;53:613–20.
33. Gleicher N, Weghofer A, Lee IH, Barad DH. FMR1 genotype with autoimmunity-associated polycystic ovary-like phenotype and decreased pregnancy chance. PLoS One. 2010;5:e15303.
34. Biancalana V, Glaeser D, McQuaid S, Steinbach P. EMQN best practice guidelines for the molecular genetic testing and reporting of fragile X syndrome and other fragile X-associated disorders. Eur J Hum Genet. 2015;23:417–25.
35. Kushnir VA, Yu Y, Barad DH, Weghofer A, Himaya E, Lee HJ, Wu YG, Shohat-Tal A, Lazzaroni-Tealdi E, Gleicher N. Utilizing FMR1 gene mutations as predictors of treatment success in human in vitro fertilization. PLoS One. 2014;9:e102274.
36. Alvarez-Mora MI, Rodriguez-Revenga L, Feliu A, Badenas C, Madrigal I, Milà M. Skewed X inactivation in women carrying the FMR1 Premutation and its relation with fragile-X-associated tremor/ataxia syndrome. Neurodegener Dis. 2016;16:290–2.

9

Dysregulated erythropoietin-producing hepatocellular receptor A2 (EphA2) is involved in tubal pregnancy via regulating cell adhesion of the Fallopian tube epithelial cells

Huan Jiang[1], Xiao-Yi Yang[2] and Wei-Jie Zhu[2*]

Abstract

Background: Tyrosine kinase receptor erythropoietin-producing hepatocellular receptor A2 (EphA2) is abundant in the endometrium and plays a role in the establishment of eutopic implantation. A similar molecular mechanism may exist between uterine implantation and tubal implantation, therefore EphA2 involvement in tubal pregnancy is suspected. Due to the limited availability of human Fallopian tube specimens, EphA2 expression in human Fallopian tube epithelium remains largely unknown.

Methods: A total of 31 women with tubal pregnancy and 41 non-pregnant women with benign uterine diseases were enrolled in this study. Immunohistochemistry was used to investigate the expression pattern of EphA2 in the Fallopian tube epithelium of non-pregnant women ($n = 29$) and women with tubal pregnancy ($n = 17$). The changes of EphA2 and its activated form, phosphorylated-EphA2 (Pho-EphA2), in the Fallopian tube epithelium from non-pregnant women ($n = 12$) and women with tubal pregnancy ($n = 14$) were compared by quantitative RT-PCR and western blot assay.

Results: EphA2 was expressed throughout the Fallopian tube epithelium, including the isthmus, the ampulla and the infundibulum. EphA2 concentration remained unchanged throughout the whole menstrual cycle, irrespective of menstrual phases and tubal regions. EphA2 mRNA in the Fallopian tube epithelium did not differ between normal women and women with tubal pregnancy ($P > 0.05$). With respect to the protein level, a significantly higher ratio of EphA2 over Pho-EphA2 was shown in women with tubal pregnancy ($P < 0.05$).

Conclusions: EphA2 is widely expressed in human Fallopian tube epithelium in a temporospatial-independent manner. Dysregulated EphA2 and its phosphorylation-dependent regulatory mechanism may unexpectedly enhance the cell adhesion activity of the Fallopian tube epithelial cells, leading to a mis-contact between the Fallopian tube epithelium and the embryo.

Keywords: Receptor, EphA2, Cell adhesion, Fallopian tube, Pregnancy, Tubal

* Correspondence: tzhuwj@jnu.edu.cn
[2]Institute of Reproductive Immunology, College of Life Science and Technology, Jinan University, 601# Huangpu Da Dao Xi, Guangzhou City 510632, People's Republic of China
Full list of author information is available at the end of the article

Background

An ectopic pregnancy is a pathological event characterized by embryo implantation occurring outside the uterine cavity. Fallopian tube localization accounts for roughly 98% of all human ectopic pregnancies [1]. Tubal damage as a result of surgery or infection (especially Chlamydia trachomatis), smoking and in vitro fertilization are the dominant risk factors for tubal ectopic pregnancies [1]. However, tubal pregnancy is now thought to be a consequence of molecular dysregulation [1]. One major reason underlying this phenomenon is that adhesion molecules such as integrins and mucin 1, etc., which mediate blastocyst adhesion to the uterine wall, are also expressed in the Fallopian tube epithelium [2]. Unexpected molecular changes may afford an opportunity for the undue remain of embryo in the Fallopian tube [2, 3]. Cell adhesion molecules are abundant in human epithelial cells and crucial for intercellular adhesion. It is presumed that cell adhesion activity of the Fallopian tube epithelial cells is under the fine control of cell adhesion molecules and that changes in their concentrations can alter the cell adhesion of the Fallopian tube epithelium, leading to false recognition between mother and fetus [4–6]. Therefore, it is rational to propose that cell adhesion molecules expressed in the Fallopian tube epithelium may actively participate in the pathogenesis of tubal pregnancy.

Erythropoietin-producing hepatocellular receptor A2 (EphA2) is a member of the largest known tyrosine kinase receptor family, which is well known to generate multiple cellular responses including cell adhesion and migration [7–10]. Activation of EphA2 is phosphorylation-dependent. Binding of EphA2 to its predominant EphrinA1 ligand enables its phosphorylation (Pho-EphA2) [11, 12]. This leads to the initiation of a downstream signaling cascade, which results in the internalization and degradation of Pho-EphA2 itself [11, 12]. It is found that EphA2 is highly localized in endometrial epithelial cells accompanied by its Ephrin ligand expressed on embryonic trophoblasts, and EphA2 is suggested to mediate the establishment of uterine implantation by regulating embryo-maternal contact [13, 14]. Furthermore, EphA2 can promote the invasion and proliferation of the human extravillous trophoblastic cells probably via regulating the ephrin-A1 ligand [15]. As a similar molecular mode may exist between uterine implantation and tubal implantation, it is reasonable to expect EphA2 involvement in tubal pregnancy. However, EphA2 expression in human Fallopian tube epithelium has not been fully documented and the role of EphA2 in tubal pregnancy remains unknown as yet.

We have previously demonstrated in vitro study that EphrinA1 could induce EphA2 activation in human fallopian tubal epithelial cells, accompanied by the up-regulation of Pho-EphA2 [16]. Moreover, we used fibronectin-coated culture plates to interact with the cultured Fallopian tube epithelial cells and found that EphA2 activation could attenuate its cell adhesion activity, which, when disrupted, may be associated with certain pathological events occurred in the Fallopian tube, such as tubal pregnancy [16]. However, the expression pattern of EphA2 in human Fallopian tube epithelium remains presently unknown. Therefore, the present study was undertaken to investigate the EphA2 expression in human Fallopian tube epithelium by immunohistochemical analysis. Considering the involvement of EphA2 activation in regulating cell adhesion activity of the Fallopian tube epithelial cells, the changes of EphA2 and its activated form, Pho-EphA2, in the Fallopian tube epithelium were further compared between non-pregnant women and women with tubal pregnancy using quantitative reverse transcription-polymerase chain reaction (qRT-PCR) and western blot assay, aiming to elucidate the roles of EphA2 and its phosphorylation-dependent mechanism in the molecular pathogenesis of tubal pregnancy.

Methods

Specimen collection of human fallopian tubes

Thirty-one women who had been diagnosed as tubal pregnancy and undergone surgeries in the First Affiliated Hospital of Jinan University, PR China were collected, and 41 non-pregnant women who had undergone hysterectomies for benign uterine diseases were set as controls. Informed consent was attained from each patient and ethical approval for this study was obtained from the Local Research Ethics Committee. All the enrolled subjects should meet the following criteria: (1) a normal history of fertility and regular menses; (2) a definitive date of the last menstrual period; and (3) no use of exogenous hormonal drugs or intrauterine devices in the 6 months preceding the surgery. Women with tubal pregnancy who were determined to have morphological abnormalities in the Fallopian tubes or benign uterine diseases such as uterine leiomyoma, adenomyosis and endometriosis after surgical operations were excluded.

Among all the enrolled subjects, the Fallopian tube samples from 17 tubal pregnant women (mean age 27.7 ± 3.7 years; range 26–34 years; gestational weeks 8.5 ± 0.9) and 29 non-pregnant women (control) (mean age 37.6 ± 3.8 years; range 35–45 years) were paraffin embedded and used for immunohistochemistry. Each Fallopian tube sample with tubal pregnancy was further divided into 2 portions, implantation site ($n = 17$) and non-implantation site ($n = 17$), according to the distance apart from the gestational sac. The implantation site was defined as the circumference originating 5 mm from the gestation sac, while the non-implantation site was 10 mm outside the gestation sac [17]. The controls were further divided into 4 groups based on the corresponding endometrial morphology [18]: early-stage of the prolifera-tive phase (days 1–5; $n = 8$), mid- and late-stages of the proliferative phase (days 7–14; $n = 6$), early-stage of the secretory phase (days 15–18; $n = 7$) and mid- and late-stages of the secretory phase (days 19–28; $n = 8$). All of the paraffin blocks were cut and prepared for immuno-histochemical staining.

Fresh Fallopian tube samples obtained from the other 14 tubal pregnant women (mean age 28.9 ± 4.1 years; range from 28 to 37 years; gestational weeks 8.9 ± 0.9 weeks) and 12 non-pregnant women (mean age 40.3 ± 4.2 years; range from 35 to 46 years) were used for qRT-PCR and western blot analysis. Each Fallopian tube tissue with tubal preg-nancy was similarly classified into implantation site and non-implantation site. Samples used for mRNA analysis were immersed into Trizol solution, and all fresh specimens were frozen at $-70\ °C$ until analysis.

Immunohistochemistry

The paraffin-embedded materials were cut into 4-μm-thick sections. These sections were deparaffinized and boiled in citrate buffer solution for 15 min in an oven. After washing with phosphate-buffered saline (PBS), the sections were immersed into 3% hydrogen peroxide for 10 min to quench endogenous peroxidase activity. Afterwards, mouse anti-human EphA2 monoclonal antibody (1:200; ab118882; Abcam, Cambridge, UK) was applied overnight at 4 °C according to the EnVision™ system (Zhongshan Gold-enbridge Biotechnology Co., Ltd., Beijing, China). The sections were washed in PBS and incubated for 30 min with horse radish peroxidase (HRP)-conjugated goat anti-mouse IgG (BM2101; Dako Cytomatin, Glostrup, Denmark). Diaminobenzidine (DAB) substrate-chromogen system (Zhongshan Goldenbridge Biotechnology Co., Ltd., Beijing, China) was used as the color-developing substrate. The slides were applied in two 5-min incubations and then counter-stained with hematoxylin. Normal gastric mucosa with known presence of EphA2 served as a positive control. The primary antibody was replaced with non-immune mouse serum IgG to serve as a negative control. All slides were viewed under an E200 microscope (Nikon, Tokyo, Japan). Sections were quantified over ten randomly selected fields of view. Positive unit (PU) assessed by the QW550 image analysis system (Leica, Wetzlar, German) was used to describe the EphA2 expression [19, 20]. The formula was $PU = 100\ (Ga - Gb)/Gmax$. Ga and Gb were the average gray scale of positive staining and background, respectively. Gmax was the maximum gray scale of image analytical system.

Quantitative RT-PCR

Total RNA was extracted from the fresh Fallopian tube samples using Trizol total RNA extraction reagent (Takara, Dalian, China). Agarose gel electrophoresis was used to ascertain the quality of the RNA products by the presence of 28S rRNA, 18S rRNA and 5S rRNA bands, with a 2:1 ratio of 28S rRNA to 18S rRNA. cDNA was reverse transcribed from the extracted RNA using RT kit (Takara, Dalian, China). The primers used for EphA2 were 5′-AAGACCCTGGCTGACTTT-3′ (forward) and 5′-GTTCACCTGGTCCTTGAGT-3′ (reverse), while the primers for 18sRNA were 5′-CCTGGATACCGCAGCT AGGA-3′ (forward) and 5′-CCTGGATACCGCAGCTA GGA-3′ (reverse). Real time RT-PCR was carried out using an ABI 7300 real-time PCR system (ABI, Carlsbad, USA) with 5 μl diluted cDNA and 0.5 μl primers. The pro-grammed thermocycler included 40 cycles of predenatura-tion at 95 °C for 10 min, followed by denaturation at 95 °C for 15 s, annealing at 60 °C for 15 s, and extension at 72 °C for 30 s. All reactions were performed in triplicate. Relative quantification of EphA2 mRNA was calculated using the comparative Ct method ($\Delta\Delta Ct = \Delta Ct_{EphA2} - \Delta Ct_{18sRNA}$).

Western blot

The total protein content extracted from the fresh Fallopian tube samples was resolved by sodium dodecylsulfate-poly-acrylamide gel electrophoresis (SDS-PAGE), after which the proteins were transferred to nitrocellulose mem-branes. The membranes were blocked for 2 h in 10% bo-vine serum albumin (BSA) (DingguoChangsheng Biotechnology Co., Ltd., Beijing, China) at room temperature, followed by incubation at 4 °C overnight with the primary antibodies, rabbit anti-human polyclonal anti-bodies against EphA2 and Pho-EphA2 (1:1000; 6997S and 6347S; Cell signaling technology Co., Ltd., Boston, USA) and mouse anti-human monoclonal antibody against glyc-eraldehyde phosphate dehydrogenase (GAPDH) (1:1000; sc-59,540; Santa Cruz, California, USA). After washing, the membranes were then incubated for 1 h with the ap-propriate HRP-conjugated secondary antibodies, goat anti-rabbit IgG (1:800; A0208; Beyotime Biotechnology Co., Ltd., Shanghai, China) or rabbit anti-mouse IgG (1:1000; D031402; Dako Cytomatin, Glostrup, Denmark). Protein bands were identified using ECL (Pierce, Rock-ford, USA). The bands were semi-quantified using Bio-Rad Quantity One software. EphA2 was normalized to GADPH, and Pho-EphA2 was normalized to EphA2.

Statistical analysis

All statistical analyses were carried out using SPSS V.14. (SPSS, Chicago, USA). Differences among groups were determined by one-way analysis of variance (ANOVA) followed by Student–Newman–Keuls (SNK) multiple-comparison test. Results were presented as mean ± standard deviation (SD). P values < 0.05 were considered statistically significant.

Results

EphA2 expressions in human fallopian tube epithelia of non-pregnant women

Immunohistochemistry confirmed that EphA2 was present throughout the Fallopian tube epithelium, embracing the isthmus, the ampulla and the infundibulum. EphA2 showed stronger staining on the apical membrane of both the ciliated cells and the secretory cells as well as the cilia. The cytoplasm of the ciliated cells and the secretory cells showed positive staining of EphA2, but the staining intensities in the cytoplasm were weaker than those on the apical membranes (Fig. 1a and b). No staining was detected in the interstitial cells. No significant differences of the staining intensities could be found among different sites of the Fallopian tube during the same menstrual phase or among different menstrual phases at the same tubal region ($P > 0.05$) (Table 1).

Changes of EphA2 and pho-EphA2 in human fallopian tube epithelia of women with tubal pregnancy

Immunohistochemical staining confirmed the presence of EphA2 in the Fallopian tube epithelia of women with tubal pregnancy, including the implantation site and the non-implantation site (Fig. 2a, b and c). The strongest staining of EphA2 was noted in the implantation group (10.16 ± 3.59), compared with that in the non-implantation group (8.03 ± 2.49) and the control group (6.20 ± 2.72) ($P < 0.05$). With regard to the latter two groups, the EphA2 staining intensities were similar ($P > 0.05$) (Fig. 2d).

Western blot analysis revealed positive bands of EphA2 and Pho-EphA2 in both the implantation group and the non-implantation group (Fig. 3a). Similar to the results obtained from immunohistochemical assessment, the implantation group had a significantly increased level of EphA2 (2.08 ± 0.87) compared to that in the non-implantation group (1.41 ± 0.64) and the control group (1.44 ± 0.62) ($P < 0.05$). As for Pho-EphA2, a remarkably decreased level was seen in the implantation group (0.51 ± 0.25) compared to that in the non-implantation group (0.79 ± 0.37) and the control group (0.78 ± 0.35) ($P < 0.05$). However, both EphA2 and Pho-EphA2 levels did not differ between the non-implantation group and the control group ($P > 0.05$) (Fig. 3b).

EphA2 mRNA in human fallopian tube epithelia between non-pregnant women and women with tubal pregnancy

The EphA2 mRNA levels were similar among the implantation site, the non-implantation site and the Fallopian tube from non-pregnant women (control), with the corresponding values referring to 1.94 ± 0.51, 1.85 ± 0.74 and 2.02 ± 0.55, respectively ($P > 0.05$) (Fig. 4).

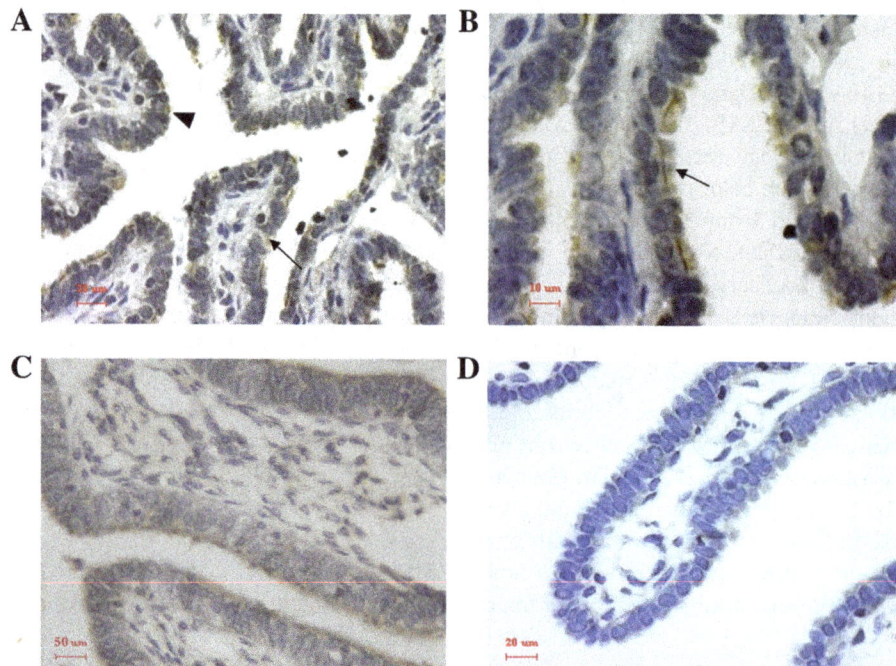

Fig. 1 EphA2 immunostaining (brown) on the Fallopian tube epithelium during normal menstrual cycle. **a** EphA2 was expressed on the apical membrane (triangle) and in the cytoplasm (arrow) of the tubal epithelial cells, including the ciliated cells and the secretory cells, while the staining intensities in the cytoplasm were weaker than those on the apical membranes. There was no staining evident in the interstitial cells. **b** EphA2 was present in the cilia of the ciliated cells (arrow). **c** Stronger stains were shown on the apical membranes of the tubal epithelial cells. **d** Negative control

Table 1 EhpA2 expressions in human Fallopian tube epithelia

Menstrual cycle phases	Exact menstrual cycle days	N	The Fallopian tube sites		
			Isthmus	Ampulla	infundibulum
Early-stage of proliferative phase	Days 1–5	8	4.57 ± 2.38	6.15 ± 2.23	5.16 ± 2.47
Mid- and late-stages of proliferative phase	Days 7–14	6	6.43 ± 3.02	7.02 ± 3.15	6.29 ± 2.36
Early-stage of secretive phase	Days 15–18	7	6.57 ± 3.29	6.54 ± 3.07	6.21 ± 2.98
Mid- and late-stages of secretive phase	Days 19–28	8	5.43 ± 2.59	5.91 ± 2.54	5.73 ± 2.65

Positive unit (PU) values were determined by immunohistochemistry technique, and data were presented as mean ± standard deviation (SD). $P > 0.05$, compared between the two groups in the same line

Discussion

To the best of our knowledge, this is the first study to compare the expressions of EphA2 in human Fallopian tube epithelia between non-pregnant women and women with tubal pregnancy. Acted like the endometrium, the morphology of the Fallopian tube epithelium could similarly respond to a menstrual cycle [21, 22]. Therefore, in the present study, the normal Fallopian tube samples were categorized according to the corresponding endometrial morphology, and EphA2 was revealed to widely

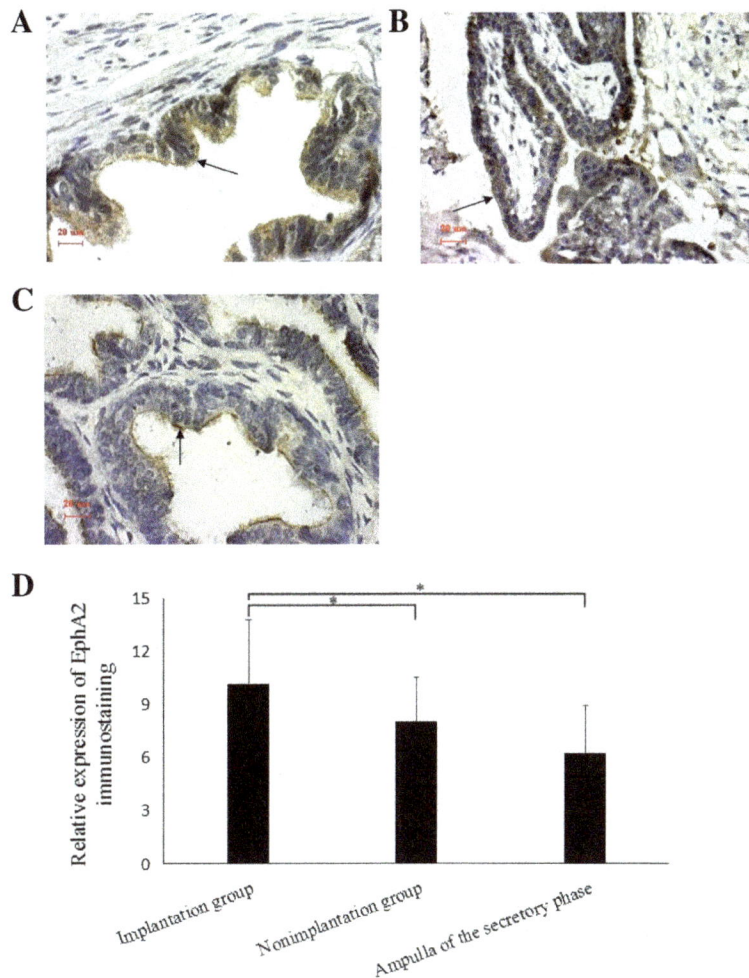

Fig. 2 EphA2 immunostaining (brown) on the Fallopian tube epithelium during tubal pregnancy. **a** EphA2 was present in the epithelial cells located in the implantation site of tubal pregnancy (arrow). **b** EphA2 was present in trophoblast cells found in the implantation site (arrow). **c** EphA2 was present in the non-implantation site of tubal pregnancy, and a stronger staining was evident on the cytomembrane (arrow) than that in the cytoplasm. **d** EphA2 expressions on the Fallopian tube epithelia with tubal pregnancy ($n = 17$) and the secretory Fallopian tube epithelia of normal controls ($n = 15$). EphA2 expression in the implantation group presented with the highest-level, compared with that in the non-implantation group and the control group ($P < 0.05$). EphA2 expressions in the latter two groups did not differ ($P > 0.05$)

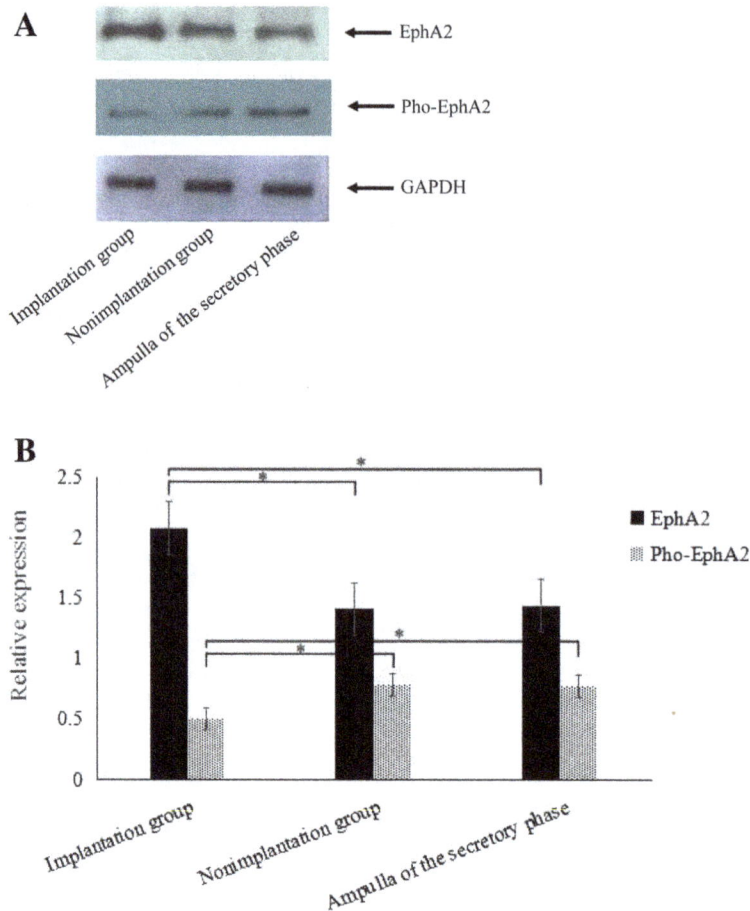

Fig. 3 Comparisons of EphA2 and Pho-EphA2 protein expression between the samples derived from the normal Fallopian tubes of the secretory phase (control) ($n = 12$) and the tubal pregnant tissues, which were further divided into the implantation group ($n = 14$) and the non-implantation group ($n = 14$). **a** Western blot showed positive bands of EphA2 and Pho-EphA2 in both the implantation and non-implantation groups of tubal pregnancy. **b** The highest EphA2 accompanied by the lowest Pho-EphA2 was detected in the implantation group, compared with that in the non-implantation group and the control group ($P < 0.05$). EphA2 and Pho-EphA2 protein expressions in samples of the latter two groups were similar ($P > 0.05$)

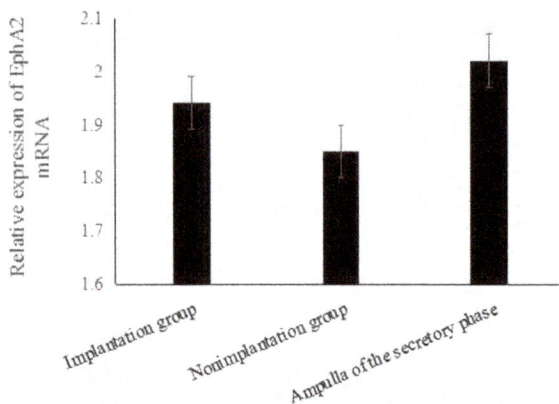

Fig. 4 EphA2 mRNA levels did not differ among the control group ($n = 12$), the implantation group ($n = 14$) and the non-implantation group ($n = 14$) ($P > 0.05$)

express in human Fallopian tube epithelium in a temporospatial-independent manner. An increased EphA2 accompanied by a decreased Pho-EphA2 was noted in the Fallopian tube epithelium with tubal pregnancy. EphA2 activation is autophosphorylation-dependent and the elevated Pho-EphA2, induced by EphA2 activation, could attenuate the cell adhesion activity of human Fallopian tube epithelial cells [16]. Combined with the present data, it is speculated that the aberrant EphA2 in the Fallopian tube epithelium with tubal pregnancy, as indicated by a decreased ratio of Pho-EphA2 over EphA2, may unexpectedly enhance cell adhesion activity the of Fallopian tube epithelial cells, leading to a mis-contact between the Fallopian tube epithelium and the embryo.

Investigation of pathological events occurring within the Fallopian tube necessitates considerations of the tubal microenvironment, of which the homeostasis is largely regulated by the molecules expressed on the Fallopian tube epithelium. Tubal pregnancy is currently accepted to be a direct consequence of molecular causes, considering that molecules capable of mediating cell adhesion have been confirmed to play a critical role in the pathogenesis of tubal pregnancy [23]. Eph receptor tyrosine kinases as well as their ligands, ephrins, are important regulators in cell-to-cell interaction and have been proven to play crucial roles in cell migration and adhesion during embryonic development in mammals [24]. EphA2 is abundant in human endometrial epithelial cells and its ligand ephrin is expressed in the blastocysts. A previous study revealed that the Eph-ephrin A system could regulate the initial embryo-maternal contact during the cross-talk period that preceded embryo implantation in the endometrium [14]. Similar regulatory mechanism may exist in the process of tubal implantation. However, evidence pertaining to the role of EphA2 in tubal pregnancy is scarce. The present study revealed that EphA2 was presented in both the ciliated and secretory cells of the Fallopian tube epithelia, and a temporospatial-independent pattern of EphA2 expression was noted. The levels of EphA2 in the Fallopian tube epithelia remained unchanged throughout the whole menstrual cycle, irrespective of menstrual phase or Fallopian tube region. The morphology and physiology of the Fallopian tube epithelium, including the ciliated and secretory cells, can be regulated by sex hormones fluctuating with the menstrual cycle [21]. Such a temporospatial-independent pattern may, in a sense, imply that sex hormones have no impact on EphA2 expression in the Fallopian tube epithelium.

It is well-recognized that overexpression of EphA2 is merely presented in malignant cells, but in non-transformed epithelial cells, EphA2 displays a relatively low level of expression [25–27]. Similar to this pattern, EphA2 was noted to be less abundant in the normal Fallopian tube epithelial cells in contrast to a significant increase in those from women with tubal pregnancy. One possible explanation for this phenomenon may be that EphA2 and its regulatory mechanism are initiated improperly under certain pathological conditions. Moreover, EphA2 is reported to not only function as a marker in transformed cells, but also possess the property to aggravate the malignant progression. Overexpression of EphA2 in non-transformed mammary epithelial cells is sufficient to promote a malignant phenotype [27]. Thus, we tended to speculate that the overexpression of EphA2 presented in the Fallopian tube epithelium may represent its active participation in tubal pregnancy via increasing the cell adhesion activity of the Fallopian tube epithelial cells but not only a simple result caused by tubal implantation.

An increased level of EphA2 was shown in the implantation group compared with that in the non-implantation group and the control group by western blot. However, it

seemed a paradox that we failed to find any discrepancy in EphA2 mRNA in the Fallopian tube samples among these three groups. Previous studies concerning the linkage between EphA2 and malignant tumors indicated that an elevated EphA2 found in malignant tumors was a result of deficient phosphorylation of EphA2 itself, leading to the consequent blockage of EphA2 degradation. In other words, insufficient Pho-EphA2 could accordingly give rise to an excessive storage of EphA2 [28, 29]. This conclusion may shed some light on the present data. The presence of increased EphA2 was accompanied by a decrease in Pho-EphA2, implying that the homeostasis of EphA2 in the Fallopian tube epithelium was hampered during tubal pregnancy, and the increased level of EphA2 may occur on the basis of insufficient phosphorylation of EphA2 itself. The activation of EphA2 is coupled with its autophosphorylation, characterized by an elevated ratio of Pho-EphA2 over EphA2, which could attenuate the cell adhesion activity of the Fallopian tube epithelial cells [16]. In the present study, a decreased ratio of Pho-EphA2 over EphA2 was detected in the implantation site of the Fallopian tube epithelium. We hypothesized that this may disclose an inactivated state of EphA2, which would on the contrary unexpectedly enhance the cell adhesion activity of the Fallopian tube epithelium. Thereafter, a false recognition between fetus and mother may be evoked to take place within the specific site of the Fallopian tube epithelium.

Ciliary motion is closely associated with female fecundity by regulating the processes of ovum pickup and transport [30]. Altered activity of cilia was reported to play a pivotal role in the pathogenesis of tubal pregnancy, based on the fact that women presenting with decreased cilia consequently suffered from tubal pregnancy [31]. EphA2/Ephrin-A1 signaling could attenuate cell adhesion activity of the Fallopian tube epithelial cells [16]. EphA2 was shown in the cilia of the tubal ciliated cells, suggesting a possibility that EphA2 may have some implications in the modulation of ciliary activity by regulating cell adhesion. However, the precise mechanisms about how the inactivated EphA2, characterized in the present study as an increased ratio of EphA2 over Pho-EphA2, influenced the ciliary motion still need to be further elucidated.

There are still certain limitations in the present study we need to take into consideration. Firstly, there were a limited number of samples included in this study which may weaken the strength of our evidence. Secondly, there were some age differences between non-pregnant women and women with tubal pregnancy since it is difficult to obtain Fallopian tube specimens from normal young non-pregnant women for ethical reasons. Lastly, Fallopian tube samples from women with tubal pregnancy can only be collected after an implantation event has occurred, making it difficult to directly identify the causal linkage between EphA2 and tubal pregnancy.

Many efforts have been made to clarify the mechanisms responsible for EphA2 activation during pathological events, yet there is still largely unexplored [32–34]. EphA2 activation can suppress tumor cell growth and hence EphA2 has been established as a therapeutic target for malignant tumors by hindering the progression of tumor invasion [35]. Known to be one of the key molecules responsible for regulating cell adhesion activity, it is plausible to assume that EphA2 activation and its downstream signaling could also be established as a molecular target in medical therapy for tubal pregnancy by decreasing cell adhesion activity of the Fallopian tube epithelial cells to avoid the mis-recognition at the maternal-fetal interface.

Conclusions

In conclusion, we have demonstrated that EphA2 is expressed in human Fallopian tube epithelium in a temporospatial-independent manner. EphA2 and its phosphorylation-dependent regulatory mechanism seem to be activated only under pathological conditions. The presence of a reduced Pho-EphA2 accompanied by an elevated EphA2, a state that may be recognized as EphA2 inactivation, maybe involved in the molecular pathogenesis of tubal pregnancy through up-regulating cell adhesion activity of the Fallopian tube epithelial cells. A better understanding of EphA2 and its signal pathways is of significance to illustrate the molecular pathogenesis of tubal pregnancy. Further investigations with larger samples are necessary to complement our present study.

Abbreviations

BSA: Bovine serum albumin; DAB: Diaminobenzidine; EphA2: Erythropoietin-producing hepatocellular receptor A2; GAPDH: Glyceraldehyde phosphate dehydrogenase; HRP: Horse radish peroxidase; PBS: Phosphate-buffered saline; Pho-EphA2: Phosphorylated EphA2; PU: Positive unit; qRT-PCR: Quantitative reverse transcription-polymerase chain reaction; SDS-PAGE: Sodium dodecylsulfate-polyacrylamide gel electrophoresis

Acknowledgments

We would like to thank Dr. Ling-Juan Wu and Dr. Richard Daniel, CBCB, Newcastle University, UK, for critical reading of this manuscript.

Authors' contributions

HJ and XYY contributed equally to this study. HJ, XYY and WJZ contributed to the conception and design of this study. XYY acquired the data. HJ and XYY performed the data analysis. All authors assisted in interpretation of data. HJ drafted the manuscript and WJZ revised it critically. All authors read and gave final approval of the manuscript.

Competing interests

The authors declare that they have no competing interests.

Author details

[1]Department of Reproductive Endocrinology, Longgang District Maternal and Child Healthcare Hospital, 6# Ailong Road, Longgang Central District, Shenzhen City 518172, People's Republic of China. [2]Institute of Reproductive Immunology, College of Life Science and Technology, Jinan University, 601# Huangpu Da Dao Xi, Guangzhou City 510632, People's Republic of China.

References

1. Shaw JL, Dey SK, Critchley HO, Horne AW. Current knowledge of the aetiology of human tubal ectopic pregnancy. Hum Reprod Update. 2010;16(4):432–44.
2. Brito LR, Guedes Neto EP, Furich DG, Savaris RF. MUC1 (VPM654 and EPR1023) expression in mucosa of fallopian tubes with ectopic pregnancy is altered. Appl Immunohistochem Mol Morphol. 2016;24(8):569–74.
3. Zhang JR, Li SD, Wu XP. Eutopic or ectopic pregnancy: a competition between signals derived from the endometrium and the fallopian tube for blastocyst implantation. Placenta. 2009;30(10):835–9.
4. Bowen JA, Hunt JS. The role of integrins in reproduction. Proc Soc Exp Biol Med. 2000;223(4):331–43.
5. Makrigiannakis A, Karamouti M, Petsas G, Makris N, Nikas G, Antsaklis A. The expression of receptivity markers in the fallopian tube epithelium. Histochem Cell Biol. 2009;132(2):159–67.
6. Utreras E, Ossandon P, Acuna-Castillo C, Varela-Nallar L, Muller C, Arraztoa JA, Cardenas H, Imarai M. Expression of intercellular adhesion molecule 1 (ICAM-1) on the human oviductal epithelium and mediation of lymphoid cell adherence. J Reprod Fertil. 2000;120(1):115–23.
7. Carter N, Nakamoto T, Hirai H, Hunter T. EphrinA1-induced cytoskeletal reorganization requires FAK and p130(cas). Nat Cell Biol. 2002;4(8):565–73.
8. Davy A, Aubin J, Soriano P. Ephrin-B1 forward and reverse signaling are required during mouse development. Genes Dev. 2004;18(5):572–83.
9. Zhao C, Irie N, Takada Y, Shimoda K, Miyamoto T, Nishiwaki T, Suda T, Matsuo K. Bidirectional ephrinB2-EphB4 signaling controls bone homeostasis. Cell Metab. 2006;4(2):111–21.
10. Lim BK, Matsuda N, Poo MM. Ephrin-B reverse signaling promotes structural and functional synaptic maturation in vivo. Nat Neurosci. 2008;11(2):160–9.
11. Nasreen N, Mohammed KA, Lai Y, Antony VB. Receptor EphA2 activation with ephrinA1 suppresses growth of malignant mesothelioma (MM). Cancer Lett. 2007;258(2):215–22.
12. Lema Tome CM, Palma E, Ferluga S, Lowther WT, Hantgan R, Wykosky J, Debinski W. Structural and functional characterization of monomeric EphrinA1 binding site to EphA2 receptor. J Biol Chem. 2012;287(17):14012–22.
13. Goldman-Wohl D, Greenfield C, Haimov-Kochman R, Ariel I, Anteby EY, Hochner-Celnikier D, Farhat M, Yagel S. Eph and ephrin expression in normal placental development and preeclampsia. Placenta. 2004;25(7):623–30.
14. Fujii H, Tatsumi K, Kosaka K, Yoshioka S, Fujiwara H, Fujii S. Eph-ephrin a system regulates murine blastocyst attachment and spreading. Dev Dyn. 2006;235(12):3250–8.
15. Yang Y, Min J. Effect of ephrin-A1/EphA2 on invasion of trophoblastic cells. J Huazhong Univ Sci Technolog Med Sci. 2011;31(6):824–7.
16. Yang XY, Zhu WJ, Jiang H. Activation of erythropoietin-producing hepatocellular receptor A2 attenuates cell adhesion of human fallopian tube epithelial cells via focal adhesion kinase dephosphorylation. Mol Cell Biochem. 2012;361(1–2):259–65.
17. Lam PM, Briton-Jones C, Cheung CK, Leung SW, Cheung LP, Haines C. Increased messenger RNA expression of vascular endothelial growth factor and its receptors in the implantation site of the human oviduct with ectopic gestation. Fertil Steril. 2004;82(3):686–90.
18. Noyes RW, Hertig AT, Rock J. Dating the endometrial biopsy. Am J Obstet Gynecol. 1975;122(2):262–3.

19. Murray TJ, Fowler PA, Abramovich DR, Haites N, Lea RG. Human fetal testis: second trimester proliferative and steroidogenic capacities. J Clin Endocrinol Metab. 2000;85(12):4812–7.

20. Harrison JL, Adam CL, Brown YA, Wallace JM, Aitken RP, Lea RG, Miller DW. An immunohistochemical study of the localization and developmental expression of ghrelin and its functional receptor in the ovine placenta. Reprod Biol Endocrinol. 2007;5:25.

21. Zhu J, Xu Y, Rashedi AS, Pavone ME, Kim JJ, Woodruff TK, Burdette JE. Human fallopian tube epithelium co-culture with murine ovarian follicles reveals crosstalk in the reproductive cycle. Mol Hum Reprod. 2016;22(11):756–67.

22. Bauersachs S, Rehfeld S, Ulbrich SE, Mallok S, Prelle K, Wenigerkind H, Einspanier R, Blum H, Wolf E. Monitoring gene expression changes in bovine oviduct epithelial cells during the oestrous cycle. J Mol Endocrinol. 2004;32(2):449–66.

23. Kemp B, Kertschanska S, Kadyrov M, Rath W, Kaufmann P, Huppertz B. Invasive depth of extravillous trophoblast correlates with cellular phenotype: a comparison of intra- and extrauterine implantation sites. Histochem Cell Biol. 2002;117(5):401–14.

24. Fujiwara H, Yoshioka S, Tatsumi K, Kosaka K, Satoh Y, Nishioka Y, Egawa M, Higuchi T, Fujii S. Human endometrial epithelial cells express ephrin A1: possible interaction between human blastocysts and endometrium via Eph-ephrin system. J Clin Endocrinol Metab. 2002;87(12):5801–7.

25. Coffman KT, Hu M, Carles-Kinch K, Tice D, Donacki N, Munyon K, Kifle G, Woods R, Langermann S, Kiener PA, Kinch MS. Differential EphA2 epitope display on normal versus malignant cells. Cancer Res. 2003;63(22):7907–12.

26. Kinch MS, Carles-Kinch K. Overexpression and functional alterations of the EphA2 tyrosine kinase in cancer. Clin Exp Metastasis. 2003;20(1):59–68.

27. Walker-Daniels J, Hess AR, Hendrix MJC, Kinch MS. Differential regulation of EphA2 in normal and malignant cells. Am J Pathol. 2003;162(4):1037–42.

28. Miao H, Burnett E, Kinch M, Simon E, Wang B. Activation of EphA2 kinase suppresses integrin function and causes focal-adhesion-kinase dephosphorylation. Nat Cell Biol. 2000;2(2):62–9.

29. Brantleysieders DM, Zhuang G, Hicks D, Fang WB, Hwang Y, Cates JM, Coffman K, Jackson D, Bruckheimer E, Muraokacook RS. The receptor tyrosine kinase EphA2 promotes mammary adenocarcinoma tumorigenesis and metastatic progression in mice by amplifying ErbB2 signaling. J Clin Invest. 2008;118(1):64–78.

30. Noreikat K, Wolff M, Kummer W, Kolle S. Ciliary activity in the oviduct of cycling, pregnant, and muscarinic receptor knockout mice. Biol Reprod. 2012;86(4):120.

31. Lyons RA, Saridogan E, Djahanbakhch O. The reproductive significance of human fallopian tube cilia. Hum Reprod Update. 2006;12(4):363–72.

32. Dohn M, Jiang J, Chen X. Receptor tyrosine kinase EphA2 is regulated by p53-family proteins and induces apoptosis. Oncogene. 2001;20(45):6503–15.

33. Kikawa KD, Vidale DR, Van Etten RL, Kinch MS. Regulation of the EphA2 kinase by the low molecular weight tyrosine phosphatase induces transformation. J Biol Chem. 2002;277(42):39274–9.

34. Saito T, Masuda N, Miyazaki T, Kanoh K, Suzuki H, Shimura T, Asao T, Kuwano H. Expression of EphA2 and E-cadherin in colorectal cancer: correlation with cancer metastasis. Oncol Rep. 2004;11(3):605–11.

35. Noblitt LW, Bangari DS, Shukla S, Mohammed S, Mittal SK. Immunocompetent mouse model of breast cancer for preclinical testing of EphA2-targeted therapy. Cancer Gene Ther. 2005;12(1):46–53.

10

The preclinical evaluation of immunocontraceptive vaccines based on canine zona pellucida 3 (cZP3) in a mouse model

Ying Wang, Yijie Li, Beibei Zhang and Fuchun Zhang[*]

Abstract

Background: Stray dogs are the reservoirs and carriers of rabies and are definitive hosts of echinococcosis. To control the overpopulation of stray dogs, zona pellucida 3 (ZP3), a primary receptor for sperm, is a potential antigen for developing contraceptive vaccines.

To enhance the immune responses and contraceptive effects of canine ZP3 (cZP3), dog gonadotropin-releasing hormone (GnRH) and a T cell epitope of chicken ovalbumin (OVA) were selected to construct two fusion proteins with cZP3, ovalbumin-GnRH-ZP3 (OGZ) and ovalbumin-ZP3 (OZ), and their contraceptive effects were evaluated in mice.

Methods: The synthesized DNA sequences of *OGZ* and *OZ* were cloned into plasmid pET-28a respectively. The fusion proteins OGZ and OZ were identified by SDS-PAGE and Western blot. Mice were immunized with OGZ, OZ and cZP3, and the infertility rates were monitored. Mice immunized with mouse ZP3 (mZP3) or adjuvant alone were used as positive control and negative control, respectively. cZP3- and GnRH-specific antibodies (Abs) were detected by ELISA. The bindings of the Abs to oocytes were detected by indirect immunofluorescence assay. The paraffin sections of mice ovaries were observed under microscope for analyzing pathological characteristics.

Results: SDS-PAGE and Western blot analyses showed that the two fusion proteins OGZ and OZ were correctly expressed. ELISA results showed that OGZ vaccine induced both cZP3- and GnRH-specific Abs, and OZ vaccine induced cZP3-specific Ab, which lasted for up to 168 days. The levels of follicle stimulating hormone (FSH) and estradiol (E2) in sera were significantly decreased in OGZ immunized mice. Indirect immunofluorescence results showed that Abs induced by cZP3 and mZP3 could bind to the mouse ZP and dog ZP each other. Compared with the adjuvant group, all vaccine immunized groups significantly decreased the fertility rate and mean litter size. Interestingly, the fertility rate in OGZ-immunized group is the lowest, and only 1 mouse out of 10 mice is fertile. Histological analysis of murine ovarian sections indicated that most of the infertile mice in the immunized groups lacked mature follicles as well as accompanied by inflammatory infiltration. Meanwhile, immunization with OGZ decreased the number of corpora lutea in the infertile mice.

Conclusions: The fusion protein OGZ resulted in the lowest fertility rate and the least mean litter size in the immunized mice. OGZ might be a promising antigen for developing a new contraceptive vaccine for stray dog controlling.

Keywords: Dog, Zona pellucida 3, GnRH, Fusion protein, Contraceptive vaccine

* Correspondence: fuchunzhangxju@126.com
Xinjiang Key Laboratory of Biological Resources and Genetic Engineering, College of Life Science and Technology, Xinjiang University, 666, Shengli Road, Urumqi 830046, China

Background

Nowadays, the overpopulation of stray dogs has seriously affected peoples' daily lives as well as city's environmental sanitation. Stray dogs in Xinjiang, China, are the reservoirs and carriers of rabies, and they are definitive hosts of echinococcosis. Therefore, it is urgent to develop effective contraceptive vaccines to control stray dog's population. Zona pellucida 3 (ZP3), as the primary receptor of sperm on egg cell and an inducer of the acrosome reaction, plays a key role during fertilization [1–4]. Extensive studies have demonstrated that contraceptive vaccines based on ZP3 can limit the population of mice [5–7], koalas [8], gray kangaroos [9], and rabbits [10]. Recombinant canine ZP3 (cZP3) can also induce infertility in female dogs [11]. In this study, cZP3 of 35~350aa containing the major B-cell epitopes was selected as the basic antigen for immunocontraception.

To enhance the contraceptive efficacy of cZP3, canine gonadotropin-releasing hormone (GnRH) was selected as another antigen. GnRH plays an important role in vertebrate fertilization. It is a decapeptide produced by hypothalamus. Immunization with GnRH can produce contraceptive effects in both males and females [12–14]. Several commercial GnRH-based contraceptive vaccines have been developed, and these vaccines appear to have different functions in different animal species [15–17]. Thus, canine GnRH was selected as the second antigen for preparing a fusion protein vaccine. In addition, a T-cell epitope (QAVHAAHAEINE) of chicken ovalbumin (OVA) was added to the N -terminal of the fusion protein to further enhance the immune responses [18].

In this study, we chose cZP3 as the basic antigen for constructing two fusion proteins that encompassed a T cell epitope of OVA and, or GnRH. The contraceptive efficacy of the two fusion proteins were evaluated in female mice. The related Ab levels and the binding of Abs on ZP3 of oocytes were conducted to explain the mechanisms underlying the contraceptive effect.

Methods

Animals

All animal experiments in this study were approved by the Animal Ethics Committee of Xinjiang University. Treatment and care of animals were conducted strictly according to the guidelines, and all efforts were made to minimize damages to the animals. All mice were maintained under constant room temperature (21 ± 2 °C) with a photoperiod of D 12: 12. Mice had free access to food and water. No mice died during the experiments.

Construction, expression and purification of the fusion proteins

Two recombinant fragments *OGZ* and *OZ* were constructed. For *OGZ*, canine GnRH (G) and cZP3 (23~

350 aa) (Z) nucleotide sequences were retrieved from GenBank (XP_850859.2 and NM 001003224.1). A T-cell epitope of chicken ovalbumin (O) was added to the 5′-end of the recombinant fragment. A flexible linker (Gly-Gly-Gly-Gly-Ser) (GGGS) was inserted to separate each component in the fusion protein (Fig. 1a). *OZ* recombinant fragment was constructed same as OGZ except for missing the GnRH and the second GGGS (Fig. 1a). The synthesized DNA sequences were codon-optimized for *E. coli* expression, and the expressed fusion proteins were named as OGZ and OZ, respectively. The nucleic acid fragments of *OGZ* and *OZ*, were digested with *Eco*R I and *Bam*H I, and cloned into pET28a vector respectively. The recombinant plasmids pET28a-OGZ and pET28a-OZ were transformed into *E. coli* BL21 (DE3) cells respectively. The expressional conditions were optimized by testing different combination of factors, including isopropyl β-D-1-thiogalactopyranoside (IPTG) concentration (0.1, 0.3, 0.5, 0.8, 1, 1.5 and 2 mmol/L), induction time (4 h, 6 h and 8 h) and temperature (25 °C, 30 °C and 37 °C). Finally, the optimal induction conditions in 1 L LB medium for OGZ or OZ expression was as follows: 10 mL overnight culture was inoculated into 1 L LB medium and cultured at 37 °C with shaking at 250 r/min. When OD_{600} reached between 0.4~0.6, 1 mM IPTG was added into the culture. The culture was continually incubated at 37 °C for 4 h. Cell pellets were harvested by centrifugation at 5000 r/min for 15 min and washed once with phosphate buffered saline (PBS). Then, the pellets were re-suspended in PBS (100 mg/2 mL, containing 20 μL protease inhibitor cocktail) and sonicated in an ice bath for 20 min at 5 s intervals. The cell lysate was harvested by centrifugation at 10000 r/min for 15 min, and the pellets were resuspended in 20 mL binding buffer (20 mM Tris-HCl, pH 7.9, containing 6 M urea, 0.5 M NaCl, and 5 mM imidazole). After spinning at 10000 r/min for 20 min, the filtrated supernatant was passed through a nickel-affinity chromatography column three times and washed 20 times with a column volume of binding buffer. The fusion proteins were eluted by elution buffer (500 mM imidazole). After ultrafiltration, protein concentrations were determined using a BCA Protein Assay Kit (Thermo).

Western blot analysis of the fusion proteins OGZ and OZ

The antisera against cZP3 (23~350 aa) and GnRH were raised respectively by one subcutaneous and two intra-peritoneal injections in female mice.

The transformed *E. coli* cells were induced with IPTG to express OGZ and OZ respectively. The whole cells were collected by centrifugation at 10000 r/min for 1 min and washed once with PBS. The pellets were dissolved in SDS-PAGE loading buffer and heated at 100 °C for 5 min. The samples were then separated on a 12% SDS-PAGE gel and transferred onto PVDF membranes separately. The membranes were blocked with 5% skim milk powder

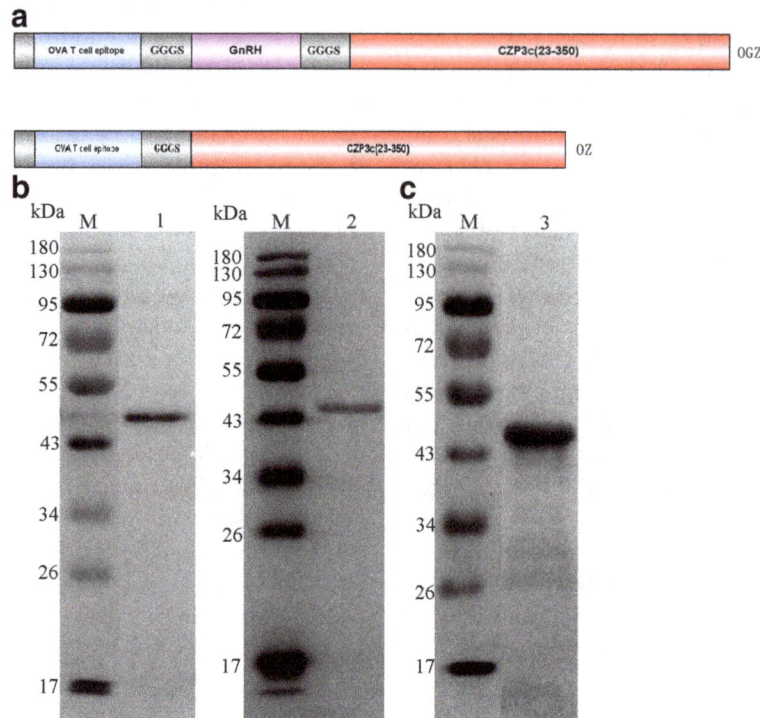

Fig. 1 Schematic representation and Western blot analysis of the fusion proteins OGZ and OZ. **a**. The main components of OGZ were T cell epitope of OVA, GnRH and cZP3. The main components of OZ were T cell epitope of OVA and cZP3. A flexible linker (GGGS) was inserted in between the components. **b**. OGZ and OZ reacted with antibodies (Abs) against cPZ3. Lane 1: OGZ, lane 2: OZ. **C**. OGZ reacted with Abs against GnRH. Lane 3: OGZ. Lane M: protein molecular weight markers

dissolved in 0.5% Tween-20 in TBS pH 7.9 (TBST) at 4 °C overnight. The membranes were then probed with different anti-sera. For OGZ and OZ, the membranes were probed with Abs against cZP3. OGZ was also probed with Abs against GnRH. After incubation at 4 °C for 2 h, the membranes were washed with TBST three times. Horseradish (HRP)-conjugated goat anti-mouse IgG was used as a second Ab. Color was developed with 3, 3′-diaminobenzidine (DAB). All reactions were terminated by adding distilled water.

Mouse immunization
Fifty female BALB/c mice (6~ 8 weeks old) were purchased from Xinjiang Medical University and were randomly divided into five groups ($n = 10$). Immunization with OGZ, OZ and cZP3 (23~ 350 aa) was designated as the antigen-specific groups. Immunization with mouse ZP3(mZP3, 21~ 361 aa) was designated as positive control. cZP3 and mZP3 proteins were previously expressed and purified in our laboratory. Freund's adjuvant injection was set as a negative control.

After the protein was emulsified with Freund's complete adjuvant, each mouse received 25 μg protein subcutaneously. The same amount of protein was given intraperitoneally as a booster dose on day 21 and 42 after administration of the first immunization. Serum

samples were collected from the retro-orbital on day 14, 35, 56, and 168 after the first immunization. 70 μL sera were collected from each mouse, and were stored at − 80 °C for later use.

Detection of the abs levels by enzyme linked immunosorbent assay (ELISA)
We detected the Ab levels of ZP3 and GnRH using ELISA. A ninety-six-well plate was coated with 100 μL ZP3 (4 μg/mL) and incubated at 4 °C overnight. The plate was blocked with blocking buffer (5% skim milk powder in PBST) at 37 °C for 1 h. After washing three times, the plate was incubated with serum (100 μL per well) diluted at 1:1000 in blocking buffer at 37 °C for 1 h. Then, the plate was incubated with the second Ab, HRP-conjugated goat anti-mouse IgG at a dilution of 1: 1000, at 37 °C for 1 h. TMB substrate solution (Thermo) (50 μl per well) was used for color development. After 15 min, the reaction was terminated by adding the same volume of 0.2 M H_2SO_4. Absorbance values were read at OD_{450} nm.

The GnRH Ab levels were detected as described above. The optimal coating concentration of GnRH was 15 μg/mL and the working concentration of the serum samples was 1:100 dilution as determined by chessboard assay.

Determination of the levels of FSH and E2 in the sera of OGZ immunized mice by ELISA

The levels of FSH and E2 in the mice sera of adjuvant and OGZ groups were determined respectively by sandwich and competitive ELISA according to the manufacturer's instructions (Elabscience, Wuhan, China). Serum samples were collected on day 14, 35 and 56 after the first immunization. The assay sensitivity was 1.56~ 100 ng/mL and 40~ 1400 pg/mL, respectively. The intra- and inter-assay of the variations for FSH and E2 was 10 and 15%, respectively.

Indirect immunofluorescence of mouse oocytes

Five 6-week-old female BALB/c mice were stimulated by intramuscular injection with 12 IU of pregnant mare serum gonadotrophin (PMSG, Ningbo Sansheng Pharamceutical, China). 46 h later, these mice were injected intramuscularly with 12 IU human chorionic gonadotropin (hCG, Ningbo SanSheng Pharamecutical, China). All the mice were sacrificed after 13 h of the injection, and the cumulus-oocyte complexes (COCs) were collected from the mice ampulla. After incubation with hyaluronidase (50 µg/mL) for 5 min, the denuded oocytes were obtained. The oocytes were blocked with blocking buffer (5% BSA in PBS) at 37 °C for 1 h, and then were transferred into the freshly diluted serum droplets (1:50) for 1 h. After the oocytes were washed several times with PBS, fluorescein isothiocyanate (FITC)-conjugated rabbit anti mouse IgG (1:200) was added, then the oocytes were incubated at 37 °C for 30 min. Finally, the oocytes were washed with PBS and observed under fluorescence microscope.

Indirect immunofluorescence of dog ovarian sections

For detecting whether the antisera of the OGZ- and OZ- immunized mice could bind to dog oocytes, we performed surgery and collected four ovaries from two Beagles. The ovaries were immediately fixed in 4% para-formaldehyde and kept at 4 °C for at least 24 h, and then were made into paraffin sections. The sections were blocked with PBS containing 10% normal rabbit sera at 37 °C for 1 h. Serum samples (from the mice of adjuvant, OGZ, OZ, mZP3 and cZP3 injection) were diluted with blocking buffer (1:50), and were added onto the sections, respectively, and kept at 4 °C overnight. The diluted FITC conjugated rabbit anti mouse IgG (1:200 in blocking buffer) was added as a second Ab. After washing, the paraffin sections were observed under fluorescence microscope.

Evaluation of the contraceptive effects in vivo

On day 56 after the primary immunization, mice in each group were divided into five cages (two mice per cage) and a healthy male mouse was put into each cage. The male mice were rotated in the cages every day. After 3 weeks, the male mouse was removed from the cage, and the litter size of each female mouse was counted. On day 168, the mating test was repeated.

Histological analysis

On day 210 after the first immunization, all of the mice were sacrificed. The ovaries from each mouse was obtained and fixed in 4% paraformaldehyde at 4 °C. After embedded with paraffin, the ovaries were cut into two consecutive sections at 5 µm thickness. The sections were stained with hematoxylin and eosin, and observed under microscope. Histopathological changes of the ovaries were graded 0 to 4 as previously described [19].

Statistical analysis

The Abs levels for FSH, E2 and GnRH were analyzed by one-way analysis of variance (one-way ANOVA) and Tukey's multiple comparison test. The Ab levels of ZP3 during the immunization were analyzed by two-way ANOVA. The correlation between the sera FSH concentration and the Ab levels of GnRH was analyzed using Pearson's correlarion coefficient. For analysis of the difference in mean litter size among each group, the data was firstly converted into square root of $x + 1$, then analyzed by one-way ANOVA and Tukey's multiple comparison test. The Ab levels and the mean litter size were presented as mean ± SEM. $P < 0.05$ was considered as significant.

Results

Purification and detection of the fusion proteins OGZ and OZ

Fusion protein OGZ was combined with canine GnRH (G), cZP3 (Z, 23~ 350 aa) and a T-cell epitope of chicken ovalbumin (O). Fusion protein OZ was combined with cZP3 (Z, 23~ 350 aa) and chicken OVA (O) (Fig. 1a). After these two proteins were expressed in *E.coli* by IPTG induction, and after proteins purification, the fusion protein OGZ and OZ showed a major band at 46 kDa and 44 kDa on SDS-PAGE gel respectively as expected (figure not shown). Western blot results confirmed these specific bands accordingly. Both OGZ and OZ could bind to the Abs against cZP3 (Fig. 1b). Besides, OGZ also bound to Abs against GnRH (Fig. 1c).

Fusion proteins induced high levels of abs against ZP3

From day 14 to day 56 after the first immunization the levels of the Ab against ZP3 in all proteins immunized mice were significantly higher than the adjuvant control group. The increase of the Ab levels was in a linear way with the time prolonging. On day 168 the Ab levels decreased greatly but still kept 5~ 10 fold of the adjuvant control (Fig. 2a). There was no significant difference among these protein groups. In addition, OGZ group could also generate high levels of Ab against GnRH and the levels also last

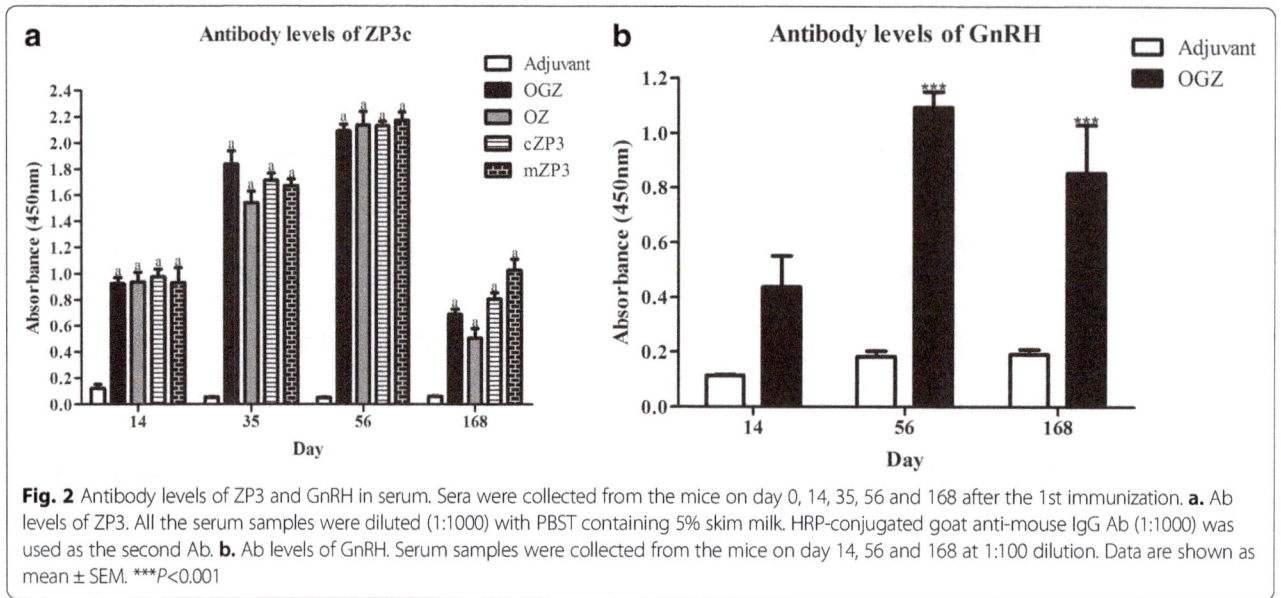

Fig. 2 Antibody levels of ZP3 and GnRH in serum. Sera were collected from the mice on day 0, 14, 35, 56 and 168 after the 1st immunization. **a.** Ab levels of ZP3. All the serum samples were diluted (1:1000) with PBST containing 5% skim milk. HRP-conjugated goat anti-mouse IgG Ab (1:1000) was used as the second Ab. **b.** Ab levels of GnRH. Serum samples were collected from the mice on day 14, 56 and 168 at 1:100 dilution. Data are shown as mean ± SEM. ***$P<0.001$

for 168 days (Fig. 2b). However, the levels of Ab against GnRH were not as high as that of ZP3.

Sera FSH and E2 levels were significantly decreased in OGZ group

The sera FSH and E2 levels in the OGZ group showed a gradual decline (Fig. 3a, b) after immunization, and for FSH it was almost undetectable on day 56 after the first immunization. The FSH concentration in the sera of OGZ group was negatively correlated with the Ab levels of GnRH (Fig. 3c) with a Pearson's correlation coefficient of − 0.6403.

Abs against fusion proteins could bind to the ZP matrix of mouse and dog

Indirect immunofluorescence assay of mice oocytes showed that the Abs against ZP3 in each vaccine immunization group could specifically bind to the ZP matrix of mice (Fig. 4a). Meanwhile the results of indirect immunofluorescence assay to dog ovarian sections suggested

the Abs against ZP3 in each vaccine group could react with the dog ZP matrix, but not with other cells in ovaries (Fig. 4b).

Immunization with OGZ and OZ both caused a decline in mice fertility

To detect the contraceptive effects of the fusion proteins, the OGZ and OZ immunized female mice were mated respectively with male mice for 3 weeks on day 56 after the first immunization. The results showed that both the fertility rate and litter size in OGZ group and OZ group decreased significantly compared to the adjuvant group, so did the mZP3 and cZP3 groups. The fertility rate decreased from 100% in the adjuvant group to 10% in OGZ group, 40% in mZP3 group and 50% in cZP3 and OZ groups (Table 1).

To detect how long the contraceptive efficacy of OGZ and OZ vaccines could last, the mating test was re-conducted on day 168. The results showed that the

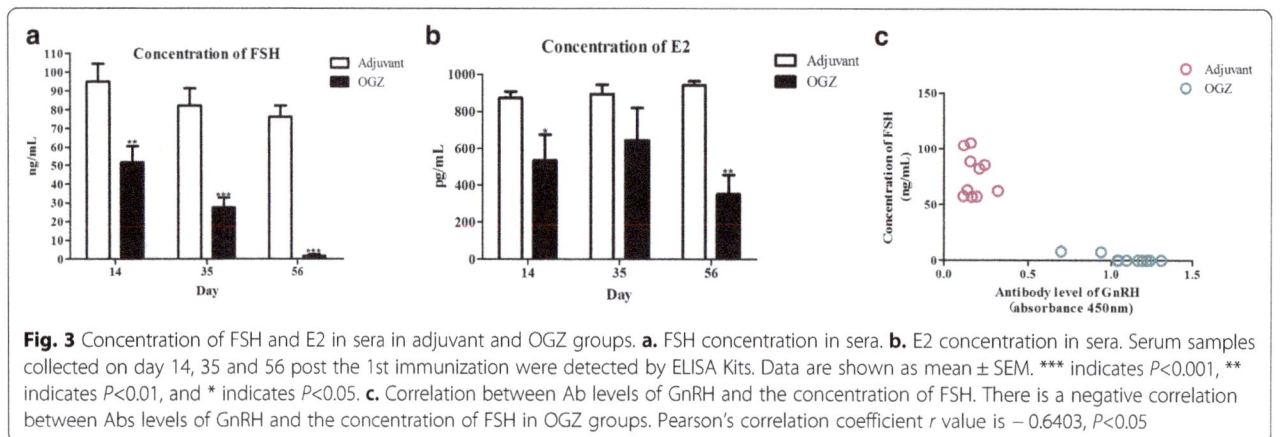

Fig. 3 Concentration of FSH and E2 in sera in adjuvant and OGZ groups. **a.** FSH concentration in sera. **b.** E2 concentration in sera. Serum samples collected on day 14, 35 and 56 post the 1st immunization were detected by ELISA Kits. Data are shown as mean ± SEM. *** indicates $P<0.001$, ** indicates $P<0.01$, and * indicates $P<0.05$. **c.** Correlation between Ab levels of GnRH and the concentration of FSH. There is a negative correlation between Abs levels of GnRH and the concentration of FSH in OGZ groups. Pearson's correlation coefficient r value is − 0.6403, $P<0.05$

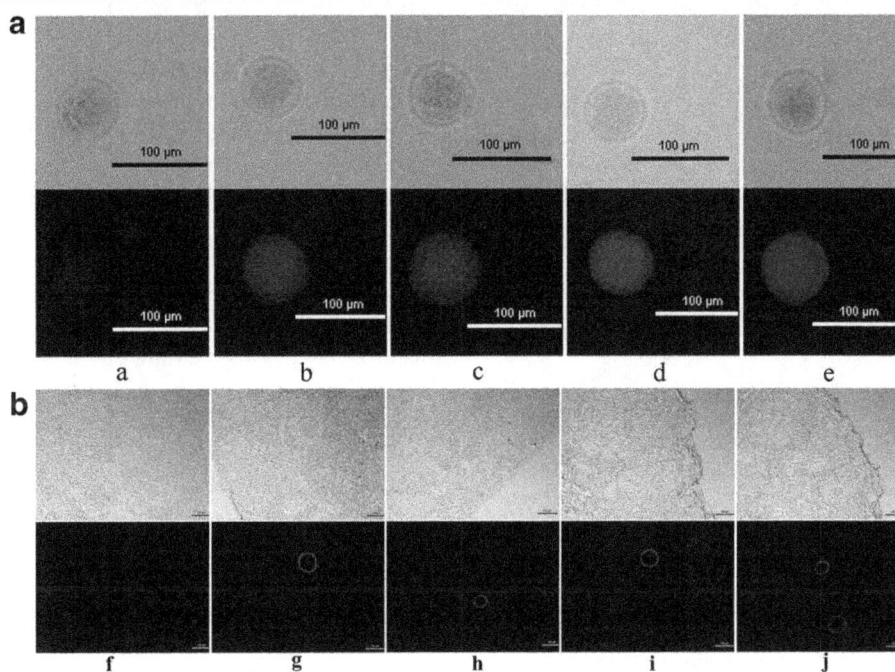

Fig. 4 Abs against ZP3 could react with mouse and dog ZP in the indirect immnofluorescence assay. **a**. Abs against ZP3 react with mouse oocytes. **a**, **b**, **c**, **d** and **e** represent adjuvant, OGZ, OZ, cZP3 and mZP3, respectively. **b**. Abs against ZP3 reacted with sections of dog ovaries. **f**, **g**, **h**, **i** and **j** represent the adjuvant, OGZ, OZ, cZP3 and mZP3, respectively. The top panel is in bright field, the bottom panel is in fluorescent field

fertility rate and litter size in each group increased slightly compared to the first mating, but still kept a significant decrease compared to the adjuvant group. The fertility rate decreased from 100% in the adjuvant group to 10% in the OGZ group and 50% in OZ, cZP3 and mZP3 groups (Table 2).

The average litter size in OZ group was 2.3, similar to the groups of mZP3 which was 2 and cZP3 which was 2.2, and all of them were very significantly lower than the

adjuvant group which was 7 (Table 1). The OGZ group had the least average litter size of 0.4 (out of 10 mice only 1 produced 4 pubs). The results in the second mating test showed similar effects (Table 2). These results suggested that these protein vaccines effectively decreased the litter size of the immunized mice, and OZ, cZP3 and mZP3 had similar moderate effect, while OGZ had very strong effect.

The scatter diagrams about the Ab levels of ZP3 and the litter size in each mouse (Fig. 5) showed that all of the

Table 1 Contraceptive effects of the recombinant proteins in the first mating test

Antigen	Fertility rate (%)[a]	Mean litter size[b]	Average Abs levels	P^c
Adjuvant	100% (10/10)	7 ± 0.516	0.050 ± 0.004[d]	
			0.183 ± 0.02[e]	
OGZ	10% (1/10)	0.4 ± 0.4	2.092 ±0 .162 [d]	***
			1.095 ± 0.056 [e]	
OZ	50% (5/10)	2.3 ± 0.883	2.138 ±0 .334 [d]	**
cZP3	50% (5/10)	2.2 ± 0.772	2.134 ±0 .103 [d]	**
mZP3	40% (4/10)	2 ± 0.907	2.215 ±0 .156 [d]	***

[a]Fertility rate: number of the fertile mice/total number of the mated mice in each group
[b]Mean litter size of mice: total number of pups in each group/total number of the mated mice in each group
[c]Mean litter size in each group vs adjuvant group;* represents $P < 0.05$; ** represents $P < 0.01$; *** represents $P < 0.005$
[d]Average Abs levels of cZP3
[e]Average Abs levels of GnRH

Table 2 Contraceptive effects of the recombinant proteins in the second mating test

Antigen	Fertility rate (%) [a]	Mean litter size [b]	Average Abs levels	P^c
Adjuvant	100% (10/10)	6.1 ± 0.924	0.058 ± 0.003 [d]	
			0.191 ± 0.018 [e]	
OGZ	10% (1/10)	0.2 ± 0.2	0.691 ± 0.039 [d]	***
			0.854 ± 0.176 [e]	
OZ	50% (5/10)	2.5 ± 0.86	0.506 ± 0.073 [d]	*
cZP3	50% (5/10)	2.6 ± 0.884	0.808 ± 0.047 [d]	*
mZP3	50% (5/10)	2.7 ± 0.920	1.028 ± 0.084 [d]	*

[a]Fertility rate: number of the fertile mice/total number of the mated mice in each group
[b]Mean litter size of mice: total number of the pups in each group/total number of the mated mice in each group
[c]Mean litter size in each group vs adjuvant group;* represents $P < 0.05$; ** represents $P < 0.01$;*** represents $P < 0.005$
[d]Average Abs levels of cZP3
[e]Average Abs levels of GnRH

mice in the protein groups had higher Ab levels than the adjuvant control, and the litter size was smaller than the adjuvant (Table 1 and Table 2). However, the difference in the litter size among the individuals in each group was great, for OZ, cZP3 and mZP3 groups, the range were 6, suggesting that random factors had influence on a mouse's litter size apart from the main factor of the contraceptive vaccine. This situation was even evidence in the adjuvant group (Fig. 5), the range was 11. Due to the data severely deviated from normal distribution, Pearson's correlation analysis were not applicable.

Immunization with OGZ and OZ led to pathological changes in mice ovaries

To investigate whether immunization with the fusion proteins could affect mice ovarian morphology, the mice ovaries were collected, and sections were made for observation. We found that, compared with the adjuvant group, most of the infertile mice immunized with protein vaccines had abnormal follicular development, which led to immature follicles. In additon, these ovaries were also accompanied by inflammatory cell infiltration in the atretic follicles and/or the growing and mature follicles. The number of corpora lutea in the infertile mice receiving OGZ also decreased. Most of the fertile mice in these protein immunization groups showed no significant changes in the number of corpora lutea (Fig. 6).

Discussion

In face of the overpopulation of stray dogs, developing a safe and effective contraceptive vaccine is in need. ZP3, due to the vital function in the fertilization process, is considered as a promising target for such a vaccine. In order to induce a stronger immune response, two recombinant fragments OGZ and OZ were constructed. The fusion proteins OGZ and OZ were correctly expressed in *E.coli*.

Both of the mature fragment of mZP3 and cZP3 induced strong immune responses in female mice and lead to infertility as expected. OGZ and OZ also induced strong

immune responses, there were no significant differences in the anti-ZP3 Ab levels among the protein immunization groups. Compared to cZP3, mZP3 encompassed all the epitopes on mice ZP matrix, however, it did not elicit the highest Ab level as predicted (Fig. 2a). This is probably because cZP3 has stronger immunogenicity than mZP3 to mouse and stimulated stronger immune responses [20]. This result suggested that in developing contraceptive vaccines for controlling mammalians heterologous ZP3 might be more prospective. Additionally, the anti-GnRH Ab level was lower than that of anti-ZP3 (Fig. 2b), and this was probably due to the differences in the coating antigen. The Ab levels detected by ELISA with fusion proteins as coating antigens are usually higher than synthetic peptides as coating antigens, and this difference is similar to the results of previous studies [21, 22].

The protein vaccines showed significant contraceptive effects on the immunized female mice. Both the fertility rate and litter size decreased significantly in comparing with the adjuvant group. The effect of OGZ was profound, in the first mating test, 9 out of the 10 mice gave no birth, the only fertilized one only produced 4 pubs which was lower than the average litter size which was 2~ 2.3 in the other ZP3 protein groups. These results suggested that OGZ vaccine not only blocked ZP3 but also blocked GnRH, thus led to the highest infertility rate (9/10) than OZ(5/10), cZP3(5/10) and mZP3(4/10).

The Abs against GnRH bind to GnRH to prevent GnRH from interacting with the receptors, which, in turn, disturb the hypothalamic-pituitray-gonad axis and inhibit downstream hormonal activities, such as the secretion of FSH and E2 [23, 24]. FSH stimulates the production of E2, and a decrease in FSH concentration could suppress the synthesis of E2. In this study, Abs against GnRH in the female mice were adequate for interacting with GnRH and resulting in the decrease of E2 concentration. Compared to adjuvant, the sera FSH and E2 levels in OGZ group were remarkably reduced (Fig. 3a, b). These results were similar to other studies in which immunization with GnRH caused a significant

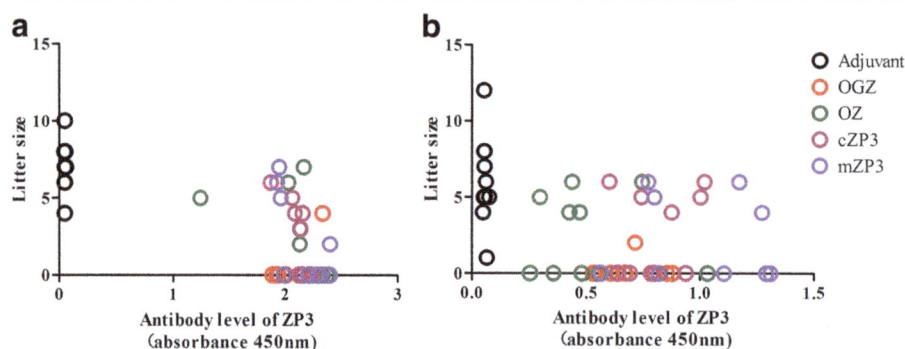

Fig. 5 Scatter diagram of the antibody levels of cZP3 in each mouse and the litter size of each mouse after the first mating (**a**) and the second mating (**b**)

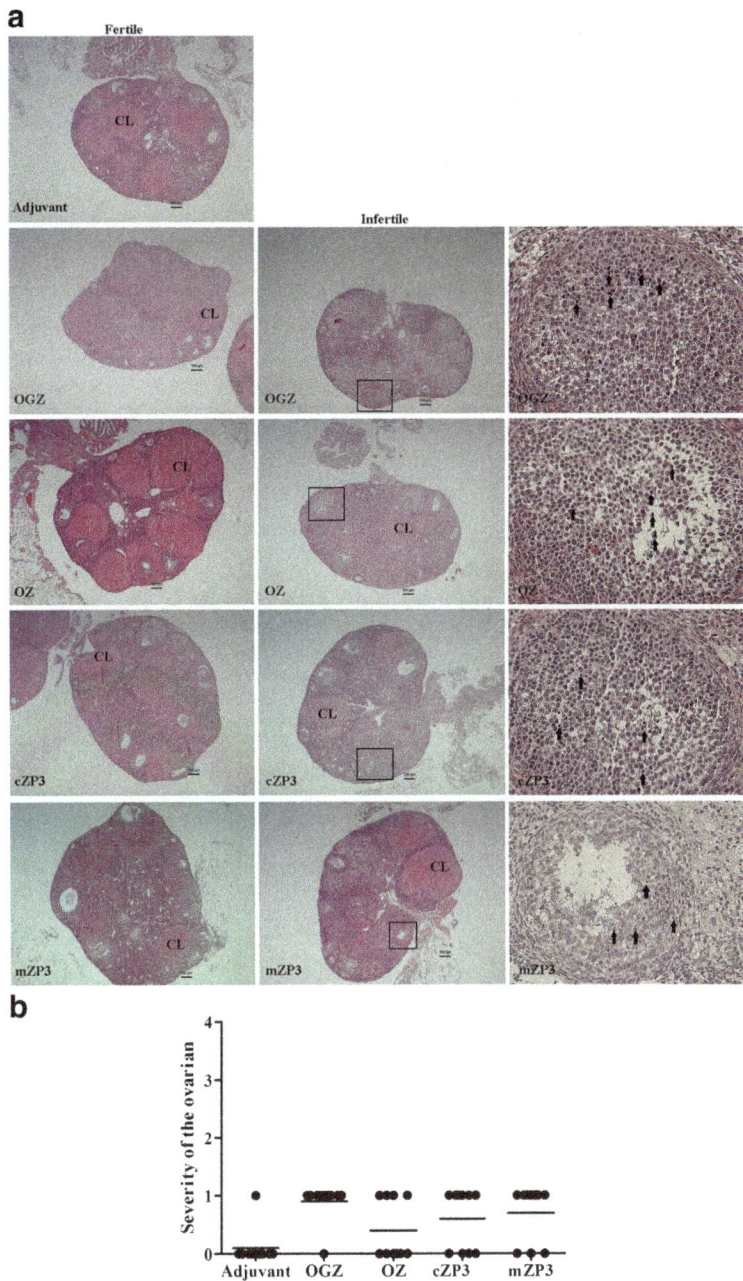

Fig. 6 Histological analysis of the ovaries of the mice immunized with different ZP3 vaccines. Mice ovaries were collected on day 210 after the first immunization. The paraffin sections were observed after HE staining. **a.** Histological analysis of the ovaries of the fertile and infertile mice in each group. The magnified(200×)image of the black box are on the right. Black arrows indicate inflammatory cell infiltration. CL represents corpus luteum. **b.** Severity of the ovarian lesions in different immunized groups

reduction in FSH and E2 concentration [21–27]. Lower concentration of FSH and E2 possibly resulted in ovary dysfunction and infertility.

The results of the indirect immunofluorescence assay showed that the Abs against cZP3 had the affinity to ZP matrix of mice and dogs. This may be attribute to the sequence similarity of cZP3 and mZP3, they shared 65% identity [28].

A large body of evidence indicates that ZP3 induces infertility via two mechanisms: (1) sufficient anti-ZP3 Abs bind to ZP matrix and block the sperm-egg interactions; (2) ovarian dysfunction mediated by inflammatory cell infiltration and anti-ZP3 Abs [29–34]. In this study, most of the infertile mice showed aberrant development of ovarian follicles, which had inflammatory cell infiltration and lack of mature follicles (Fig. 6a). The normal ovarian functions were interfered with Abs against ZP3 and/or inflammatory cells, which might lead to infertility. Our results agreed with this explanation.

Other studies report that ovaries receiving GnRH present a decrease in the number of corpora lutea in the infertile mice, and that lead to follicular dysplasia [24, 35–37]. Our results in OGZ group were in accord with those studies. The decrease in the number of corpora lutea and mature follicles was consistent with the decreases in sera FSH and E2 concentrations in the OGZ immunization group. These findings indicate that the Abs against cZP3 and GnRH worked together to lead to serious infertility with only 10% fertility rate and an average of 0.4 litter size in the OGZ group.

Conclusions

The results in this study showed that fusion protein OGZ had very stronger effect on reducing the fertility rate and litter size of the immunized mice than cZP3 and mZP3 by inducing high Abs levels of anti-ZP3 Abs and anti-GnRH Abs which not only blocked ZP3 but also blocked GnRH. OGZ immunization also caused pathological changes in ovary, which led to ovarian dysfunction and further increased infertility. Thus, the fusion protein OGZ could be a promising candidate for developing contraceptive vaccines for stray dogs controlling.

Acknowledgements
We would like to thank Prof Ji Ma for her assistance in statistical analysis.

Funding
The study was financially supported by grant from the Science and Technology projects aid to Xinjiang (No. 201591134). The funders had no role in study design, data collection and analysis, decision to publish and preparation of the manuscript.

Authors' contributions
YW and YJL designed this study. YW and BBZ performed the laboratory work. YW did the data analysis. YW and FCZ drafted and revised the manuscript. All authors have read and approved the final manuscript.

Competing interests
The authors declare that they have no competing interests.

References

1. Bansal P, Chakrabarti K, Gupta SK. Functional activity of human ZP3 primary sperm receptor resides toward its C- terminus. Biol Reprod. 2009;81(1):7–15.
2. Bleil JD, Wassarman PM. Mammalian sperm-egg interaction: indentification of a glycoprotein in mouse egg zonae pellucidae possedding receptor activity for sperm. Cell. 1980;20(3):873–82.
3. Hinsch E, Aires VA, Hedrich F, Oehninger S, Hinsch KD. A synthetic decapeptide from a conserved ZP3 protein domain induces the G protein-regulated acrosme reaction in bovine spermatozona. Theriogenology. 2005;63(6):1682–94.
4. Jungnickel MK, Sutton KA, Wang Y, Florman HM. Phosphoinositede-dependent pathways in mouse sperm are regulated by egg ZP3 and drive the acrosome reaction. Dev Biol. 2007;304(1):116–26.
5. Yu MF, Fand WN, Xiong GF, Yang Y, Peng JP. Evidence for the inhibition in vitro by anti-ZP3 antisera derived from DNA vaccine. Vaccine. 2011;29(31): 4933–9.
6. Zhang A, Li J, Zhao G, et al. Intranasal co-administration with the mouse zona pellucida 3 ecpressing construct and its coding protein induces contraception in mice. Vaccine. 2011;29(39):6785–92.
7. Li J, Jin H, Zhang A, Li Y, Wang B, Zhang F. Enhanced contraceptive response by co-immunization of DNA and protein vaccines encoding the mouse zona pellucida 3 with minimal oophoritis in mouse ovary. J Gene Med. 2007;9(12):1095–103.
8. Kitchener AL, Kay DJ, Walters B, et al. The immune response and fertility of koalas (Phascolarctos cinereus) immunised with procine zonae pellucidae or recombinant brushtail possum ZP3 protein. J Reprod Immunol. 2009;82(1):40–7.
9. Kitchener AL, Harman A, Kay DJ, McCartney CA, Mate KE, Rodger JC. Immunocontraception of eastern Grey kangaroos (Macropus giganteus) with recombinant brushtail possum (Trichosurus vulpecula) ZP3 protein. J Reprod Immunol. 2009;79(2):156–62.
10. Mackenzie SM, McLaughlin EA, Perkins HD, et al. Immunocontraceptive effects on female rabbits infected with recombinant myxoma virus expressing rabbit ZP2 or ZP3. Biol Reprod. 2006;74(3):511–21.
11. Srivastave N, Santhanam R, Sheela P, et al. Evaluation of the immunocontraceptive potential of Escherichia coli-expressed recombinant dog ZP2 and ZP3 in a homologous animal model. Reproduction. 2002; 123(6):847–57.
12. Goodwin D, Simerska P, Chang C, et al. Active immunization of mice with GnRH lipopetide vaccine candidates: importance of T helper or multi-dimer GnRH epitope. Bioorg Med Chem. 2014;22(17):4848–54.
13. Robbins SC, Jelinski MD, Stotish RL. Assessment of the immunological efficacy of two differntnt doses of recombinant GnRH vaccine in domestic male and female cats (Felis catus). J Reprod Immunol. 2004;64(1–2):107–19.
14. Levy JK, Miller LA, Cynda Crawford P, Ritchey JW, Ross MK, Fagerstone KA. GnRH immnocontraception of male cats. Theriogenology. 2004;62(6):1116–30.
15. Miller LA, Gionfriddo JP, Fagerstone KA, Rhyan JC, Killian GJ. The sigle-shot GnRH immunocontraceptive vaccine (GonaCon) in white-tailed deer: comparison of several GnRH preparations. Am J Repord Immunol. 2008; 60(3):214–23.
16. Brunius C, Zamaratskaia G, Andersson K, et al. Early immunocastration of male pigs with Improvac®-effect on boar taint, hormones and reproductive organs. Vaccine. 2011;29(51):9514–20.
17. Levy JK, Friary JA, Miller LA, Tucker SJ, Fagerstone KA. Long-term fertility control in female cats with GonaCon™, a GnRH immunocontraceptive. Theriogenology. 2011;76(8):1517–25.
18. Chambers RS, Johnston SA. High-level generation of polyclonal antibodies by genetic immunization. Nat Biotechnol. 2003;21(9):1088–92.
19. Tung K, Agersborg S, Bagavant H, Garza K, Wei K. Autoimmune ovarian disease induced by immunization with zona pellucida (ZP3) peptide. Curr Protoc Immunol. 2002; Chapter 15: Unit 15.17
20. Shrestha A, Wadhwa N, Gupta SK. Evaluation of recombinant fusion protein comprising dog zona pellucida glycoprotein-3 and Izumo and individual fragments as immunogens for contraception. Vaccine. 2014;32(5):564–71.
21. Arukha AP, Minhas V, Shrestha A, Gupta SK. Contraceptive efficacy of recombinant fusion protein comprising zona pellucida glycoprotein-3 fragment and gonadotropin releasing hormone. J Rrpord Immunol. 2016; 114:18–26.
22. Minhas V, Shrestha A, Wadhwa N, Singh R, Gupta SK. Novel sperm and gonadotropin-releasing hormone-based recombinant fusion protein:

achievement of 100% contraceptive efficacy by co-immunization of male and female mice. Mol Reprod Dev. 2016;83(12):1048–59.

23. Bauer A, Lacorn M, Danowski K, Claus R. Effects of immunization against GnRH on gonadotropins, the GH-IGF-I-axis and metabolic parameters in barrows. Animal. 2008;2(8):1215–22.

24. Robbins SC, Jelinski MD, Stotish RL. Assessment of the immunological and biological efficacy of two different doses of a recombinant GnRH vaccine in domestic male and female cats (Felis catus). J Reprod Immunol. 2004;64(1–2):107–19.

25. Dalin AM, Andresen O, Malgren L. Immunization against gnRH in mature mares: antibody titers, ovarian function, hormonal levels and oestrous behavior. J Vet Med A Physiol Pathol Clin Med. 2002;49(3):125–31.

26. Bishop DK, Wettemann RP, Yelich JV, Spicer LJ. Ovarian response after gonadotropin treatment of heifers immunized against gonadotropin-releasing hormone. J Anim Sci. 1996;74(5):1092–7.

27. Liu Y, Tian Y, Zhao X, et al. Immunization of dogs with recombinant GnRH-1 suppresses the development of reproductive function. Theriogenology. 2015;83(3):314–9.

28. Gupta N, Shrestha A, Panda AK, Gupta SK. Production of tag-free recombinant fusion protein encompassing promiscuous T cell epitope of tetanus toxoid and dog zona pellucida glycoprotein-3 for contraceptive vaccine development. Mol Biotechnol. 2013;54(3):853–62.

29. Henderson CJ, Braude P, Aitken RJ. Polyclonal antibodies to a 32-kDa deglycosylated polypeptide from porcine zonae pellucidae will prevent human gamete interaction in vitro. Gamete Res. 1987;18(3):251–65.

30. Henderson CJ, Hulme MJ, Aitken RJ. Contraceptive potential of antibodies to the zona pellucida. J Reprod Fertil. 1988;83(1):325–43.

31. Henderson CJ, Hulme MJ, Aitken RJ. Analysis of the biological properties of antibodies raised against intact and deglycosylated porcine zonea pellucidae. Gamete Res. 1987;16(4):323–41.

32. Lloyd ML, Papadimitriou Jm, O'Leary S, Robertson SA, Shellam GR. Immunoglobulin to zona pellucida 3 mediates ovarian damage and infertility after contraceptive vaccination in mice. JAutoimmun 2010; 35(1): 77–85.

33. Li J, Jin H, Zhang F, et al. Treatment of autoimmune ovarian disease by co-administration with mouse zona pellucida protein 3 and DNA vaccine through induction of adaptive regulatory T cells. J Gene Med. 2008;10(7):810–20.

34. Monnier-Barbarino P, Forges T, Faure GC, Béné MC. Ovarian autoimmunity and ovarian pathologies: antigenic targets and diagnostic significance. J Gynecol Obstet Biol Reprod (Paris). 2005;34(7 Pt 1):649–57.

35. McNeilly AS, Jonassen JA, Fraser HM. Suppression of follicular development after chronic LHRH immunoneutralization in the ewe. J Reprod Fertil. 1986; 76(1):481–90.

36. Jinshu X, Jingjing L, Duan P, et al. A synthetic gonadotropin-releasing hormone (GnRH) vaccine for control of fertility and hormone dependent diseases without any adjuvant. Vaccine. 2005;23(40):4834–43.

37. Killian G, Miller L, Rhyan J, Doten H. Immunocontraception of Florida feral swine with a single-dose GnRH vaccine. Am J Reprod Immunol. 2006;55(5):378–84.

11

Docosahexaenoic acid (DHA) effects on proliferation and steroidogenesis of bovine granulosa cells

Virginie Maillard[1,2*†], Alice Desmarchais[1†], Maeva Durcin[1], Svetlana Uzbekova[1] and Sebastien Elis[1]

Abstract

Background: Docosahexaenoic acid (DHA) is a n-3 polyunsaturated fatty acid (PUFA) belonging to a family of biologically active fatty acids (FA), which are known to have numerous health benefits. N-3 PUFAs affect reproduction in cattle, and notably directly affect follicular cells. In terms of reproduction in cattle, n-3 PUFA-enriched diets lead to increased follicle size or numbers.

Methods: The objective of the present study was to analyze the effects of DHA (1, 10, 20 and 50 μM) on proliferation and steroidogenesis (parametric and/or non parametric (permutational) ANOVA) of bovine granulosa cells in vitro and mechanisms of action through protein expression (Kruskal-Wallis) and signaling pathways (non parametric ANOVA) and to investigate whether DHA could exert part of its action through the free fatty acid receptor 4 (FFAR4).

Results: DHA (10 and 50 μM) increased granulosa cell proliferation and DHA 10 μM led to a corresponding increase in proliferating cell nuclear antigen (PCNA) expression level. DHA also increased progesterone secretion at 1, 20 and 50 μM, and estradiol secretion at 1, 10 and 20 μM. Consistent increases in protein levels were also reported for the steroidogenic enzymes, cytochrome P450 family 11 subfamily A member 1 (CYP11A1) and hydroxy-delta-5-steroid dehydrogenase, 3 beta- and steroid delta-isomerase 1 (HSD3B1), and of the cholesterol transporter steroidogenic acute regulatory protein (StAR), which are necessary for production of progesterone or androstenedione. FFAR4 was expressed in all cellular types of bovine ovarian follicles, and in granulosa cells it was localized close to the cellular membrane. TUG-891 treatment (1 and 50 μM), a FFAR4 agonist, increased granulosa cell proliferation and MAPK14 phosphorylation in a similar way to that observed with DHA treatment. However, TUG-891 treatment (1, 10 and 50 μM) showed no effect on progesterone or estradiol secretion.

Conclusions: These data show that DHA stimulated proliferation and steroidogenesis of bovine granulosa cells and led to MAPK14 phosphorylation. FFAR4 involvement in DHA effects requires further investigation, even if our data might suggest FFAR4 role in DHA effects on granulosa cell proliferation. Other mechanisms of DHA action should be investigated as the steroidogenic effects seemed to be independent of FFAR4 activation.

Keywords: Bovine, Gene expression, Lipid, N-3 PUFA, DHA, Folliculogenesis, MAPK, AKT, AMPK, Signaling pathways, Free fatty acid receptor 4 (FFAR4)

* Correspondence: virginie.maillard@inra.fr
†Equal contributors
[1]UMR PRC, CNRS, IFCE, INRA, Université de Tours, 37380 Nouzilly, France
[2]INRA Centre Val de Loire, Physiologie de la Reproduction et des Comportements, 37380 Nouzilly, France

Background

N-3 polyunsaturated fatty acids (PUFAs) belong to a family of biologically active fatty acids (FAs) and are known to have numerous health benefits [1]. The most well-known members are alpha-linolenic acid (ALA), eicosapentaenoic acid (EPA) and docosahexaenoic acid (DHA). These are essential FAs, as mammals cannot produce ALA, the precursor of n-3 PUFA. Furthermore, DHA, the longest-chain member of this family, has a 22-carbon chain (C22:6) and can theoretically be produced from shorter-chain members of this family. As the efficiency of the desaturation reaction is low, the most extensive source of DHA is the diet, cold-water fish in particular [2, 3]. DHA is reported to exert pleiotropic effects at both central and peripheral levels, including the brain, heart and immune system [4–6].

Among their physiological roles, n-3 PUFAs affect reproduction in cattle [7, 8]. The feeding of diets supplemented with n-3 PUFAs (enriched in ALA) was shown to increase calving rate in dairy cows [9–11]. At the uterus level, n-3 PUFAs reduced prostaglandin F2 alpha (PGF2α) secretion from endometrial cells [12–15]. Moreover, n-3 PUFA dietary supplement in cows was reported to exert effects at the ovarian level. Indeed, a n-3 PUFA-enriched diet led to an increased cleavage rate or a trend to increased blastocyst rate after in vivo maturation [16, 17] and n-3 PUFA supplementation during in vitro maturation also led to increased blastocyst rates [18, 19]. In addition, dietary ALA supplementation led to an increase in the size of the pre-ovulatory follicles [9], in number of total follicles [16] or small follicles [17], to larger corpus luteum size and higher plasma progesterone levels [20, 21]. Dietary fish oil supplementation, containing both EPA and DHA, also led to an increased number of large follicles [11]. Dietary DHA improved resumption of estrous cyclicity and pregnancy at first artificial insemination [22]. These data suggest that n-3 PUFAs could favorably affect folliculogenesis by having direct effects on follicular cells, in addition to the already described effects on the oocyte. Nevertheless, several studies reported no effect of n-3 PUFA diet on female reproduction [21, 23], or even a deleterious effect leading to a more unfavorable uterine environment for sustaining pregnancies and reduced fertility in cows [24].

There are several mechanisms by which n-3 PUFAs could exhibit multiple physiological roles in organism development and diseases [25]: indirect actions on cells by influencing metabolite, hormone concentration, or other factors as oxidation of LDL and oxidative stress, direct actions on cells via receptors, sensors or cell membrane fatty acid composition (membrane order, lipid rafts, etc.) (reviewed in [26]). Most of the studies of n-3 PUFA mechanisms concern the inflammatory process [27]. Indeed, n-3 PUFAs were shown to affect cytokine expression, especially inflammatory cytokines (TNF, IL-1β, IL-6 and IL-8), and to simultaneously help produce inflammatory resolving metabolites (resolvins, protectins, maresins) [26, 28]. Feeding with a n-3 PUFA-enriched diet results in the membrane lipid composition being enriched in n-3 PUFA. Eicosanoids (prostaglandins, leukotrienes, thromboxanes and lipoxins) produced from n-3 PUFAs (for example, 3-series prostaglandins) are therefore increased and, conversely, eicosanoids produced from arachidonic acid (for example, 2-series prostaglandins) are reduced [28]. This decrease in 2-series prostaglandins induced a less inflammatory environment because 3-series prostaglandins are less inflammatory [29]. N-3 PUFAs were also reported to act through intracellular sensors such as peroxisome proliferator-activated receptors (PPARs) and nuclear factor kappa B and thus to modulate their target gene expression [26]. By affecting the membrane lipid composition, n-3 PUFAs are also able to increase membrane fluidity and to promote lipid raft formation and organization (reviewed in [30]), and therefore signaling pathways. N-3 PUFAs are also reported to act through free fatty acid receptors, FFAR1 and FFAR4, located in the membrane and activate their signaling pathways [31]. Indeed, FFAR4 can modulate signaling of mitogen-activated protein kinases MAPK1/3 (alias ERK 1/2) and MAPK14 (alias p38), and protein kinase B (Akt) [32, 33], which are already known to be involved in bovine granulosa cell (GC) proliferation and steroidogenesis [34–38].

In the present study, we choose to focus solely on DHA. Indeed, recent in vivo studies focused on algae oil supplementation, containing mainly DHA and no EPA (substitute of fish oil which does not exhibit the limitation of fish oil: limited resources and competition with human diet) [22, 39, 40]. Studying solely DHA effects is therefore a relevant step to understand its mechanism of action granulosa cells. We hypothesize that DHA could stimulate steroidogenesis in bovine GC and that it could exert part of its activity through the membrane receptor, FFAR4. The objective of the present study was therefore to examine the effects of DHA on proliferation and steroidogenesis of bovine GCs. We then investigated FFAR4 expression in GCs and reported its expression in ovarian follicles and in GCs. We thus investigated whether supplementation of the culture medium with a FFAR4 agonist, TUG-891 [41], could reproduce the effects of DHA in GCs. Treatment with DHA and TUG-891 was performed during GC culture, followed by examination of cell proliferation, progesterone and estradiol secretion, gene and protein expression, and signaling pathways.

Methods

Ethics

No experiments with living animals were performed.

Chemicals and antibody

Customized anti-FFAR4 antibody was produced from a rabbit immunized against a peptide designed from the second extracellular loop (179–194 amino acids) of the bovine sequence (Accession number: NP_001315586.1). Serum from immunized rabbit underwent affinity purification and antibody concentration was measured by enzyme-linked immunosorbent assay (ELISA; Agro-Bio, La Ferté Saint-Aubin, France). This customized antibody enabled detection of a 42 kDa band by western blot in lung tissue extract (Additional file 1: Figure S1). Lung tissue was used to validate the antibody, as in other species, namely mice and humans, the level of expression of FFAR4 protein is reported to be higher in this tissue than in other tissues, such as adipose tissue, intestine and liver [42].

DHA was obtained from Sigma-Aldrich (Saint Quentin Fallavier, France) and TUG-891 from Tocris (Bio-Techne Europe, Lille, France). Unless otherwise stated in the text, all other chemicals were obtained from Sigma-Aldrich (Saint Quentin Fallavier, France). Primary antibodies used are indicated in Additional file 2: Table S1. Horseradish peroxidase (HRP)-conjugated anti-rabbit and anti-mouse were purchased from Perkin Elmer (Courtaboeuf, France) and biotinylated horse anti-mouse and anti-rabbit IgG were from Vector Laboratories (Clinisciences, Nanterre, France). Alexa Fluor 488-conjugated donkey anti-rabbit IgG was purchased from Jackson ImmunoResearch (Newmarket, United Kingdom). Dimethyl sulfoxide (DMSO) 1/2000 was used as the control treatment as it is used as a solvent for DHA and TUG-891.

Biological material

Ovarian cortex were carefully dissected from 5 bovine ovaries collected from a local slaughterhouse. Theca cells were retrieved from healthy follicles of 5 bovine ovaries (local slaughterhouse): once the follicle is carefully dissected and opened, the inside of the follicle is gently scraped and washed in PBS to remove granulosa cells and cumulus-oocyte complex. Cumulus cells (without oocyte) were recovered as previously described [19] from 20 ovaries, briefly cumulus-oocyte complexes were sorted out after follicular punctures and oocytes were dissociated from cumulus cells by mechanical aspiration and removed. GCs were collected according the same protocol as when performing cell culture experiment (described in the following section). In the case of GC culture, antral follicles with a diameter of 2 to 6 mm were used. Ovaries exhibiting very large corpora lutea were excluded from the samples to avoid contamination of our granulosa cell samples from growing follicles with luteinized granulosa cells (originating from these corpora lutea) during ovary punctures. Lung tissue was collected from one cow (local slaughterhouse).

Isolation and culture of granulosa cells

Follicles from bovine ovaries were punctured using an 18G needle linked to a vacuum pump and a 50-mL falcon tube, enabling the collection of follicular fluid which contained GCs. GCs were then washed in modified McCoy's 5A serum-free medium containing: L-glutamine (3 mM), HEPES (20 mM; pH 7.6), bovine serum albumin (BSA; essentially fatty acid free; 0.1%), penicillin-streptomycin (120×10^3 UI/L penicillin; 120 mg/L streptomycin), amphotericin B (50 µg/L), bovine insulin (1.74 nM), bovine apo-transferrin (5 mg/L), selenium (0.12 µM) and 4-androsten-11β-ol-3,17-dione (96 nM). After centrifugation and washes in medium, suspended cells were dropped off on a Percoll density medium (50% Percoll, 50% medium) and GCs were purified by centrifugation (300 g). Recovered GCs were incubated in serum-free modified McCoy's 5A medium in the appropriate cell density and plates according to the assays as described below. From the beginning of the culture, cells were cultured in the presence or absence of test reagents for different durations depending on the biological function of interest. Cultures were performed in a water-saturated atmosphere containing 5% CO_2 in air at 38 °C. The use of culture media without fetal bovine serum and a short culture duration limited the differentiation of GCs, which retained the round shape exhibited in vivo. Under the culture conditions used in this experiment, GCs still exhibited steroidogenic activity and were able to proliferate. The Additional file 3: Figure S2 presents the experiment design of the present work.

Immunohistochemistry

Bovine ovaries were embedded in paraffin and serially sectioned at a thickness of 7 µm using a microtome. Adjacent sections were deparaffinized in toluene, rehydrated and incubated in antigen unmasking solution (1% in water; Vector Laboratories) for 2 min in a microwave (850 W), left to cool for 1 h at room temperature, and washed twice in phosphate buffered saline (PBS) for 5 min. Endogenous peroxidase activity was quenched by treating sections with 0.3% hydrogen peroxide in PBS containing 0.1% triton for 30 min at 4 °C. After two 5-min washes in PBS, sections were incubated in PBS containing BSA (2%) and goat serum (5%) for 1 h at room temperature and quickly washed in PBS with BSA (0.1%). Sections were incubated overnight at 4 °C in PBS with BSA (0.5%) with primary rabbit antibodies against bovine FFAR4 (19 µg/mL; customized antibody; Agro-Bio) or with the pre-immunized serum (similar IgG concentration; Agro-Bio) from the same rabbit (negative control). After four 5-min washes in PBS with Tween 20 (0.1%), sections were then incubated with secondary biotinylated horse anti-mouse and anti-rabbit IgG (1:700

dilution) in PBS with BSA (0.5%) for 1 h at room temperature. After four 5-min washes in PBS with Tween 20 (0.1%), sections were incubated in a ready-to-use avidine and biotinylated horseradish peroxidase solution (Vectastain® Elite® ABC kit, Vector Laboratories) for 30 min at room temperature, according to the manufacturer's instructions. After three 5-min washes in PBS with Tween 20 (0.1%), immunostaining was developed by incubating sections in 50 mM Tris-HCl (pH 7.8) containing 0.4 mg/ml 3,3'-diaminobenzidine tetrahydrochloride dehydrate (DAB) and 0.007% hydrogen peroxide for 5 min at room temperature. Sections were then dehydrated and mounted using Depex. Immunospecific staining (brown) was observed using an Axioplan Zeiss transmission microscope coupled with a 10× objective with a numerical aperture of 0.03 or a 40× objective with a numerical aperture of 0.75. Images were generated with a numerical camera piloted by the Software Spot (version 5.2 for Windows; Diagnostic Instruments, Inc., MicroMecanique, Evry, France).

Immunofluorescence

After collection and washes, as described above, GCs were incubated on a 8-well chamber slide (Lab-Tek® Nunc, Thermo-Fisher Scientific, Courtaboeuf, France) for 48 h. Cells were then washed in Tris-buffer saline (TBS), fixed in PBS containing paraformaldehyde (4%) for 20 min and washed in TBS-0.1% BSA for 3 min at room temperature. After blocking in TBS containing BSA (1%) and horse serum (5%) for 1 h at room temperature, GCs were incubated overnight at 4 °C in TBS containing BSA (1%) and horse serum (5%) with primary rabbit antibodies against bovine FFAR4 (9. 5 μg/mL; customized antibody) or the pre-immunized serum (similar IgG concentration) of the same rabbit (negative control). Other GCs were incubated in the same conditions with primary rabbit antibodies against human FFAR4 (20 μg/mL; Aviva Systems Biology) or rabbit IgG (similar concentration) as a negative control. After three 10-min washes in TBS containing BSA (0.1%), sections were then incubated with secondary Alexa Fluor 488-conjugated donkey anti-rabbit IgG (1:800 dilution) in TBS containing BSA (0.1%) for 1.5 h at room temperature. Then, GCs were washed in TBS containing BSA (0.1%) (three 10-min washes), and incubated in TBS with 1 μg/mL Hoechst 33,258 for 15 min at room temperature to stain nuclei. Sections were then mounted using Moviol® and fluorescence was observed under a Zeiss confocal microscope LSM700 (Carl Zeiss Microscopy GmbH, Munich, Germany) using an oil 40× objective with a numerical aperture of 1.3 or an oil 63× objective with a numerical aperture of 1.4 and the appropriate filters. Images were

captured using Zen 2012 software (black edition version 8.0, Carl Zeiss Microscopy GmbH).

GC proliferation

Cell proliferation was determined by measurement of ^{3}H-thymidine incorporation into bovine GCs after 24 h of culture, as previously described [43] with some modifications. Briefly, GCs (2.5×10^5 viable cells/250 μL media/well) were cultured in 48-well dishes in modified McCoy's 5A media containing ^{3}H-thymidine (0.25nCi/μL corresponding to 18.5 kBq/mL; Perkin Elmer, Courtaboeuf, France) in the presence or absence of DHA (1, 10, 20 or 50 μM) or TUG-891 (1, 10 or 50 μM). Cultures were maintained at 38 °C in air containing 5% CO_2. After culture for 24 h, excess thymidine was removed by washing twice with PBS (200 μL/well). Cells were then fixed with cold 50% trichloroacetic acid (100 μL/well) for 15min and lysed using 0.5 M NaOH (250 μL/well) for 10 min at room temperature. Radioactivity was counted using Ultima Gold MV scintillation fluid (Perkin Elmer) and a β-photomultiplier C2900 (Perkin Elmer). The results are expressed as mean ± SEM of 13 independent cultures (cells from one culture came from several follicles originating from several ovaries (around 10 follicles per ovary, and 15 ovaries per cultures) and each culture came from a specific batch of ovaries), with four replicates of each treatment. Data are expressed as disintegrations per minute (dpm).

Progesterone assay

GCs were cultured in 96-well dishes (1×10^5 viable cells/150 μL media/well) in modified McCoy's 5A medium in the presence or absence of DHA (1, 10, 20 or 50 μM) or TUG-891 (1, 10 or 50 μM) for 48 h. Supernatants and cells were separately stored at $- 20$ °C until progesterone analysis and protein assays (BCA protein quantification kit;Interchim, Montluçon, France), respectively. The concentration of progesterone was determined in the culture media using an ELISA protocol, as described previously [44]. For progesterone concentrations ranging from 0.25 to 32 ng/mL, the intra-assay coefficient of variation (CV) averaged $< 10\%$. Progesterone secreted in each well was normalized by the protein concentration of the same well. The results are expressed as the amount of progesterone (ng/mL) secreted per 48 h per protein amount (μg/mL) per well. Data, representing 12 independent cultures (as described in GC-proliferation section) with each treatment conducted in quadruplicate, are expressed as mean ± SEM and as ng of secreted progesterone per μg of protein.

Estradiol assay

GCs were cultured in 96-well dishes (1×10^5 viable cells/150 μL media/well) in modified McCoy's 5A medium in the presence or absence of DHA (1, 10, 20 or 50 μM) or TUG-891 (1, 10 or 50 μM) for 48 h. Supernatants and cell layer were separately stored at − 20 °C until estradiol analysis and protein assays (BCA protein quantification kit), respectively. The concentration of estradiol in the culture media was determined using the DIAsource E2-EASIA Kit (DIAsource, Louvain-la-Neuve, Belgium), in accordance with the manufacturer's recommendations. Briefly, 50 μL of spent medium was used for the assay and the competition between unlabeled estradiol (present in the culture media) and labeled estradiol (provided by the kit) lasted overnight at 4 °C. For estradiol concentrations ranging from 1.56 to 50 pg/mL, the inter-assay CVs averaged 15%. Estradiol was normalized as described for progesterone. Data, represented six independent cultures with each treatment conducted in quadruplicate, are expressed as mean ± SEM as pg of secreted estradiol per μg of protein.

Fatty acid analysis
GCs were cultured in 48-well dishes (2.5×10^5 viable cells/250 μL media/well) in modified McCoy's 5A medium in the presence or absence of DHA (1, 10 or 50 μM) for 15 h. Supernatants were removed. Cells with the same treatment (pool of 12 wells) were isolated in PBS 1X and stored at − 80 °C until lipid analysis. Lipids were extracted and analyzed as previously described [45]. Briefly, total lipids were extracted twice from granulosa cells with ethanol/chloroform (1:2, v/v). Before extraction, 1,2-diheptadecanoyl-sn-gycero-3-phosphocholine (GPC di-17:0) was added as internal standard. Lipids were trans-methylated with toluene-methanol (2:3, v/v) and boron trifluoride in methanol (14%) at 100 °C for 90 min in screw-capped tubes. After addition of 1.5 mL K2CO3 in 10% water, the resulting fatty acid methyl esters (FAME) were extracted by 2 mL of isooctane. The FAMEs were analyzed by gas chromatography with a HP6890 instrument equipped with a fused silica capillary BPX70 SGE column (60×0.25 mm). The vector gas was hydrogen. Temperatures of the Ross injector and the flame ionization detector were set at 230 °C and 250 °C, respectively. FAMEs were identified by making a comparison of their relative retention times with those of commercial standards. Fatty acid composition is expressed as the mole percentage of total fatty acids. The results are expressed as means ± SEM ($n = 4$ per treatment).

Protein extraction and western blot analysis
In order to validate the FFAR4 antibody designed against the bovine protein, proteins were extracted from lung tissue. Moreover, on GC, assays were conducted for proliferating cell nuclear antigen (PCNA), for steroidogenic enzymes, cytochrome P450 family 11 subfamily A member 1 (CYP11A1 alias cholesterol side-chain cleavage)

and hydroxy-delta-5-steroid dehydrogenase, 3 beta- and steroid delta-isomerase 1 (HSD3B1 alias 3β-HSD), and for the cholesterol transporter steroidogenic acute regulatory protein (StAR). GCs were cultured in 48-well dishes (2.5×10^5 viable cells/250 μL media/well) in modified McCoy's 5A medium in the presence or absence of DHA for 15 h. Five independent experiments were performed for HSD3B1, StAR, CYP11A1 after DHA 20 μM treatment and six independent experiments for PCNA after DHA 10 μM treatment.

Cell signaling pathway assays were conducted for AMP-activated protein kinaseα (AMPKα), MAPK14, MAPK1/3 and Akt as these pathways are of interest to explore GC functions. Indeed, these pathways are involved in both cellular proliferation and steroidogenesis, the functions investigated in the present study. GCs were cultured in 48-well dishes (2.5×10^5 viable cells/ 250 μL media/well) in modified McCoy's 5A medium. After 15 h, 100 μL supernatant was removed and replaced with 100 μL fresh modified McCoy's 5A medium in the presence or absence of DHA (10 or 50 μM final concentration in well) or TUG-891 (1, 10 or 50 μM final concentration in well) for 5, 10, 30 or 60 min. Four independent experiments were performed.

With all assays, analyses were performed on total protein extracts from cultured GCs or from lung tissue in the case or FFAR4 validation. Total proteins were extracted from GCs on ice in lysis buffer (10 mM Tris (pH 7.4), 150 mM NaCl, 1 mM EDTA, 2 mM EGTA, 0.5% Nonidet P40, 1% Triton X 100) containing phosphatase inhibitors (10 mM sodium fluoride, 12 mM sodium dihydrogen phosphate, 2 mM sodium orthovanadate). In the case of lung tissue, proteins were extracted on ice after 2 h lysis buffer action in order to favor membrane receptor extraction. Lysates were centrifuged for 30 min at 4 ° C at 16000 g for GC proteins and 6000 g (to favor membrane receptor recovery) for lung proteins. The protein concentration in the supernatants was determined using a colorimetric assay (kit BC Assay protein quantification; Interchim, Montluçon, France) and proteins were denatured in Laemmli buffer for 5 min at 95 °C. Protein lysates (15 μg GC or 150 μg lung) were subjected to electrophoresis on 4–12% acrylamide gel (Life technologies, Saint-Aubin, France) and electrotransferred onto 0.45-μm nitrocellulose membranes (Pall Corporation, VWR International, France). After blocking with 5% non-fat dry milk powder (NFDMP) in TBS-0.1% Tween-20 (TBST) for 90 min at room temperature, blots were incubated with appropriate primary antibodies (for final dilutions, see Table 1) in TBST with 5% NFDMP at 4 °C overnight. The membranes were then washed in TBST and incubated with the appropriate HRP-conjugated

Table 1 Primer sequences for real-time reverse transcription–polymerase chain reaction

Abbrev.	Gene	Accession no.	Forward primer	Reverse primer	bp	E %
FFAR4	Free fatty acid receptor 4	XM_865266	GGGTTCCTTTTCGATGTGAA	GCCGTGACTCTTTGGAGAAG	166	94
GPX4	Glutathione peroxidase 4	NM_174770	CGATACGCCGAGTGTGGTTTAC	ACAGCCGTTCTTGTCAATGAGG	261	96
GLUT1	Solute carrier family 2 (facilitated glucose transporter), member 1	NM_174602	CTGATCCTGGGTCGCTTCAT	ACGTACATGGGCACAAAACCA	68	113
NFkB	Nuclear factor of kappa light polypeptide gene enhancer in B-cells 1	NM_001076409.1	GCACCACTTATGACGGGACT	CCATGTCCAGAGGAGTGGTT	195	89
PPARA	Peroxisome proliferator-activated receptor alpha	NM_001034036.1	CCTACGGGAATGGCTTCATA	GCACAATACCCTCCTGCATT	219	97
PPARG	Peroxisome proliferator-activated receptor gamma	Y12419/Y12420	CCCTGGCAAAGCATTTGTAT	ACTGACACCCCTGGAAGATG	222	88
RPL19	Ribosomal protein L19	BC102223	AATCGCCAATGCCAACTC	CCCTTTCGCTTACCTATACC	156	94
RPS9	Ribosomal protein S9	BC148016	GGAGACCCTTCGAGAAGTCC	GGGCATTACCTTCGAACAGA	180	100
SREBF1	Sterol regulatory element binding transcription factor 1	AB355703.1	ACCGCTCTTCCATCAATGAC	TTCAGCGATTTGCTTTTGTG	190	97

Abbrev gene abbreviation, *bp* product size in base pair, *E* primer efficiency

secondary antibody (final dilution 1:5000) in TBST with 5% NFDMP for 2 h at room temperature. The signal of specific bands, detected by ECL (West Dura; Thermo-Fisher Scientific, Courtaboeuf, France), was quantified using a charge-coupled device camera GeneGnome (Syngene, Cambridge, United Kingdom) with Genesys 1.5.4 software (Syngene). The analysis of signal intensity was performed using Gene-Tools 4.01 software (Syngene). Results for PCNA, HSD3B1, StAR and CYP11A1 expression levels are expressed as the fold change between controls and DHA treatment. Results of MAPK14, AMPKα, Akt and MAPK1/3 phosphorylation are expressed as the ratio of phosphorylated protein to total protein, normalized by the control value at the same time-point, and with time 0 min being equal to 1 (for reference).

Gene expression analysis in GCs

GCs were cultured in 48-well dishes (2.5×10^5 viable cells/250 µL media/well) in modified McCoy's 5A medium in the presence or absence of DHA (1, 10, 20 or 50 µM) or TUG-891 (1, 10 or 50 µM) for 8 h. After removal of the medium, cells were recovered using 200 µl/well of TriZol reagent (Invitrogen, Cergy Pontoise, France), immediately frozen and stored until analysis. An additional condition, consisting in GC collected from ovaries and then immediately frozen and stored until analysis was also constituted and named in vivo GC. Total RNA was extracted from GCs according to the manufacturer's instructions. RNA concentration was determined using a NanoDrop ND-1000 spectrophotometer (Nyxor Biotech, Paris, France). DNAse treatment and reverse transcription (RT) was performed on 1 µg of total RNA extracted from GCs using Maxima First Strand cDNA Synthesis kit (Thermo-Fisher Scientific) according to the manufacturer's recommendations.

Real-time PCR reactions were carried out on a CFX96 (Bio-Rad, Marnes-la-Coquette, France) in 20 µL volumes containing primers, each at a final concentration of 150 nM (Table 1), 5 µL of the diluted RT reaction (10 ng cDNA per reaction) and qPCR Mastermix Plus for Sybr Green I (Bio-Rad) according to the manufacturer's instructions. As expression of *FFAR4* and *FFAR1* in ovarian tissue is low, real-time RT-PCR were performed on 50 ng cDNA per reaction. The efficiency of the primers (Table 2) and standard curve for each gene were calculated from serial dilutions of the corresponding cDNA fragment obtained as a template. Relative gene expression levels were determined in ten independent GC samples for each treatment. The geometric mean of two housekeeping genes, Ribosomal protein L19 (*RPL19*) and Ribosomal protein S9 (*RPS9*), was used to normalize gene expression. The relative amounts of gene transcripts (R) were calculated according to the equation: $R = \frac{(E_{gene}^{-Ct\ gene})}{(\text{geometric mean } (E_{RPS9}^{-Ct\ RPS9}; E_{RPL19}^{-Ct\ RPL19}))}$, where E is the primer efficiency and Ct the cycle threshold.

Statistical analysis

Statistical analyses were performed for GC proliferation, steroidogenesis, gene expression, protein expression, GC lipid composition taking into account treatment effect and replica effect. Concerning cell signaling, the time effect and replica effect were analyzed. GC proliferation, progesterone secretion, estradiol secretion, GC lipid composition and cell signaling were compared between the groups. A one-way ANOVA was used when distribution and variance enabled performance of a parametric study (Shapiro test, Levene test, Rcmdr package), with Tukey's post hoc comparison (R package multcomp

Table 2 Fatty acid composition from total lipids of bovine granulosa cells after 15 h treatment with DHA

Fatty acids (mole % of total fatty acids)	Control [a]	DHA1 µM	DHA 10 µM	DHA 50 µM
	$n = 5$	$n = 4$	$n = 4$	$n = 3$
Saturates				
16:0	31.50 ± 7.48	40.16 ± 9.38	44.12 ± 11.60	48.45 ± 7.44
18:0	10.68 ± 2.25	13.36 ± 3.03	15.04 ± 3.89	16.24 ± 2.60
Monounsaturates				
16:1 n-7	2.32 ± 0.55	3.03 ± 0.72	3.33 ± 0.91	3.52 ± 0.68
18:1 n-7	8.93 ± 2.17	11.51 ± 2.85	12.36 ± 3.72	12.22 ± 3.01
18:1 n-9 cis	29.99 ± 7.18	38.91 ± 9.08	42.49 ± 11.58	43.03 ± 7.86
n-6 PUFA				
18:2 n-6 cis	6.05 ± 1.29	7.87 ± 1.81	8.59 ± 2.33	8.41 ± 2.07
20:4 n-6	8.85 ± 2.12	11.87 ± 3.08	13.02 ± 3.99	11.24 ± 4.10
n-3 PUFA				
18:3 n-3	0.51 ± 0.12	0.66 ± 0.15	0.74 ± 0.18	0.67 ± 0.17
20:5 n-3	0.98 ± 0.25	1.34 ± 0.31	1.60 ± 0.38	1.37 ± 0.42
22:5 n-3	7.03 ± 1.72	9.33 ± 2.28	10.04 ± 2.90	7.79 ± 3.31
22:6 n-3 (DHA)	0.84 ± 0.16	2.17 ± 0.04 *	10.27 ± 0.11 *	23.05 ± 6.58 *

Granulosa cells (GC) (2.5×10^5 viable cells/250 µL media/well) were cultured into 48-well dishes in modified McCoy's 5A media in the presence or absence of DHA (1, 10 or 50 µM). After 15 h culture, supernatants were removed and cells with the same treatment (12 wells) were pooled and stored under nitrogen gas at −80 °C until the total lipid extraction. The fatty acid analysis was performed by gas chromatography by the Plateforme de Lipidomique Fonctionnelle (INSA, Villeurbanne, France). The relative amount of each fatty acid is expressed as the area of each fatty acid peak, relative to the total area for all fatty acids (mole%). The results are expressed as means ± SEM ($n = 4$ per treatment). [a] Control corresponds to the serum-free modified McCoy's 5A medium supplemented with DMSO (1:2000) as carrier solvent of DHA. The prepared mediums with the different concentrations of DHA were all adjusted for DMSO at 1:2000. * indicates a significant difference with control condition (Kruskal-Wallis test with Tukey's multiple comparison test as post-hoc test, $p < 0.05$)

[46]). A non-parametric ANOVA (permutational ANOVA) was used when distribution was not normal and variance was not homogenous (R package lmPerm [47]), with a Tukey's post-hoc test (R package nparcomp [48]), R version 3.3.1 [49]). Gene expression was analyzed using K-sample Fisher Pitman permutation test with a Monte Carlo approximation (Rcmdr package) with the treatment as a fixed factor and the replica as a random factor, with Tukey's post hoc comparison (R package nparcomp). Protein expression levels of PCNA, HSD3B1, StAR and CYP11A1 were analyzed using the Kruskal-Wallis test (Shapiro test, Levene test, Rcmdr package). A p-value of ≤0.05 was considered to indicate a significant difference and $0.05 < p ≤ 0.10$ a tendency.

Results
FFAR4 expression
Both *FFAR1* and *FFAR4* mRNA were detectable at a low level in several ovarian compartments, such as the cortex and theca, granulosa and cumulus cells (Additional file 4: Figure S3). An antibody was designed against a peptide from the second extracellular loop of the FFAR4 bovine protein. The signal corresponding to the 42 kDa band was extinguished by increasing the quantity of peptide used to prepare the antibody, demonstrating that the band corresponded to FFAR4 (Additional file 1: Figure S1). The protein FFAR4 was detected by both

immunohistochemistry (brown labelling, Fig. 1) on bovine ovarian follicles and immunofluorescence (green fluorescence, Fig. 2) on cultured bovine GCs, using the bovine FFAR4 antibody. FFAR4 protein was present in all cellular types of follicles with small and large antrum. FFAR4 protein immunofluorescence seemed to exhibit a peripheral labelling close to the cellular membrane in some GCs and the intensity and presence of the staining was variable in GCs cultured in vitro (Fig. 2). The precise localization of the labelling to the cellular membrane is not obvious in all cells. This signal is similar to FFAR4 immunofluorescence in bovine GCs, obtained using a commercial antibody design against a peptide of the human protein sharing 89% identity with the bovine FFAR4 sequence (Additional file 5: Figure S4).

Cellular proliferation
DHA significantly increased basal cellular proliferation at 10 µM (1.9-fold increase; $p < 0.0001$) and 50 µM (1.8-fold increase; $p < 0.0001$) compared to the control (Fig. 3). A similar increase in GC proliferation was also observed with TUG-891 at 1 µM (1.7-fold increase; $p = 0.014$) and 50 µM (2.2-fold increase; $p < 0.0001$; Fig. 3).

Steroidogenesis
DHA significantly increased basal progesterone secretion at 20 µM (1.3-fold increase; $p < 0.0001$) and 50 µM (1.2-

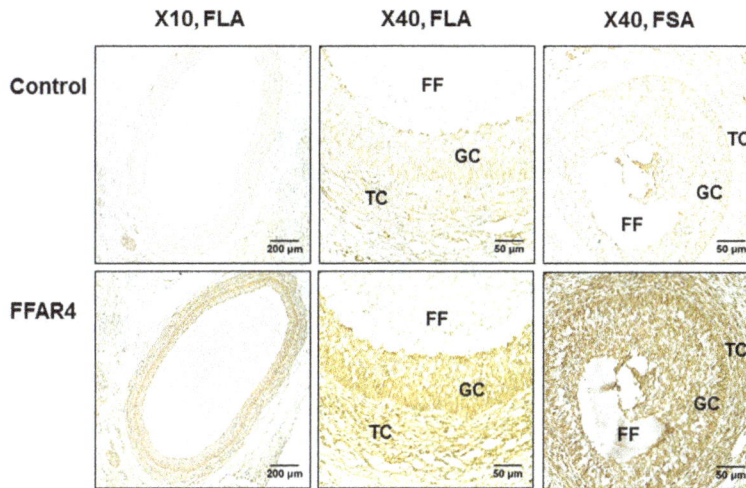

Fig. 1 Expression of free fatty acid receptor 4 (FFAR4) in bovine ovarian follicles by immunohistochemistry. Immunohistochemistry was performed on sections of ovarian follicles. FFAR4 (brown labeling) was immunodetected in ovarian follicles with large (FLA) or small (FSA) antrum (customized FFAR4 rabbit antibody, Agro-Bio). Pre-immunized rabbit serum was used as the control with the same secondary antibody as for FFAR4 detection. Bars = 200 µm and 50 µm for 10× and 40× microscope objectives, respectively. FF - follicular fluid, GC – granulosa cells, TC – theca cells

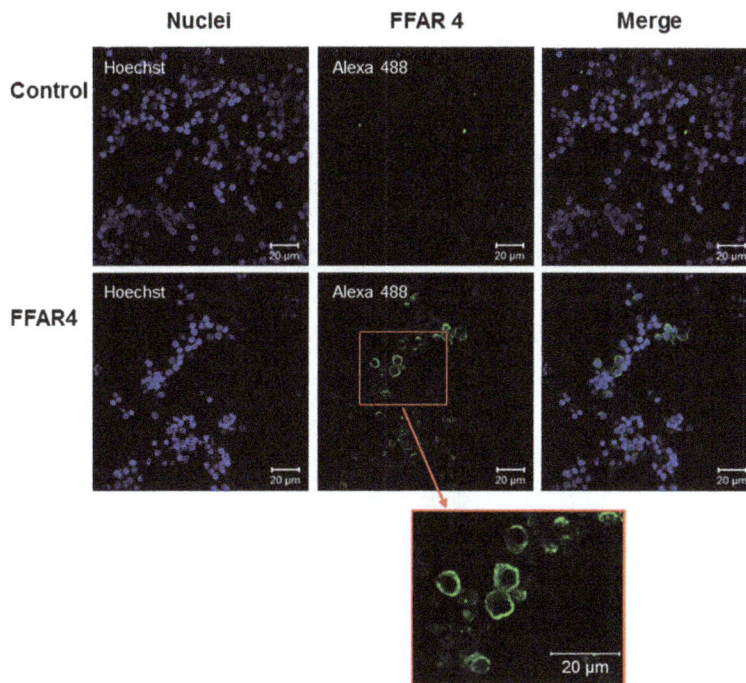

Fig. 2 Expression and localization of free fatty acid receptor 4 (FFAR4) in bovine granulosa cells by immunofluorescence. Immunofluorescence was performed on granulosa cells (GCs) after in vitro culture. Briefly, recovered GCs after follicle puncture and GC washing were incubated in serum-free modified McCoy's 5A medium (2.5×10^5 viable cells/well on a 8-well chamber slide (Lab-Tek® Nunc) for 48 h. Cultures were performed in a water-saturated atmosphere containing 5% CO_2 in air at 38°C. FFAR4 (green fluorescence) was immunodetected in GCs (customized FFAR4 rabbit antibody, Agro-Bio). Pre-immunized rabbit serum was used as the control with the same secondary antibody as for FFAR4 detection. Nuclei were stained with Hoechst 33,258 (blue fluorescence). The picture framed in red is a magnification of the area framed in red from the original image. Bars = 20 µm

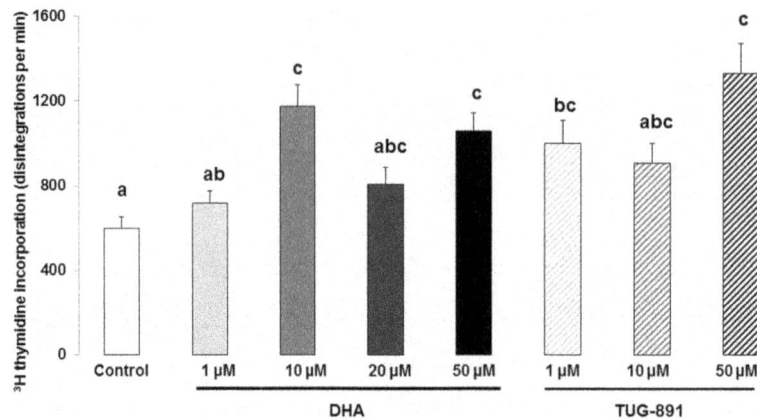

Fig. 3 Synthesis of DNA in bovine granulosa cells: ^{3}H-thymidine incorporation after 24 h treatment with DHA or TUG-891. Effects of DHA or TUG-891 on cell proliferation were assessed by measurement of ^{3}H-thymidine incorporation in bovine granulosa cells after 24 h culture in enriched McCoy's 5A media with various doses of DHA (1, 10, 20 and 50 μM) or TUG-891 (1, 10 and 50 μM), as described in Material and Method section. The chemical DMSO alone (1/2000) was used as a negative control due to its use as a solvent for DHA and TUG-891. The data are expressed as disintegrations per minute. Results represent 13 independent cultures with each treatment conducted in four replicates and are presented as mean ± SEM. Bars with different superscripts are significantly different ($p < 0.05$)

fold increase; $p = 0.028$) compared to the control (Fig. 4). With regard to the effect of TUG-891, no significant effect was observed on progesterone secretion at any concentration (Fig. 4).

DHA significantly increased basal estradiol secretion at 10 μM (1.2-fold increase; $p = 0.030$) and 20 μM (1.3-fold increase; $p < 0.0001$) compared to the control (Fig. 5). No effect of TUG-891 on estradiol secretion was reported at any concentration (Fig. 5).

Protein expression

PCNA expression level was analyzed by western blotting in GCs after 15 h in the presence or absence of DHA

(10 μM; Fig. 6a Additional file 6: Figure S6), as this dose exhibited the highest significant effect on GC proliferation. DHA showed a tendency to increase PCNA expression levels (1.9-fold increase; $p = 0.055$). Expression levels of the steroidogenic enzymes, HSD3B1 and CYP11A1, and the cholesterol transporter StAR, were analyzed by western blotting in GCs after 15 h in the presence or absence of DHA (20 μM; Fig. 6b-d, respectively, Additional file 6: Figure S6), as this dose exhibited the highest significant effect on GC progesterone and estradiol secretion. DHA showed a significant 1.88-fold increase in HSD3B1 expression ($p = 0.028$), a significant 1.67-fold increase in StAR expression ($p = 0.016$) and a

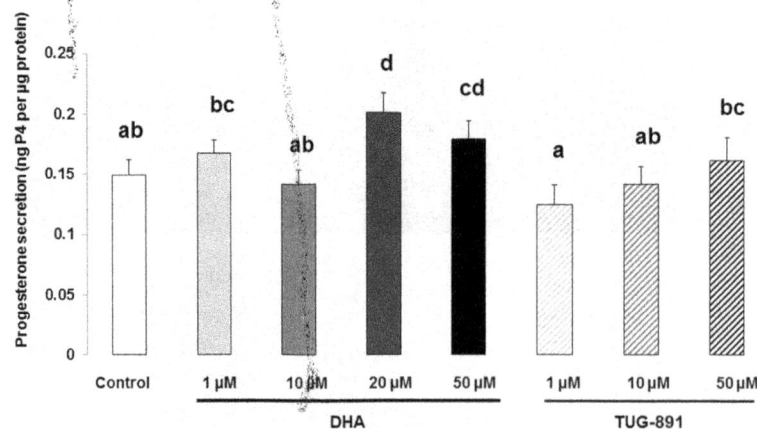

Fig. 4 Progesterone secretion from bovine granulosa cells after 48 h treatment with DHA or TUG-891. Effects of DHA or TUG-891 on progesterone secretion were assessed in culture media of bovine granulosa cells cultured for 48 h in enriched McCoy's 5A media with various doses of DHA (1, 10, 20 and 50 μM) or TUG-891 (1, 10 and 50 μM), as described in Material and Method section. The chemical DMSO alone (1/2000) was used as a negative control due to its use as a solvent for DHA and TUG-891. Progesterone secretion was normalized with the protein concentration in each well and expressed as ng progesterone (P4) per μg protein. Results of 12 independent cultures, with each treatment conducted in quadruplicate, are presented as mean ± SEM. Bars with different superscripts are significantly different ($p < 0.05$)

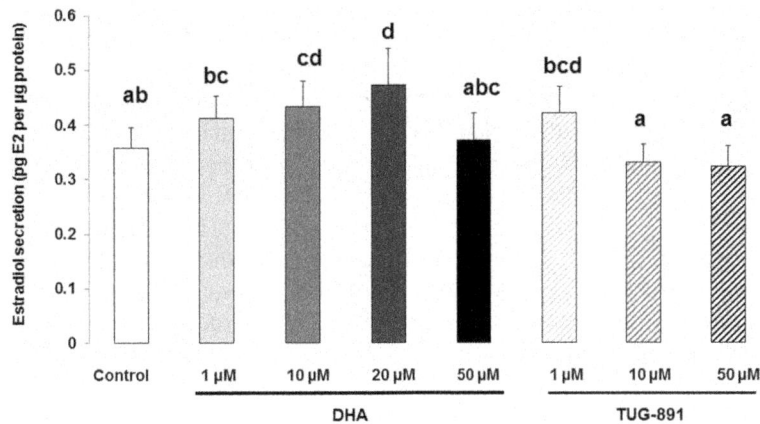

Fig. 5 Estradiol secretion from bovine granulosa cells after 48 h treatment with DHA or TUG-891. Effects of DHA or TUG-891 on estradiol secretion were assessed in culture media of bovine granulosa cells cultured for 48 h in enriched McCoy's 5A media with various doses of DHA (1, 10, 20 and 50 μM) or TUG-891 (1, 10 and 50 μM), as described in Material and Method section. The chemical DMSO alone (1/2000) was used as a negative control due to its use as a solvent for DHA and TUG-891. Estradiol secretion was normalized with the protein concentration in each well and expressed as pg estradiol (E2) per μg protein. Results of six independent cultures, with each treatment conducted in quadruplicate, are presented as mean ± SEM. Bars with different superscripts are significantly different ($p < 0.05$)

significant 2-fold increase in CYP11A1 expression ($p = 0.047$).

Gene expression

Gene expression of several candidate genes previously reported to be involved in n-3 PUFA effects: *GLUT1* (involved in glucose metabolism), *GPX4* (involved in oxidative stress), *PPARA*, *PPARG* and *SREBF1*, 3 transcription factors (involved in lipid metabolism) and *FFAR4* (membrane receptor able to bind DHA and *NFκB*, a signaling molecule reported to be involved in DHA action) (Fig. 7). Four genes showed a significant condition effect: *GPX4* ($p = 0.026$), *NFκB* ($p = 0.003$), *PPARA* ($p = 0.050$) and *SREBF1* ($p = 0.015$). *GPX4*, *PPARA* and *NFκB* exhibited a significant 2.6-

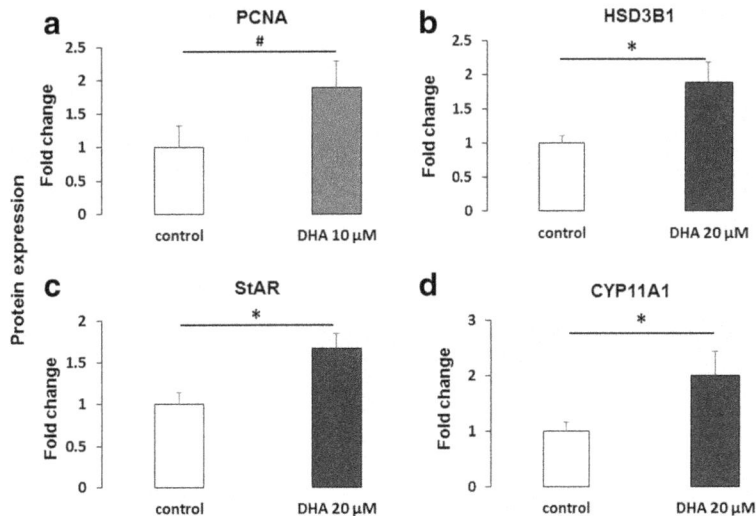

Fig. 6 Protein expression of (**a**) proliferating cell nuclear antigen (PCNA), (**b**) hydroxy-delta-5-steroid dehydrogenase, 3 beta- and steroid delta-isomerase 1 (HSD3B1), (**c**) steroidogenic acute regulatory protein (StAR) and (**d**) cytochrome P450 family 11 subfamily A member 1 (CYP11A1) after 15 h treatment with DHA. Effects of DHA treatment on protein levels were assessed in bovine granulosa cells after 15 h culture in enriched McCoy's 5A media in presence or absence of DHA 10 or 20 μM. The chemical DMSO alone (1/2000) was used as a negative control due to its solvent activity on DHA. Protein extracts were separated by electrophoresis on 4–12% (w:v) SDS-polyacrylamide gel. After electrotransfer to nitrocellulose membranes, the proteins were probed with anti-PCNA (**a**), anti-HSD3B1 (**b**), anti-StAR (**c**) or anti-CYP11A1 (**d**) antibodies. The blots were stripped and re-probed with antibodies against Vinculin (VCL). Results of at least five independent experiments are presented. Bands on the blots were quantified and the total protein / VCL protein ratio was calculated. Results are expressed relative to the control as mean ± SEM of five independent experiments for HSD3B1, StAR, CYP11A1 and six independent experiments for PCNA. * indicates significant difference ($p < 0.05$) and # indicates tendency ($p < 0.10$)

fold increase ($p = 0.004$), 5.4-fold increase ($p = 0.004$), and 4.5-fold increase ($p = 0.018$), respectively, in expression with TUG-891 (10 µM) compared to the control. NFκB also exhibited a significant 4.3-fold increase in expression with DHA 50 µM compared to the control ($p = 0.028$). No other treatments caused any difference in gene expression compared to controls.

Cell signaling pathways

MAPK14, AMPKα, Akt and MAPK1/3 pathways were investigated after 5, 10, 30 or 60 min in the presence or absence of DHA (10 or 50 µM) or TUG-891 (1, 10 or 50 µM, Fig. 8, Additional file 7: Figure S5 and Additional file 8: Figure S7). The non parametric ANOVA showed a significant treatment effect for Akt ($p = 0.005$), AMPKα ($p = 0.001$), MAPK1/3 ($p = 0.048$) and MAPK14 ($p < 0.001$). Only for MAPK14 phosphorylation, a significant time effect was reported ($p < 0.001$), and significant time by treatment interaction were reported for MAPK14 ($p < 0.0001$), MAPK1/3 ($p = 0.040$) and AMPKα ($p = 0.008$). The significant time by treatment interaction meant that the cells did not respond similarly across time to all doses of DHA and TUG-891. We therefore analyzed the effect of time for each treatment used.

The main changes were observed on MAPK14 pathway (Fig. 8a and Additional file 7: Figure S5A). Treatment with DHA (10 µM) led to a significant 8.7-fold increase in MAPK14 phosphorylation at 30 min compared to the control ($p = 0.007$; Fig. 8a). Treatment with DHA (50 µM) led to significant 5.4-fold and 8.4-fold increases in MAPK14 phosphorylation at 5 min ($p = 0.035$) and 30 min ($p = 0.001$), respectively; a similar tendency was observed at 10 min (5.0-fold increase; $p = 0.054$, Additional file 5: Figure S4A). Treatment with TUG-891 (1 µM and 50 µM) led to significant 7.5-fold and 22.5-fold increases in MAPK14 phosphorylation at 30 min, respectively, compared to the control ($p = 0.026$ and 0.024, respectively; Fig. 8a; Additional file 5: Figure S4A). Treatment with TUG-891 (10 µM) led to a significant 7.6-fold increase in MAPK14 phosphorylation at 10 min compared to the control ($p = 0.031$); a similar tendency was observed at 5 min (6.0-fold increase; $p = 0.091$; Additional file 5: Figure S4A). Whilst no effect was observed on Akt and AMPKα phosphorylation after DHA treatment at 10 µM   (Fig. 8c) or 50 µM (data not shown), treatment with TUG-891 (1 µM) resulted in a significant 5.3-fold increase in Akt phosphorylation at 5 min ($p = 0.020$; Fig. 8c) and a 13.2-fold increase in AMPKα phosphorylation at 5 min ($p = 0.029$; Fig. 8b) compared to the control. Moreover, treatment with TUG-891 (50 µM) led to a significant 5.8-fold increase in AMPKα phosphorylation at 30 min ($p = 0.039$); a similar tendency was observed at 60 min (5.5-fold increase; $p = 0.053$; Additional file 7: Figure S5B). Finally, no effect was observed on MAPK1/3

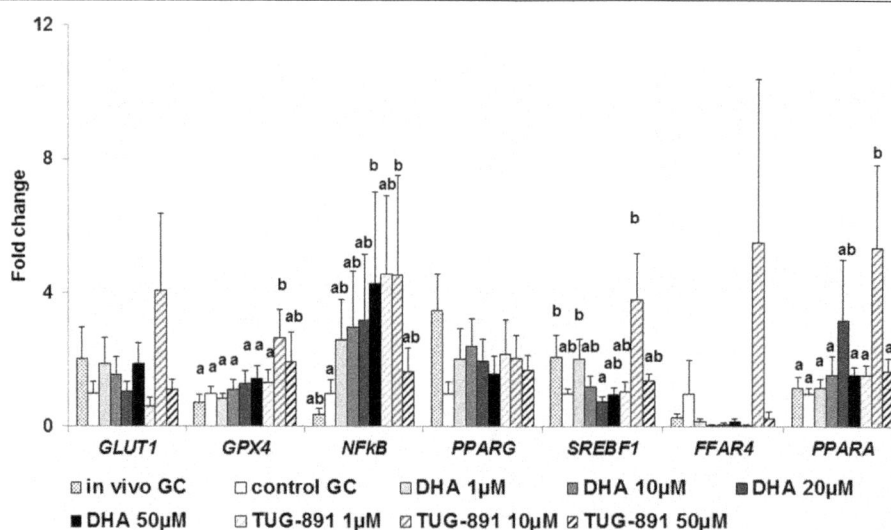

Fig. 7 Gene expression in bovine granulosa cells before or after 8 h treatment with DHA or TUG-891. Effects of DHA or TUG-891 on mRNA expression of solute carrier family 2 member 1 (*GLUT1*), glutathione peroxidase 4 (*GPX4*), nuclear factor of kappa light polypeptide gene enhancer in B-cells 1 (*NFkB*), peroxisome proliferator-activated receptor gamma (*PPARG*), sterol regulatory element binding transcription factor 1 (*SREBF1*), free fatty acid receptor 4 (*FFAR4*) and PPAR alpha (*PPARA*) were assessed in bovine granulosa cells (GC) before or after 8 h culture in enriched McCoy's 5A media with various doses of DHA (1, 10, 20 and 50 µM) or TUG-891 (1, 10 and 50 µM), as described in Material and Method section. The chemical DMSO alone (1/2000) was used as a negative control due to its use as a solvent for DHA and TUG-891. Total mRNA was extracted from GC and reverse-transcribed, and real-time RT-PCR was performed. The geometric mean of two housekeeping genes (*RPL19*- ribosomal protein L19 and *RPS9*- ribosomal protein S9) was used to normalize gene expression. Results of 10 independent cultures are presented as mean ± SEM. Bars with different superscripts are significantly different ($p < 0.05$)

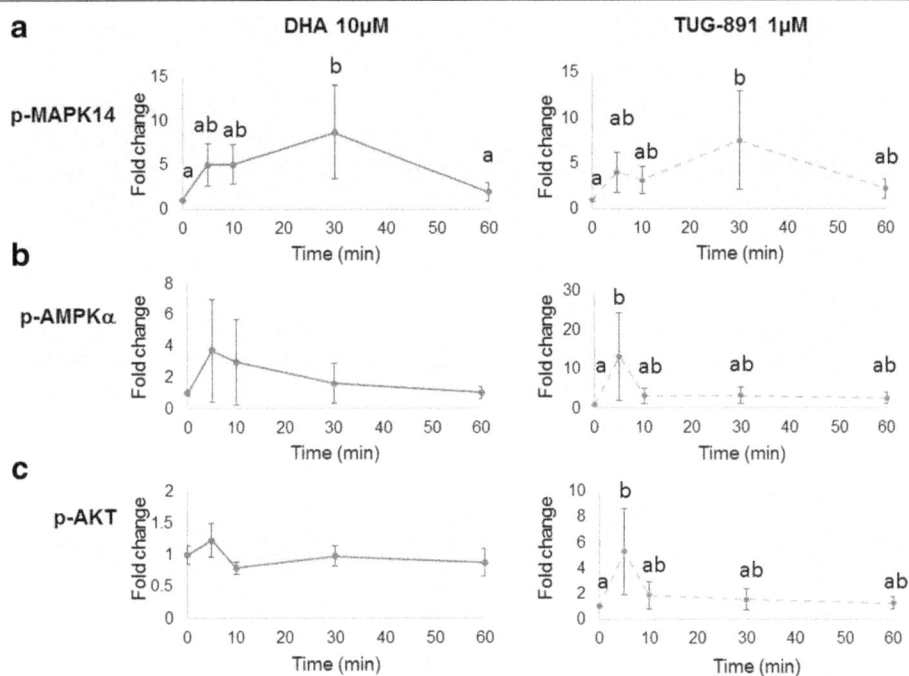

Fig. 8 Signaling pathways in bovine granulosa cells after DHA or TUG-891 treatment. Effects of DHA or TUG-891 on phosphorylation of (**a**) mitogen-activated protein kinase 14 (MAPK14), (**b**) AMP-activated protein kinasea (AMPKα) and (**c**) protein kinase B (Akt) signaling pathways were assessed in bovine granulosa cells cultured for 15 h in enriched McCoy's 5A media with 10 μM DHA or 1 μM TUG-891, as described in Material and Method section for 5, 10, 30 and 60 min. Protein extracts were separated by electrophoresis on 4–12% (w:v) SDS-polyacrylamide gel. After electrotransfer to nitrocellulose membranes, the proteins were probed with anti-phosphorylated (p-)MAPK14 (**a**), anti-p-AMPKα (**b**) or anti-p-AKT1/2/3 (**c**) antibodies. The blots were stripped and re-probed with antibodies against MAPK14, AMPKα or Akt, respectively. Bands on the blots were quantified. Results of four independent experiments are presented as the ratio of p-protein to total protein, normalized by the ratio observed in control at each time and expressed as mean ± SEM of four independent experiments, with time 0 min being equal to 1 (for reference). Bars with different superscripts are significantly different ($p < 0.05$)

phosphorylation with DHA (10 or 50 μM) or TUG-891 (1 or 10 μM) (data not shown). Only a transient, albeit significant, increase in MAPK1/3 phosphorylation was observed after 5 min treatment with TUG-891 at 50 μM (1.6-fold increase; $p = 0.021$; Additional file 7: Figure S5C).

DHA incorporation in granulosa cells

Fatty acid composition was analysed in GC after DHA treatment on total fatty acids (Table 2). DHA 1 μM led to a significant 2.6-increase ($p < 0.032$) 10 μM led to a significant 12-fold increase ($p < 0.0055$) and DHA 50 μM led to a significant 27-fold increase ($p < 0.0016$) in DHA lipid composition. No other difference in FA lipid composition was reported between groups.

Discussion

In the present study, we investigated the effect of DHA treatment on bovine GCs in culture. For the first time, we showed that the addition of 10 μM and 50 μM DHA increased cellular proliferation, that the addition of 20 μM and 50 μM DHA increased progesterone secretion and that the addition of 10 μM and 20 μM DHA

increased estradiol secretion. We also performed experiments to decipher the possible mechanisms of DHA action on GC functions. We showed that DHA increased PCNA, StAR and steroidogenic enzyme HSD3B1 and CYP11A1 protein expression and MAPK14 phosphorylation. We also reported, for the first time, the mRNA and protein expression of FFAR4 in bovine GCs and showed that FFAR4 activation by the FFAR4 agonist TUG-891 led to a similar increase in cellular proliferation and MAPK14 phosphorylation as with DHA treatment. However, TUG-891 treatment did not lead to increases in steroid secretion.

DHA increased in vitro granulosa cell proliferation

We reported here that DHA (10 and 50 μM) increased cellular proliferation of GCs in vitro. This finding is relevant to the increase in PCNA expression that we also observed after DHA treatment. Indeed, PCNA is involved in both DNA synthesis and repair [50]. Such effects of n-3 PUFAs on GC proliferation have already been reported in ovine cells in vitro [51]. Moreover, our in vitro results are also consistent with in vivo n-3 PUFA dietary supplementation data previously reported for bovine animals. Indeed, n-3 PUFA-enriched diets have resulted in increases in the pre-ovulatory follicle size [9, 10], and the number of total follicles [16], small follicles [17], medium follicles [52, 53] and large follicles [11] in bovine animals. These data are consistent with a stimulatory effect of n-3 PUFAs on GC proliferation, which is the crucial step involved in the increase in size of the entire follicle. Indeed, an increase in follicle numbers corresponds to increase in follicles that are detectable by ultrasonographic examination (> 2–3 mm). The increase of follicles of this size is a consequence of follicles < 2 mm growth and of the proliferation of their GCs.

DHA increased in vitro granulosa cell steroidogenesis

With regard to steroidogenesis, we reported here that DHA increased secretion of both progesterone and estradiol. This finding is consistent with increases in the protein expression level of the steroidogenic enzymes, HSD3B1, CYP11A1 and of the carrier StAR that we observed. Indeed, StAR protein is essential for the initial and rate-limiting step in steroid biosynthesis, namely transfer of hydrophobic cholesterol from the outer mitochondrial membrane to the inner mitochondrial membrane (reviewed in [54]), the location of another enzyme crucial to steroid biosynthesis, CYP11A1. This enzyme converts cholesterol into pregnenolone [55]. The HSD3B1 enzyme is a required step in the conversion of pregnenolone into progesterone [56] or in theca cells to further obtain androstenedione [57], the latter being a necessary precursor in estradiol synthesis. Moreover, such stimulating effects of n-3 PUFAs on steroidogenesis have already been described for ovine GCs in vitro, involving both progesterone and estradiol secretion [51]. The increase in progesterone and estradiol observed after DHA treatment is also consistent with our previous results, which showed a stimulatory effect of DHA on progesterone secretion from bovine cumulus cells, originating from GCs [19]. N-3 PUFAs have also been shown to increase progesterone secretion from ovine theca cells in vitro [58] and follicular fluid progesterone concentration (from follicles 4–7 mm diameter) in vivo, in ewes fed with a n-3 PUFA-enriched diet [51]. Furthermore, in agreement with the increase in StAR protein level measured in the present study, Waters et al. previously showed that a n-3 PUFA-enriched diet led to increased *StAR* gene expression in another bovine reproductive compartment, the endometrium [59]. In mouse Leydig tumor cells, inhibition of PTGS2 activity (an enzyme required for prostaglandin biosynthesis) is known to facilitate cAMP-induced steroidogenesis via increased StAR protein expression [60]. N-3 PUFAs are known to be potent inhibitors of PTGS2 activity [61]; this may explain the increase in StAR protein expression reported in the present study, following DHA treatment

of GCs. The increased estradiol effect observed after DHA treatment indicates that DHA might also affect cytochrome P450 aromatase and/or 17β-HSD protein expression levels, as both of these enzymes are necessary for conversion of androstenedione (supplied in our culture media) to estradiol [62]. However, this hypothesis would require further investigation. Finally, examination of steroidogenic enzyme activities would clarify whether DHA affects expression levels only or also the activities of these enzymes.

DHA mechanisms of action through FFAR4

For the first time, we showed in the present study that FFAR4 is expressed in bovine granulosa cells. To our knowledge, granulosa expression of FFAR4 has not yet been reported in other species. Only a few published papers have reported FFAR4 expression in bovine tissues, namely adipose tissue [63, 64]. In other species, FFAR4 is expressed in adipose tissue, spleen and intestine in pigs [65], while in human and rodents, its expression is more widely reported in additional tissues (immune cells, pancreatic cells, lung, muscle, liver and placenta) [42, 66–69]. We demonstrated here that FFAR4 is localized in the vicinity of the cellular membrane in GCs, as expected for a G protein-coupled receptor. This expression of FFAR4 in bovine GCs indicates that long chain fatty acids, including DHA, could act on GCs, at least in part, via this receptor. However, it should be noted that not all cultured GCs were shown to express FFAR4.

Activation of FFAR4 by TUG-891 (1 and 50 μM) mirrored the effect of DHA on GC proliferation, but not on progesterone and estradiol secretion, suggesting that DHA effects on cell proliferation could occur through FFAR4 activation. Indeed, TUG-891 is a specific and potent agonist of FFAR4 [41, 70]. Thus, the effects observed after TUG-891 treatment could be related to FFAR4 activation. It has already been reported that DHA could exert effects through FFAR4 stimulation in adipocytes [71], in macrophages [72] or in cardia cells [73]. Of note, a linear dose response was not reported in the present study, notably concerning GC proliferation (DHA 20 μM). This observation could suggest that the DHA dose response followed a U-shaped (for example) response pattern [74]. It is also possible that, at higher concentration, other DHA mechanisms could occur, potentially counteracting the FFAR4 effect on proliferation.

Moreover, several effects, such as the ability of DHA to inhibit responsiveness of macrophages to endotoxin, inhibition of IκB kinase phosphorylation, IκB phosphorylation and degradation, and inhibition of production of TNF, IL-6 and MCP-1, that have already been demonstrated, were abolished in FFAR4 knockdown cells [28, 75]. In our study, we observed an increase in MAPK14 phosphorylation in GCs after

DHA supplementation (10 and 50 μM), and a similar increase after TUG-891 treatment (1, 10 and 50 μM). As shown in the published literature, MAPK14 (p38 MAPK) may be involved in follicle stimulating hormone (FSH)-induced estradiol secretion in rat and mouse GCs [37, 38], but was also demonstrated to be involved in GC proliferation in a culture model of hamster pre-antral follicles stimulated with transforming growth factor β1 (TGFβ1) [76]. Thus, these results suggest that FFAR4 activation leads to the activation of this MAPK14 signaling pathway, which might play a role in DHA effects on bovine GC proliferation. However, additional experiments would be needed to demonstrate that DHA could activate FFAR4 in bovine GCs, involving investigation of, for example, plasmid transfection, FFAR4 overexpression and inhibition, and intracellular calcium measurement.

No effect of TUG-891 treatment was reported on GC steroidogenesis, suggesting that DHA effects on progesterone and estradiol secretion are independent of FFAR4 activation. Several other mechanisms of action have already been proposed for DHA: modification of cellular membrane lipid composition (fluidity, raft formation); regulation of eicosanoid production (for example, prostaglandins and leukotrienes); transcription factor expression (PPARG and SREBF1, for example) or signaling pathways, such as NFκB [26, 28, 30]. In this study, we evidenced a significant increase in cellular DHA level from total lipids after 1 μM, 10 μM and 50 μM DHA treatment. It is thus possible that DHA affected steroidogenesis by one of these mechanisms and not by activating FFAR4.

The study of candidate gene expression that was performed here showed no modification of canonical genes (PPARG, PPARA, SREBF1) following DHA treatment, except for PPARA with the highest DHA dose used, DHA50 μM. Similar absence of effects on PPARG have already been reported in other studies, as in this study [77]. Nevertheless, TUG-891 treatment has already been reported to modify PPARG transcription after several days of culture in 3T3L1 [71]. In this study, we analyzed GC gene expression after 8 h of TUG-891 stimulation, which might be too brief a period to enable transcription modifications to occur immediately after FFAR4 stimulation. The only differences observed in gene expression are upregulations of GPX4 (glutathione peroxidase 4), NFκB (nuclear factor kappa B) and PPARA (peroxisome proliferator-activated receptor alpha) expression after TUG-891 treatment (10 μM). GPX4 is a phospholipid hydroperoxidase that protects cells against membrane lipid peroxidation. Such a mechanism has already been described for DHA in murine hippocampal cells [78]. By increasing GPX4 expression, DHA is able to protect the cell from oxidative damage resulting of non-enzymatic

peroxidation of membrane phospholipids. It is possible that this mechanism is associated with FFAR4 activation, as we found a similar increase in GPX4 expression after TUG-891 treatment. DHA is able to bind PPARG and PPARA and can consequently increase insulin sensitivity [26]. Through binding to PPARG, DHA could inhibit activation of NFκB, a key transcription factor involved in inflammatory pathways [26]. Moreover, the inhibitory effect of DHA on NFkB can also occur via the FA receptor FFAR4 [28]. The increased NFkB mRNA expression reported after DHA 50 μM and TUG 10 μM in the present study is thus surprising and NFκB activation, which was not investigated in the present study, should be studied.

Overall, despite functional differences between DHA-treated and control GCs, there were no huge changes in gene expression. In order to further investigate the effects and mechanisms of action of FFAR4 activation, experiments involving primary GC culture should be replaced by those involving GC line cultures; such cultures would enable FFAR4 overexpression and inactivation, while maintaining a GC phenotype. It is also possible that a global transcriptomic approach should be envisioned after DHA treatment in order to have a broad picture of the potential mechanisms involved. Indeed, the investigation of other genes, such as PTGS2, might have shown differences that could explain StAR regulation, for example.

Of note, the culture system used in this experiment is serum free and prevent the differentiation of granulosa cells generally occurring after about 15 h culture. It also enable to treat cells with the precise concentrations of DHA (which would be already present in culture medium if we had used serum). In the culture system used in the present paper, GC are maintaining a round shape even when platted, at least till 48 h culture (the latest endpoints in this paper), and not a fibroblastic-like shape, meaning they did not differentiate as much as when serum is used. On the other hand, this culture system also presented some disadvantages. Indeed, primary cell cultures require freshly isolating GCs for each culture, and therefore they can exhibit huge variation in response to treatment, depending on the batch of ovaries used. In this context, the use of a high number of independent culture can be compulsory, as in the present work. Moreover, in this culture system, in order to be able to set up endpoints before 48 h culture, we chose to treat cells at the beginning of the culture, meaning that both platted and non-platted cells were treated. A similar number of living cells is cultured in each well, with a varying proportion of dead cells (assessed by trypan blue staining and cell counting). Concerning proliferation assay, as floating cells are removed before the assay, only thymidine incorporated in platted cells is measured (most of floating cells being dead cells in our cell culture system). Concerning data on steroidogenesis, steroid secreted in the culture medium by both platted and non-platted cells during the cell culture are measured after 48 h. Steroid concentration are normalized by protein concentration in each well, meaning by protein amount of platted cells only. We estimated that the proportion of platted cells to viable floating cells is the same in each well for a specific batch of cells. This normalization might biased the steroid results as the concentration of steroid for a viable amount of cells might be slightly overestimated due to the normalization taking into account only platted cells. Nevertheless, we believe that this normalization would not affect differences observed between conditions.

Conclusions

The present study reported that DHA treatment during in vitro culture increased granulosa cell proliferation and PCNA expression level, suggesting an effect of this n-3 PUFA on DNA synthesis. This effect is relevant with the increase in ovarian follicular population observed after in vivo n-3 enriched diet supplementation of dairy cows. DHA supplementation also increased progesterone and estradiol secretion, together with the protein expression level of the steroidogenic enzymes HSD3B1, CYP11A1 and the cholesterol transporter StAR. Such increase in progesterone level is also reported after in vivo n-3 enriched diet supplementation of dairy cows. These effects on granulosa cell function could thus be related to the improved reproduction observed after n-3 enriched diet supplementation. TUG-891, a FFAR4 agonist, showed similar effects to DHA on GC proliferation and on MAPK14 phosphorylation, but had no effect on steroidogenesis. These data indicate that DHA might act on GC proliferation through FFAR4 activation, which, in turn, leads to MAPK14 phosphorylation. Nevertheless, FFAR4 activation by DHA remains to be demonstrated in bovine GCs. Other potential mechanisms of DHA action on steroidogenesis should be investigated, as our hypothesis of FFAR4-mediated effects on steroidogenesis was not verified.

Additional files

Additional file 1: Figure S1. Control of customized free fatty acid receptor 4 (FFAR4) antibody specificity. Protein extracts from bovine lung tissue were separated by electrophoresis on 4–12% (w:v) SDS-polyacrylamide gel. After electrotransfer to nitrocellulose membranes, the proteins were probed with anti-FFAR4 antibody (0.95 µg/mL, customized FFAR4 rabbit antibody, Agro-Bio), which was pre-incubated for 15 min with different concentrations of the bovine specific peptide (Agro-Bio) used to produce the antibody (from 0 to 2.5 µg/mL). The blots were stripped and re-probed with antibodies against vinculin (VCL) used as the loading control. (TIF 93 kb)

Additional file 2: Table S1. Characteristics of primary antibodies used for western blotting and / or immunohistochemistry or immunofluorescence. (DOCX 16 kb)

Additional file 3: Figure S2. Experiment design of the study. * Some experiments enabled to measure both progesterone and estradiol in supernatants of the same 96-well dishes. (TIF 342 kb)

Additional file 4: Figure S3. Gene expression of (A) free fatty acid receptor 1 (*FFAR1*) and (B) free fatty acid receptor 4 (*FFAR4*) in bovine ovarian cells. Total mRNA was extracted from the ovarian cortex (CX), thecal cells (TH), granulosa cells (GC) and cumulus cells (CC). Total mRNA was then reverse-transcribed and real-time RT-PCR was performed. The geometric mean of two housekeeping genes (*RPL19*- ribosomal protein L19 and *RPS9*- ribosomal protein S9) was used to normalize gene expression. Results of 2 to 4 independent samples are presented as means ± SEM. Bars with different superscripts are significantly different ($p < 0.05$). (TIF 59 kb)

Additional file 5: Figure S4. Expression and localization of free fatty acid receptor 4 (FFAR4) in bovine granulosa cells by immunofluorescence with a commercial antibody against human FFAR4. Immunofluorescence was performed on granulosa cells (GC) after in vitro culture. Briefly, recovered GCs after follicle puncture and GC washing were incubated in serum-free modified McCoy's 5A medium (2.5×10^5 viable cells/well on a 8-well chamber slide (Lab-Tek® Nunc) for 48 h. Cultures were performed in a water-saturated atmosphere containing 5% CO_2 in air at 38°C. FFAR4 (green fluorescence) was immunodetected in GC (commercial human FFAR4 rabbit antibody, Aviva Systems Biology, Clinisciences, Nanterre, France) with a similar protocol to the protocol used with the customized anti-FFAR4 antibody. The commercial anti- FFAR4 antibody was produced by using a peptide from the FFAR4 human c-terminal region, which shares 89% identity (Protein BLAST® result on NCBI website) with the *Bos taurus* FFAR4 (Accession number: NP_001315586.1) and no identity with other amino acid sequences of bovine proteome. Rabbit IgG was used as the control with the same secondary antibody as for FFAR4 detection. Nuclei were stained with Hoechst 33,258 (blue fluorescence). Fluorescence was observed under a Zeiss confocal microscope LSM700 (Carl Zeiss Microscopy GmbH, Munich, Germany) using an oil 63× objective and the appropriate filters. The images were captured using Zen 2012 software (black edition version 8.0, Carl Zeiss Microscopy GmbH). The picture framed in red is a magnification of the area framed in red from the original image. Bars = 10 µm. (TIF 132 kb)

Additional file 6: Figure S6. Protein expression of (A) proliferating cell nuclear antigen (PCNA), (B) hydroxy-delta-5-steroid dehydrogenase, 3 beta- and steroid delta-isomerase 1 (HSD3B1), (C) steroidogenic acute regulatory protein (StAR) and (D) cytochrome P450 family 11 subfamily A member 1 (CYP11A1) after 15 h treatment with DHA. Effects of DHA treatment on protein levels were assessed in bovine granulosa cells after 15 h culture in enriched McCoy's 5A media in presence or absence of DHA 10 or 20 µM. The chemical DMSO alone (1/2000) was used as a negative control due to its solvent activity on DHA. Protein extracts were separated by electrophoresis on 4–12% (w:v) SDS-polyacrylamide gel. After electrotransfer to nitrocellulose membranes, the proteins were probed with anti-PCNA (A), anti-HSD3B1 (B), anti-StAR (C) or anti-CYP11A1 (D) antibodies. The blots were stripped and re-probed with antibodies against Vinculin (VCL). The blots presented are representative of the quantification reported in Fig. 6. (TIF 180 kb)

Additional file 7: Figure S5. Signaling pathways in bovine granulosa cells after treatment with other concentrations of DHA (50 µM) or TUG-891 (10 and 50 µM). Effects of DHA or TUG-891 on phosphorylation of (A) mitogen-activated protein kinase 14 (MAPK14), (B) AMP-activated protein kinaseα (AMPKα) and (C) mitogen-activated protein kinase 1/3 (MAPK1/3) signaling pathways were assessed in bovine granulosa cells cultured for 15 h in enriched McCoy's 5A media with 50 µM DHA or with 10 or 50 µM TUG-891, as described in Material and Method section for 5, 10, 30 and 60 min. Protein extracts were separated by electrophoresis on 4–12%

(w:v) SDS-polyacrylamide gel. After electrotransfer to nitrocellulose membranes, the proteins were probed with anti-phosphorylated (p-)MAPK14 (A), anti-p-AMPKα (B) or anti-p-MAPK1/3 (C) antibodies. The blots were stripped and re-probed with antibodies against MAPK14, AMPKα, or MAPK1/3, respectively. Bands on the blots were quantified. Results of four independent experiments are presented as the ratio of p-protein to total protein, normalized by the ratio observed in control at each time and expressed as mean ± SEM, with time 0 min being equal to 1 (for reference). Bars with different superscripts are significantly different ($p < 0.05$). (TIF 99 kb)

Additional file 8: Figure S7. Signaling pathways in bovine granulosa cells after DHA or TUG-891 treatment. Effects of DHA or TUG-891 on phosphorylation of (A) mitogen-activated protein kinase 14 (MAPK14), (B) AMP-activated protein kinaseα (AMPKα) and (C) protein kinase B (Akt) signaling pathways were assessed in bovine granulosa cells cultured for 15 h in enriched McCoy's 5A media with 10 μM DHA or 1 μM TUG-891, as described in Material and Method section for 5, 10, 30 and 60 min. Protein extracts were separated by electrophoresis on 4–12% (w:v) SDS-polyacrylamide gel. After electrotransfer to nitrocellulose membranes, the proteins were probed with anti-phosphorylated (p-) MAPK14 (A), anti-p-AMPKα (B) or anti-p-AKT1/2/3 (C) antibodies. The blots were stripped and re-probed with antibodies against MAPK14, AMPKα or Akt, respectively. The blots presented are representative of the quantification reported in Fig. 8. (TIF 228 kb)

Abbreviations

Akt: Protein kinase B; ALA: Alpha-linolenic acid; AMPKα: AMP-activated protein kinaseα; BSA: Bovine serum albumin; CYP11A1: Cytochrome P450 family 11 subfamily A member 1; DAB: Diaminobenzidine tetrahydrochloride dehydrate; DHA: Docosahexaenoic acid; DMSO: Dimethyl sulfoxide; DNA: Deoxyribonucleic acid; ELISA: Enzyme-linked immunosorbent assay; EPA: Eicosapentaenoic acid; FA: Fatty acids; FAME: Fatty acid methyl ester; FFAR1: Free fatty acid membrane receptor 1; FFAR4: Free fatty acid membrane receptor 4; GC: Granulosa cells; GLUT1: Glucose Transporter Type 1; GPX4: Glutathione peroxidase 4; HRP: Horseradish peroxidase; HSD3B1: Hydroxy-delta-5-steroid dehydrogenase, 3 beta- and steroid delta-isomerase 1; IgG: Immunoglobulin G; IL-1β: Interleukine 1 beta; IL-6: Interleukine 6; IL-8: Interleukine 8; IκB: I kappa B; LDL: Low density lipoprotein; MAP K14: Mitogen-Activated Protein Kinase 14; MAPK1/3: Mitogen-Activated Protein Kinase 1/3; MCP-1: Monocyte Chemoattractant Protein-1; NFDMP: Non-fat dry milk powder; NFkB: Nuclear factor kappa B; PBS: Phosphate buffered saline; PCNA: Proliferating cell nuclear antigen; PCR: Polymerase chain reaction; PGF2α: Prostaglandin F2 alpha; PPARs: Peroxisome proliferator-activated receptors; PTGS2: Prostaglandin-Endoperoxide Synthase 2; PUFA: Polyunsaturated fatty acid; RNA: Ribonucleic acid; RPL19: Ribosomal protein L19; RPS9: Ribosomal protein S9; SEM: Standard error of the mean; SREBF1: Sterol Regulatory Element Binding Transcription Factor 1; StAR: Steroidogenic acute regulatory protein; TBS: Tris-buffer saline; TGFβ1: Transforming growth factor beta1; TNF: Tumor necrosis factor

Acknowledgements
We would like to thank the technical staff of the research (PRC) unit in INRA Val de Loire Centre (Albert Arnould and Thierry Delpuech) for collecting the ovaries.

Funding
The Institut National de la Recherche Agronomique (INRA) and « Région Centre-Val de Loire » subvention project BOVOMEGA3 financially supported this work.

Authors' contributions
AD and MD performed the experiments and analyses in this study. SU helped with preparation of the manuscript. VM performed immunofluorescence and immunohistochemistry in the study. SE and VM were involved in data analysis and were major contributors to writing the manuscript. All authors read and approved the final manuscript.

Competing interests
The authors declare that they have no competing interests.

References

1. Siriwardhana N, Kalupahana NS, Moustaid-Moussa N, Se-Kwon K. Chapter 13 - health benefits of n-3 polyunsaturated fatty acids: Eicosapentaenoic acid and docosahexaenoic acid. In: Adv Food Nutr Res. Vol. volume 65: academic press; 2012. p. 211–22.
2. Plourde M, Cunnane SC. Extremely limited synthesis of long chain polyunsaturates in adults: implications for their dietary essentiality and use as supplements. Appl Physiol Nutr Metab. 2007;32(4):619–34.
3. Baker EJ, Miles EA, Burdge GC, Yaqoob P, Calder PC. Metabolism and functional effects of plant-derived omega-3 fatty acids in humans. Prog Lipid Res. 2016;64:30–56.
4. Simopoulos AP. Omega-3 fatty acids in inflammation and autoimmune diseases. J Am Coll Nutr. 2002;21(6):495–505.
5. Deckelbaum RJ, Torrejon C. The omega-3 fatty acid nutritional landscape: health benefits and sources. J Nutr. 2012;142(3):587S–91S.
6. Calder PC. Functional roles of fatty acids and their effects on human health. J Parenter Enter Nutr. 2015;39(1 suppl):18S–32S.
7. Santos JE, Bilby TR, Thatcher WW, Staples CR, Silvestre FT. Long chain fatty acids of diet as factors influencing reproduction in cattle. Reprod Domest Anim. 2008;43(Suppl 2):23–30.
8. Gulliver CE, Friend MA, King BJ, Clayton EH. The role of omega-3 polyunsaturated fatty acids in reproduction of sheep and cattle. Anim Reprod Sci. 2012;131(1–2):9–22.
9. Ambrose DJ, Kastelic JP, Corbett R, Pitney PA, Petit HV, Small JA, Zalkovic P. Lower pregnancy losses in lactating dairy cows fed a diet enriched in alpha-linolenic acid. J Dairy Sci. 2006;89(8):3066–74.
10. Dirandeh E, Towhidi A, Zeinoaldini S, Ganjkhanlou M, Ansari Pirsaraei Z, Fouladi-Nashta A. Effects of different polyunsaturated fatty acid supplementations during the postpartum periods of early lactating dairy cows on milk yield, metabolic responses, and reproductive performances. J Anim Sci. 2013;91(2):713–21.
11. Elis S, Freret S, Desmarchais A, Maillard V, Cognié J, Briant E, Touzé J-L, Dupont M, Faverdin P, et al. Effect of a long chain n-3 PUFA-enriched diet on production and reproduction variables in Holstein dairy cows. Anim Reprod Sci. 2016;164:121–32.
12. Mattos R, Staples CR, Arteche A, Wiltbank MC, Diaz FJ, Jenkins TC, Thatcher WW. The effects of feeding fish oil on uterine secretion of PGF2alpha, milk composition, and metabolic status of periparturient Holstein cows. J Dairy Sci. 2004;87(4):921–32.
13. Caldari-Torres C, Rodriguez-Sallaberry C, Greene ES, Badinga L. Differential effects of n-3 and n-6 fatty acids on prostaglandin F2[alpha] production by bovine endometrial cells. J Dairy Sci. 2006;89(3):971–7.
14. Mattos R, Staples CR, Williams J, Amorocho A, McGuire MA. Uterine, ovarian, and production responses of lactating dairy cows to increasing dietary concentrations of menhaden fish meal. J Dairy Sci. 2002;85(4):755–64.
15. Dirandeh E, Towhidi A, Pirsaraei ZA, Hashemi FA, Ganjkhanlou M, Zeinoaldini S, Roodbari AR, Saberifar T, Petit HV. Plasma concentrations of PGFM and uterine and ovarian responses in early lactation dairy cows fed omega-3 and omega-6 fatty acids. Theriogenology. 2013;80(2):131–7.
16. Moallem U, Shafran A, Zachut M, Dekel I, Portnick Y, Arieli A. Dietary alpha-linolenic acid from flaxseed oil improved folliculogenesis and IVF performance in dairy cows, similar to eicosapentaenoic and docosahexaenoic acids from fish oil. Reproduction. 2013;146(6):603–14.
17. Zachut M, Dekel I, Lehrer H, Arieli A, Arav A, Livshitz L, Yakoby S, Moallem U. Effects of dietary fats differing in n-6:n-3 ratio fed to high-yielding dairy

cows on fatty acid composition of ovarian compartments, follicular status, and oocyte quality. J Dairy Sci. 2010;93(2):529–45.

18. Marei WF, Wathes DC, Fouladi-Nashta AA. The effect of linolenic acid on bovine oocyte maturation and development. Biol Reprod. 2009; 81(6):1064–72.

19. Oseikria M, Elis S, Maillard V, Corbin E, Uzbekova S. N-3 polyunsaturated fatty acid DHA during IVM affected oocyte developmental competence in cattle. Theriogenology. 2016;85:1625–34.

20. Petit HV, Twagiramungu H. Conception rate and reproductive function of dairy cows fed different fat sources. Theriogenology. 2006;66(5):1316–24.

21. Childs S, Carter F, Lynch CO, Sreenan JM, Lonergan P, Hennessy AA, Kenny DA. Embryo yield and quality following dietary supplementation of beef heifers with n-3 polyunsaturated fatty acids (PUFA). Theriogenology. 2008; 70(6):992–1003.

22. Sinedino LDP, Honda PM, Souza LRL, Lock AL, Boland MP, Staples CR, Thatcher WW, Santos JEP. Effects of supplementation with docosahexaenoic acid on reproduction of dairy cows. Reproduction. 2017;153(5):707–23.

23. Ponter AA, Guyader-Joly C, Nuttinck F, Grimard B, Humblot P. Oocyte and embryo production and quality after OPU-IVF in dairy heifers given diets varying in their n-6/n-3 fatty acid ratio. Theriogenology. 2012;78(3):632–45.

24. Hutchinson IA, Hennessy AA, Waters SM, Dewhurst RJ, Evans ACO, Lonergan P, Butler ST. Effect of supplementation with different fat sources on the mechanisms involved in reproductive performance in lactating dairy cattle. Theriogenology. 2012;78(1):12–27.

25. Riediger ND, Othman RA, Suh M, Moghadasian MH. A systemic review of the roles of n-3 fatty acids in health and disease. J Am Diet Assoc. 2009; 109(4):668–79.

26. Calder PC. Mechanisms of action of (n-3) fatty acids. J Nutr. 2012;142(3): 592S–9S.

27. Calder PC. Fatty acids and inflammation: the cutting edge between food and pharma. Eur J Pharmacol. 2011;668(Suppl 1):S50–8.

28. Calder PC. Marine omega-3 fatty acids and inflammatory processes: effects, mechanisms and clinical relevance. Biochim et Biophys Acta (BBA) - Molecular and Cell Biology of Lipids. 2015;1851(4):469–84.

29. Bagga D, Wang L, Farias-Eisner R, Glaspy JA, Reddy ST. Differential effects of prostaglandin derived from ω-6 and ω-3 polyunsaturated fatty acids on COX-2 expression and IL-6 secretion. Proc Natl Acad Sci U S A. 2003;100(4):1751–6.

30. Shaikh SR. Biophysical and biochemical mechanisms by which dietary N-3 polyunsaturated fatty acids from fish oil disrupt membrane lipid rafts. J Nutr Biochem. 2012;23(2):101–5.

31. Miyamoto J, Hasegawa S, Kasubuchi M, Ichimura A, Nakajima A, Kimura I. Nutritional signaling via free fatty acid receptors. Int J Mol Sci. 2016;17(4):450.

32. Prihandoko R, Alvarez-Curto E, Hudson BD, Butcher AJ, Ulven T, Miller AM, Tobin AB, Milligan G. Distinct phosphorylation clusters determine the signaling outcome of free fatty acid receptor 4/G protein-coupled receptor 120. Mol Pharmacol. 2016;89(5):505–20.

33. Gao B, Huang Q, Jie Q, Lu WG, Wang L, Li XJ, Sun Z, Hu YQ, Chen L, et al. GPR120: a bi-potential mediator to modulate the osteogenic and adipogenic differentiation of BMMSCs. Sci Rep. 2015;5:14080.

34. Gómez BI, Gifford CA, Hallford DM, Hernandez Gifford JA. Protein kinase B is required for follicle-stimulating hormone mediated beta-catenin accumulation and estradiol production in granulosa cells of cattle. Anim Reprod Sci. 2015;163:97–104.

35. Silva JM, Hamel M, Sahmi M, Price CA. Control of oestradiol secretion and of cytochrome P450 aromatase messenger ribonucleic acid accumulation by FSH involves different intracellular pathways in oestrogenic bovine granulosa cells in vitro. Reproduction. 2006;132(6):909–17.

36. Ryan KE, Glister C, Lonergan P, Martin F, Knight PG, Evans AC. Functional significance of the signal transduction pathways Akt and Erk in ovarian follicles: in vitro and in vivo studies in cattle and sheep. J Ovarian Res. 2008;1(1):2.

37. Du XH, Zhou XL, Cao R, Xiao P, Teng Y, Ning CB, Liu HL. FSH-induced p38-MAPK-mediated dephosphorylation at serine 727 of the signal transducer and activator of transcription 1 decreases Cyp1b1 expression in mouse granulosa cells. Cell Signal. 2015;27(1):6–14.

38. Inagaki K, Otsuka F, Miyoshi T, Yamashita M, Takahashi M, Goto J, Suzuki J, Makino H. p38-mitogen-activated protein kinase stimulated steroidogenesis in granulosa cell-oocyte cocultures: role of bone morphogenetic proteins 2 and 4. Endocrinology. 2009;150(4):1921–30.

39. Abughazaleh AA, Potu RB, Ibrahim S. Short communication: the effect of substituting fish oil in dairy cow diets with docosahexaenoic acid-

micro algae on milk composition and fatty acids profile. J Dairy Sci. 2009;92(12):6156–9.

40. Boeckaert C, Vlaeminck B, Dijkstra J, Issa-Zacharia A, Van Nespen T, Van Straalen W, Fievez V. Effect of dietary starch or micro algae supplementation on rumen fermentation and milk fatty acid composition of dairy cows. J Dairy Sci. 2008;91(12):4714–27.

41. Hudson BD, Shimpukade B, Mackenzie AE, Butcher AJ, Pediani JD, Christiansen E, Heathcote H, Tobin AB, Ulven T, et al. The pharmacology of TUG-891, a potent and selective agonist of the free fatty acid receptor 4 (FFA4/GPR120), demonstrates both potential opportunity and possible challenges to therapeutic agonism. Mol Pharmacol. 2013;84(5):710–25.

42. Hirasawa A, Tsumaya K, Awaji T, Katsuma S, Adachi T, Yamada M, Sugimoto Y, Miyazaki S, Tsujimoto G. Free fatty acids regulate gut incretin glucagon-like peptide-1 secretion through GPR120. Nat Med. 2005;11(1):90–4.

43. Tosca L, Chabrolle C, Uzbekova S, Dupont J. Effects of metformin on bovine granulosa cells steroidogenesis: possible involvement of adenosine 5' monophosphate-activated protein kinase (AMPK). Biol Reprod. 2007;76(3):368–78.

44. Canepa S, Laine AB, A., Fagu C, Flon C, Monniaux D: Validation d'une methode immunoenzymatique pour le dosage de la progesterone dans le plasma des ovins et des bovins. Les Cahiers Techniques de L'INRA 2008; 64:19–30.

45. Lefils J, Géloën A, Vidal H, Lagarde M, Bernoud-Hubac N. Dietary DHA: time course of tissue uptake and effects on cytokine secretion in mice. Br J Nutr. 2010;104(9):1304–12.

46. Hothorn T, Bretz F, Westfall P. Simultaneous inference in general parametric models. Biom J. 2008;50(3):346–63.

47. Wheeler B: lmPerm: Permutation tests for linear models. 2010.

48. Konietschke F, Placzek M, Schaarschmidt F, Hothorn LA. Nparcomp: an R software package for nonparametric multiple comparisons and simultaneous confidence intervals. J Stat Softw. 2015;64(9):1–17.

49. R_Core_Team. R: a language and environment for statistical computing. Vienna: R-project; 2015.

50. Choe KN, Moldovan G-L. Forging ahead through darkness: PCNA, still the principal conductor at the replication fork. Mol Cell. 2017;65(3):380–92.

51. Wonnacott KE, Kwong WY, Hughes J, Salter AM, Lea RG, Garnsworthy PC, Sinclair KD. Dietary omega-3 and -6 polyunsaturated fatty acids affect the composition and development of sheep granulosa cells, oocytes and embryos. Reproduction. 2010;139(1):57–69.

52. Moussavi ARH, Gilbert RO, Overton TR, Bauman DE, Butler WR. Effects of feeding fish meal and n-3 fatty acids on ovarian and uterine responses in early lactating dairy cows. J Dairy Sci. 2007;90(1):145–54.

53. Robinson RS, Pushpakumara PG, Cheng Z, Peters AR, Abayasekara DR, Wathes DC. Effects of dietary polyunsaturated fatty acids on ovarian and uterine function in lactating dairy cows. Reproduction. 2002;124(1):119–31.

54. Stocco DM, Zhao AH, Tu LN, Morohaku K, Selvaraj V. A brief history of the search for the protein(s) involved in the acute regulation of steroidogenesis. Mol Cell Endocrinol. 2017;441:7–16.

55. Rodgers RJ. Steroidogenic cytochrome P450 enzymes and ovarian steroidogenesis. Reprod Fertil Dev. 1990;2(2):153–63.

56. Bao B, Garverick HA. Expression of steroidogenic enzyme and gonadotropin receptor genes in bovine follicles during ovarian follicular waves: a review. J Anim Sci. 1998;76(7):1903–21.

57. Benkert AR, Young M, Robinson D, Hendrickson C, Lee PA, Strauss KA. Severe Salt-Losing 3β-Hydroxysteroid Dehydrogenase Deficiency: Treatment and Outcomes of HSD3B2 c.35G>A Homozygotes. J Clinical Endocrinol Metabol. 2015;100(8):E1105–15.

58. Hughes J, Kwong WY, Li D, Salter AM, Lea RG, Sinclair KD. Effects of omega-3 and -6 polyunsaturated fatty acids on ovine follicular cell steroidogenesis, embryo development and molecular markers of fatty acid metabolism. Reproduction. 2011;141(1):105–18.

59. Waters SM, Coyne GS, Kenny DA, MacHugh DE, Morris DG. Dietary n-3 polyunsaturated fatty acid supplementation alters the expression of genes involved in the control of fertility in the bovine uterine endometrium. Physiol Genomics. 2012;44(18):878–88.

60. Wang X, Dyson MT, Jo Y, Stocco DM. Inhibition of Cyclooxygenase-2 activity enhances steroidogenesis and steroidogenic acute regulatory gene expression in MA-10 mouse Leydig cells. Endocrinology. 2003; 144(8):3368–75.

61. Ringbom T, Huss U, Stenholm Å, Flock S, Skattebøl L, Perera P, Bohlin L. COX-2 inhibitory effects of naturally occurring and modified fatty acids. J Nat Prod. 2001;64(6):745–9.

62. Pavone ME, Bulun SE. Aromatase inhibitors for the treatment of endometriosis: a review. Fertil Steril. 2012;98(6):1370–9.

63. Elis S, Desmarchais A, Freret S, Maillard V, Labas V, Cognié J, Briant E, Hivelin C, Dupont J, et al. Effect of a long-chain n-3 polyunsaturated fatty acid–enriched diet on adipose tissue lipid profiles and gene expression in Holstein dairy cows. J Dairy Sci. 2016;99(12):10109–27.

64. Agrawal A, Alharthi A, Vailati-Riboni M, Zhou Z, Loor JJ. Expression of fatty acid sensing G-protein coupled receptors in peripartal Holstein cows. J Anim Sci Biotechnol. 2017;8(1):20.

65. Song T, Peng J, Ren J, H-k W, Peng J. Cloning and characterization of spliced variants of the porcine G protein coupled receptor 120. Biomed Res Int. 2015;2015:813816.

66. Gotoh C, Hong YH, Iga T, Hishikawa D, Suzuki Y, Song SH, Choi KC, Adachi T, Hirasawa A, et al. The regulation of adipogenesis through GPR120. Biochem Biophys Res Commun. 2007;354(2):591–7.

67. Miyauchi S, Hirasawa A, Iga T, Liu N, Itsubo C, Sadakane K, Hara T, Tsujimoto G. Distribution and regulation of protein expression of the free fatty acid receptor GPR120. Naunyn Schmiedeberg's Arch Pharmacol. 2009;379(4):427–34.

68. Cornall LM, Mathai ML, Hryciw DH, McAinch AJ. Diet-induced obesity up-regulates the abundance of GPR43 and GPR120 in a tissue specific manner. Cell Physiol Biochem. 2011;28(5):949–58.

69. Lager S, Ramirez VI, Gaccioli F, Jansson T, Powell TL. Expression and localization of the omega-3 fatty acid receptor GPR120 in human term placenta. Placenta. 2014;35(7):523–5.

70. Shimpukade B, Hudson BD, Hovgaard CK, Milligan G, Ulven T. Discovery of a potent and selective GPR120 agonist. J Med Chem. 2012;55(9):4511–5.

71. Song T, Zhou Y, Peng J, Tao Y-X, Yang Y, Xu T, Peng J, Ren J, Xiang Q, et al. GPR120 promotes adipogenesis through intracellular calcium and extracellular signal-regulated kinase 1/2 signal pathway. Mol Cell Endocrinol. 2016;434:1–13.

72. Anbazhagan AN, Priyamvada S, Gujral T, Bhattacharyya S, Alrefai WA, Dudeja PK, Borthakur A. A novel anti-inflammatory role of GPR120 in intestinal epithelial cells. Am J Physiol Cell Physiol. 2016;310(7):C612–21.

73. Li X, Ballantyne LL, Che X, Mewburn JD, Kang JX, Barkley RM, Murphy RC, Yu Y, Funk CD. Endogenously generated Omega-3 fatty acids attenuate vascular inflammation and Neointimal hyperplasia by interaction with free fatty acid receptor 4 in mice. J Am Heart Assoc: Cardiovasc Cerebrovasc Dis. 2015;4(4):e001856.

74. Calabrese EJ, Baldwin LA. U-shaped dose-responses in biology, toxicology, and public health. Annu Rev Public Health. 2001;22:15–33.

75. Oh DY, Talukdar S, Bae EJ, Imamura T, Morinaga H, Fan W, Li P, Lu WJ, Watkins SM, et al. GPR120 is an omega-3 fatty acid receptor mediating potent anti-inflammatory and insulin-sensitizing effects. Cell. 2010;142(5):687–98.

76. Yang P, Roy SK. Transforming growth factor B1 stimulated DNA synthesis in the granulosa cells of preantral follicles: negative interaction with epidermal growth factor. Biol Reprod. 2006;75(1):140–8.

77. Vaidya H, Cheema SK. Arachidonic acid has a dominant effect to regulate lipogenic genes in 3T3-L1 adipocytes compared to omega-3 fatty acids. Food Nutr Res. 2015;59 https://doi.org/10.3402/fnr.v3459.25866.

78. Casañas-Sánchez V, Pérez JA, Fabelo N, Quinto-Alemany D, Díaz ML. Docosahexaenoic (DHA) modulates phospholipid-hydroperoxide glutathione peroxidase (Gpx4) gene expression to ensure self-protection from oxidative damage in hippocampal cells. Front Physiol. 2015;6:203.

12

Alleviation of endoplasmic reticulum stress protects against cisplatin-induced ovarian damage

Yuping Wu[1], Congshun Ma[2], Huihui Zhao[1], Yuxia Zhou[1], Zhenguo Chen[3*] ⓘ and Liping Wang[1*]

Abstract

Background: Cisplatin (CDDP), a widely used chemotherapeutic agent, can induce excessive granulosa cell apoptosis, follicle loss and even premature ovarian insufficiency (POI). However, the mechanism remains elusive, although some studies have indicated the involvement of endoplasmic reticulum stress (ERS). The aim of our study was to investigate the possible mechanism ERS in CDDP-induced granulosa cell apoptosis and follicle loss.

Methods: A POI mouse model was generated by CDDP. The ovaries samples were collected and processed for isobaric tags for relative and absolute quantification analysis (iTRAQ) to screen out our interested proteins of HSPA5 and HSP90AB1, and the decline in their expression were verified by a real-time quantitative PCR and a western blotting assay. In vitro, human granulosa cells, KGN and COV434 cells were transfected with siRNA targeting *HSPA5* and *HSP90AB1* and then treated with CDDP, or treated with CDDP with/without CDDP+ 4-phenylbutyric acid (4-PBA) and 3-methyladenine (3-MA). The levels of ERS, autophagy and apoptosis were evaluated by western blotting, DALGreen staining and flow cytometry. In vivo, ovaries from mice that received intraperitoneal injections of saline, CDDP, CDDP+ 4-PBA and CDDP+ 3-MA were assayed by immunofluorescence, hematoxylin and eosin (H&E) staining for follicle counting, and terminal-deoxynucleotidyltransferase-mediated dUTP nick end labeling (TUNEL) staining for cell apoptosis assay. The plasma hormone levels were measured by an enzyme-linked immunosorbent assay (ELISA) kit.

Results: We have clarified the relationships between ERS, autophagy, and apoptosis in CDDP-induced granulosa cell apoptosis, both in vitro and in vivo. Alleviating ERS by inhibiting HSPA5 and HSP90AB1 attenuated CDDP-induced autophagy and apoptosis. 4-PBA treatment significantly attenuated CDDP-induced cell autophagy and apoptosis in cultured KGN and COV434 cells. However, inhibiting cell autophagy with 3-MA negligibly restored the CDDP-induced changes in ERS and apoptosis. In vivo experiments also demonstrated that treatment with 4-PBA, but not 3-MA, prevented CDDP-induced ovarian damage and hormone dysregulation.

Conclusions: CDDP-induced ERS could promote autophagy and apoptosis in granulosa cells, causing excessive follicle loss and endocrine disorders. Alleviation of ERS with 4-PBA, but not of autophagy with 3-MA, protect against CDDP-induced granulosa cell apoptosis and ovarian damage. Thus, 4-PBA can be used to protect the ovary during chemotherapy in women.

Keywords: Cisplatin, Endoplasmic reticulum stress, Granulosa cell apoptosis, Ovarian damage, 4-PBA

---

* Correspondence: czg1984@smu.edu.cn; wlilyu@hotmail.com
[3]Department of Cell Biology, School of Basic Medical Sciences, Southern Medical University, Guangzhou 510515, China
[1]Department of Obstetrics and Gynecology, Nanfang Hospital, Southern Medical University, Guangzhou 510515, China
Full list of author information is available at the end of the article

Background

Premature ovarian insufficiency (POI), previously called premature ovarian failure (POF), is described as the cessation of ovarian function before the age of 40 years [1]. The diagnosis is based on oligo- or amenorrhea for at least 4 months and an elevated follicle-stimulating hormone (FSH) level of > 25 IU/l on two occasions > 4 weeks apart [2]. The decline in ovarian functions is related to the loss of the resting follicles and the reduced biological competence of atresia follicles [3]. The orchestrated cross-talk between the oocytes and the surrounding granulosa cells is necessary for folliculogenesis [4]. Therefore, the loss of homeostasis in granulosa cells often leads to POI [5].

Chemotherapeutic treatments frequently causes ovarian damage [6]. Cisplatin (CDDP) is an anticancer agent widely used alone or in combination with other chemotherapeutic agents, and has been a key component of first-line chemotherapy against broad range of cancers [7]. However, nonselective distribution of the drug between normal and tumor tissue causes severe side effects [8]. CDDP can induce DNA damage and cell apoptosis, reduce follicle reserve and decrease steroidogenic activity, and even impairs female reproduction [9]. Previous studies have demonstrated various signaling pathways that participate in CDDP-induced apoptosis on granulosa cells. Several members of the Wnt signaling pathway were found to be downregulated in granulosa cells after exposure to CDDP, and restoration of β-catenin signaling protected granulosa cells from the injury induced by CDDP [10]. CDDP can also damage the DNA of granulosa cells by upregulation p63 and activated c-Abl-de pendant pathway [11]. Additionally, p53 can induce granulosa cell apoptosis after CDDP treatment, by the transactivation of pro-apoptotic genes such as *Bax30*, *NOXA* and *PUMA*, or by relocating at the mitochondrion [12]. However, the detailed mechanisms underlying the ovarian damage caused by CDDP are still unclear.

After the discovery of the death receptor signaling and mitochondrial pathways, it was demonstrated that endoplasmic reticulum stress (ERS) can lead to apoptosis [13]. ERS occurs when mutant proteins disrupt protein folding in the ER, and ERS activates a signaling network called "the unfolded protein response" (UPR) [14]. Excessive and persistent ERS leads to cell dysfunction or even death [15, 16]. Recently, several studies have suggested that ERS promotes cell apoptosis and is related to follicular atresia, for which an ERS-mediated mechanism of cell autophagy and apoptosis has been proposed [16, 17]. In contrast, another study suggested that ERS inhibits autophagy [18]. Therefore, the exact effects of ERS on cell fate and its role in CDDP-induced ovarian damage remain to be clarified.

In this study, we generated a mouse model of POI with the intraperitoneal injection of CDDP for 7 days. The whole mouse ovaries were then subjected to proteomic screening using isobaric tags for relative and absolute quantification (iTRAQ) analysis. The results showed that two ERS-related proteins, 78-kDa glucose-regulated protein (HSPA5, GRP78, or BiP) and heat shock protein HSP90-beta (HSP90AB1, HSP84, or TSTA) were strongly associated with CDDP-induced ovarian damage. We then found that both of them were predominantly expressed in the granulosa cells from secondary and antral follicles. Thus, we hypothesize that HSPA5 and HSP90AB1 play key roles in CDDP-induced granulosa cell apoptosis and ovarian damage. Therefore, we designed in vitro and in vivo experiments using small interfering RNAs (siRNAs) directed against *HSPA5* and *HSP90AB1* and an inhibitor of ERS, 4-phenylbutyric acid (4-PBA), to clarify the roles of ERS in CDDP-induced cell autophagy, granulosa cell apoptosis and ovarian damage.

Methods

Animals

Six-week-old wild-type female C57BL/6 J mice were from the Southern Medical University Animal Center (Guangzhou, China). The mice were housed in a temperature- and humidity-controlled animal facility and maintained on a 12-h light/dark cycle. They were acclimated for 5 days before the experiment, with free access to a commercial rodent diet and tap water. All animal experiments were approved by the Southern Medical University Committee on the Use and Care of Animals and were performed in accordance with the Committee's guidelines and regulations.

POI model

Twenty mice were randomly and evenly divided into two groups. The experimental group received intraperitoneal injections of CDDP (2.5 mg/kg/d in saline) (Sigma-Aldrich, Shanghai, China) for 7 consecutive days, and the control group were injected with saline. This dosage was according to a previous study [19] and our preliminary results showing that this is the minimum dose causing significant morphological changes within 7 days when compared with the control group. After anesthesia induced with 10% chloral hydrate, the mice were killed and their ovaries rapidly dissected. Ovaries of three mice randomly selected from each group were subjected to a proteomic analysis with iTRAQ (Fitgene Biotech, Guangzhou, China). The remaining ovaries were used for real-time quantitative PCR (qPCR) and a western blotting analysis. Ovaries for histological examination were fixed in 4% formaldehyde.

Protein preparation

The frozen ovaries were grinded by liquid nitrogen and then lysed in 500 μl of LC3 SDS lysis buffer (Add 1× PMSF before use) containing 7 M Urea, 2 M Thiourea,

20 mM Tris base and 0.2% SDS. Then the samples were sonicated and centrifuged to collect the supernatant. Every 250 µL of supernatant was precipitated overnight at − 20 °C with 1 mL acetone. After discarding the acetone and air drying, the resulting pellet was dissolved in lysate L3 (no SDS). Then the sample was sonicated on ice and centrifuged at 12,000×g for 20 min at 4 °C, the supernatant was collected. Protein concentration was estimated by the Bradford method (Fitgene Biotech, Guangzhou, China).

Trypsin digestion and iTRAQ labeling

iTRAQ labeling was performed according to the manufacturer's protocol (Applied Biosystems, Sciex). Briefly, 200 µg of each protein sample was reduced with TCEP Reducing Reagent at 60 °C for 1 h, and alkylated with MMTS Cysteine-Blocking Reagent at room temperature for 30 min. Then, proteins were digested with trypsin (Promega, USA) at 37 °C at a ratio of 1:50 (enzyme-to-substrate) overnight. Each sample was labeled separately with two of the eight available tags (control: 114 and 116 tags; cisplatin: 117 and 119 tags). All labeled peptides were pooled together.

High-pH reversed-phase chromatography

The Ultimate 3000 HPLC system (Dionex, USA) equipped with a 2.00-mm-inner diameter *100-mm-long Gemini-NX 3u C18110Acolumns (Phenomenex, USA) was used for High-pH fractionation. Peptides were loaded onto the column and washed isocratically at 95% eluent A (20 mM HCOONH4, 2 M NaOH) (pH 10). The iTRAQ-tagged peptides fractionation was performed using a linear binary gradient from 15 to 50% B (20 mM HCOONH 4, 2 M NaOH, 80% ACN) (pH 10) at 0.2 ml/min for more than 45 min. Finally, the column was washed at 90% B for 10 min and returned to 95% A for 10 min. Set the UV detector was at 214/280 nm, and fractions were collected every 1 min. 10 fractions were pooled and dried by vacuum centrifuge for subsequent nano-reversed phase liquid chromatography (nano-LC) fractionation.

RPLC-MS/MS analysis

The fraction was resuspended in loading buffer (0.1% FA, 2% ACN) and separated with an Ultimate 3000 nano-LC system equipped with a C18 reverse phase column (100-µm inner diameter, 10-cm long, 3-µm resin from MichromBioresources, Auburn, CA). Separate the peptides with the following parameters: 1) mobile phase A:0.1% FA, 5% ACN, dissolved in water; 2) mobile phase B: 0.1% FA, 95% ACN; 3) flow rate: 300 nl/min; 4) gradient: B-phase increased from 5 to 40%, 70 min. Then, the LC eluent was subject to Q Exactive (Thermo Fisher) in an information dependent acquisition mode. MS spectra were acquired across the mass range of 400–1250 m/z in high resolution mode (> 30,000) using 250 ms accumulation time per spectrum. A maximum of 20 precursors per cycle were chosen for fragmentation from each MS spectrum with100 ms minimum accumulation time for each precursor and dynamic exclusion for 20 s. Tandem mass spectra were recorded in high sensitivity mode (resolution > 15,000) with rolling collision energy on and iTRAQ reagent collision energy adjustment on.

Tissue collection and morphological analysis

The ovaries were fixed in 4% formaldehyde for 24 h, embedded in paraffin wax, sectioned at 4 µm thickness, and mounted on glass slides for hematoxylin and eosin (H&E) staining. At least five sections (taken 100 µM apart) from an ovary and 5 ovaries from each group were photographed for follicle assessment. A follicle was deemed present if the oocyte contained a germinal vesicle, and was counted and classified according to its health and developmental stage, as a healthy (including primordial, primary, secondary, and antral follicle) or atresia follicle, according to previously described criteria [20].

Immunofluorescence

For the immunofluorescence analysis, the sections were incubated with the antibodies summarized in Additional file 1: Table S1, followed by incubation with Alexa-Fluor-488-labeled secondary antibodies (Molecular Probes, MA, USA) and 4′,6-diamidino-2-phenylindole (Invitrogen, Carlsbad, CA, USA) to visualize the nuclei. The immunofluorescent images were obtained using FluoView FV1000 confocal microscopy (Olympus, Tokyo, Japan).

TUNEL analysis

Cell apoptosis in the follicles was evaluated in sections using a terminal-deoxynucleotidyltransferase-mediated dUTP nick end labeling (TUNEL) assay for the situ visualization of DNA fragmentation with the commercial DeadEnd™ Fluorometric TUNEL System (Promega, Madison, WI, USA). Images were obtained with a FluoView FV1000 confocal microscope. Every 25th section in 5 ovaries from each group were analyzed, and the level of apoptosis was expressed as the total number of apoptotic cells on five sections from an ovary of each mouse.

Serum hormone measurement with enzyme-linked immunosorbent assays (ELISAs)

The mice were anesthetized to collect their blood via cardiocentesis. The blood samples were centrifuged at 3000×g for 10 min and the serum collected. The plasma levels of FSH and estradiol (E2) hormone were measured with ELISA kits (Elabscience Biotechnology, Wuhan, China).

Real-time quantitative PCR

Total ovarian RNA was purified with TriGene Reagent, and then processed to cDNA with the RETRO-script Reverse Transcription Kit, and amplified and quantified with the RealStar Power SYBR Kit (all from GenStar BioSolutions, Beijing, China) with a StepOne-Plus Real-Time PCR System (Applied Biosystems, Waltham, MA, USA). The gene-specific primers (San-gong Biotech, Shanghai, China) for qPCR were: For *Hspa5*, forward: 5′-ACTTGGGGACCACCTATTC CT-3′, reverse: 5′-GTTGCCCTGATCGTTGGCTA-3′; for *Hsp90ab1*, forward: 5′- GTCCGCCGTGTGTT CATCAT-3′, reverse: 5′-GCACTTCTTGACGATGTT CTTGC-3′. The expression of *Hspa5* and *Hsp90ab1* were normalized to that of glyceraldehyde 3-phosphate dehydrogenase (*Gapdh*).

Western blotting

Ovaries were homogenised in lysis buffer and boiled in sodium dodecyl sulfate (SDS) loading buffer. The protein extracts were then subjected to 6–12% SDS-PAGE and electrotransferred to nitrocellulose membranes (GE Healthcare Life Sciences, Beijing, China). The membranes were blocked with 5% nonfat dry milk for 1 h at room temperature, washed, and incubated with the indicated primary antibody at 4 °C overnight. The membranes were further washed, incubated with Peroxidase-AffiniPure Goat Anti-Rabbit or -Mouse IgG (H + L) (Jackson ImmunoResearch, West Grove, PA, USA) for 1 h at room temperature, washed again, and finally visualized with an enhanced chemiluminescence kit (PerkinElmer, Waltham, MA, USA). The primary antibodies used for the immunoblotting analysis are summarized in Additional file 1: Table S1.

In vivo inhibitor treatment

Seventy-two mice were evenly and randomly divided into four groups, which received intraperitoneal injections of 0.9% saline as control group, and experimental groups were intraperitoneal injections of CDDP (2.5 mg/kg/d), CDDP + 4-PBA (2.5 + 150 mg/kg/d, respectively) [21], and CDDP + 3-methyladenine (3-MA; 2.5 + 10 mg/kg/d), respectively [22] (4-PBA and 3-MA were from Sigma-Aldrich), for 1, 3 and 7 days. The mice were euthanized at the indicated time points, and their ovaries were isolated for histological analysis and a western blotting assay.

Cell culture and related assays

Cell culture

KGN cell line (a generous gift from Prof. Yiming Mu, Chinese PLA General Hospital, China), which was established from a human ovarian granulosa cell tumor [23], and COV434 cell line (a generous gift from Prof. Hongyan Yang, Second Affiliated Hospital of Guangzhou University of Traditional Chinese Medicine, China), immortalized granulosa cells derived from a solid granulosa cell tumor [24], were cultured with Dulbecco's Modified Eagle's Medium/Ham's F12 (Invitrogen) supplemented with 10% fetal bovine serum (FBS, Gibco by Invitrogen). The cells were maintained in a subconfluent state at 37 °C during all the experiments in an atmosphere of 5% CO_2/95% humidified air.

siRNA transfection

KGN and COV434 cells (1×10^5) were seeded in 12-well plates for 24 h, and then transfected with siRNA (GenePharma, Shanghai, China) targeting *HSPA5* and *HAP90AB1* mRNAs using Lipofectamine 3000 (Invitrogen). After 48 h, the cells were exposed to CDDP (50 μM) for the indicated times for western blotting. The siRNA sequences were: *HSPA5*: sense: 5′-UGUUGGUGGCUCGACUCGAUT-3′, antisense: 5′-UCGAGUCGAGCCACCAACAAG-3′; *HSP90AB1*: 5′-AGUAAACUAAGGGUGUCAAUT-3′, antisense: 5′-UUGACACCCUUAGUUUACUGC-3′. Nonspecific siRNA sequences were used as the negative controls (NC): sense: 5′-UUCUCCGAACGUGUCACGUTT-3′, antisense: 5′-ACGUGACACGUUCGGAGAATT-3′.

Cell apoptosis analysis with flow cytometry

Apoptotic cells were measured with an Annexin V/ propidium iodide (PI) apoptosis analysis kit (Sungene Biotech, Tianjin, China). Briefly, 1×10^6 cells were seeded in six-well plates and then incubated with the indicated chemicals for the indicated times. After the cells were washed with cold phosphate-buffered saline, they were collected by centrifugation and the cell concentration was adjusted to 1×10^6/mL with binding buffer. Annexin V solution (5 μL) was added to the tubes and incubated for 10 min, followed by incubation with 5 μL of PI solution for another 5 min. The whole operation was performed at room temperature and protected from light. The final fluorescence was measured with a flow cytometer (Beckman Coulter, Brea, CA, USA), and a CytExpert software was used for data acquisition (1×10^4 events per sample). The percentages of cells in four classes were determined: viable (annexin V^{neg}, PI^{neg}), early apoptosis (annexin V^{pos}, PI^{neg}), late apoptosis (annexin V^{pos}, PI^{pos}), and necrosis (annexin V^{neg}, PI^{pos}).

Autophagy detection with DALGreen staining

Cells were plated in confocal dishes and cultured at 37 °C with 1 mL of a 0.6 μM DALGreen [25] (Dojindo Laboratories, Shanghai, China) working solution for 30 min. After the cells were washed twice with culture medium, they were incubated with 50 μM CDDP, with or without 5 mM 4-PBA [26] or 5 mM 3-MA [27]. 8 h later, cells were washed twice with Hanks' HEPES buffer and observed with a FluoView FV1000 confocal microscope.

Cells with more than three DALGreen-positive foci were considered to be autophagy-positive cells.

Statistical analysis

The peptide data were analyzed using Protein Pilot Software 4.0 (AB SCIEX, CA), and the parameters were set as follows: Cys alkylation: MMTS; ID focus: biological modifications; Digestion: typsin; Database: Uniprot_-MOUSE; Search effort: thorough ID. All experiments were performed at least in duplicate. Data are presented as means ± SD, and differences between groups were analyzed with an independent-samples t-test and among groups with one-way ANOVA followed by the SNK test (SPSS 25.0, SPSS Inc., Chicago, IL, USA). If the data were not normally distributed, the nonparametric Mann-Whitney test was used. A $\chi 2$ test was used for rate comparisons. $p < 0.05$ was considered statistically significant.

Results

Ovarian HSPA5 and HSP90AB1 protein levels were significantly reduced in the CDDP-induced POI model

To investigate the molecular changes underlying CDDP-induced ovarian damage, we generated a mouse model of POI by injecting mice intraperitoneally with CDDP for 7 days, and then subjecting their ovaries to proteomic screening with an iTRAQ analysis. The expression levels of 214 proteins were significantly upregulated (fold change ≥1.5) and the levels of 180 proteins were significantly downregulated (fold change ≥ − 1.5) (Additional file 1: Table S2). Of these 394 differentially expressed proteins, HSPA5 and HSP90AB1, two well-established markers for ERS and UPR [14], were of our particular interest, because they were downregulated 2.5-fold and 2.3-fold, respectively, in the CDDP-treated ovaries (Table 1). Furthermore, a STRING analysis showed that both of them were at the core of signaling network (Additional file 1:Figure S1). To confirm this proteomic result, we used qPCR to show that the relative mRNA expression of $Hspa5$ and $Hsp90ab1$ was significantly lower in the CDDP group than in the control group (Fig. 1a). Western blotting further confirmed the reduction in their protein levels in the CDDP group (Fig. 1b, c). Although the proteomic analysis indicated a more dramatic decline in the protein levels of FADS2 and HSD11B2, which, however, were not confirmed by western blotting (Additional file 1:Figure S2). These results

Table 1 iTRAQ analysis showed reduced HSPA5 and HSP90AB1 expression in a CDDP-induced POI model

Name	Gene Name	Fold Change[a]
78 kDa glucose-regulated protein	GN=HSPA5	−2.5
Heat shock protein HSP 90-beta	GN=HSP90AB1	−2.3

[a]"-" = Downregulated in the CDDP-treated ovaries. $n = 3$

indicated that ERS was strongly associated with CDDP-induced ovarian damage.

Inhibition of ERS attenuates CDDP-induced granulosa cells autophagy and apoptosis

We next characterized the expression profiles of HSPA5 and HSP90AB1 in the CDDP-treated ovaries with immunofluorescence. Both HSPA5 and HSP90AB1 were predominantly localized to the cytoplasm around the nucleic of granulosa cells from secondary and antral follicles, modestly expressed in those from primary follicles, while hardly present in those of from primordial follicles (Fig. 2a), indicating that ERS in granulosa cells may play a role in CDDP-induced follicle loss. Therefore, two human granulosa tumor cell lines, KGN and COV434, were used for an in vitro study. CDDP at 50 µM significantly decreased the proteins expression of HSPA5 and HSP90AB1 in KGN cells at 24 h,thus we treated cells with the dose in the following cell experiments (Fig. 2b). CDDP (50 µM) induced time-dependent changes in HSPA5 and HSP90AB1 protein levels in the KGN cells, with an increase at 4 h, which were then decreased at 24 h (Fig. 2c), indicating that ERS was induced upon exposure to CDDP. Autophagy related 12 (ATG12) is positively involved in the assembly of the autophagosome. P62 binds to polyubiquitinated proteins and LC3 on the autophagosomal membrane to target aggregates to the autophagosomes for degradation, and its expression negatively correlates with autophagosome formation [28]. CDDP treatment induced a time-dependent increase in the expression of ATG12 and a reduction in P62, and also an increase in cleaved PARP protein, a marker of cell apoptosis (Fig. 2d). Interestingly, when either the $HSPA5$ or $HSP90AB1$ gene was knocked down with RNA interference (RNAi), the levels of both ATG12 and cleaved PARP proteins were greatly reduced (Fig. 2d). This finding suggested that ERS induced cell autophagy and apoptosis in response to excessive CDDP treatment. This was verified by introducing 4-PBA, an ERS inhibitor, into CDDP-treated cells, where it significantly relieved CDDP-induced ERS, cell autophagy, and cell apoptosis (Fig. 2e). A flow-cytometric analysis of annexin V/PI staining further confirmed that CDDP-induced cell apoptosis was largely prevented by 4-PBA ($P < 0.05$, Fig. 2f, g). These results together demonstrated that the alleviation of ERS attenuated CDDP-induced cell autophagy and apoptosis.

Suppressing autophagy with 3-MA neither reduced CDDP-induced cell apoptosis nor alleviated ERS

We next examined whether inhibiting autophagy protected cells from CDDP-induced apoptosis. DALgreen staining showed that although both 3-MA and 4-PBA efficiently reduced the production of CDDP-induced

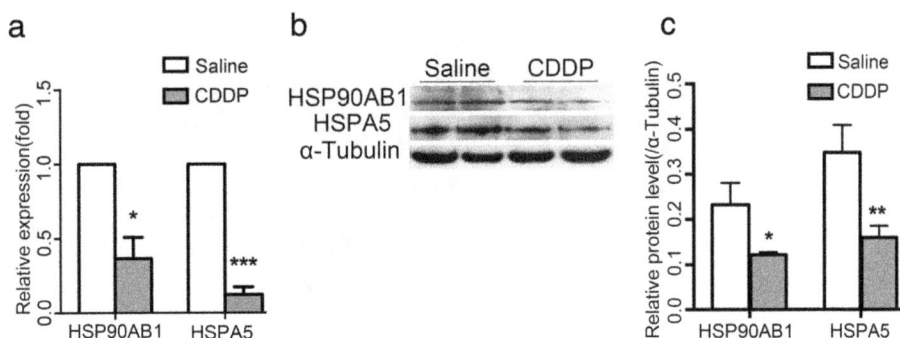

Fig. 1 CDDP decreases the expressions of HSPA5 and HSP90AB1 in ovaries. **a** qPCR showed that both mRNA levels of *Hspa5* and *Hsp90ab1* were decreased in CDDP-treated ovaries. **b** western blotting showed that both protein levels of HSPA5 and HSP90AB1 were decreased in CDDP-treated ovaries. **c** Quantification of the results in b. Protein levels were normalized to that of Tubulin. Data are presented as mean ± SD. n = 3, * P < 0.05, ** P < 0.01, *** P < 0.001

autophagosomes ($P < 0.05$) (Fig. 3a, b). Western blotting also showed that 3-MA alleviated CDDP-induced autophagy level by reducing the expression of ATG12 and by increasing that of P62, whereas the protein levels of cleaved PARP, HSPA5, and HSP90AB1 remained stable (Fig. 3c). The finding that 3-MA negligibly reduced CDDP-induced cell apoptosis was further supported by the results of flow cytometry ($p > 0.05$, Fig. 3d, e). These findings collectively suggested that lowering the autophagy level with 3-MA neither reduced cell apoptosis nor alleviated ERS during CDDP treatment.

Effects of 4-PBA and 3-MA on CDDP-induced POI in vivo

We then compared the protective effects of 4-PBA and 3-MA against CDDP-induced ovarian damage in vivo. Female mice were treated with CDDP combined with 4-PBA or 3-MA for 1, 3, or 7 days. A histological examination showed that the morphologies of follicles at different stages of development were parallel across all the groups on day 1, except that the healthy follicles in CDDP group decreased, compared with the saline group (($P < 0.05$, Fig. 4a-c). By day 3, the CDDP-treated group had significantly fewer healthy follicles and more atresia follicles than the saline-treated group ($P < 0.01$), which was predominantly attributable to the loss of primordial and antral follicles (Fig. 4b, c). By day 7, the longer exposure to CDDP seriously damaged the healthy follicles and produced excessive atresia follicles than the saline-treated group (both $P < 0.01$). Besides primordial and antral follicles, more secondary follicles were damaged, whereas the primary follicles appeared not susceptible. We speculate that it is associated with follicular recruitment and CDDP-induced granulosa cell apoptosis in growing follicles. The more granulosa cells in the growing population of follicles, the more susceptible they were to CDDP. These data support a previous report that chemotherapeutic agents over activate the primordial follicles and damage the growing population

of follicles, leading to the premature depletion of follicle reserves [29]. As expected, 4-PBA, but not 3-MA, markedly ameliorated CDDP-induced follicle loss and preserved more healthy follicles by protecting follicles from atresia (Fig. 4b, c). Consistent with this, a TUNEL assay showed that CDDP-induced granulosa cell apoptosis peaked on day 3 ($P < 0.01$), and was markedly ameliorated by 4-PBA ($P < 0.05$) but not by 3-MA ($P > 0.05$, Fig. 5a, b). By day 7, the intensity of granulosa cell apoptosis had decreased in the CDDP group compared to the 3rd day, and 4-PBA slightly reduced the number of apoptotic cells (Fig. 5a, b). Consistent with the histological results, hormone measurements with ELISAs showed that exposure to CDDP for 7 days clearly reduced the plasma E_2 content, and especially, increased the FSH level (both $P < 0.01$, Fig. 5c), which is considered as the most important biochemical indicator of POI in clinical. The 4-PBA treatment clearly-inhibited the CDDP-induced increase in FSH, but not the reduction in E_2, whereas and the 3-MA treatment had negligible effects on these changes (Fig. 5c). We propose that the secretion of FSH is affected by the negative feedback of E_2 and FSH receptors, the production of E_2 decreased due to excessive granulosa cell apoptosis induced by CDDP, which in turn stimulates the secretion of FSH from pituitary. 4-PBA reduced granulosa cell apoptosis and may preserve FSH receptors, therefore, the secretion of FSH was not increased significantly. Furthermore, an immunoblotting analysis of whole-mount ovarian proteins showed that in vivo treatment with 4-PBA blocked the increases in the protein levels of ATG12 and cleaved PARP, but not of HSPA5 and HSP90AB1during CDDP treatment (Fig. 5d). This may indicate different responses to 4-PBA between in vivo and in vitro. The CDDP-induced increase in cleaved PARP was resistant to 3-MA treatment, although 3-MA reduced the protein level of ATG12 and increased P62 (Fig. 5d). These results together provided in vivo evidence supporting the notion that the alleviation of ERS attenuated CDDP-induced granulosa cell death and ovarian damage.

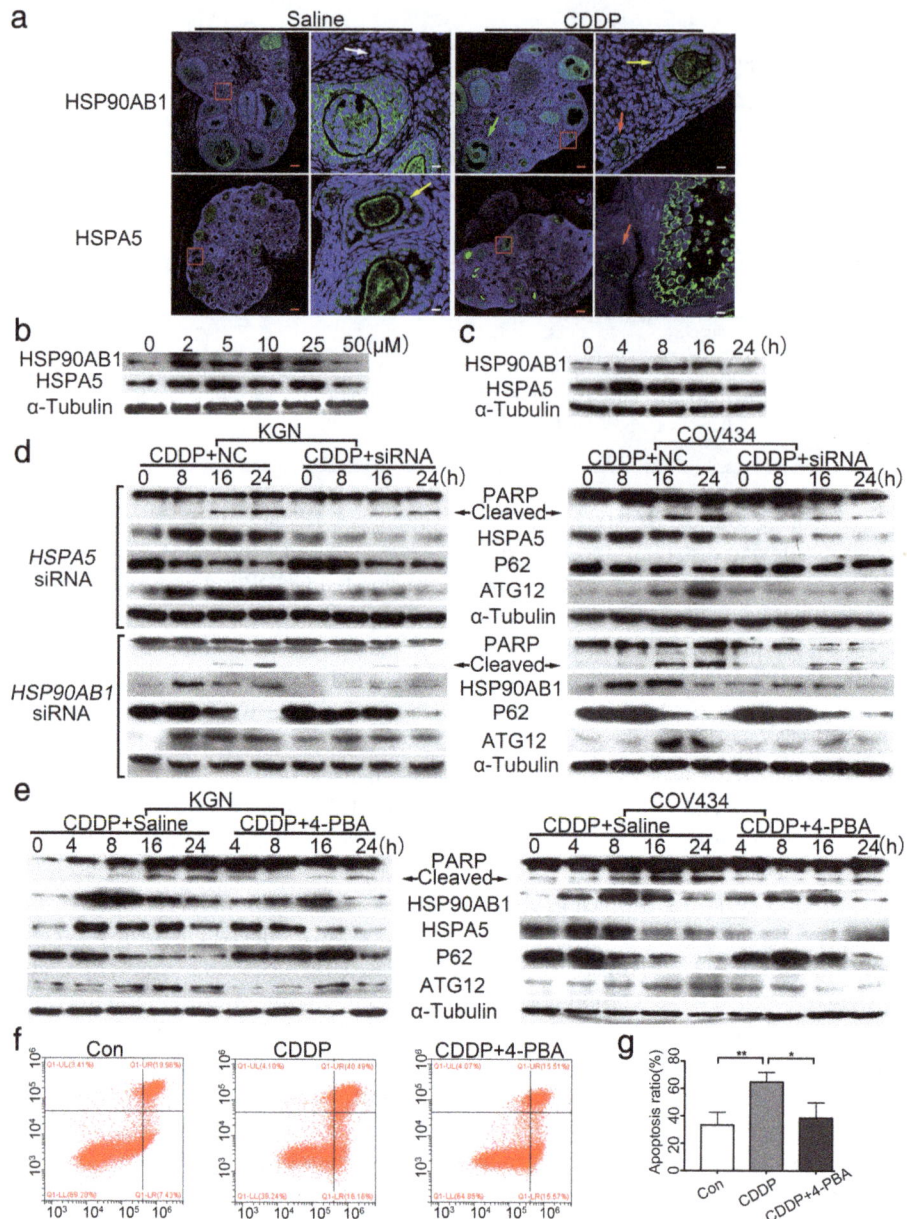

Fig. 2 Inhibition of ERS depresses CDDP-induced ERS, autophagy and apoptosis in granulosa cells. **a** Immunofluorescence of HSP90AB1 and HSPA5 in the saline and CDDP-treated ovaries. Nuclei were stained with DAPI. White arrow indicates primordial follicle; red, primary follicle; yellow, secondary follicle; green, antral follicle. Red scale bars = 80 μm, White scale bars = 10 μm (**b**) Immunoblotting of HSP90AB1 and HSPA5 in the KGN cells treated with CDDP at indicated concentrations (0, 2, 5, 10, 25 and 50 μM) for 24 h. **c** Immunoblotting of HSP90AB1 and HSPA5 in the KGN cells treated with CDDP at 50 μM for indicated times (0, 4, 8, 16, 24 h). **d** KGN and COV434 cells were transfected with HSPA5 and HSP90AB1-specific siRNA and NC-siRNA respectively for 48 h, and then treated with 50 μM CDDP for indicated times. Immunoblotting was carried out to detect the protein levels of ERS-, autophagy- and apoptosis-related genes. **e** KGN and COV434 cells were treated with 50 μM CDDP with/without 5 mM 4-PBA for indicated times. ERS, autophagy and apoptosis levels were detected by western blot. **f** KGN cells were treated with 50 μM CDDP with/without 5 mM 4-PBA for 24 h and then stained with Annexin V-FITC and PI. Both cells at early (annexin V^{pos}; PI^{neg}) and late apoptotic stages (annexin V^{pos}; PI^{pos}) were counted. **g** Quantification of the results in f. * $P < 0.05$, ** $P < 0.01$

Discussion

In this study, we established the central role of ERS in CDDP-induced granulosa cell apoptosis. Reducing ERS by knocking down the expression of either the *HSPA5* or *HSP90AB1* gene with RNAi or by introducing the ERS inhibitor 4-PBA significantly attenuated CDDP-induced cell autophagy and apoptosis in cultured KGN and COV434 cells. However, inhibiting cell autophagy with 3-MA negligibly blocked the changes in ERS and apoptosis induced by CDDP (Fig. 6). Our in vivo experiments

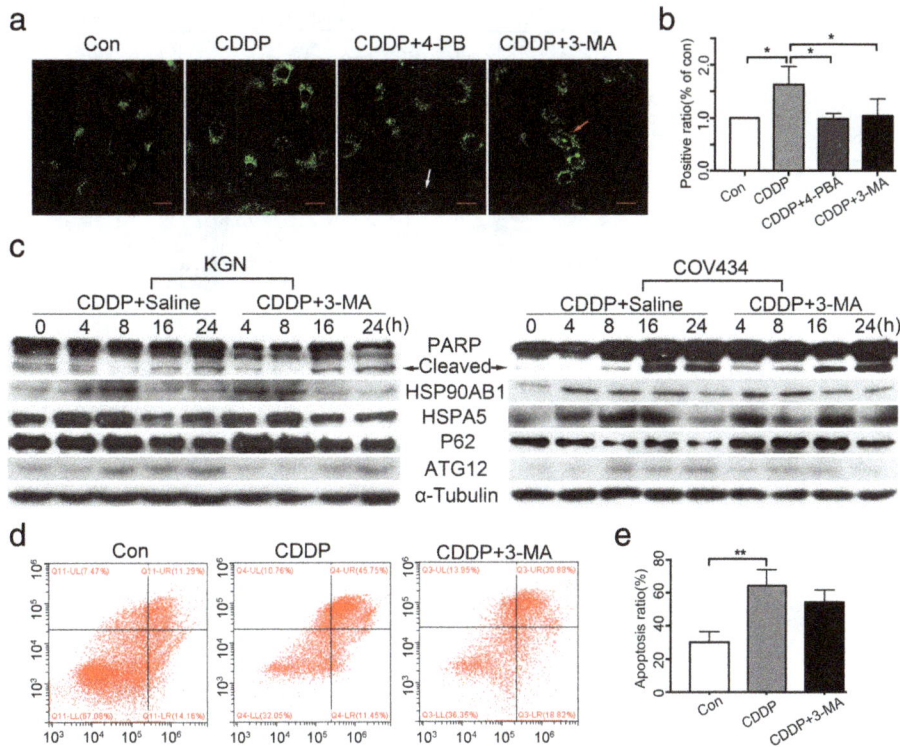

Fig. 3 Suppressing autophagy hardly alleviates CDDP-induced cell apoptosis or ERS. **a** Autophagy levels in KGN cells after indicated treatments by DALGreen staining. Positive autophagosomes were observed by fluorescence microscopy. White arrow indicates autophagosome-negative cell and the red indicates autophagsome-positive cell. Scale bars = 80 μm. **b** Quantification of the positive phagosomes in a. **c** KGN and COV434 cells were treated with 50 μM CDDP with/without 5 mM 3-MA for indicated times. ERS, autophagy and apoptosis levels were detected by western blotting. **d** KGN cells were treated with 50 μM CDDP with/without 5 mM 3-MA for 24 h and then stained with Annexin V-FITC and PI. **e** Quantification of the results in d. * $P < 0.05$

also demonstrated that in vivo treatment with 4-PBA, but not 3-MA, prevented CDDP-induced follicle loss and hormone dysregulation. Therefore, the alleviation of ERS protects against cisplatin-induced granulosa cell apoptosis and ovarian damage.

Our results clearly demonstrated that ERS was an important switch in the decision of the granulosa cell fate during CDDP treatment. An iTRAQ analysis revealed a notable decline in both the HSPA5 and HSP90AB1 proteins, which was confirmed with real time quantitative PCR and immunoblotting. However, in vitro experiments using either KGN or COV434 cells showed that the levels of both the HSPA5 and HSP90AB1 proteins increased at 4 h, and declined at 24 h after treatment with CDDP. These changes in response to CDDP treatment prompted us to infer that CDDP induced misfolded or unfolded proteins accumulated on the ER, and activated the UPR to upregulate ER chaperones such as HSPA5 and HSP90AB1, which degraded the misfolded or unfolded proteins [30]. Autophagy was subsequently prompted to degrade the denature proteins and damaged organelles in autolysosomes,

manifested as an increase in ATG12 and a decrease in P62 at 8 h after treatment with CDDP. This may be a protective mechanism by which ERS maintains cellular homeostasis, possibly by triggering prosurvival cellular events. However, when stress persists, ERS elements are impaired and cellular homeostasis is perturbed, ultimately leading to apoptosis [31], as indicated in the results that cleaved PARP increased and ERS-related proteins HSPA5 and HSP90AB1 decreased. 4-PBA reduced granulosa cell apoptosis by alleviating the prolonged or excessive ERS in granulosa cell, depressing the expression of HSPA5 and HSP90AB1, attenuating the autophagy level. It is interesting to note that although the expression of HSPA5 and HSP90AB1 is weak in primordial follicles, PBA treatment also effectively preserves primordial follicles, meaning that CDDP may acts in primordial and developed follicles via different mechanisms, and ERS may not be the only target for PBA.

We also investigated whether cell autophagy was one of the mechanisms by which ERS maintained cellular homeostasis. Autophagy degrades destructive substances and dysfunctional organelles to maintain

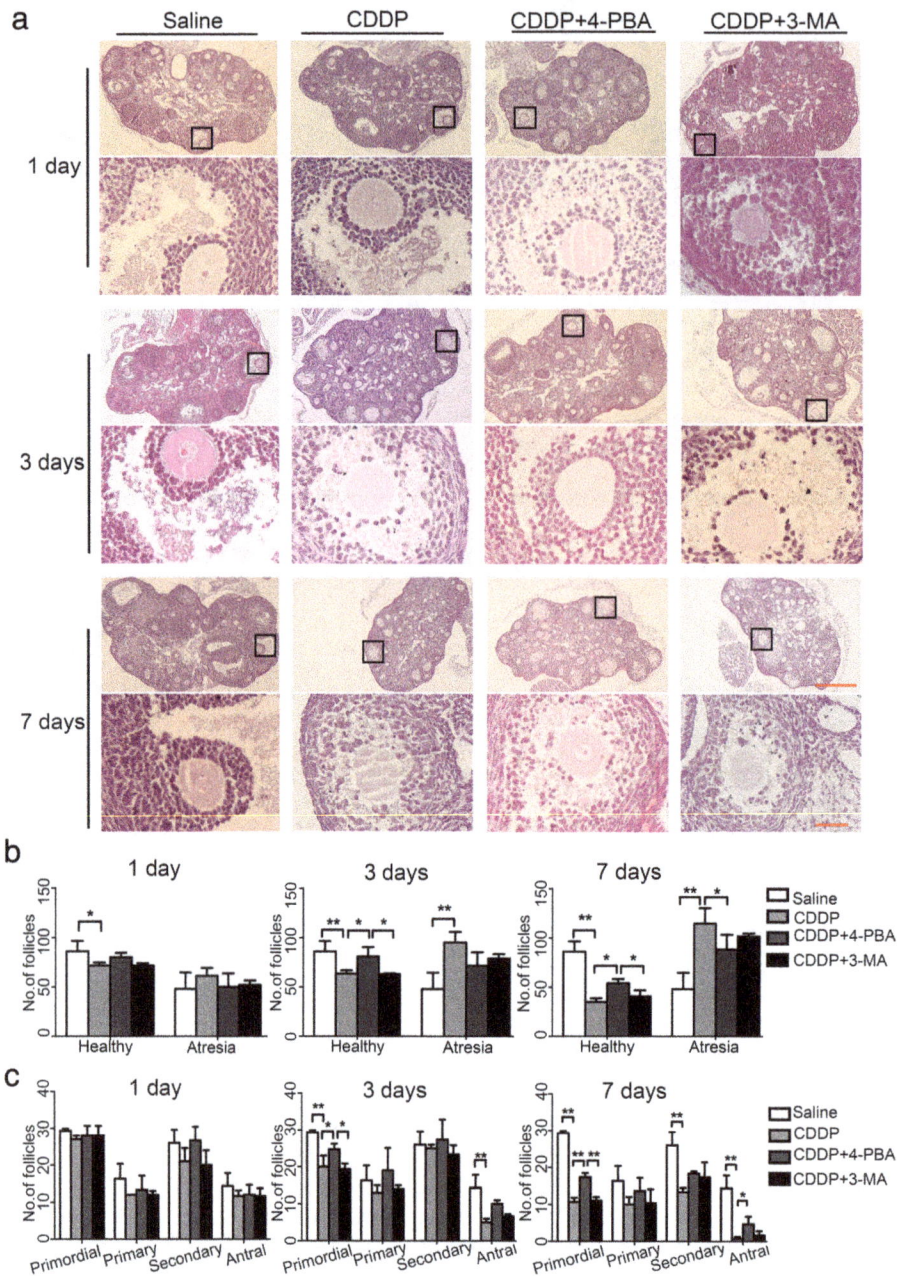

Fig. 4 Effects of 4-PBA and 3-MA on ovarian histology in CDDP-treated mice. Mice were treated with saline, CDDP, and CDDP with 4-PBA or 3-MA for 1 day, 3 days and 7 days, respectively. **a** H&E staining showed the ovarian histology in each group. Five sections (taken 100 μm apart) from an ovary were photographed for follicle assessment. Scale bars = 40 μm (upper panels) and 4 μm (lower panels). **b** Comparison of the total number of healthy and atresia follicles among groups. Healthy follicles include healthy primordial, primary, secondary and antral follicles. **c** Comparison of the number of healthy primordial, primary, secondary and antral follicles among groups. $n = 5$, * $P < 0.05$, ** $P < 0.01$

cellular homeostasis. In cultured KGN and COV434 cells, exposure to CDDP induced ERS as early as 4 h, which was followed by autophagy at about 8–16 h, and finally excessive apoptosis at about 24 h. Therefore, we hypothesized that CDDP-induced ERS stimulated autophagy, which in turn degraded damaged ER elements to maintain the survival of the cell. However, excessive or prolonged ERS and autophagy will ultimately lead to apoptosis. This hypothesis is supported by the finding that the suppression of ERS, either with siRNA targeting *HSPA5* or *HSP90AB1* or with 4-PBA, significantly inhibited cell autophagy and apoptosis, which eventually alleviated follicle loss. However, although 3-MA reduced the level of autophagy, it negligibly attenuated ERS or apoptosis. A previous study indicated that ERS inhibits autophagy

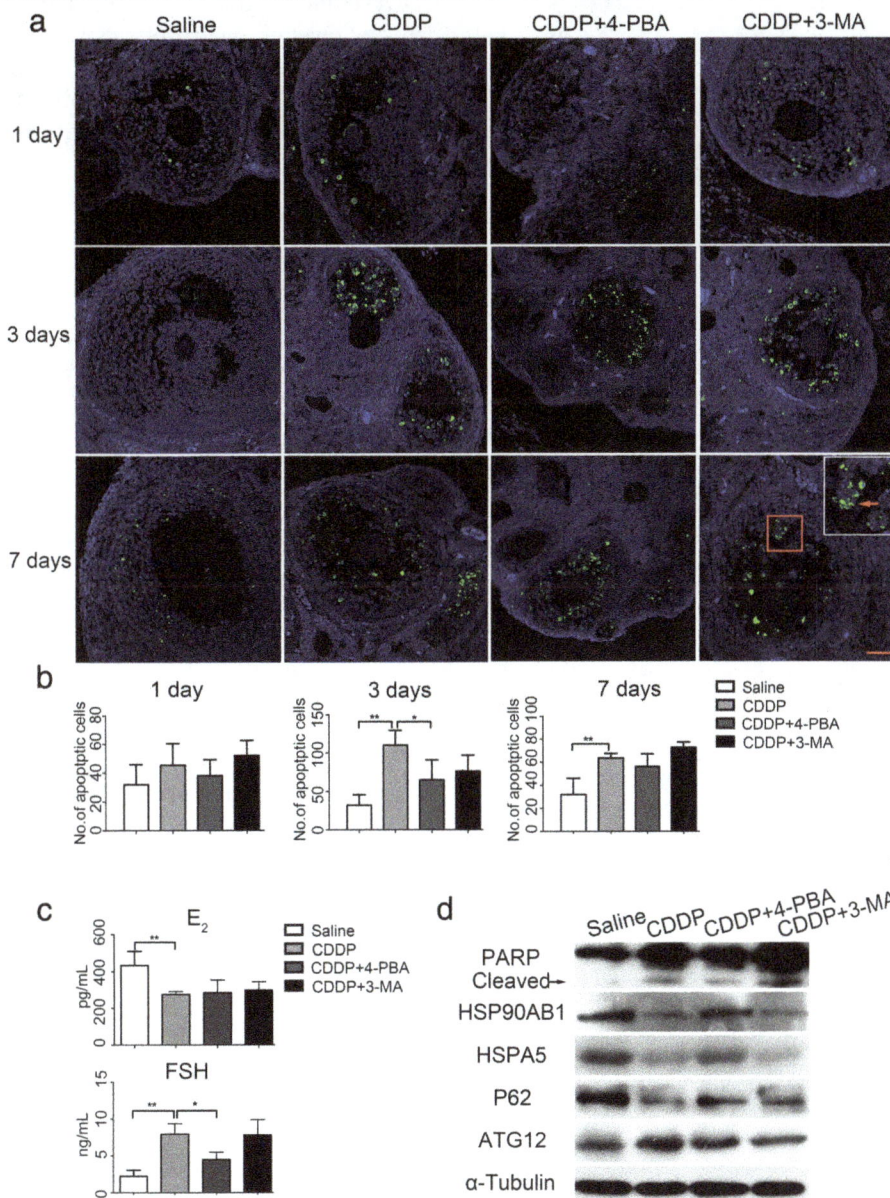

Fig. 5 Effects of 4-PBA and 3-MA on ovarian function in CDDP-treated mice. **a** Granulosa cell apoptosis in ovarian sections from each group was measured by fluorescent TUNEL staining. Green fluorescences indicate TUNEL-positive apoptotic cells (red arrow). The level of apoptosis is present as the total number of apoptotic granulosa cell on five sections (taken 100 μm apart) from an ovary. Scale bars =40 μm. **b** Quantification of TUNEL-positive apoptotic cells in each group. **c** Plasma E_2 and FSH levels by ELISA in mice with indicated treatment for 7 days. **d** Immunoblotting of the protein levels of ERS-, autophagy- and apoptosis-related proteins in each group. Protein extractions were from mice with indicated treatment for 7 days. $n = 5$, * $P < 0.05$, ** $P < 0.01$

[18] and another study showed that CDDP combined with an autophagy inhibitor or an ERS inhibitor increased the apoptosis of human lung cancer cells [32]. We suspect that these discrepancies may be attributable to the different doses of CDDP used, the different cell types examined, and therefore the different sensitivities of the cells to CDDP.

Various rescue methods have been tested to restore chemotherapy-induced ovarian damage, including human amniotic epithelial cells [33], co-treatment with a gonadotropin-releasing hormone agonist [34], melatonin treatment [19], and umbilical cord mesenchymal stem cells [35, 36]. However, the effectiveness has not been confirmed in the ovarian function and fertility when these treatments have been applied in clinical practice. As far as we know, this is the first report to demonstrate a relationship between ERS, autophagy, and apoptosis both in vitro and *vivo*. In vitro, 4-PBA alleviated ERS

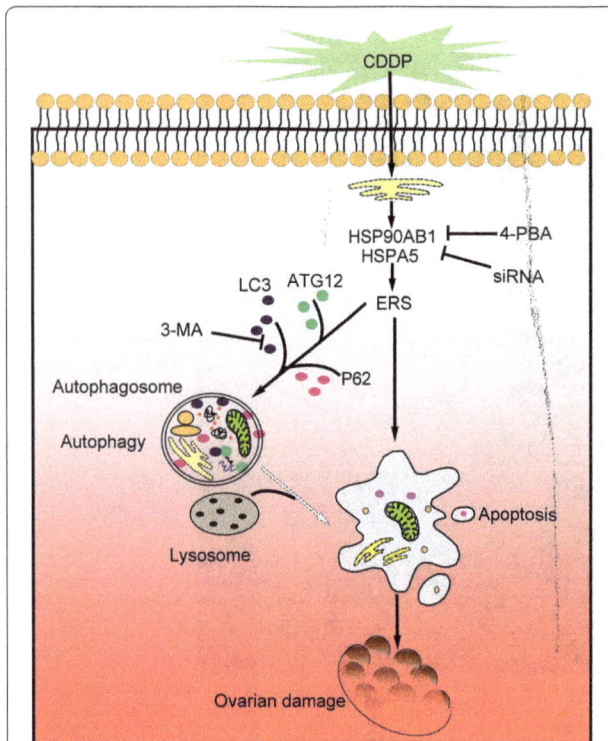

Fig. 6 A schematic mechanism of ERS in CDDP-induced ovarian damage. Exogenous CDDP increases the accumulation misfolded proteins in ER in granulosa cells, which subsequently enhance HSPA5 and HSP90AB1 expressions, leading to activation of ERS. ERS promotes cell autophagy and apoptosis. Excessive granulosa cell apoptosis induces follicular atresia contributing to ovarian dysfunction. 4-PBA can alleviate ERS, suppress cell autophagy and apoptosis, preserve follicles, and thus prevent against CDDP-induced ovarian damage

CDDP-induced granulosa cell apoptosis and ovarian damage. Overall, our results can be used as a reference point in determining the underlying pathophysiology of ovarian injury induced by chemotherapeutic treatments and may provide potential pharmacotherapeutic options.

Abbreviations
3-MA: 3-methyladenine; 4-PBA: 4-phenylbutyric acid; CDDP: Cisplatin; E2: Estradiol; ELISAs: Enzyme-linked immunosorbent assays; ERS: Endoplasmic reticulum stress; FBS: Fetal bovine serum; FSH: Follicle-stimulating hormone; H&E: Hematoxylin and eosin; HSP90AB1: Heat shock protein HSP 90-beta; HSPA5: 78-kDa glucose-regulated protein; iTRAQ: Isobaric tags for relative and absolute quantification; PI: Propidium iodide; POF: Premature ovarian failure; POI: Premature ovarian insufficiency; qPCR: Real-time quantitative PCR; RNAi: RNA interference; TUNEL: Terminal-deoxynucleotidyltransferase-mediated dUTP nick end labeling; UPR: The Unfolded protein response

Acknowledgements
We are grateful to Prof. Hongyan Yang and Prof. Yiming Mu for kindly providing the granulosa cells lines.

Funding
The study was financially supported by grant from the National Natural Science Foundation of China (No. 81571389).

Authors' contributions
LPW and ZGC designed the experiments. YPW conducted the experiments and the statistical analysis with help from CSM, HHZ and YXZ. YPW and ZGC wrote the manuscript. All of the authors read and approved the final manuscript.

Competing interests
The authors declare that they have no competing interests.

Author details
[1]Department of Obstetrics and Gynecology, Nanfang Hospital, Southern Medical University, Guangzhou 510515, China. [2]Reproductive Medicine Center, Guangdong Provincial Family Planning Special Hospital, Guangzhou 510699, China. [3]Department of Cell Biology, School of Basic Medical Sciences, Southern Medical University, Guangzhou 510515, China.

and attenuated ERS-induced autophagy and apoptosis in granulosa tumor cells. In a mouse model, 4-PBA played a protective role against CDDP-induced ovarian dysfunction. Based on these results, we considered that ERS plays a vital role in regulating the growth of granulosa cell and the development of the ovary. Therefore, 4-PBA could be an effective agent for relieving CDDP-induced ovarian damage, while the present evidences do not support that relieving autophagy can attenuate ERS or apoptosis. A previous study showed that 3-MA led to the simultaneous attenuation of autophagy and apoptosis, but did not affect cell necrosis [37]. This discrepancy reminded us that rescuing ovarian injury by inhibiting autophagy should be undertaken with caution.

Conclusions

In summary, we have clarified the relationships between ERS, autophagy, and apoptosis in CDDP-induced granulosa cell apoptosis and ovarian damage, both in vitro and in vivo. Alleviating ERS attenuated CDDP-induced autophagy and apoptosis. The 4-PBA largely attenuates

References
1. Goswami D, Conway GS. Premature ovarian failure. Hum Reprod Update. 2005;11:391–410.
2. European Society for Human R, embryology guideline group on POI, Webber L, Davies M, Anderson R, Bartlett J, Braat D, cartwright B, Cifkova R, de Muinck Keizer-Schrama S, et al. ESHRE guideline: management of women with premature ovarian insufficiency. Hum Reprod. 2016;31:926–37.

3. Tatone C, Amicarelli F. The aging ovary--the poor granulosa cells. Fertil Steril. 2013;99:12–7.

4. Uyar A, Torrealday S, Seli E. Cumulus and granulosa cell markers of oocyte and embryo quality. Fertil Steril. 2013;99:979–97.

5. Adhikari D, Liu K. Molecular mechanisms underlying the activation of mammalian primordial follicles. Endocr Rev. 2009;30:438–64.

6. Bines J, Oleske Dm Fau-Cobleigh MA, Cobleigh MA. ovarian function in premenopausal women treated with adjuvant chemotherapy for breast cancer. J Clin Oncol. 1995;14:1718–29.

7. Bae KH, Tan S, Yamashita A, Ang WX, Gao SJ, Wang S, Chung JE, Kurisawa M. Hyaluronic acid-green tea catechin micellar nanocomplexes: fail-safe cisplatin nanomedicine for the treatment of ovarian cancer without off-target toxicity. Biomaterials. 2017;148:41–53.

8. Duan X, He C, Kron SJ, Lin W. Nanoparticle formulations of cisplatin for cancer therapy. Wiley Interdiscip Rev Nanomed Nanobiotechnol. 2016;8:776–91.

9. Chatterjee R, Helal M, Mobberley M, Ryder T, Bajoria R: Impaired steroidogenesis and apoptosis of granulosa-luteal cells in primary culture induced by cis-platinum. Am J Obstet Gynecol 2014, 210:252 e251–257.

10. Sanchez AM, Giorgione V, Vigano P, Papaleo E, Candiani M, Mangili G, Panina-Bordignon P. Treatment with anticancer agents induces dysregulation of specific Wnt signaling pathways in human ovarian luteinized granulosa cells in vitro. Toxicol Sci. 2013;136:183–92.

11. Morgan S, Lopes F, Gourley C, Anderson RA, Spears N. Cisplatin and doxorubicin induce distinct mechanisms of ovarian follicle loss; imatinib provides selective protection only against cisplatin. PLoS One. 2013;8:e70117.

12. Manousakidi S, Guillaume A, Pirou C, Bouleau S, Mignotte B, Renaud F, Le Floch N. FGF1 induces resistance to chemotherapy in ovarian granulosa tumor cells through regulation of p53 mitochondrial localization. Oncogenesis. 2018;7:18.

13. Yang Z, Liu Y, Liao J, Gong C, Sun C, Zhou X, Wei X, Zhang T, Gao Q, Ma D, Chen G. Quercetin induces endoplasmic reticulum stress to enhance cDDP cytotoxicity in ovarian cancer: involvement of STAT3 signaling. FEBS J. 2015;282:1111–25.

14. Schroder M, Kaufman RJ. ER stress and the unfolded protein response. Mutat Res. 2005;569:29–63.

15. Zhang R, Wang R, Chen Q, Chang H. Inhibition of autophagy using 3-methyladenine increases cisplatin-induced apoptosis by increasing endoplasmic reticulum stress in U251 human glioma cells. Mol Med Rep. 2015;12:1727–32.

16. Gan PP, Zhou YY, Zhong MZ, Peng Y, Li L, Li JH. Endoplasmic reticulum stress promotes autophagy and apoptosis and reduces chemotherapy resistance in mutant p53 lung Cancer cells. Cell Physiol Biochem. 2017;44:133–51.

17. Sun Z, Zhang H, Wang X, Wang QC, Zhang C, Wang JQ, Wang YH, An CQ, Yang KY, Wang Y, et al. TMCO1 is essential for ovarian follicle development by regulating ER ca(2+) store of granulosa cells. Cell Death Differ. 2018;

18. Lee H, Noh JY, Oh Y, Kim Y, Chang JW, Chung CW, Lee ST, Kim M, Ryu H, Jung YK. IRE1 plays an essential role in ER stress-mediated aggregation of mutant huntingtin via the inhibition of autophagy flux. Hum Mol Genet. 2012;21:101–14.

19. Jang HLO, Lee Y, Yoon H, Chang EM, Park M, Lee JW, Hong K, Kim JO, Kim NK, Ko JJ, Lee DR, Yoon TK, Lee WS, Choi Y. Melatonin prevents cisplatin-induced primordial follicle loss via suppression of PTEN/AKT/FOXO3a pathway activation in the mouse ovary. J Pineal Res. 2016;60:336–47.

20. Chen ZG, Luo LL, Xu JJ, Zhuang XL, Kong XX, Fu YC. effects of plant polyphenols on ovarian follicular reserve in aging rats. Biochem Cell Biol. 2010;88:737–45.

21. Wang C, Zhang S, Ma R, Zhang X, Zhang C, Li B, Niu Q, Chen J, Xia T, Li P, et al. Roles of endoplasmic reticulum stress, apoptosis and autophagy in 2,2',4,4'-tetrabromodiphenyl ether-induced rat ovarian injury. Reprod Toxicol. 2016;65:187–93.

22. Liu YM, Lv J, Zeng QL, Shen S, Xing JY, Zhang YY, Zhang ZH, Yu ZJ. AMPK activation ameliorates D-GalN/LPS-induced acute liver failure by upregulating Foxo3A to induce autophagy. Exp Cell Res. 2017;358:335–42.

23. Xu L, Sun H, Zhang M, Jiang Y, Zhang C, Zhou J, Ding L, Hu Y, Yan G. MicroRNA-145 protects follicular granulosa cells against oxidative stress-induced apoptosis by targeting Kruppel-like factor 4. Mol Cell Endocrinol. 2017;452:138–47.

24. Rehnitz J, Alcoba DD, Brum IS, Hinderhofer K, Youness B, Strowitzki T, Vogt PH. FMR1 and AKT/mTOR signalling pathways: potential functional interactions controlling folliculogenesis in human granulosa cells. Reprod BioMed Online. 2017;35:485–93.

25. Iwashita H, Sakurai HT, Nagahora N, Ishiyama M, Shioji K, Sasamoto K, Okuma K, Shimizu S, Ueno Y. Small fluorescent molecules for monitoring autophagic flux. FEBS Lett. 2018;592:559–67.

26. Cui Y, Zhao D, Sreevatsan S, Liu C, Yang W, Song Z, Yang L, Barrow P, Zhou X. Mycobacterium bovis induces endoplasmic reticulum stress mediated-apoptosis by activating IRF3 in a murine macrophage cell line. Front Cell Infect Microbiol. 2016;6:182.

27. Sun X, Li L, Ma HG, Sun P, Wang QL, Zhang TT, Shen YM, Zhu WM, Li X. Bisindolylmaleimide alkaloid BMA-155Cl induces autophagy and apoptosis in human hepatocarcinoma HepG-2 cells through the NF-kappaB p65 pathway. Acta Pharmacol Sin. 2017;38:524–38.

28. Mathew R, Karp CM, Beaudoin B, Vuong N, Chen G, Chen HY, Bray K, Reddy A, Bhanot G, Gelinas C, et al. Autophagy suppresses tumorigenesis through elimination of p62. Cell. 2009;137:1062–75.

29. Morgan S, Anderson RA, Gourley C, Wallace WH, Spears N. How do chemotherapeutic agents damage the ovary? Hum Reprod Update. 2012;18:525–35.

30. Rath E, Berger E, Messlik A, Nunes T, Liu B, Kim SC, Hoogenraad N, Sans M, Sartor RB, Haller D. Induction of dsRNA-activated protein kinase links mitochondrial unfolded protein response to the pathogenesis of intestinal inflammation. Gut. 2012;61:1269–78.

31. Senft D, Ronai ZA. UPR, autophagy, and mitochondria crosstalk underlies the ER stress response. Trends Biochem Sci. 2015;40:141–8.

32. Shi S, Tan P, Yan B, Gao R, Zhao J, Wang J, Guo J, Li N, Ma Z. ER stress and autophagy are involved in the apoptosis induced by cisplatin in human lung cancer cells. Oncol Rep. 2016;35:2606–14.

33. Zhang Q, Bu S, Sun J, Xu M, Yao X, He K, Lai D. Paracrine effects of human amniotic epithelial cells protect against chemotherapy-induced ovarian damage. Stem Cell Res Ther. 2017;8:270.

34. Beck-Fruchter R, Weiss A, Shalev E. GnRH agonist therapy as ovarian protectants in female patients undergoing chemotherapy: a review of the clinical data. Hum Reprod Update. 2008;14:553–61.

35. Wang S, Yu L, Sun M, Mu S, Wang C, Wang D, aY Y. The therapeutic potential of umbilical cord mesenchymal stem cells in mice premature ovarian failure. Biomed Res Int. 2013;

36. Song D, Zhong Y, Qian C, Zou Q, Ou J, Shi Y, Gao L, Wang G, Liu Z, Li H, et al. Human umbilical cord mesenchymal stem cells therapy in cyclophosphamide-induced premature ovarian failure rat model. Biomed Res Int. 2016;2016:1–13.

37. Carlisle RE, Brimble E, Werner KE, Cruz GL, Ask K, Ingram AJ, Dickhout JG. 4-Phenylbutyrate inhibits tunicamycin-induced acute kidney injury via CHOP/GADD153 repression. PLoS One. 2014;9:e84663.

13

The VEGF and PEDF levels in the follicular fluid of patients co- treated with LETROZOLE and gonadotropins during the stimulation cycle

Jigal Haas[1,2,3*], Rawad Bassil[1,2], Noa Gonen[1,2], Jim Meriano[1,2], Andrea Jurisicova[1,2] and Robert F. Casper[1,2]

Abstract

Background: Previous studies have shown that androgens, in addition to serving as precursors for ovarian estrogen synthesis, also have a fundamental role in primate ovarian follicular development by augmentation of FSH receptor expression on granulosa cells. Recent studies have shown that aromatase inhibitor, letrozole, improves ovarian response to FSH in normal and poor responder patients, possibly by increasing intraovarian androgen levels. Studies in mice also showed an effect of letrozole to increase pigment epithelium-derived factor (PEDF) and to lower vascular epithelial growth factor (VEGF), which might be expected to reduce the risk of ovarian hyperstimulation syndrome (OHSS) with stimulation. The aim of this study was to compare the VEGF and PEDF levels in the follicular fluids of normal responders treated with letrozole and gonadotropins during the ovarian stimulation with patients treated with gonadotropins only.

Methods: A single center, prospective clinical trial. We collected follicular fluid from 26 patients, on a GnRH antagonist protocol, dual triggered with hCG and GnRH agonist. The patients in one group were co-treated with letrozole and gonadotropins during the ovarian stimulation and the patients in the other group were treated with gonadotropins only. VEGF, PEDF, estrogen, progesterone and testosterone levels were measured by ELISA kits.

Results: The age of the patients, the total dose of gonadotropins and the number of oocytes were comparable between the two groups. In the follicular fluid, the estrogen levels (2209 nmol/l vs. 3280 nmol/l, $p = 0.02$) were significantly decreased, and the testosterone levels (246.5 nmol/l vs. 40.7 nmol/l, $p < 0.001$) were significantly increased in the letrozole group compared to the gonadotropin only group. The progesterone levels (21.4 μmol/l vs. 17.5 $p = $ NS) were comparable between the two groups.
The VEGF levels (2992 pg/ml vs. 1812 pg/ml $p = 0.02$) were significantly increased and the PEDF levels (9.7 ng/ml vs 17.3 ng/ml $p < 0.001$) were significantly decreased in the letrozole group.

Conclusions: Opposite to observations in the mouse, we found that VEGF levels were increased and PEDF levels were decreased in the follicular fluid in patients treated with letrozole during the stimulation cycles. Further investigation is required to determine if patients treated with letrozole during the IVF stimulation protocol are at increased risk for developing OHSS as a result of these findings.

Keywords: Letrozole, VEGF. PEDF

* Correspondence: jigalh@hotmail.com
[1]Division of Reproductive Sciences, University of Toronto,
Lunenfeld-Tanenbaum Research Institute, Mount Sinai Hospital, Toronto,
Canada
[2]TRIO fertility partners, 655 Bay St 11th floor, Toronto, ON M5G 2K4, Canada
Full list of author information is available at the end of the article

Background

The addition of the aromatase inhibitor, letrozole, to gonadotropin stimulation has been an accepted treatment for oocyte retrieval in women with breast cancer and has been demonstrated to result in lower serum estrogen levels [1, 2] an endocrine response that is considered to be favourable in these women who may have estrogen sensitive tumors. In normal women undergoing IVF, lowering serum and follicular estrogen levels could also be potentially beneficial by lowering the risk of ovarian hyperstimulation syndrome (OHSS) since a correlation has been observed between administration of letrozole and lowering the incidence of OHSS [3].

A previous study in a rat model of OHSS [4] demonstrated that treatment with a single dose of letrozole on the hCG trigger day, reduced ovarian diameter, reduced VEGF levels and increased the levels of pigment epithelium derived factor (PEDF). VEGF has been identified as one of the prime causative factors in OHSS while PEDF has been shown to decrease the angiogenic activity of VEGF [5]. These combined results might be expected to reduce the risk of OHSS.

In addition, supraphysiologic levels of estrogen are believed to have a negative effect on oocyte quality [6] and embryo implantation [7] with subsequent adverse pregnancy outcomes [8, 9] and therefore, lowering estrogen levels by adding letrozole could be beneficial in normal women undergoing IVF by increasing implantation and reducing pregnancy complications.

More recently, it has also been observed that breast cancer patients undergoing IVF with the addition of letrozole have an increase in the number of oocytes recovered compared to controls [1, 2]. Several studies have shown that letrozole, improves ovarian response to FSH in normal and poor responder patients, possibly by increasing intraovarian androgen levels (1–3, 11–13). Previous studies have shown that androgens, in addition to serving as precursors for ovarian estrogen synthesis, also have a fundamental role in primate ovarian follicular development by augmentation of FSH receptor expression on granulosa cells [10].

The objective of this study was to measure VEGF and PEDF levels as well as estrogen and testosterone levels in the follicular fluids of normal responder women treated with letrozole and gonadotropins throughout the entire ovarian stimulation for IVF and to compare the results with the follicular fluid levels in patients treated with gonadotropins only.

Methods
Ethical approval

The study was approved by the Mount Sinai Hospital ethics review committee, and all couples were required to sign a written informed consent after the provision of complete information.

This study included a total of 26 IVF cycles performed in 26 normal responders treated at our institution between June, 2016 and March, 2017. Patients with PCOS or POR by Bologna criteria were excluded from the study.

The study group included patients on a GnRH antagonist protocol treated with daily letrozole 5 mg together with gonadotropins, from the first day of ovarian stimulation until the trigger day. The control group included patients matched by age, infertility diagnosis and starting gonadotropin dose, on the same GnRH antagonist protocol, treated with gonadotropins only during the stimulation. All the patients included in the study had a dual trigger with hCG and GnRH agonist for final oocyte maturation. The study was not randomized and the decision whether to co-treat with letrozole was made by each treating physician independently.

The decision to administer letrozole was not made for the sake of this study. The treating physicians made this treatment decision independently of the study.

Stimulation protocols

Gonadotropin treatment (with or without letrozole) was initiated on the 3rd day of menses with the use of recombinant FSH (Gonal F, EMD Serono). Once the leading follicle had reached a size of 13 mm, or E2 levels exceeded 1200 pmol/L, co-treatment with a GnRH antagonist 0.25 mg/day (Orgalutran, Merck) and recombinant LH (Luveris, Serono) or highly purified human menopausal gonadotropin (Menopur, Ferring) was commenced. Follicle growth and hormone levels were serially monitored by ultrasound and blood tests until the dominant follicles reached an average diameter of 18–20 mm. At that point human chorionic gonadotropin (10,000 IU Pregnyl; Merck, Kirkland, Quebec) and GnRH agonist (0.5 mg Suprefact; Sanofi-Aventis, Canada) were administered subcutaneously to trigger ovulation. Thirty-six hours later oocyte retrieval was performed under transvaginal guided ultrasound and needle aspiration.

The follicular fluid (FF) was obtained at the time of oocyte retrieval for the IVF procedure. Only the first follicle from each ovary was collected avoiding blood clots, and only FF from mature full sized follicles (≥16 mm) was included in the study. Only one single follicular fluid sample per patient was included in the study.

After isolation of the oocyte, the clear follicular fluid was centrifuged at 500 g for 10 min at room temperature to separate out cellular contents and debris and was then transferred to sterile tubes and frozen at − 80 °C until analysis. The follicular fluid was analyzed for testosterone, estradiol, progesterone by an automated assay (Vitros), and VEGF (Cedarlane; CL76149K) and

PEDF (Chemicon;CYT 420) concentrations were measured by commercial ELISA using an ELISA kits according to the manufacturer's instructions. We measured follicular fluid progesterone concentrations as a possible way to ensure similar ovarian stimulation in each group.

Comparisons were performed using the paired two-tailed student's t-test. A $P < 0.05$ was considered statistically significant.

Results

The age of the patients, the total dose of gonadotropins and the number of oocytes were comparable between the two groups (Table 1). In the follicular fluid, the mean estrogen level (2209 nmol/l vs. 3280 nmol/l, $p = 0.02$) was significantly decreased, and the mean testosterone level (246.5 nmol/l vs. 40.7 nmol/l, $p < 0.001$) was significantly increased in the letrozole co-treated group compared to the gonadotropin only group. The mean follicular fluid progesterone level (21.4 µmol/l vs. 17.5 µmol, $p = NS$) was comparable between the two groups (Table 2).

The mean VEGF level (2992 pg/ml vs. 1812 pg/ml $p = 0.02$) was significantly increased and the mean PEDF level (9.7 ng/ml vs 17.3 ng/ml p < 0.001) was significantly decreased in the letrozole group (Table 3).

None of the patients in the study group or in the control group developed early or late OHSS.

Discussion

In contrast to observations in mice, we found that VEGF levels were increased and PEDF levels were decreased in the follicular fluids of patients treated with letrozole during the stimulation cycles, despite a significant suppression of estradiol concentration in follicular fluid. In the

Table 2 The hormone levels in the follicular fluid from patients co-treated with letrozole and gonadotropins vs. gonadotropins only

	Letrozole group (13)	Control group (13)	P
Estrogen(nmol/l)	2009 ± 1034	3280 ± 1371	0.01
Testosterone(nmol/l)	246.5 ± 153.2	40.7 ± 14.3	< 0.001
Progesterone(µmol/l)	21.4 ± 8.3	17.5 ± 10.3	0.3

murine model, letrozole was administered only at the trigger day and not during the ovarian stimulation whereas in our current study, the patients were treated during the entire ovarian stimulation, which might explain the differences between the VEGF and PEDF levels observed.

Similarly to the murine findings, He et al. demonstrated a decrease in the VEGF serum levels after treatment with letrozole in the luteal phase. He found a dose dependent decrease in the levels of VEGF with increasing doses of letrozole administered in the luteal phase [11]. The findings of He et al. suggested that letrozole could decrease the risk of OHSS although it is not clear if the effect on VEGF and PEDF secretion was a direct action of letrozole or an indirect effect through a reduction in estradiol levels.

A randomized controlled study in hyper-responder patients which aimed to compare the efficacy of letrozole to aspirin during the luteal phase in primary prevention of early ovarian hyperstimulation syndrome showed a lower incidence of OHSS in women receiving letrozole compared with aspirin [3]. In contrast to previous studies, the patients treated with letrozole had higher levels of VEGF in the serum compared to the patients not treated with letrozole. The authors hypothesized that the mechanism of lower incidence of OHSS was independent of

Table 1 Characteristics of the IVF cycles for patients co-treated with letrozole compared to the control group

	Letrozole group (n = 13)	Without letrozole (n = 13)	P value
Age (years)	36.3 ± 3.9	35.8 ± 3.7	NS
AMH (pmol/l)	14.26 ± 7.7	16.4 ± 6.7	NS
FSH	7.3 ± 1.6	6.6 ± 1.9	NS
Etiology for infertility	Unexplained-8 Male factor-3 Mechanical-0 Fertility preservation-2	Unexplained-7 Male factor-3 Mechanical-1 Fertility preservation- 2	NS
Length of stimulation (days)	9.4 ± 1.8	10.7 ± 1.7	NS
Dosage of gonadotropins	3085 ± 633	3294 ± 917	NS
Oocytes (n)	11.7 ± 5.7	12.1 ± 6.1	NS
2PN(n)	6.6 ± 5.1	7.6 ± 4.4	NS
Blastocysts (n)	3.1 ± 2.2	2.9 ± 1.9	NS
Blastocyst rate (blast/2PN)	46.9%	38.1%	NS
E2 levels (pmol/l)	1032 ± 375	8069 ± 3068	0.001
Ongoing Pregnancy rate	5/11 (45.4%)	4/11(36.3%)	NS

Table 3 The VEGF and PEDF levels in the follicular fluid from patients co-treated with letrozole and gonadotropins vs. gonadotropins only

	Letrozole group (13)	Control group (13)	p
VEGF (pg/ml)	2992 ± 431.7	1812 ± 462.4	0.02
PEDF (ng/ml)	9.7 ± 5.7	17.3 ± 8.4	< 0.001

VEGF but rather due to the induction of a luteolytic effect and lower estradiol concentrations which reduced the risk of early-onset OHSS (5).

Although we didn't measure the VEGF or PEDF levels in the serum, we found increased VEGF and PEDF levels in the follicular fluid of letrozole treated patients at the time of oocyte retrieval. In the follicular phase, letrozole reduces serum estrogen levels which results in reduced negative feedback on gonadotrophin secretion from the hypothalamus-pituitary axis [12–14]. By lowering serum estrogen concentrations in the early follicular phase, letrozole causes secretion of more FSH and LH, which acts directly on the granulosa cells and may be responsible for the increased secretion of VEGF. In addition, we found higher intrafollicular levels of testosterone in the letrozole group. We believe that the androgen increase may have a positive effect on follicular development, oocyte maturation and implantation. Since androgens have been shown to increase FSH receptor expression in both murine [15] and primate models [16, 17] it is possible that the increased VEGF level could also be influenced by the impact of increased androgen levels on the granulosa cell responsiveness to FSH in the letrozole treated group.

Previous studies demonstrated [18, 19] that women who did not conceive had higher FF VEGF concentrations than women achieving a clinical pregnancy. A negative correlation was observed between FF VEGF concentrations, peak estradiol levels and number of oocytes retrieved. Friedman et al. [20] showed increased VEGF levels in the FF from patients with advanced age compared with younger women. They hypothesized that the higher VEGF concentrations resulted from relative follicular hypoxia which is a stimulant for VEGF production.

As published previously by our group [21], we found a higher number of oocytes, zygotes and blastocysts in women co-treated with letrozole compared to matched patients treated with gonadotropins only. We hypothesize that in normal responders co treated with letrozole the pathophysiology increasing VEGF levels is different and not related to follicular hypoxia. We believe that by lowering serum estrogen concentrations in the early follicular phase, letrozole causes secretion of more FSH and LH, which acts directly on the granulosa cells and may be responsible for the increased secretion of VEGF.

VEGF binds to specific receptors located in endothelial cells called VEGF-R1 (Flt-1) and VEGF-R2. Soluble VEGF-R1 is a naturally produced receptor capable of binding and sequestering VEGF and is able to reduce the level of free, active VEGF [22].

Jakimiuk et al. [23] demonstrated that VEGF/ sFlt-1 ratio in FF on the day of oocyte retrieval in women undergoing IVF procedure, regardless of the type of stimulation protocol, might predict the risk of developing OHSS.

The sFlt-1 contribute to the amount of free, biological active VEGF in FF and later in serum by binding VEGF and thereby depleting the amount of free circulating biological active VEGF.

In our study we didn't measure sFlt-1 levels in the FF and therefore it's still speculative whether free circulating VEGF levels were different between the groups.

Tropea et al. [24], cultured human luteal phase with androgens and demonstrated that different doses of androgens significantly increased VEGF secretion. By culturing the cells with aromatase inhibitor, VEGF levels decreased. We think it's difficult to compare those results with our current study because in our study the patients were treated with letrozole which causes secretion of LH and FSH from the pituitary gland in contrast to the cultured granulosa cells which are not affected by those changes. Another major difference is that the granulosa cells were cultured in the luteal phase whereas in our study the patients were treated with letrozole in the follicular phase and the granulosa cells in the follicular phase may respond differently than in the luteal phase to androgens in terms of VEGF production.

In the letrozole group the estrogen levels in the follicular fluid were significantly lower and more similar to the estrogen levels in the natural cycle compared to estrogen levels in the gonadotropins only group [25]. Previous studies have demonstrated a reduced pregnancy rate with increasing E2/ oocyte ratio [6, 26] and therefore we assume that treatment with letrozole which reduces the serum and intrafollicular estrogen concentrations, may have a positive effect on the oocyte quality and embryo development.

Although none of the patients in our study group developed OHSS, we think that further investigation is required to determine if patients treated with letrozole during the IVF stimulation protocol are at increased risk for developing OHSS as a result of our new findings demonstrating increased VEGF levels and decreased PEDF levels after treatment with letrozole.

We conclude that co-treatment with gonadotropins and letrozole during the follicular phase increase the VEGF levels and decrease the PEDF levels in the follicular fluid. Whether co-treatment with letrozole during the follicular phase may increase the incidence of OHSS is still unknown and further studies should be performed to evaluate this risk.

Abbreviations
ET: Embryo transfer; FET: Frozen embryo transfer; FSH: Follicle stimulating hormone; IVF: In vitro fertilization; OHSS: Ovarian hyperstimulation; PEDF: Pigment epithelium-derived factor; VEGF: Vascular epithelial growth factor

Authors' contributions
JH designed and conducted the study and wrote the initial draft of the manuscript. RB, JM, AJ, NG and RC helped with the study design, data analysis, interpretation and manuscript editing. RB, AJ and NG performed the proteins and hormones measurements. All authors read and approved the final manuscript.

Competing interest
The authors declare that they have no competing interests.

Author details
[1]Division of Reproductive Sciences, University of Toronto, Lunenfeld-Tanenbaum Research Institute, Mount Sinai Hospital, Toronto, Canada. [2]TRIO fertility partners, 655 Bay St 11th floor, Toronto, ON M5G 2K4, Canada. [3]Department of Obstetrics and Gynecology, Sheba Medical Center, Sackler School of Medicine, Tel-Aviv University, Tel-Hashomer, Israel.

References
1. Pereira N, Hancock K, Cordeiro CN, Lekovich JP, Schattman GL, Rosenwaks Z. Comparison of ovarian stimulation response in patients with breast cancer undergoing ovarian stimulation with letrozole and gonadotropins to patients undergoing ovarian stimulation with gonadotropins alone for elective cryopreservation of oocytesdagger. Gynecol Endocrinol. 2016;32:823–6.
2. Quinn MM, Cakmak H, Letourneau JM, Cedars MI, Rosen MP: Response to ovarian stimulation is not impacted by a breast cancer diagnosis. Hum Reprod. 2017;32(3):568-74.
3. Mai Q, Hu X, Yang G, Luo Y, Huang K, Yuan Y, Zhou C. Effect of letrozole on moderate and severe early-onset ovarian hyperstimulation syndrome in high-risk women: a prospective randomized trial. Am J Obstet Gynecol. 2017;216:42 e41–10.
4. Sahin N, Apaydin N, Toz E, Sivrikoz ON, Genc M, Turan GA, Cengiz H, Eskicioglu F. Comparison of the effects of letrozole and cabergoline on vascular permeability, ovarian diameter, ovarian tissue VEGF levels, and blood PEDF levels, in a rat model of ovarian hyperstimulation syndrome. Arch Gynecol Obstet. 2016;293:1101–6.
5. Chuderland D, Ben-Ami I, Kaplan-Kraicer R, Grossman H, Ron-El R, Shalgi R. The role of pigment epithelium-derived factor in the pathophysiology and treatment of ovarian hyperstimulation syndrome in mice. J Clin Endocrinol Metab. 2013;98:E258–66.
6. Orvieto R, Zohav E, Scharf S, Rabinson J, Meltcer S, Anteby EY, Homburg R. The influence of estradiol/follicle and estradiol/oocyte ratios on the outcome of controlled ovarian stimulation for in vitro fertilization. Gynecol Endocrinol. 2007;23:72–5.
7. Imudia AN, Goldman RH, Awonuga AO, Wright DL, Styer AK, Toth TL. The impact of supraphysiologic serum estradiol levels on peri-implantation embryo development and early pregnancy outcome following in vitro fertilization cycles. J Assist Reprod Genet. 2014;31:65–71.
8. Ishihara O, Araki R, Kuwahara A, Itakura A, Saito H, Adamson GD. Impact of frozen-thawed single-blastocyst transfer on maternal and neonatal outcome: an analysis of 277,042 single-embryo transfer cycles from 2008 to 2010 in Japan. Fertil Steril. 2014;101:128–33.
9. Wennerholm UB, Henningsen AK, Romundstad LB, Bergh C, Pinborg A, Skjaerven R, Forman J, Gissler M, Nygren KG, Tiitinen A. Perinatal outcomes of children born after frozen-thawed embryo transfer: a Nordic cohort study from the CoNARTaS group. Hum Reprod. 2013;28:2545–53.
10. Weil S, Vendola K, Zhou J, Bondy CA. Androgen and follicle-stimulating hormone interactions in primate ovarian follicle development. J Clin Endocrinol Metab. 1999;84:2951–6.
11. He Q, Liang L, Zhang C, Li H, Ge Z, Wang L, Cui S. Effects of different doses of letrozole on the incidence of early-onset ovarian hyperstimulation syndrome after oocyte retrieval. Syst Biol Reprod Med. 2014;60:355–60.
12. Kamat A, Hinshelwood MM, Murry BA, Mendelson CR. Mechanisms in tissue-specific regulation of estrogen biosynthesis in humans. Trends Endocrinol Metab. 2002;13:122–8.
13. Naftolin F, MacLusky NJ, Leranth CZ, Sakamoto HS, Garcia-Segura LM. The cellular effects of estrogens on neuroendocrine tissues. J Steroid Biochem. 1988;30:195–207.
14. Naftolin F, Romero R. H2-receptor antagonists and sexual differentiation. Gastroenterology. 1984;87:248–9.
15. Laird M, Thomson K, Fenwick M, Mora J, Franks S, Hardy K. Androgen stimulates growth of mouse Preantral follicles in vitro: interaction with follicle-stimulating hormone and with growth factors of the TGFbeta superfamily. Endocrinology. 2017;158:920–35.
16. Gervasio CG, Bernuci MP, Silva-de-Sa MF, Rosa ESAC. The role of androgen hormones in early follicular development. ISRN Obstet Gynecol. 2014;2014:818010.
17. Nielsen ME, Rasmussen IA, Kristensen SG, Christensen ST, Mollgard K, Wreford Andersen E, Byskov AG, Yding Andersen C. In human granulosa cells from small antral follicles, androgen receptor mRNA and androgen levels in follicular fluid correlate with FSH receptor mRNA. Mol Hum Reprod. 2011;17:63–70.
18. Friedman CI, Seifer DB, Kennard EA, Arbogast L, Alak B, Danforth DR. Elevated level of follicular fluid vascular endothelial growth factor is a marker of diminished pregnancy potential. Fertil Steril. 1998;70:836–9.
19. Ocal P, Aydin S, Cepni I, Idil S, Idil M, Uzun H, Benian A. Follicular fluid concentrations of vascular endothelial growth factor, inhibin a and inhibin B in IVF cycles: are they markers for ovarian response and pregnancy outcome? Eur J Obstet Gynecol Reprod Biol. 2004;115:194–9.
20. Friedman CI, Danforth DR, Herbosa-Encarnacion C, Arbogast L, Alak BM, Seifer DB. Follicular fluid vascular endothelial growth factor concentrations are elevated in women of advanced reproductive age undergoing ovulation induction. Fertil Steril. 1997;68:607–12.
21. Haas J, Bassil R, Meriano J, Samara N, Barzilay E, Gonen N, Casper RF. Does daily co-administration of letrozole and gonadotropins during ovarian stimulation improve IVF outcome? Reprod Biol Endocrinol. 2017;15:70.
22. Sela S, Natanson-Yaron S, Zcharia E, Vlodavsky I, Yagel S, Keshet E. Local retention versus systemic release of soluble VEGF receptor-1 are mediated by heparin-binding and regulated by heparanase. Circ Res. 2011;108:1063–70.
23. Jakimiuk AJ, Nowicka MA, Zagozda M, Koziol K, Lewandowski P, Issat T. High levels of soluble vascular endothelial growth factor receptor 1/sFlt1 and low levels of vascular endothelial growth factor in follicular fluid on the day of oocyte retrieval correlate with ovarian hyperstimulation syndrom regardless of the stimulation protocol. J Physiol Pharmacol. 2017;68:477–84.
24. Tropea A, Lanzone A, Tiberi F, Romani F, Catino S, Apa R. Estrogens and androgens affect human luteal cell function. Fertil Steril. 2010;94:2257–63.
25. von Wolff M, Kollmann Z, Fluck CE, Stute P, Marti U, Weiss B, Bersinger NA. Gonadotrophin stimulation for in vitro fertilization significantly alters the hormone milieu in follicular fluid: a comparative study between natural cycle IVF and conventional IVF. Hum Reprod. 2014;29:1049–57.
26. Yang JH, Chen HF, Lien YR, Chen SU, Ho HN, Yang YS. Elevated E2: oocyte ratio in women undergoing IVF and tubal ET. Correlation with a decrease in the implantation rate. J Reprod Med. 2001;46:434–8.

14

Analysis of human sperm DNA fragmentation index (DFI) related factors: a report of 1010 subfertile men in China

Jin-Chun Lu[1,2†]⊙, Jun Jing[1†], Li Chen[1], Yi-Feng Ge[1], Rui-Xiang Feng[2], Yuan-Jiao Liang[1] and Bing Yao[1*]

Abstract

Background: Many factors may lead to sperm DNA damage. However, it is little known that the correlations of sperm DNA damage with obesity-associated markers, and reproductive hormones and lipids levels in serum and seminal plasma.

Methods: In our prospective study, a total of 1 010 subfertile men, aged from 18 to 50 years old, were enrolled from August 2012 through June 2015. Their obesity-associated markers, semen parameters, sperm acrosomal enzyme activity, seminal plasma biochemical markers, and reproductive hormones and lipids levels in serum and seminal plasma were detected. Sperm DNA fragmentation index (DFI) was determined by sperm chromatin structure assay. The correlations between DFI and each of the above-mentioned variables were analyzed.

Results: Spearman correlation analysis showed that sperm DFI was positively related to age and abstinence time ($P<0.001$). Sperm DFI was also positively related to semen volume and percent of abnormal sperm head ($P<0.001$), while negatively related to sperm concentration, progressive motility (PR), sperm motility, total normal-progressively motile sperm count (TNPMS), percent of normal sperm morphology (NSM), percent of intact acrosome and acrosomal enzyme activity ($P<0.001$). Sperm DFI was positively related to seminal plasma zinc level ($P<0.001$) but unrelated to seminal plasma total α-glucotase, γ-glutamyl transpeptidase (GGT) and fructose levels. There was no any correlation between sperm DFI and obesity-associated markers such as body mass index (BMI), waist-to-hip ratio (WHR), waist circumference (WC) and waist-to-height ratio (WHtR), and serum lipids levels, but there was positive correlation between sperm DFI and seminal plasma triglyceride (TG) and total cholesterol (TC) levels ($P<0.001$). Sperm DFI was positively related to serum luteinizing hormone (LH) and follicle stimulating hormone (FSH) levels and seminal plasma FSH and estradiol (E2) levels ($P<0.001$), but unrelated to serum and seminal plasma testosterone (T) levels. The multivariate regression analysis for the variables which were significantly correlated with sperm DFI in Spearman correlation analysis showed that age, semen volume, sperm concentration, progressive motility, TNPMS and intact acrosome were independently correlated with sperm DFI.

Conclusions: There are many potential factors associated with sperm DFI, including age, abstinence time, spermatogenesis and maturation, seminal plasma lipids and reproductive hormones levels. However, the potential effects of seminal plasma lipids and reproductive hormones on sperm DNA damage need still to be demonstrated by the studies with scientific design and a large size of samples.

Keywords: Sperm DNA fragmentation index, Male infertility, Obesity-associated marker, Lipids, Reproductive hormone

* Correspondence: 2424572228@qq.com
†Equal contributors
[1]The Reproductive Medical Centre, Nanjing Jinling Hospital, Nanjing University School of Medicine, 305 Zhongshan East Road, Nanjing 210002, Jiangsu, China
Full list of author information is available at the end of the article

Background

Through searches of "sperm" and "DNA fragmentation index" in PubMed from 2002 to August 2015, we retrieved over 200 literatures associated with sperm DNA fragmentation index (DFI). Comprehensive analyses of these literatures indicated that since the detection of sperm DNA damage was performed in 2002, it had been applied in some clinical andrology laboratories. The detection of sperm DNA damage, as an important supplement to semen routine examination strategies, may predict the outcomes of natural conception and *in vitro* fertilization, monitor the damage of sperm DNA induced by environmental pollutants and medical interventions, and evaluate the sperm DNA damage related to male reproductive system diseases and their treatments [1]. The factors related to sperm DNA damage included age, environmental pollutants such as organophosphorus and organochloride pesticides, plasticizer, heavy metals such as lead, carcinogens such as polycyclic aromatic hydrocarbons (c-PAHs) and zearalenone (ZEA), male reproductive system diseases or systemic diseases such as varicocele, infection, tumor, spermatogenesis and maturation dysfunction, spinal cord injury and endocrine disorders, seasons and temperature, lifestyle, abstinence time, semen refrigeration, semen handling *in vitro*, and certain medications [2]. However, controversial results remain.

Obesity and subfertility have become major global public health concerns. Obesity was reportedly associated with lower fertility. Our previously published data showed that, although obesity-associated markers such as body mass index (BMI), waist circumference (WC), waist-to-hip ratio (WHR) and waist-to-height ratio (WHtR) could not predict semen quality [3], the metabolism abnormality of lipids in male reproductive system may affect male fertility [4]. It raises the question of whether sperm DNA damage, as an important factor influencing sperm quality, be associated with obesity and metabolism abnormality of lipids. No data currently available address this question [5]. In this study, we comprehensively analyzed the correlations between sperm DFI and age, abstinence time, obesity-associated markers such as BMI, WC, WHR and WHtR, semen parameters such as semen volume, sperm concentration, total sperm count (TSC), sperm motility, progressive motility (PR), percent of normal sperm morphology (NSM), percent of abnormal sperm head, percent of intact acrosome, acrosomal enzyme activity and total normal-progressively motile sperm count (TNPMS), serum lipids such as total cholesterol (TC), triglyceride (TG), low density lipoprotein cholesterol (LDL-C) and high density lipoprotein cholesterol (HDL-C) levels, serum reproductive hormones such as follicle stimulating hormone (FSH), luteinizing hormone (LH), estradiol (E2), total testosterone (TT) and sex hormone binding globulin (SHBG) levels, seminal plasma biochemical markers such as total α-glucotase, γ-glutamyl transpeptidase (GGT), zinc and fructose, seminal plasma lipids such as TG, TC, LDL-C and HDL-C, and seminal plasma reproductive hormones such as FSH, E2 and testosterone in 1 010 subfertile Chinese men (The raw data for these variables were shown in Additional file 1).

Methods

Study population

Subfertile men, aged from 18 to 50 years and whose partners had not conceived within 12 months after stopping use of contraception, who attended infertility outpatient clinic at Nanjing Jinling Hospital between August 2012 and June 2015 were included in this prospective study. This study was approved by the Human Subject Committees of Nanjing Jinling Hospital (Approved number: 2012NZKY-012), and informed consent was obtained from all participants. All participants were asked to complete a questionnaire to provide information on occupation, medical and reproductive history and lifestyle factors including intake of alcohol and smoking history. Then, all participants underwent physical examination, and obesity-associated markers were measured, semen samples were collected, and fasting venous blood were drawn during 8:00 am and 10:00 am. Stringent exclusion criteria were employed to exclude regular alcohol drinkers, heavy smokers, and men with chronic diseases, urogenital infections, varicocele, azoospermia and other diseases which might lead to dysspermia, and incomplete data. One thousand and ten (1 010) men were eligible for the inclusion criteria and enrolled in this study.

Measurement of obesity-associated markers

Height and weight were measured with the participants standing without shoes and heavy outer garments. WC was measured at the level midway between the lower rib margin and the iliac crest with participants in standing position without heavy outer garments and with empty pockets, breathing out gently. Hip circumference was recorded as the maximum circumference over the buttocks. BMI was calculated as weight divided by height squared (kg/m^2). WHR was calculated as the ratio of WC over the hip circumference. WHtR was calculated as the ratio of WC over height.

With regard to the current Chinese men criteria [6], a BMI under 18.5 kg/m^2 was considered underweight; BMI between 18.5 and 23.99 kg/m^2 as normal weight; BMI between 24 and 27.99 kg/m^2 as overweight; and BMI ≥ 28 kg/m^2 as obesity. Generalized obesity and abdominal obesity were defined using WHO Asia Pacific guidelines with WC cutoff as ≥ 90 cm [7], WHR cutoff as ≥ 0.9 [8], and WHtR cutoff as ≥0.5 [9].

Analysis of semen parameters

Semen specimens were collected by masturbation after a period of 2–7 days of sexual abstinence and were kept to liquefy at 37 °C for 30 min. After liquefaction, semen volume was measured by weighing the sample, sperm concentration, total motility and PR were analyzed using a computer-aided sperm analysis (CASA) system (CFT-9201; Jiangsu Rich Life Science Instrument Co., Ltd., Nanjing, China) [10], and sperm morphology was evaluated using Diff-Quik staining, and NSM, percent of abnormal sperm head, percent of intact acrosome and TNPMS (semen volume × sperm concentration × PR × NSM) were calculated. Here TNPMS represents the spermatozoa with motility and normal morphology, and it is a determinative factor for male fertility. For each specimen, at least 200 spermatozoa were counted and analyzed in each replicate. If the difference between the two replicates was acceptable (within 95% confidence interval), the average results of sperm concentration, total motility, PR and NSM were reported. If the difference was too high, two new aliquots from the semen sample were repeatedly assessed [11]. Based on a colorimetric method, the determination of acrosomal enzyme activity was performed strictly according to the manufacturer's instruction. The kit was purchased from Nanjing Xindi Biological Pharmaceutical Engineering Co., Ltd. (Nanjing, China).

Detection of sperm DFI

Sperm DFI was assessed by the sperm chromatin structure assay (SCSA). The SCSA kit was purchased from CellPro Biotech Co., Ltd. (Ningbo, China). The determination of sperm DFI was performed strictly according to the manufacturer's instruction. In brief, semen samples were treated for 30 s with 400 µl of a solution of 0.1 % Triton X-100, 0.15 mol/L NaCl, and 0.08 mol/L HCl, pH 1.2. After 30 s, 1.2 ml of staining buffer (6 µg/ml acridine orange [AO], 37 mmol/L citric acid, 126 mmol/L Na_2HPO_4, 1 mmol/L disodium EDTA, 0.15 mol/L NaCl, pH 6.0) was admixed to the test tube. The sample was placed into the FACS Calibur flow cytometer (Becton Dickinson, San Jose, CA) with the sample flowing to establish optimal sheath/sample flow, and then at exactly 3 min AO staining measurements were taken. A minimum of 5 000 cells from two aliquots of each sample were acquired and analyzed by FACS scan interfaced with a data analysis software (DFIView 2010 Alpha11.15, CellPro Biotech, Ningbo, China). After completion of the sample analysis, the cytogram (red *vs* green fluorescence) and histogram (total cells *vs* DFI) plots as well as DFI readings were generated. A mean of the two sperm DFI values was reported. The variability of the replicate DFI measures was less than 5%.

Determination of seminal plasma biochemical markers

After liquefaction, routine analysis of each semen sample was performed, and the remaining semen samples were centrifuged at 12 000 g for 5 min. The upper layer seminal plasma was collected for the determination of biochemical markers. Commercially available kits for the determinations of seminal plasma GGT, total α-glucotase, zinc and fructose were purchased from Nanjing Xindi Biological Pharmaceutical Engineering Co., Ltd. (Nanjing, China). The determinations were carried out using the Olympus AU400 automatic biochemistry analyzer (Olympus Optical Co. Ltd., Japan), and performed strictly according to the manufacturer's instruction [12–15].

Determinations of serum lipids and reproductive hormones

Fasting venous blood samples were centrifuged at 3 000 g for 5 min to isolate serum for the detections of lipids and reproductive hormones levels. Commercially available kits for the determinations of TG, TC, LDL and HDL were purchased from Shanghai Zhicheng Biotechnology Co., Ltd., China. Calibration and quality control products were purchased from Randox Laboratories Ltd., Northern Ireland, United Kingdom. The determinations of serum lipids were carried out using the Olympus AU400 automatic biochemistry analyzer (Olympus Optical Co. Ltd., Japan). The sample with higher lipid level exceeding the linear range of the kit was diluted with normal saline and the diluted volume was calculated.

Commercially available kits for the determinations of FSH, LH, TT, E2 and SHBG were purchased from Beckman Coulter, Inc., USA. Serum TT, LH, FSH, E2 and SHBG levels were determined by chemiluminescence assay using an automated Unicel Dxi 800 Access Immunoassay System (Beckman Coulter, Inc., USA). The assay sensitivities were 0.35 nmol/L for TT, 0.2 IU/L for LH, 0.2 IU/L for FSH, 73 pmol/L for E2 and 0.33 nmol/L for SHBG. The intra-assay coefficients of variation (CV) for LH, FSH, TT, E2 and SHBG were all less than 5%, and the inter-assay CVs were all less than 8%.

Determinations of seminal plasma lipids and reproductive hormones

After liquefaction, the routine analysis of each semen sample was performed, and the remaining was centrifuged at 12 000 g for 5 min. The upper layer seminal plasma was collected for the determinations of lipids and reproductive hormones [4]. Commercially available kits for the determinations of TG, TC, LDL and HDL were purchased from Shanghai Zhicheng Biotechnology Co., Ltd., China. Calibration and quality control products were purchased from Randox Laboratories Ltd.,

Northern Ireland, United Kingdom. Determination of lipids in seminal plasma was carried out using the Olympus AU400 automatic biochemistry analyzer (Olympus Optical Co. Ltd., Japan). For lower LH level in seminal plasma, we didn't obtain its information. So, we only determined seminal plasma FSH, TT and E2 levels. Commercially available kits for the determinations of FSH, TT and E2 were purchased from Beckman Coulter, Inc., USA. Seminal plasma FSH, TT and E2 levels were determined by chemiluminescence assay using an automated Unicel Dxi 800 Access Immunoassay System (Beckman Coulter, Inc., USA). The sample with higher or lower level exceeding the linear range of the kit was diluted with normal saline or added sample size.

Statistical analysis

All data analyses were conducted using SPSS 11.0 software (SPSS Inc., Chicago, IL, USA). First, nonparametric tests (one-sample Kolmogorov–Smirnov test) were used to determine whether analyzed parameters were normally distributed. If the parameter was consistent with normal distribution, correlations between sperm DFI and age, obesity-associated markers, semen parameters, seminal plasma biochemical markers, and serum and seminal plasma lipids and reproductive hormones levels were examined by Pearson test. If the parameter was consistent with skewed distribution, correlations were examined by Spearman's rho test. The variables which were significantly correlated with sperm DFI in Spearman's rho test were further assessed by the multivariate logistic regression analysis. The differences among different groups and between two groups with different number of samples were assessed by one-way ANOVA test and independent-samples t test, respectively. P-value < 0.05 was considered statistically significant.

Results

The results of obesity-associated markers and sperm DFI were obtained from all of 1 010 subfertile men. The numbers of men with intact and effective semen parameters (32 men with 100% of spermatia or 100% of teratospermia were excluded), seminal plasma biochemical markers, serum lipids, serum reproductive hormones, seminal plasma lipids and seminal plasma reproductive hormones were 978, 959, 974, 954, 887 and 396, respectively. Table 1 showed the mean, standard deviation and range of all these variables. The representative figure of sperm DFI was shown in Fig. 1.

Next, we analyzed the correlations between sperm DFI and age, obesity-associated markers, semen parameters, seminal plasma biochemical markers, serum lipids and reproductive hormones, and seminal plasma lipids and reproductive hormones in subfertile men. All these variables were consistent with skewed distribution, so the

correlations between these variables were analyzed by Spearman's rho test, and the obtained results were shown in Table 2. The results showed that Sperm DFI was positively related to age and abstinence duration (P<0.001). Sperm DFI was also positively related to semen volume and percentage of abnormal sperm head (P<0.001), while negatively related to sperm concentration, progressive motility, sperm motility, percentage of normal sperm morphology, TNPMS, percentage of intact acrosome sperm and acrosomal enzyme activity (P<0.001). Sperm DFI was positively related to seminal plasma zinc but unrelated to seminal plasma total α-glucotase, GGT and fructose levels. There was no any significant correlation between sperm DFI and obesity-associated markers such as BMI, WC, WHR and WHtR, and serum lipids levels. However, sperm DFI was positively related to seminal plasma TG and TC levels. Sperm DFI was also positively related to serum LH and FSH levels and seminal plasma FSH and estradiol levels, but unrelated to serum and seminal plasma testosterone levels.

Although Spearman correlation analysis found that many variables were correlated with sperm DFI, some of them may be confounders. Therefore, we further performed the multivariate regression analysis to assess the variables which were significantly correlated with sperm DFI in Spearman's rho test. It was found that age, semen volume, sperm concentration, progressive motility, TNPMS and intact acrosome were independently correlated with sperm DFI (Table 3).

In addition, for further verifying the correlations of sperm DFI with obesity-associated markers, we set different groups according to the criteria of obesity, and compared sperm DFI based on the dichotomized analyses for BMI, WC, WHR and WHtR (Table 4). We found that there was no any significant difference in sperm DFI among different groups, demonstrating again that sperm DFI was not correlated with obesity-associaited markers.

Discussion

The determination of sperm DNA damage, as an important supplement to semen routine determination strategies, has been applied in some clinical andrology laboratories worldwide. What factors may lead to sperm DNA damage remains one of the major concerns. There were increasingly accumulated evidence for the correlation between obesity and male subfertility. It was reported that obesity was closely related to male subfertility [16]. Obesity and related abnormal lipids metabolism and the change of reproductive hormones might lead to the decrease of sperm quality [3, 4]. However, it has little reports whether obesity and related abnormal lipids metabolism and reproductive hormones may lead to the increase of sperm DNA

Table 1 The mean, standard deviation and range of the investigated parameters in 1 010 subfertile men

Variables	Number	Mean (SD)	Range
Age (years)	1010	28.89 (4.60)	18-50
DFI (%)	1010	18.61 (12.46)	1.61-85.78
BMI (kg/m^2)	1010	23.98 (3.08)	17.36-41.03
WC (cm)	1010	82.14 (9.27)	60-131
WHR	1010	0.86 (0.06)	0.70-1.13
WHtR	1010	0.47 (0.05)	0.34-0.74
Abstinence time (day)	1010	4.28 (1.72)	1-20
Semen volume (ml)	978	3.79 (1.42)	1.1-12
Sperm concentration (10^6/ml)	978	60.78 (51.97)	0.67-340.44
Total sperm count (10^6/ejaculate)	978	220.95 (199.10)	1.35-1364.86
Progressive motility (%)	978	32.29 (12.93)	0.91-81.60
Sperm motility (%)	978	45.37 (19.22)	1.51-98.89
Normal sperm morphology (%)	978	4.52 (2.01)	0.41-17.56
TNPMS (10^6/ejaculate)	978	3.81 (5.00)	0.01-45.20
Abnormal head (%)	978	67.84 (7.86)	11.10-95.15
Intact acrosome (%)	978	57.00 (10.61)	8.18-83.11
Acrosomal enzyme activity (IU/10^6 sperm)	978	48.46 (15.69)	15.13-127.65
Seminal plasma total α-glucotase (U/ml)	959	416.93 (191.90)	48.66-1019.84
Seminal plasma GGT (U/ml)	959	2436.08 (836.43)	17.62-4477.56
Seminal plasma fructose (mmol/L)	959	14.24 (7.18)	3.48-53.83
Seminal plasma zinc (mmol/L)	959	2.62 (1.16)	0.14-7.62
Serum TG (mmol/L)	974	1.65 (1.48)	0.05-23.34
Serum TC (mmol/L)	974	4.39 (0.93)	0.54-12.19
Serum LDL (mmol/L)	974	2.59 (0.73)	0.02-5.77
Serum HDL (mmol/L)	974	1.22 (0.26)	0.67-3.04
Serum LH (IU/L)	954	4.25 (2.13)	0.98-25.45
Serum FSH (IU/L)	954	4.84 (2.55)	1.14-26.43
Serum testosterone (nmol/L)	954	13.14 (4.06)	1.80-30.41
Serum estradiol (pmol/L)	954	108.74 (48.63)	3.0-331.0
Serum SHBG (nmol/L)	954	26.02 (10.92)	5.7-70.7
Seminal plasma TG (mmol/L)	887	0.14 (0.11)	0.01-0.90
Seminal plasma TC (mmol/L)	887	0.85 (0.51)	0.01-3.11
Seminal plasma LDL (mmol/L)	887	0.66 (0.34)	0.01-2.70
Seminal plasma HDL (mmol/L)	887	0.32 (0.21)	0.01-1.64
Seminal plasma FSH (IU/L)	396	0.29 (0.26)	0.10-2.13
Seminal plasma testosterone (nmol/L)	396	4.44 (2.15)	1.18-14.57
Seminal plasma estradiol (pmol/L)	396	276.17 (90.61)	62.06-505.73

TNPMS Total normal-progressively motile spermatozoa count, *SHBG* sex hormone-binding globulin

damage. Based on these, we prospectively investigated the correlations between sperm DFI and obesity-associated markers, serum and seminal plasma lipids and reproductive hormones, as well as, age, abstinence time and semen parameters.

First, as expected, our results showed that sperm DFI was positively related to age and abstinence time in subfertile men, which was consistent with other reports [17–19]. Moreover, it was reported that sperm DFI in men with age ≤ 35 years was significantly lower than that in men with age between 36-39 years and above 40 years, and no significant difference in the latter two [17, 18], indicating that the proportion of sperm with DNA damage increased with increasing age, and that the best

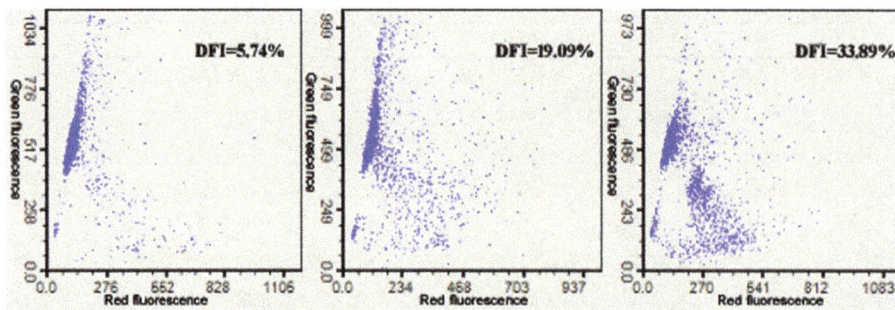

Fig. 1 Sperm DFI detected by flow cytometry. Sperm DFI was assessed by the sperm chromatin structure assay (SCSA). In brief, semen samples were treated for 30 s with 400 µl of a solution of 0.1 % Triton X-100, 0.15 mol/L NaCl, and 0.08 mol/L HCl, pH 1.2. After 30 s, 1.2 ml of staining buffer (6 µg/ml acridine orange [AO], 37 mmol/L citric acid, 126 mmol/L Na_2HPO_4, 1 mmol/L disodium EDTA, 0.15 mol/L NaCl, pH 6.0) was admixed to the test tube. The sample was placed into the FACS Calibur flow cytometer with the sample flowing to establish optimal sheath/sample flow, and then at exactly 3 min AO staining measurements were taken. A minimum of 5 000 cells from two aliquots of each sample were acquired and analyzed by FACS scan interfaced with a data analysis software. After completion of the sample analysis, the cytogram (red *vs* green fluorescence) and DFI readings were generated.

child-bearing age in males would be before 35 years old. In addition, in order to guarantee sperm quality, the abstinence time in males should not too long.

Next, we investigated the correlations between sperm DFI and semen parameters and seminal plasma biochemical markers. Similar to others' results [20–22], we found that sperm DFI was positively related to semen volume and percent of abnormal head sperm ($P<0.001$), while negatively related to sperm concentration, PR, sperm motility, TNPMS, percent of normal sperm morphology, percent of intact acrosome and acrosomal enzyme activity ($P<0.001$). It was reported that sperm DFI was independent of and could predict male fertility better than routine semen parameters [23]. Our data showed that sperm DFI was almost significantly related to all parameters reflecting semen quality, especially TNPMS, indicating that sperm DNA damage might be key factor leading to the decrease of semen quality, that is, abnormal semen parameters.

We found that sperm DFI was positively related to seminal plasma zinc level ($P<0.001$), but unrelated to seminal plasma total α-glucosidase, GGT and fructose levels. Seminal plasma total α-glucosidase, GGT and fructose levels may be used to evaluate the secretory function of epididymis, prostate and seminal vesicle, indicating that the auxiliary gonad might be less effect on sperm DNA damage, and that sperm DNA damage might be existed before sperm transferred into epididymis. It was reported that zinc played an important role not only in normal testis development but also in spermatogenesis and the maintenance of sperm motility [24, 25]. However, the excess of zinc in seminal plasma may accumulate in sperm, produce adverse effect on sperm DNA quality [26], and reduce sperm motility and survival [25]. It is indicated that the excess of seminal plasma zinc might lead to sperm DNA damage, and that the supplement of zinc in clinic should be appropriate.

Further investigations on the relationship between obesity-associated markers and sperm DFI showed that there was no any correlation between sperm DFI and BMI, WC, WHR and WHtR. Moreover, there was no any correlation between sperm DFI and serum lipids levels. This was consistent with our early investigation results, that is, obesity-associated markers could not predict semen quality in subfertile men [3], and there was no any correlation between serum lipids levels and semen parameters [4]. Furthermore, recently, Bandel *et al.* [5] found that there was no any correlation between BMI and sperm DNA integrity, which was similar to our results. However, we found that sperm DFI was positively related to seminal plasma TG and TC levels. As observed in our early study [4], unlike lipids levels in serum, TG, TC, LDL and HDL levels in seminal plasma were all negatively related to some of semen parameters. Likewise, this study demonstrated that the increase of seminal plasma TG and TC levels might lead to increased sperm DFI, indicating that the elevated lipids levels in seminal plasma might have adverse effect on sperm quality. However, the detail mechanism needs to be further elucidated.

As obesity could lead to the change of reproductive hormones, we also investigated the correlations between sperm DFI and seminal plasma reproductive hormones levels. The results showed that sperm DFI was positively related to not only serum LH and FSH levels but also seminal plasma FSH and E2 levels ($P<0.001$), but unrelated to serum and seminal plasma testosterone. Our early investigations had demonstrated that serum LH and FSH levels were negatively correlated with sperm concentration and percent of normal sperm morphology [3]. Moreover, it was reported that the change of serum LH and FSH levels had adverse effect on male fertility [27], and that serum FSH level was the risk factor of

Table 2 Non-parametric (Spearman) correlation coefficients (r) for relationships between sperm DFI and other parameters

Variables	Number	DFI	
		r	P value
Age	1010	0.115	<0.001
BMI	1010	-0.051	0.108
WC	1010	-0.065	0.050
WHR	1010	-0.009	0.785
WHtR	1010	-0.057	0.068
Abstinence time	1010	0.171	<0.001
Semen volume	978	0.145	<0.001
Sperm concentration	978	-0.115	<0.001
Total sperm count	978	-0.054	0.091
Progressive motility	978	-0.474	<0.001
Sperm motility	978	-0.487	<0.001
Normal sperm morphology	978	-0.222	<0.001
TNPMS	978	-0.288	<0.001
Abnormal head	978	0.184	<0.001
Intact acrosome	978	-0.191	<0.001
Acrosomal enzyme activity	978	-0.307	<0.001
Seminal plasma total α-glucotase	959	0.089	0.057
Seminal plasma GGT	959	0.080	0.063
Seminal plasma fructose	959	0.002	0.957
Seminal plasma zinc	959	0.137	<0.001
Serum TG	974	0.026	0.411
Serum TC	974	-0.007	-0.820
Serum LDL	974	-0.005	-0.865
Serum HDL	974	0.008	0.814
Serum LH	954	0.134	<0.001
Serum FSH	954	0.113	<0.001
Serum estradiol	954	-0.039	0.234
Serum testosterone	954	-0.042	0.194
Serum SHBG	954	0.038	0.239
Seminal plasma TG	887	0.136	<0.001
Seminal plasma TC	887	0.131	<0.001
Seminal plasma LDL	887	0.013	0.695
Seminal plasma HDL	887	-0.064	0.058
Seminal plasma FSH	396	0.184	<0.001
Seminal plasma estradiol	396	0.099	0.048*
Seminal plasma testosterone	396	-0.039	0.433

TNPMS Total normal-progressively motile spermatozoa count, SHBG sex hormone-binding globulin. *: P<0.05. Sperm DFI was positively related to age and abstinence time. Sperm DFI was also positively related to semen volume and the percentage of abnormal sperm head, while negatively related to sperm concentration, progressive motility, sperm motility, the percentage of normal sperm morphology, TNPMS, the percentage of intact acrosome sperm and acrosomal enzyme activity. Sperm DFI was positively related to seminal plasma zinc but unrelated to seminal plasma α-glucotase, GGT and fructose levels. There was no any significant correlation between sperm DFI and obesity-associated markers such as BMI, WC, WHR and WHtR, and serum lipids levels. However, sperm DFI was positively related to seminal plasma TG and TC levels. Sperm DFI was also positively related to serum LH and FSH levels and seminal plasma FSH and estradiol levels, but unrelated to serum and seminal plasma testosterone levels

Table 3 The multivariate regression analysis of the variables correlated with sperm DFI in Spearman correlation (n=298)

Variables	Odds Ratio	95% CI	P value
Age	0.865	0.785-0.954	0.004
Abstinence time	0.926	0.719-1.193	0.551
Semen volume	0.548	0.390-0.771	0.001
Sperm concentration	0.978	0.962-0.994	0.008
Progressive motility	1.173	1.041-1.323	0.009
Sperm motility	0.985	0.907-1.069	0.713
Normal sperm morphology	0.716	0.487-1.051	0.088
TNPMS	1.307	1.012-1.687	0.040
Abnormal head	0.996	0.947-1.048	0.876
Intact acrosome	1.082	1.006-1.163	0.033
Acrosomal enzyme activity	0.996	0.975-1.019	0.750
Seminal plasma zinc	1.229	0.705-2.142	0.466
Serum LH	0.976	0.768-1.239	0.839
Serum FSH	1.086	0.888-1.328	0.422
Seminal plasma TG	1.677	0.046-60.819	0.778
Seminal plasma TC	0.807	0.224-2.913	0.744
Seminal plasma FSH	0.455	0.075-2.752	0.391
Seminal plasma estradiol	0.987	0.970-1.003	0.111

TNPMS Total normal-progressively motile spermatozoa count. Age, semen volume, sperm concentration, progressive motility, TNPMS and intact acrosome were independently correlated with sperm DFI

Table 4 Comparison of sperm DFI based on the dichotomized analyses for BMI, WHR, WC and WHtR

Variables		Number	DFI (%)
BMI (kg/m²)	<18.5	20	17.60 ± 10.61
	18.5-23.99	507	18.91 ± 12.43
	24-27.99	389	18.63 ± 12.77
	≥28	94	17.17 ± 11.76
	F		0.556
	P		0.644
WC (cm)	<90	807	18.76 ± 12.50
	≥90	203	18.04 ± 12.33
	t		0.548
	P		0.459
WHR	<0.9	747	18.75 ± 12.54
	≥0.9	263	18.24 ± 12.26
	t		0.321
	P		0.571
WHtR	<0.5	686	19.00 ± 12.71
	≥0.5	324	17.80 ± 11.91
	t		2.037
	P		0.154

sperm DFI [28], which demonstrated that serum FSH and LH levels might have adverse effect on sperm maturation, and might interfere sperm DNA integrity. In addition, we also detected the reproductive hormones levels in seminal plasma, and found that sperm DFI was also positively related to seminal plasma FSH and E2 levels, indicating that the higher FSH and E2 levels in local genital tract likewise had adverse effect on sperm DNA integrity. All these demonstrated that reproductive hormones levels might influence on the integrity of sperm chromatin and then on sperm fertilizing ability [29].

Although Spearman correlation analysis found that many variables were correlated with sperm DFI, the multivariate regression analysis for the variables which were significantly correlated with sperm DFI in Spearman's rho test showed that only age, semen volume, sperm concentration, progressive motility, TNPMS and intact acrosome were independently correlated with sperm DFI. Due to the less semen volume for each sample, not all the parameters of each sample investigated in the study were detected. A total of 298 samples were analyzed all the parameters. Perhaps it was the lower size of samples that led to the difference in the results between Spearman correlation analysis and multivariate regression analysis. Therefore, whether sperm DFI is correlated with abstinence time, sperm motility, normal sperm morphology, abnormal head, acrosomal enzyme activity, serum LH and FSH, and seminal plasma zinc, TG, TC, FSH and estradiol should be further demonstrated by a large size of samples.

In the future, the mechanisms that independent correlation factors lead to sperm DNA damage should be clarified, while the potential correlation factors should be further demonstrated. The key goal to investigate sperm DFI-related factors is to prevent sperm DNA damage during spermatogenesis and sperm maturation. Therefore, the intervention experiments to some correlation factors may verify their effects on sperm DNA damage.

Conclusions

In conclusion, there are many potential factors associated with sperm DFI, including age, abstinence time, spermatogenesis and maturation, seminal plasma lipids and reproductive hormones levels. However, the potential effects of seminal plasma lipids and reproductive hormones on sperm DNA damage need still to be demonstrated by the studies with scientific design and a large size of samples.

Abbreviations

DFI: sperm DNA fragmentation index; SCSA: sperm chromatin structure assay; AO: acridine orange; TSC: total sperm count; PR: progressive motility;

TNPMS: total normal-progressively motile sperm count; NSM: percent of normal sperm morphology; CASA: computer-aided sperm analysis; BMI: body mass index; WHR: waist-to-hip ratio; WC: waist circumference; WHtR: waist-to-height ratio; TG: triglyceride; TC: total cholesterol; LDL-C: low density lipoprotein cholesterol; HDL-C: high density lipoprotein cholesterol; GGT: γ-glutamyl transpeptidase; SHBG: sex hormone binding globulin; FSH: follicle stimulating hormone; E2: estradiol; T: testosterone; TT: total testosterone; c-PAHs: polycyclic aromatic hydrocarbons; ZEA: zearalenone

Acknowledgements
None.

Funding
This study was supported by State Key Development Program for Basic Research of China (2013CB945200).

Authors' contributions
J-CL and JJ had full access to all of the data in the study and take responsibility for the integrity of the data and the accuracy of the data analysis. BY contributed to the study concept and design. All authors contributed to the acquisition, analysis, and interpretation of data. J-CL and JJ provided the statistical analysis. J-CL and BY performed the drafting of the manuscript. The funding was obtained by BY. All authors read and approved the final manuscript.

Competing interests
The authors declare that they have no competing interests.

Author details
[1]The Reproductive Medical Centre, Nanjing Jinling Hospital, Nanjing University School of Medicine, 305 Zhongshan East Road, Nanjing 210002, Jiangsu, China. [2]Department of Laboratory Science, Nanjing Hospital, Jiangsu Corps, The Armed Police Force, PLA, Nanjing 210028, Jiangsu, China.

References
1. Lu JC. Clinical application values and existed issues in the determination of sperm DNA damage. Chin Med J. 2015;95:2989–93.
2. Lu JC. Related factors of sperm DNA damage: Advances in studies. Zhonghua Nan Ke Xue. 2015;21:675–80.
3. Lu JC, Jing J, Dai JY, Zhao AZ, Yao Q, Fan K, et al. Body mass index, waist-to-hip ratio, waist circumference and waist-to-height ratio cannot predict male semen quality: A report of 1231 subfertile Chinese men. Andrologia. 2015;47:1047–54.
4. Lu JC, Jing J, Yao Q, Fan K, Wang GH, Feng RX, et al. Relationship between lipids levels of serum and seminal plasma and semen parameters in 631 Chinese subfertile men. PLoS One. 2016;11:e0146304.
5. Bandel I, Bungum M, Richtoff J, Malm J, Axelsson J, Pedersen HS, et al. No association between body mass index and sperm DNA integrity. Hum Reprod. 2015;30:1704–13.
6. Cai L, Liu A, Zhang Y, Wang P. Waist-to-height ratio and cardiovascular risk factors among Chinese adults in Beijing. PLoS One. 2013;8:e69298.

7. Jia WP, Lu JX, Xiang KS, Bao YQ, Lu HJ, Chen L. Prediction of abdominal visceral obesity from body mass index, waist circumference and waist-hip ratio in Chinese adults: receiver operating characteristic curves analysis. Biomed Environ Sci. 2003;16:206–11.

8. Alberti KG, Zimmet PZ. Definition, diagnosis and classification of diabetes mellitus and its complications. Part 1. Diagnosis and classification of diabetes mellitus provisional report of a WHO consultation. Diabet Med. 1998;15:539–53.

9. Raman R, Rani PK, Gnanamoorthy P, Sudhir RR, Kumaramanikavel G, Sharma T. Association of obesity with diabetic retinopathy: Sankara Nethralaya Diabetic Retinopathy Epidemiology and Molecular Genetics Study (SN-DREAMS Report no. 8). Acta Diabetol. 2010;47:209–15.

10. Lu JC, Huang YF, Lü NQ. Computer-aided sperm analysis: Past, present and future. Andrologia. 2014;46:329–38.

11. World Health Organization. Laboratory manual for the examination and processing of human semen. 5th ed. Geneva: World Health Organization; 2010.

12. Lu JC, Lu KG, Zhang HY, Feng RX. Establishment and evaluation of automatic method for seminal plasma γ-L-glutamyl transpeptidase detection. Zhonghua Nan Ke Xue. 2013;19:1077–81.

13. Zhang HY, Lu JC, Lu KG, Feng RX. Establishment and evaluation of an automatic method for seminal plasma α-glucosidase detection. Zhonghua Nan Ke Xue. 2014;20:886–9.

14. Lu JC, Lu KG, Zhang HY, Feng RX. Establishment and evaluation of automatic assay on level of seminal plasma zinc. Chin J Androl. 2015;29:31–5.

15. Lu JC, Lu KG, Zhang HY, Feng RX. Evaluation of rate method for detection of seminal plasma fructose. Chin J Clin Lab Sci. 2015;33:6–8.

16. Cabler S, Agarwal A, Flint M, du Plessis SS. Obesity: Modern man's fertility nemesis. Asian J Androl. 2010;12:480–9.

17. Bojar I, Witczak M, Wdowiak A. Biological and environmental conditionings for a sperm DNA fragmentation. Ann Agric Environ Med. 2013;20:865–8.

18. Das M, Al-Hathal N, San-Gabriel M, Phillips S, Kadoch IJ, Bissonnette F, et al. High prevalence of isolated sperm DNA damage in infertile men with advanced paternal age. J Assist Reprod Genet. 2013;30:843–8.

19. Håkonsen LB, Spano M, Bonde JP, Olsen J, Thulstrup AM, Ernst E, et al. Exposures that may affect sperm DNA integrity: Two decades of follow-up in a pregnancy cohort. Reprod Toxicol. 2012;33:316–21.

20. Alkhayal A, San Gabriel M, Zeidan K, Alrabeeah K, Noel D, McGraw R, et al. Sperm DNA and chromatin integrity in semen samples used for intrauterine insemination. J Assist Reprod Genet. 2013;30:1519–24.

21. Venkatesh S, Singh A, Shamsi MB, Thilagavathi J, Kumar R, Mitra DK, et al. Clinical significance of sperm DNA damage threshold value in the assessment of male infertility. Reprod Sci. 2011;18:1005–13.

22. Chi HJ, Chung DY, Choi SY, Kim JH, Kim GY, Lee JS, et al. Integrity of human sperm DNA assessed by the neutral comet assay and its relationship to semen parameters and clinical outcomes for the IVF-ET program. Clin Exp Reprod Med. 2011;38:10–7.

23. Xue X, Wang WS, Shi JZ, Zhang SL, Zhao WQ, Shi WH, et al. Efficacy of swim-up versus density gradient centrifugation in improving sperm deformity rate and DNA fragmentation index in semen samples from teratozoospermic patients. J Assist Reprod Genet. 2014;31:1161–6.

24. Atig F, Raffa M, Habib BA, Kerkeni A, Saad A, Ajina M. Impact of seminal trace element and glutathione levels on semen quality of Tunisian infertile men. BMC Urol. 2012;12:6.

25. Khan MS, Zaman S, Sajjad M, Shoaib M, Gilani G. Assessment of the level of traceelement zinc in seminal plasma of males and evaluation of its role in male infertility. Int J Appl Basic Med Res. 2011;l:93–6.

26. García-Contreras A, De Loera Y, García-Artiga C, Palomo A, Guevara JA, Herrera-Haro J, et al. Elevated dietary intake of Zn-methionate is associated with increased sperm DNA fragmentation in the boar. Reprod Toxicol. 2011; 3l:570–3.

27. Miranda-Contreras L, Gómez-Pérez R, Rojas G, Cruz I, Berrueta L, Salmen S, et al. Occupational exposure to organophosphate and carbamate pesticides affects sperm chromatin integrity and reproductive hormone levels among Venezuelan farm workers. J Occup Health. 2013;55:195–203.

28. Smit M, Romijn JC, Wildhagen MF, Weber RF, Dohle GR. Sperm chromatin structure is associated with the quality of spermatogenesis in infertile patients. Fertil Steril. 2010;94:1748–52.

29. Richthoff J, Spano M, Giwercman YL, Frohm B, Jepson K, Malm J, et al. The impact of testicular and accessory sex gland function on sperm chromatin integrity as assessed by the sperm chromatin structure assay (SCSA). Hum Reprod. 2002;17:3162–9.

15

Elective egg freezing and its underlying socio-demography: a binational analysis with global implications

M. C. Inhorn[1]* ⓘ, D. Birenbaum-Carmeli[2], J. Birger[3], L. M. Westphal[4], J. Doyle[5], N. Gleicher[6], D. Meirow[7], M. Dirnfeld[8], D. Seidman[7], A. Kahane[9] and P. Patrizio[10]

Abstract

Background: What are the underlying socio-demographic factors that lead healthy women to preserve their fertility through elective egg freezing (EEF)? Many recent reviews suggest that women are intentionally postponing fertility through EEF to pursue careers and achieve reproductive autonomy. However, emerging empirical evidence suggests that women may be resorting to EEF for other reasons, primarily the lack of a partner with whom to pursue childbearing. The aim of this study is thus to understand what socio-demographic factors may underlie women's use of EEF.

Methods: A binational qualitative study was conducted from June 2014 to August 2016 to assess the socio-demographic characteristics and life circumstances of 150 healthy women who had undertaken at least one cycle of elective egg freezing (EEF) in the United States and Israel, two countries where EEF has been offered in IVF clinics over the past 7–8 years. One hundred fourteen American women who completed EEF were recruited from 4 IVF clinics in the US (2 academic, 2 private) and 36 women from 3 IVF clinics in Israel (1 academic, 2 private). In-depth, audio-recorded interviews lasting from 0.5 to 2 h were undertaken and later transcribed verbatim for qualitative data analysis.

Results: Women in both countries were educated professionals (100%), and 85% undertook EEF because they lacked a partner. This "lack of a partner" problem was reflected in women's own assessments of why they were single in their late 30s, despite their desires for marriage and childbearing. Women themselves assessed partnership problems from four perspectives: 1) women's higher expectations; 2) men's lower commitments; 3) skewed gender demography; and 4) self-blame.

Discussion: The "lack of a partner" problem reflects growing, but little discussed international socio-demographic disparities in educational achievement. University-educated women now significantly outnumber university-educated men in the US, Israel, and nearly 75 other societies around the globe, according to World Bank data. Thus, educated women increasingly face a deficit of educated men with whom to pursue childbearing.

Conclusion: Among healthy women, EEF is a technological concession to gender-based socio-demographic disparities, which leave many highly educated women without partners during their prime childbearing years. This information is important for reproductive specialists who counsel single EEF patients, and for future research on EEF in diverse national settings.

Keywords: Socio-demography, Reproductive epidemiology, Oocyte cryopreservation, Fertility preservation, Single women, Men as partners, Gender, Education, United States, Israel

* Correspondence: marcia.inhorn@yale.edu
[1]Department of Anthropology, Yale University, 10 Sachem Street, New Haven, CT 06511, USA
Full list of author information is available at the end of the article

Background

During the second decade of the new millennium, oocyte cryopreservation via vitrification has gained increasing international acceptance as a method of fertility preservation, not only for women facing fertility-threatening medical conditions [1, 2], but also for healthy women who hope to preserve their future reproductive potential [3, 4]. In the growing literature on the non-medical uses of oocyte cyropreservation, the terms "social egg freezing," "nonmedical egg freezing," "elective oocyte cryopreservation," "elective fertility preservation," and "oocyte banking for anticipated gamete exhaustion" have all been forwarded [5, 6]. Here, we suggest that "elective egg freezing" (EEF) be added to the glossary of accepted terms [7], because it may most closely mirror women's preferred usage, per the study results described below.

Most recent reviews of oocyte cryopreservation suggest that women are undertaking EEF primarily to "delay," "defer," or "postpone" their fertility for educational and career purposes, thereby achieving reproductive autonomy [8], and forestalling age-related fertility decline [9–12]. However, it is unclear from these recent overviews whether postponement of fertility through EEF is intentional and planned, and whether the achievement of career advancement or reproductive autonomy are women's primary EEF goals.

Emerging survey data among women who have completed EEF in the United States [13, 14], Belgium [15], and Australia [16, 17] paint a somewhat different picture. In three of these reports [14–16], women specifically listed "lack of a partner" as their primary reason for undergoing EEF. In the Australian study in particular, women were contacted by mail up to 15 years after completing EEF, but 90% of women had yet to use their stored oocytes. Most reported that they were still hoping to find a partner, thereby avoiding single parenthood [16]. In one of the US studies undertaken in the San Francisco Bay Area, women who had undergone EEF on average 2 years before completing an anonymous survey reported significant anxiety, depression, loneliness, and hopelessness about their reproductive futures in the absence of current male partners [13]. One in six women also experienced regret for having undertaken EEF, for reasons that remain unclear in the study.

To date, only one, small-scale, interview-based study has explored the motivations of Euro-American women who undertook EEF, including 23 in the UK [18], as well as 7 in the US, and 1 in Norway [19–21]. All of these women were heterosexual, educated (68% with postgraduate degrees or other professional qualifications), and most were in professional or managerial roles (74%). Although all of these women were hoping to be in committed relationships, 84% were single when they undertook EEF, generally toward the end of their peak reproductive life span (average age: 37).

As noted in these reports, more empirical research is clearly needed to assess the socio-demographic profiles, specific life circumstances, and reproductive outcomes of women who have undertaken EEF [16, 18]. In particular, qualitative research based on in-depth interviews with women themselves is needed to understand women's reasons for undertaking EEF, including whether it is being used primarily for planned fertility postponement (i.e., in achieving educational or career goals during the 20s or early 30s), or whether EEF is being used primarily for fertility preservation in the absence of a committed reproductive partner (i.e., in the mid- to late-30s and early 40s).

Methods

To answer this question, we conducted a large-scale, interview-based, qualitative study to assess women's motivations for EEF. The study was designed to be binational and comparative across two countries, the United States and Israel, where clinical use of oocyte vitrification occurred early following removal of the experimental label in January 2011 in Israel and October 2012 in the US. American and Israeli women who had completed at least one cycle of EEF were invited to participate in in-depth, semi-structured, qualitative interviews regarding their EEF motivations and experiences. The theoretical framework of the study was thus largely person-centered and experiential [22]. However, detailed and relevant socio-demographic data were also collected from the women during interviews. Thus, socio-demographic profiles of study participants could be constructed, and EEF variables (e.g., education, career, financial stability, partnership status) and outcomes (e.g., number of cycles, egg stored, eggs used) assessed.

Between June 2014 and August 2016, 150 women volunteered to participate for this study—114 in the US and 36 in Israel. Women were recruited from 7 IVF clinics, 4 in the US (2 academic, 2 private) and 3 in Israel (1 academic, 2 private). In the US, women received study flyers by email or during clinic appointments. In Israel, women were invited by clinic staff to participate. Those women interested in volunteering for the study were then contacted by the first and second authors, both of whom are medical anthropologists with extensive experience in interviewing IVF clinic patients.

Women in both countries signed written informed consent forms, agreeing to participate in a confidential, audio-recorded interview at a time and location of their choosing. American women were interviewed by the first author in English, while Israeli women were interviewed by the second author in Hebrew. Because the American women were recruited from IVF clinics on both the East (e.g., New Haven, New York, Baltimore and Washington, DC) and West coasts (e.g., San Francisco Bay Area and Silicon Valley), approximately half of the interviews were carried out in person or by skype, and the rest by phone. In Israel, all but three interviews were conducted in person, primarily in Tel Aviv and Haifa. Interviews generally lasted 1 h, although they ranged in length from 0.5 to 2 h.

An identical interview schedule (which was also translated into Hebrew) was used to conduct interviews in both countries. Interviews were semi-structured, with both closed- and open-ended questions. All women were asked a brief series of socio-demographic questions (i.e., age, birthplace, current residence, education, employment, relationship status, ethnicity, religion), as well as reproductive history questions (i.e., menarche, contraception, reproductive health).

Open-ended questions focused on ten major themes: 1) knowledge and awareness of EEF; 2) motivations to undertake EEF; 3) EEF support systems in place; 4) EEF financing; 5) physical and emotional responses to the EEF process; 6) perceptions of EEF outcomes; 7) egg storage and future disposition; 8) retrospective reflections following EEF completion; 9) future hopes and plans for motherhood; and 10) final EEF thoughts and recommendations. The second theme regarding women's motivations to undertake EEF is of particular interest in this paper, given the lack of consensus in the existing literature about why otherwise healthy women are pursuing EEF.

In this study, all interviews were audio-recorded and transcribed verbatim, with Hebrew interviews then translated into English by a professional translator. Detailed case summaries were then written by the two medical anthropologist interviewers after each transcription was completed. These summaries were shared and reviewed prior to qualitative data analysis, in order to agree upon a common coding scheme. Transcriptions and case summaries were then uploaded into Dedoose, a software program designed for qualitative data analysis. Dedoose allowed for key word searching and the identification of common themes and patterns emerging from the extensive interview data. Socio-demographic information collected during the interviews was also entered into Excel files for descriptive statistical analysis. The research protocol and data management plan were approved by academic Institutional Review Boards and by the ethics committees of all the collaborating IVF clinic sites.

Results

The socio-demographic characteristics of the 150 women in the study, as well as their motivations for undertaking EEF, are supported by qualitative findings, in which women themselves provided nuanced insights on their life circumstances and motivations for EEF.

Socio-demographic findings

In-depth interviews revealed striking similarities between American and Israeli women who had completed EEF. As shown in Table 1, about three-quarters (73%) of the women

Table 1 Elective Egg Freezing in the US and Israel: Characteristics of Study Participants and Their EEF Cycles

Characteristics	United States		Israel		Total	
	n	%	n	%	n	%
Age at EEF						
25–29	1	< 1	0	0	1	1
30–34	19	17	7	19	26	17
35–39	83	73	27	75	110	73
> 40	11	10	2	6	13	9
Total	*114*	*100*	*36*	*100*	*150*	*100*
Year of EEF						
Experimental (2000–2010/11)	17	15	0	0	17	11
Clinical Approval (2011/12–2016)	97	85	36	100	133	89
Total	*114*	*100*	*36*	*100*	*150*	*100*
No. EEF Cycles						
1	65	57	21	58	86	57
2	35	31	11	30	46	31
3	10	9	1	3	11	8
< 3	4	3	1	3	5	3
Unrevealed[a]	0	0	2	6	2	1
Total	*114*	*100*	*36*	*100*	*150*	*100*
Total No. Eggs Stored						
< 5	7	6	7	19	14	9
5–10	25	22	11	31	36	24
11–15	20	17	5	14	25	17
16–20	25	22	6	17	31	21
21–25	18	16	2	6	20	14
26–30	7	6	1	3	8	5
31–35	6	5	2	5	8	5
36–40	3	3	0	0	3	2
> 40	3	3	0	0	3	2
Unrevealed[a]	0	0	2	5	2	1
Total	*114*	*100*	*36*	*100*	*150*	*100*

[a]For religious and cultural reasons

in both countries froze their eggs in their late 30s (ages 35–39), with the remainder in their early 30s (17%) or early 40s (9%). The average age for EEF in the US was 36.6, and 36.2 in Israel. Only one woman in the study froze her eggs before age 30 (an American woman who was 29).

More than half of the women (57%) undertook only one EEF cycle, and one-third (31%) undertook two cycles. These figures did not vary significantly between the two countries, although slightly more women in the US (12%) than in Israel (6%), undertook a third or higher-order cycle. On average, nearly 18 eggs per woman were retrieved and frozen among the US group, versus 13 in Israel.

As shown in Table 2, women who froze their eggs in both countries were highly educated. Only four women had *not*

Table 2 Educational Achievement and Relationship Status of Women Undertaking Elective Egg Freezing (EEF) in the US and Israel

	US		ISRAEL		TOTAL	
	n	%	n	%	n	%
HIGHEST DEGREE						
High School	0	0	1	3	1	1
Associates Degree (2-Year)	1	1	0	0	1	1
Professional Arts Performance	2	2	0	0	2	1
Bachelors	23	20	14	39	37	25
Masters	52	45	13	36	65	43
MD	16	14	7	19	23	15
PhD	11	10	1	3	12	8
JD	8	7	0	0	8	5
MD-PhD	1	1	0	0	1	1
Total N	114	100	36	100	150	100
RELATIONSHIP STATUS AT TIME OF EEF						
Single						
Being Single	59	51	25	70	84	56
Divorced or Divorcing	19	17	6	17	25	17
Broken Up	16	14	2	5	18	12
TOTAL SINGLE	*94*	*82*	*33*	*91*	*127*	*85*
Partnered (Unstable)						
Relationship Too New or Uncertain	6	5	1	3	7	5
Partner Refuses to Have Children	2	2	0	0	2	1
Partner Has Multiple Partners	2	2	0	0	2	1
TOTAL UNSTABLE PARTNERSHIPS	*10*	*9*	*1*	*3*	*11*	*7*
Partnered (Stable)						
Not Ready to Have Children	10	9	2	5	12	8
TOTAL STABLE PARTNERSHIPS	*10*	*9*	*2*	*0*	*12*	*8*
Total N	114	100	36	100	150	100

graduated from college due to successful careers in the performing arts or military. The rest of the women had considerable educational achievements. One-quarter of the women had completed bachelors' degrees (25%), and the rest had earned advanced degrees, including master's degrees (43%), medical degrees (15%), doctoral degrees (8%), and law degrees (5%). More than 10% of the American women had dual graduate degrees (e.g., MD-PhD, MD-MPH, MPP-PhD). More than half (58%) had attended Ivy League universities or other "elite" US academic institutions.

Given these high levels of education, both the American and Israeli women in this study were professional women, whose careers were devoted to, among others, the health fields, basic and applied sciences, government and law, diplomacy and foreign service, academia, business management, information and technology,

entrepreneurship, media and communications, human resources, the arts, the military, and beyond.

As shown in Table 2, 85% of these highly educated professional women were single at the time of EEF, either because they had no partner, were divorced, or had recently broken up from long-term relationships. Only one of these women had born a child from a prior relationship, which had ended. All of the other unpartnered women were childless at the time of EEF. Among the 15% of women who were partnered at the time of EEF, half of these relationships were unstable for the reasons outlined in Table 2. Only 10 (7%) of the women in this study, all of whom were American, were stably partnered at the time of EEF with men who hoped to have children with them in the future, even though most of the men were "not ready" yet.

Table 3 describes the post-EEF life circumstances of women at the time of our interviews. More than three-quarters of women (78%) were still single, while 22% were partnered (with either the same or a new partner). Seven percent of the partnered women had gone onto marry. However, as shown in Table 3, there were often significant differences in age, education, and reproductive history among women and their partners (e.g., a 38-year-old woman with a 55-year-old divorced man with children, or a woman ER physician with a high-school-educated paramedic). Only 7% of women described themselves as being in "equal" partnerships in terms of their partners' education, age, and reproductive history (i.e., no children from a prior relationship).

As also shown in Table 3, some women, whether partnered or not, decided to have children, with or without their frozen eggs. Twelve women in the study (10 American, 2 Israeli) had born children and six were currently pregnant at the time of the interviews. Few of these women had relied on their frozen eggs to become pregnant. Only 10 (6%) of the 150 women interviewed, all of them American, had pursued reproduction using frozen oocytes. Eight women had thawed all their eggs in an attempt to become pregnant, but only one had delivered a child and one had learned that she was pregnant at the time of the interview. The overall usage of frozen eggs remained low, as did the rate of frozen-egg conceptions.

Qualitative findings

The socio-demographic findings above suggest that the lack of a stable partnership is the primary motivation among highly educated professional women in both the US and Israel. This result is supported by qualitative findings from women's interviews. Women in the study routinely explained that they had been unable to find a stable, committed relationship with a man who also wanted to have children with them. Women often explained that throughout their educational and career-building years, they had attempted to find a compatible male partner,

Table 3 Relationship Status and Reproductive Outcomes Following Elective Egg Freezing (EEF) among Study Participants in the US and Israel

	US		ISRAEL		TOTAL	
	n	%	n	%	n	%
Years Elapsed Since EEF Undertaken						
Same year	40	35	1	3	41	27
1 year	28	25	12	33	40	26
2 years	21	18	13	36	34	23
3 years	12	11	6	17	18	12
4 years	7	6	3	8	10	7
5 or more years (5–11)	6	5	0	0	6	4
Wouldn't reveal date of EEF	0	0	1	3	1	< 1
Total	*114*	*100*	*36*	*100*	*150*	*100*
Relationship Status Following EEF (@ Time of Interview)						
Still Single	89	78	27	75	116	78
Partnered	17	15	6	17	23	15
Married	8	7	3	8	11	7
TOTAL	*114*	*100*	*36*	*100*	*150*	*100*
Status of Those Women Partnered/Married						
Equal Partnership (Education, Age, No Children from Prior Relationship)	6	5	5	14	11	7
Partner Divorced without Children	1	1	0	0	1	1
Partner Divorced with Children	7	6	2	5	9	6
Partner Significantly Younger	3	3	1	3	4	3
Partner Significantly Older/Retired	2	2	1	3	3	2
Partner Significantly Less Educated	1	1	0	0	1	.5
Partner Significantly Less Educated/Divorced	1	1	0	0	1	.5
Partner Significantly Less Educated/Divorced with Children	1	1	0	0	1	.5
Partner Significantly Less Educated/Younger	1	1	0	0	1	.5
Partner with Alcohol or Legal Issues	2	2	0	0	2	1
TOTAL AND PERCENT OF TOTAL N	*25*	*22*	*9*	*25*	*34*	*22*
Pregnancy and Live Birth Outcomes Post EEF (@ Time of Interview)						
Child Born from Frozen Oocyte Conception	1	1	0	0	1	.5
Child Born from Natural Conception (No Frozen Oocytes Used)	3	2	1	3	4	3
Child Born from Donor Sperm (Single Mother by Choice, No Frozen Oocytes Used)	2	2	1	3	3	2
Child Born from IUI, IVF or Surrogacy (No Donor Sperm, No Frozen Oocytes Used)	4	3	0	0	4	3
Currently Pregnant from Frozen Oocyte	1	1	0	0	1	.5
Currently Pregnant from Natural Conception	2	2	1	3	3	2
Currently Pregnant from Donor Sperm (Single Mother by Choice, No Frozen Oocytes Used)	0	0	2	5	2	1
TOTAL AND PERCENT OF TOTAL N	*13*	*11*	*5*	*14*	*18*	*12*
Women Who Had Used Frozen Oocytes (by Time of Interview)						
All Oocytes Thawed, One Live Birth, One Blastocyst Remaining	1	1	0	0	1	.5
All Oocytes Thawed, Currently Pregnant, 24 Embryos Remaining	1	1	0	0	1	.5
All Oocytes Thawed, No Fertilization	8	7	0	0	8	5
TOTAL AND PERCENT OF TOTAL N	*10*	*9*	*0*	*0*	*10*	*6*

with whom they could build a family. When they had been unable to find one, they had pursued EEF, usually in their mid- to late 30s, but sometimes in their early 40s, in an effort to preserve their remaining reproductive potential.

In fact, in our study of 150 American and Israeli women, only one woman—who was American, and at age 30, the second youngest woman in the study—told us that she had explicitly used EEF to postpone her fertility "en route" to becoming a successful entrepreneur. Another American woman, age 33, was happy to have finally passed the difficult Foreign Service exam; she froze her eggs before her deployment to Latin America, where her career was just taking off. With the exception of these two women, the rest of the women in this study, both American and Israeli, did not pursue EEF for career-related purposes—as a means of postponing childbearing on the way to a better job or professional advancement. Rather, EEF was being used late in women's reproductive lives because of ongoing reproductive partnership obstacles.

During interviews, both American and Israeli women often volunteered their insights—and considerable frustrations—over having to defer motherhood due to the lack of a partner. Women offered a variety of experiential perspectives on the lack of a partner problem in their own lives and for educated women more generally. Women's assessments could be summarized and categorized in four main ways:

Women's higher expectations
Women in this study addressed generational changes in women's expectations for egalitarian partnerships. Women described how their parents, especially mothers, had encouraged them to "have it all," and thus they had been raised to believe in gender equality and egalitarian relationships at home and at work. Thus, they hoped not to "settle" for a man who was less educated, less professionally accomplished, or less committed to similar interests and life goals. Many women in both the US and Israel said that they were still hoping to find the "right" person—the "soulmate" they were "meant" to be with. Searching for this person took time and commitment, but could prevent the fearful outcome of "settling for less" or entering into a "bad marriage."

Men's lower commitments
Having said this, women in the study, especially in the US, were skeptical about men of their generation, and whether these men shared the same desires and life goals. Women pointed out that men were not necessarily socialized in the same way to want egalitarian relationships with professional women, with whom they could balance the burdens and responsibilities of family life. Women in this study described men's increasing "commitment phobia," particularly men who were the "children of divorce" and

were not sanguine about the virtues of either marriage or fatherhood. Furthermore, women in the US portion of the study, particularly on the West coast, described the "Peter Pan" syndrome—i.e., boys (in men's bodies) who never grow up. These men were often described as not able to hold steady jobs, sometimes living with their parents (or being subsidized by them), and unable to fulfill the roles assumed by adult men in society. Furthermore, in the San Francisco Bay Area and other "progressive" cities, women described the growing phenomenon of "polyamory"—namely, millennial-generation men's desires to have multiple, open relationships with "primary" and "secondary" female partners. In short, women in this study described men's lowered commitments to fidelity, marriage, and parenthood—the trifecta often expected within traditional, heteronormative family structures.

Skewed gender demography
Beyond changing gender expectations on the part of both women and men, there was clear acknowledgment by many of the women in both countries that men of similar backgrounds—namely, single, college-educated, professionals, often with advanced degrees and high earnings—were simply hard to find. As one woman explained it succinctly, "the caliber of women is just higher than the caliber of guys." This lament was especially true among American women on the East Coast, and particularly in New York City and Washington, DC, metropolitan areas that are known (via media reports) to have higher percentages of educated women than men. Women in those cities often lamented the dearth of "available" (and heterosexual) male partners in the skewed gender landscapes in which they were living. Furthermore, women often described their difficulties in "dating down" to less educated or less successful men. They characterized such relationships as fraught with "intimidation" on the part of men, who were generally emasculated by a woman's superior professional status, living situation, or earnings.

Furthermore, because women in many societies, including the US and Israel, have traditionally been told to marry "up" (hypergamy) while men marry "down" (hypogamy) in terms of age, class, education, salary, and so on, trying to reverse this entrenched gender norm was inherently problematic on many levels, according to most women in the study. For one, they pointed out that most men were "ageist"—very reluctant to marry an older woman, especially one in her late 30s or early 40s who might place "pressure" on a partner to have children immediately.

Self-blame
Women who found themselves in this position—without partners in their mid- to late-30s—sometimes posed the "Why me?" question out loud in their interviews. Often with sadness, women expressed their amazement and

disbelief that they had somehow "ended up" without a part-ner. Yet, they often added that they knew (many) other pro-fessional women in this situation. In both countries, but particularly in Israel, women sometimes blamed themselves for not finding a partner, criticizing themselves for being too "picky," only attracted to "alpha males," or that they had let a "good one" get away. Some women surmised that they were not attractive enough to men, or had not put enough "energy" into dating (especially online dating, which was widespread in our study population).

The inability to find a partner was a source of both frus-tration and anguish among women in both countries. As one American woman, an academic physician in her mid-30s, put it, "If I found a man, I'd move to Alaska! But most men don't want relationships. They just want to meet and date. And most women won't go out with the [unedu-cated] check-stand dude, but men will. So I think I have about a .09% chance of meeting someone. And meanwhile, I was feeling like, 'OMG, my biological clock, it's ticking, it's ticking, it's ticking,' you know? So, even though I'm 1,000% happy I did it [EEF], it felt somewhat like a defeat. I felt like I gave up, because I couldn't find a man."

Discussion

To date, this is the largest interview-based study of women who have undertaken EEF, and the only one with an international comparison. As a binational study, the research was designed to assess both similarities and dif-ferences in American and Israeli women's: 1) life circum-stances, 2) socio-demographic characteristics, and 3) motivations for undertaking EEF.

In all three realms, striking similarities were found across the two groups of women. In both countries, "lack of a partner" was the primary and driving force be-hind healthy women's decisions to undergo EEF as a fer-tility preservation option. This dearth of male partners among the highly educated professional women in this study held true across both countries. It was a finding that was clearly expressed by women themselves as they reflected on their own EEF motivations and experiences.

Given this situation, an important question remains open for discussion: Namely, where are the "missing men," who should presumably want to couple with these accomplished women? Should lack of a partner be taken for granted as a "natural fact" of educated women's re-productive lives?

Here, we point to an underlying cause of this "man def-icit," one that has been carefully described and analyzed by one of us, Jon Birger [23], with particular focus on the US. Using US census data, Birger shows that there are 5.5 mil-lion university-educated women in their 20s (ages 22–29) in the US for only 4.1 million university-educated men. This is a ratio of 4:3. Between the ages of 30 and 39—when women start freezing their eggs—there are 7.4 million

university-educated American women for only 6 million university-educated American men. This is a ratio of 5:4. Adding the two groups together, there are nearly 3 million more university-educated women than university-educated men in women's prime reproductive years in America. To quote Birger ([23], p.3), "These lopsided gender ratios may add up to a sexual nirvana for heterosexual men, but for heterosexual women—especially those who put a high pri-ority on getting married and having children in wedlock—they represent a demographic time bomb."

What Birger calls a "massive undersupply" of university-educated men in America: 1) is growing over time as young women enter universities at much higher rates; 2) has reached a new high of 37% more American women than men in higher education, ac-cording to the most recent census data; 3) makes the long-term prospects for millennial-generation women decidedly worse; and 4) is particularly acute in major US cities such as Washington, DC, New York, and Miami, where university-educated women tend to cluster, but now outnumber university-educated men by the hundreds of thousands [23].

Beyond the US, this "man deficit" appears to be emer-ging around the world. As seen in Table 4, the most re-cent World Bank data from 2012 to 2016 show that women significantly outstrip men in higher education in at least 70 countries where data are available [24]. For example, this includes Australia, with 41% more women than men in higher education, as well as many other high-income countries including Belgium, France, Italy, New Zealand, Norway, Sweden, and the United King-dom. These educational disparities are also emerging in many non-Western countries, including Argentina, China, Cuba, Lebanon, Malaysia, Panama, South Africa, Thailand, and Tunisia, to name only a few.

In Israel, where part of our study was conducted, women have surpassed men at all academic levels. Between the years 1970–2013, the percent of female master's students soared from 26 to 61%, and at the doctoral level, from 19 to 52% [25]. In the 2010–2011 academic year, women com-prised 57% of undergraduates, 60% of master's students, and 52% of PhD students [26]. In the academic year 2015–2016, women undergraduate students outnumbered men by 21% (and 40%, if teachers' colleges are included). At the master's level, the gap reached 62.5% [26]. Although women are still underrepresented in fields like computer sciences, their percentage has increased dramatically in prestigious, well-remunerated fields, including medicine, engineering, architecture, physics, and law. In fact, women now make up the majority of medical and law students in Israel [27].

As shown in our study, these educational disparities are clearly "creeping into" educated women's lives. Table 3 re-veals that women who partner may make "unequal"

Table 4 Countries Where Women Significantly Outnumber Men in Higher Education[a]

No.	Country	F/M Ratio	% More Women than Men in Higher Education
1.	Albania	1.39865994	40%
2.	Algeria	1.55961001	56%
3.	Argentina	1.61947	62%
4.	Armenia	1.12863004	13%
5.	Aruba	2.26302004	126%
6.	Australia	1.40989006	41%
7.	Austria	1.20158994	20%
8.	Bahrain	1.92068005	92%
9.	Belarus	1.32676005	33%
10.	Belgium	1.31350005	31%
11.	Belize	1.60633004	61%
12.	Bermuda	2.31813002	132%
13.	Botswana	1.43773997	44%
14.	Brazil	1.39809	40%
15.	Canada[b]	1.29524887	30%
16.	Chile	1.13678002	14%
17.	China	1.18620002	19%
18.	Colombia	1.16246998	16%
19.	Costa Rica	1.30727994	31%
20.	Croatia	1.35680997	36%
21.	Cuba	1.42532003	43%
22.	Czech Republic	1.40742004	41%
23.	Estonia	1.53139997	53%
24.	Finland	1.20589006	21%
25.	France	1.22571003	23%
26.	Georgia	1.21904004	22%
27.	Guyana	2.03288007	103%
28.	Hong Kong SAR, China	1.16025996	16%
29.	Hungary	1.25191998	25%
30.	Iceland	1.71160996	71%
31.	Indonesia	1.1243	12%
32.	Ireland	1.09338999	9%
33.	Israel	1.3829	38%
34.	Italy	1.35718	36%
35.	Jamaica	1.72571003	73%
36.	Jordan	1.11230004	11%
37.	Kazakhstan	1.23714995	24%
38.	Kuwait	1.61944997	62%
39.	Latvia	1.42805004	43%
40.	Lebanon	1.15689003	16%
41.	Lithuania	1.46904004	47%

Table 4 Countries Where Women Significantly Outnumber Men in Higher Education[a] *(Continued)*

No.	Country	F/M Ratio	% More Women than Men in Higher Education
42.	Luxembourg	1.13515997	14%
43.	Macao SAR, China	1.32536995	33%
44.	Macedonia, FYR	1.24822998	25%
45.	Malaysia	1.52705002	53%
46.	Malta	1.37038004	37%
47.	Mongolia	1.38279998	38%
48.	Myanmar	1.22817004	23%
49.	Netherlands	1.10478997	10%
50.	New Zealand	1.35090995	35%
51.	Norway	1.45779002	46%
52.	Palau	1.54859996	55%
53.	Panama	1.49242997	49%
54.	Philippines	1.28163004	28%
55.	Poland	1.52178001	52%
56.	Portugal	1.13217998	13%
57.	Puerto Rico	1.40998995	41%
58.	Romania	1.23240995	23%
59.	Russian Federation	1.21165001	21%
60.	Serbia	1.33327997	33%
61.	Slovak Republic	1.54595995	55%
62.	Slovenia	1.44420004	44%
63.	South Africa	1.48450994	48%
64.	Spain	1.17773998	18%
65.	Sri Lanka	1.53942001	54%
66.	St. Lucia	1.90204	90%
67.	Sweden	1.52547002	53%
68.	Syrian Arab Republic	1.13739002	14%
69.	Thailand	1.41378999	41%
70.	Tunisia	1.65129006	65%
71.	Ukraine	1.15558004	16%
72.	United Kingdom	1.30744004	31%
73.	United States	1.36754	37%

[a]Based on the most recent World Bank data available from 2012 to 2016, as collected by the United Nations Educational, Scientific, and Cultural Organization (UNESCO) Institute for Statistics. https://data.worldbank.org/indicator/SE.ENR.TERT.FM.ZS?end=2011&name_desc=false&start=1970
[b]Statistics Canada. https://www150.statcan.gc.ca/n1/en/type/data#tables

alliances with older, younger, or divorced men, including men with children from previous relationships, and often with significantly less education. As noted earlier, this phenomenon is known in anthropological terms as hypogamy—when a person marries "down." Traditionally, women in societies around the world have tried to achieve hypergamy, or marrying "up," in an attempt to secure a better future for themselves and their children. However, as women rise educationally around the globe, and men no longer keep pace, these trends may be reversing.

In a recent report entitled "Wayward Sons: The Emerging Gender Gap in Labor Markets and Education," the authors conclude that "Although a significant minority of males continues to reach the highest echelons of achievement in education and labor markets, the median male is moving in the opposite direction" [28]. Overall, less-educated men in the US and in many other countries around the world are losing ground, not only in labor markets, but in marriage markets and parenthood, as reported by this and other studies [29].

What we see, then, are the difficult choices currently facing educated women in the US, Israel, and in many other nations regarding partnership and family formation [30, 31]. In this new era of EEF, "to freeze or not to freeze" has become the leading question among societies' most educated women [13]. Indeed, EEF is not about women who are intentionally "delaying" childbearing or "postponing" their fertility in order to "lean in" to their careers [32]. Rather, EEF appears to be a technological concession among highly educated professional women who are grappling with gender-based socio-demographic disparities well beyond their individual reproductive control. Yet, given that knowledge of the educational gender gap is not widespread, women may end up engaging in self-blame—a negative discourse that author Sarah Eckel has questioned in her book *It's Not You: The 27 (Wrong) Reasons You're Single* [33].

To date, very few in-depth studies of this highly educated, egg-freezing population have been conducted. This study is by far the largest (e.g., 150 women interviewed versus 31 in the study by Baldwin [19, 20] and Baldwin et al. [18, 21]). However, as a large, binational, qualitative study, there were some inherent design and methodological limitations that must be acknowledged in assessing the aforementioned results. First, the overall number of participants recruited in the two countries was unequal, reflecting national differences in population size and, hence, EEF uptake. Second, the American and Israeli women participating in this study were recruited from a small number of metropolitan areas, thereby limiting the generalizability of the findings. Third, in the two countries, women were recruited into the study somewhat differently, and interviewed by two different medical anthropologists in two different languages, perhaps shaping their responses in unexpected ways. Furthermore, the numbers of women who were contacted in each clinic and each country varied considerably. Thus, women who chose not to participate in the study may have differed significantly from those women who volunteered; but the rates of non-response or lack of follow-up could not be calculated because of the less controlled, qualitative study design.

All of these are sources of potential bias that could not be avoided.

Conclusion

The major finding to emerge from this binational study was the "lack of partner" problem in highly educated professional women's lives, leading them to EEF by their late 30s. A remarkable degree of consistency emerged in the findings from the two countries, as shown in Tables 1, 2, and 3. Furthermore, for a qualitative study of this nature, the sample size was quite large, and the in-depth nature of women's interviews served to increase the validity of the study findings.

Instead of achieving motherhood, this cohort of exceptional, "30-something" women found themselves in what author Melanie Notkin ([34], p. xxi) has called "otherhood"—"single and approaching the end of our fertility." Such otherhood has led to what Notkin calls "circumstantial infertility"—women waiting for love, not wanting to settle for a lesser love, but also realizing with trepidation that a loving partnership may not arrive in time for motherhood. Thus, these women's childlessness is undesired and circumstantial, rather than the result of intentional fertility "postponement" and reproductive "choice."

Given the lack of partner problem that is leading otherwise healthy women to pursue EEF, we conclude with two recommendations that seem to emerge from this study. First, it is important for IVF clinicians to become aware of, and sensitive, to the overarching lack of a partner problem facing their EEF patients. EEF patients may need different forms of social and emotional support, as well as patient-centered care, when they enter the couples-oriented world of IVF. Second, this study speaks to the need for additional qualitative research with women themselves as they both consider and undertake EEF in diverse national settings. We need to understand why some women who seek information about EEF decide against it, and why others decide to move forward, like the American and Israeli women who participated in this study. Future global empirical research of this nature will serve to facilitate worldwide comparisons of the underlying socio-demographic forces and gender-based disparities leading to the burgeoning uptake of EEF among otherwise healthy women around the globe.

Abbreviations
EEF: Elective egg freezing; IVF: In vitro fertilization

Acknowledgments
The authors would like to thank Jennifer DeChello, Jeannine Estrada, Rose Keimig, Sandee Murray, Tasha Newsome, Mira Vale, and Ruoxi Yu for various forms of editorial, study recruitment, and transcription assistance.

Funding
This study was funded by a grant from the US National Science Foundation, BCS-1356136. MCI was the PI and PP the co-PI. NSF had no role in the study design, data collection, analysis, or interpretation. NSF also played no role in

the writing of this paper, or the decision to submit this paper for publication. Those decisions were made by the authors alone. The corresponding author had full access to all of the data in the study and final responsibility for the decision to submit for publication.

Authors' contributions

MCI is the study PI, responsible for the study design, all American data collection, data analysis, and interpretation. She led the collaborative writing of this article. DB-C is responsible for all Israeli data collection, data analysis, and interpretation. She assisted in the collaborative writing of this article. JB collected the US census and World Bank data necessary for the interpretations offered in the Discussion. He compiled Table 4 and assisted in the collaborative writing of this article. LMW, JD, and NG were responsible for participants' recruitment in three different collaborating study sites in the US. They also assisted in the collaborative writing of this article. DM, MD, DS, and AK were responsible for participants' recruitment in three different collaborating study sites in Israel. They also assisted in the collaborative writing of this article. PP is the study co-PI. In addition to overseeing study design and participants' recruitment in one collaborating study site, he assisted in data analysis, interpretation, and writing, and oversaw the collaborative nature of this binational study between seven different IVF clinic sites. All authors read and approved the final manuscript.

Authors' information

MCI of Yale University and DB-C of University of Haifa are professors of medical anthropology who specialize in qualitative research with assisted reproduction patients. They are personally responsible for the in-depth interviews that form the core dataset of this paper. As the corresponding author of this paper, further information on MCI's research can be found at www.marciainhorn.com.

Competing interests

The authors declare that they have no competing interests.

Author details

[1]Department of Anthropology, Yale University, 10 Sachem Street, New Haven, CT 06511, USA. [2]Department of Nursing, University of Haifa, 3498838 Haifa, Israel. [3]Larchmont, USA. [4]Stanford Fertility and Reproductive Medicine Center, Stanford University, 1195 W. Fremont Ave, Sunnyvale, CA 94087, USA. [5]Shady Grove Fertility, 9600 Blackwell Road, Rockville, MD 20850, USA. [6]Center for Human Reproduction, 21 E. 69th Street, New York, NY 10021, USA. [7]Department of Obstetrics and Gynecology, Sheba Medical Center, IVF and Fertility Unit, 1 Emek Ha'ella St, 52621 Ramat Gan, Israel. [8]Division Reproductive Endocrinology-IVF, Department of Obstetrics & Gynecology, Carmel Medical Center, Ruth & Bruce Faculty of Medicine, Technion, 3436212 Haifa, Israel. [9]Assuta Medical Center, 13 Eliezer Mazal, 75653 Rishoon Lezion, Israel. [10]Yale Fertility Center, Yale University, 150 Sargent Drive, New Haven, CT 06511, USA.

References

1. Rashedi A, de Roo SF, Ataman LM, et al. Survey of fertility preservation options available to patients with cancer around the globe. J Glob Oncol. 2017. http://ascopubs.org/doi/pdf/10.1200/JGO.2016.008144.
2. Salama M, Woodruff TK. Anticancer treatments and female fertility: clinical concerns and role of oncologists in oncofertility practice. Expert Reviews Anticanc Ther 2017;17:687–92.
3. Mertes H. The portrayal of healthy women requesting oocyte cryopreservation. FVV Obstet Gynaecol. 2013;5:141–6.
4. Potdar N, Gelbaya TA, Nardo A. Oocyte vitrification in the 21st century and post-warming fertility outcomes: a systematic review and meta-analysis. Reprod BioMed Online. 2014;29:159–76.
5. Baldwin K, Culley L, Hudson N, Mitchell H. Reproductive technology and the life course: current debates and research in social egg freezing. Hum Fertil. 2014;17:170–9.
6. Stoop D, van der Veen F, Deneyer M, Nekkebroeck J, Tournaye H. Oocyte banking for anticipated gamete exhaustion (AGE) is a preventive intervention, neither social nor nonmedical. Reprod BioMed Online. 2014;28:548–51.
7. Zegers-Hochschild F, Adamson GD, Dyer S, et al. The international glossary of infertility and fertility care, 2017. Hum Reprod. 2017;32:1786–801.
8. Goldman KN, Grifo JA. Elective oocyte cryopreservation for deferred childbearing. Clin Obstetr Gynecol. 2016;23:458–64.
9. Argyle CE, Harper JC, Davies MC. Oocyte cryopreservation: where are we now? Hum Reprod Update. 2016;22:440–9.
10. Cobo A, Garcia-Velasco JA. Why all women should freeze their eggs. Clin Obstetr Gynecol. 2016;28:206–10.
11. Donnez J, Dolmans M-M. Fertility preservation in women. New Engl J Med. 2017;377:1657–65.
12. Gunnala V, Schattman G. Oocyte vitrification for elective fertility preservation: the past, present, and future. Clin Obstetr Gynecol. 2017;29:59–63.
13. Greenwood EA, Pasch LA, Hastie J, Cedars MI, Huddleston HG. To freeze or not to freeze: decision regret and satisfaction following elective oocyte cryopreservation. Fertil Stertil. 2018;109:1097–104.
14. Hodes-Wertz B, Druckenmiller S, Smith M, Noyes N. What do reproductive-age women who undergo oocyte cryopreservation think about the process as a means to preserve fertility? Fertil Stertil. 2014;100:1343–9.
15. Stoop D, Maes E, Polyzos NP, Verheyen G, Tournaye H, Nekkebroeck J. Does oocyte banking for anticipated gamete exhaustion influence future relational and reproductive choices? A follow-up of bankers and non-bankers. Hum Reprod. 2015;30:338–44.
16. Hammarberg K, Kirkman M, Pritchard N, et al. Reproductive experiences of women who cryopreserved oocytes for non-medical reasons. Hum Reprod. 2017;32:575–81.
17. Pritchard N, Kirkman M, Hammarberg K, McBain J, Agresta F, Bayly C, Hickey M, Peate M, Fisher J. Characteristics and circumstances of women in Australia who cryopreserved their oocytes for non-medical indications. J Reprod Infant Psychol. 2017;35:108–18.
18. Baldwin K, Culley L, Hudson N, Mitchell H, Lavery S. Oocyte cryopreservation for social reasons: demographic profile and disposal intentions of UK users. Reprod BioMed Online. 2015;31:239–45.
19. Baldwin K. "I suppose I think to myself, that's the best way to be a mother": how ideologies of parenthood shape women's use for social egg freezing technology. Sociol Res Online. 2017;22:2–15.
20. Baldwin K. Conceptualising women's motivations for social egg freezing and experience of reproductive delay. Sociol Hlth Illness 2018; doi: https://doi.org/10.1111/1467-9566.12728.
21. Baldwin K, Culley LA, Hudson N, Mitchell HL. Running out of time: exploring women's motivations for social egg freezing. J Psychosom Obstet Gynecol; doi: https://doi.org/10.1080/0167482X.2018.1460352.
22. Hollan D. The psychology of person-centered ethnography. In: Moore CC, Mathews HF, editors. The psychology of cultural experience. Cambridge: Cambridge University Press; 2001. p. 48–67.
23. Birger J. Date-onomics: how dating became a lopsided numbers game. New York: Workman Publishing; 2015.

24. World Bank. https://data.worldbank.org/indicator/SE.ENR.TERT.FM.ZS?end=
2011&name_desc=false&start=1970

25. Council for Higher Education. The higher education system in Israel; 2014. p.
31. http://che.org.il/wp-ontent/uploads/2016/10/
%D7%9E%D7%A2%D7%A8%D7%9B%D7%AA-
%D7%94%D7%94%D7%A9%D7%9B%D7%9C%D7%94-
D7%94%D7%92%D7%91%D7%95%D7%94%D7%94-
%D7%91%D7%99%D7%A9%D7%A8%D7%90%D7%9C-2014-ilovepdf-
compressed-1.pdf

26. Israel Central Bureau of Statistics. Students in universities, academic colleges
and colleges of education, by degree, sex, age, population group and
district of residence. Table. 2017;8:56.

27. Israel Central Bureau of Statistics, Yaffe Nurit. 2013. Men and Women 1990–
2011, Statistical Series 132, p. 10–11, http://www.cbs.gov.il/www/statistical/
mw2013_h.pdf.

28. Autor A, Wasserman M. 2013. Wayward sons: the emerging gender gap in
labor markets and education. https://economics.mit.edu/files/8754.

29. Edin K, Nelson TJ. Doing the best I can: fatherhood in the inner city.
Berkeley: University of California Press; 2013.

30. Allahbadia GN. Social egg freezing: developing countries are not exempt. J
Obstetr Gynecol India. 2016;66:213–7.

31. Santo EVE, Dieamant F, Petersen CG, et al. Social oocyte cryopreservation: a
portrayal of Brazilian women. JBA Assist Reprod. 2017;21:101–4.

32. Sandberg S. Lean in: women, work, and the will to lead. New York: Knopf; 2013.

33. Eckel S. It's not you: 27 (wrong) reasons why you're single. New York:
Penguin; 2014.

34. Notkin M. Otherhood: modern women finding a new kind of happiness.
Berkeley: Seal Press; 2014.

16

Allopregnanolone alters follicular and luteal dynamics during the estrous cycle

Joana Antonela Asensio[1†], Antonella Rosario Ramona Cáceres[1,2†], Laura Tatiana Pelegrina[1,2], María de los Ángeles Sanhueza[1], Leopoldina Scotti[3], Fernanda Parborell[3] and Myriam Raquel Laconi[1,2,4*]

Abstract

Background: Allopregnanolone is a neurosteroid synthesized in the central nervous system independently of steroidogenic glands; it influences sexual behavior and anxiety. The aim of this work is to evaluate the indirect effect of a single pharmacological dose of allopregnanolone on important processes related to normal ovarian function, such as folliculogenesis, angiogenesis and luteolysis, and to study the corresponding changes in endocrine profile and enzymatic activity over 4 days of the rat estrous cycle. We test the hypothesis that allopregnanolone may trigger hypothalamus - hypophysis - ovarian axis dysregulation and cause ovarian failure which affects the next estrous cycle stages.

Methods: Allopregnanolone was injected during the proestrous morning and then, the animals were sacrificed at each stage of the estrous cycle. Ovarian sections were processed to determine the number and diameter of different ovarian structures. Cleaved caspase 3, proliferating cell nuclear antigen, α-actin and Von Willebrand factor expressions were evaluated by immunohistochemistry. Luteinizing hormone, prolactin, estrogen and progesterone serum levels were measured by radioimmunoassay. The enzymatic activities of 3β-hydroxysteroid dehydrogenase, 3α-hydroxysteroid oxidoreductase and 20α-hydroxysteroid dehydrogenase were determined by spectrophotometric assays. Two-way ANOVA followed by Bonferroni was performed to determine statistical differences between control and treated groups along the four stages of the cycle.

Results: The results indicate that allopregnanolone allopregnanolone decreased the number of developing follicles, while atretic follicles and cysts increased with no effects on normal cyclicity. Some cysts in treated ovaries showed morphological characteristics similar to luteinized unruptured follicles. The apoptosis/proliferation balance increased in follicles from treated rats. The endocrine profile was altered at different stages of the estrous cycle of treated rats. The angiogenic markers expression increased in treated ovaries. As regards *corpora lutea*, the apoptosis/proliferation balance and 20α-hydroxysteroid dehydrogenase enzymatic activity decreased significantly. Progesterone levels and 3β-hydroxysteroid dehydrogenase enzymatic activity increased in treated rats. These data suggest that allopregnanolone interferes with steroidogenesis and folliculogenesis at different stages of the cycle.

Conclusion: Allopregnanolone interferes with *corpora lutea* regression, which might indicate that this neurosteroid exerts a protective role over the luteal cells and prevents them from luteolysis. Allopregnanolone plays an important role in the ovarian pathophysiology.

Keywords: Allopregnanolone, Folliculogenesis, Angiogenesis, Apoptosis, Steroidogenesis, *Corpora lutea*, Luteolysis

* Correspondence: mlaconi@yahoo.com; mlaconi@mendoza-conicet.gov.ar
†Equal contributors
[1]Laboratorio de Fisiopatología Ovárica, Instituto de Medicina y Biología Experimental de Cuyo (IMBECU - CONICET), Mendoza, Argentina
[2]Facultad de Ciencias Veterinarias y Ambientales, Universidad Juan Agustín Maza, Mendoza, Argentina
Full list of author information is available at the end of the article

Background

The brain has always been considered a target for sex steroid hormones produced by peripheral steroidogenic organs (gonads and the adrenal glands); it is now well accepted that the brain synthesizes neurosteroids *de novo*, and converts circulating steroids to neuroactive steroids [1]. Regardless of their origin, steroids affect brain function through actions at their cognate receptors, or by affecting receptors whose primary transmitter is not a steroid (e.g., GABA receptors). Allopregnanolone (3α-hydroxy-5α-pregnan-20-one, ALLO) is a neurosteroid synthesized in the brain, adrenal glands and gonads from progesterone (PG) metabolism by the action of the 3α-hydroxysteroid dehydrogenase (3α-HSD) enzyme [2]. It can also be produced *de novo* from cholesterol in the brain [3] and it acts as a potent neurosteroid that can alter membrane excitability [4, 5].

One of the most intriguing questions has been the relationship of peripheral steroids with neurosteroids. Free steroids (i.e., steroids not bound to carrier proteins) are capable of diffusing across the blood–brain barrier to bind both membrane-associated steroid receptors and intracellular receptors. Thus, levels of a particular steroid in the brain are a composite of steroids from the periphery, converted peripheral steroids, and neurosteroids. Additionally, hormonal steroids also regulate the site-specific synthesis of neurosteroid levels [6, 7] and their cognate receptors [8–10] that affect neurosteroid levels and function. ALLO is a positive allosteric modulator of GABA$_A$ receptors; in fact, ALLO enhances GABA activity at nanomolar concentrations and opens chloride channels at micromolar concentrations [5, 11–13]. Production of ALLO increases in response to stress in order to decrease pain sensitivity and restore physiologic homeostasis [14–16]. In previous works from our laboratory, ALLO reduced anxiety and inhibited lordosis, and thus it influences sexual behavior in the female rat [17, 18]. Several studies revealed that higher than physiological ALLO concentrations inhibit GnRH and sexual behavior in rats [18–22]. These findings prompted us to consider ALLO not only as a modulator of hypothalamic function but also of ovarian physiology.

Follicular development process, ovulation, *corpora lutea* (CL) formation and luteolysis are critical events that occur cyclically in the rat ovary, which are subject to a complex endocrine regulation. In previous studies, we reported that ALLO injected via intracerebroventricular (i.c.v.) during proestrous (PE) morning inhibited luteinizing hormone (LH) surge and, consequently, decreased the number of ovulated oocytes in estrous (E) rats. ALLO also increased prolactin (PRL) and PG serum levels, and decreased the number of apoptotic *nuclei* in luteal cells [22]. Furthermore, ALLO interfered with folliculogenesis process since the number of developing follicles and new CL were reduced in E treated rats. ALLO also increased the number of cystic structures and altered steroidogenesis at E stage; however, normal cyclicity was not altered [23]. While the role of ALLO is well documented in the central nervous system (CNS), the functions on the ovarian physiology remains to be fully explored.

As we found previously, ALLO affected several important ovarian parameters that might impair reproduction [22, 23]; therefore, we aim to investigate if these alterations remain throughout the next estrous cycle. We evaluated the effect of a single pharmacological dose of ALLO, injected in the PE morning, on (a) number of ovarian structures, (b) follicle and CL sizes, (c) apoptosis, proliferation and angiogenesis processes (d) LH, PRL, 17β-estradiol (E2) and PG serum levels, and (e) 3β-hydroxysteroid dehydrogenase (3β-HSD), 3α-hydroxysteroid oxidoreductase (3α-HSOR) and 20α-hydroxysteroid dehydrogenase (20α-HSD) enzymatic activities. The effects of ALLO on these parameters were evaluated on E, diestrous 1 (D1), diestrous 2 (D2) and PE stages of the cycle. The relevance of this study is that it is the first evidence of the effect of ALLO on the whole cycle and its putative pathological consequences.

Methods

Animals

Adult female Sprague Dawley rats (*Rattus norvegicus*) of 200-250 g were maintained under controlled conditions of temperature and light (12 h light/12 h darkness photoperiod). They were housed in groups of four animals *per* cage with food (standard rat chow Cargil, Córdoba, Argentina) and water available *ad libitum*. Vaginal smears from each rat were observed daily (07:00-09:00 am) with a light microscope (Zeiss, Germany) to determine the stage of the estrous cycle. Only those animals exhibiting two or more consecutive 4 or 5-day cycle were used. All protocols were previously approved by the Institutional Committee for Care and Use of Experimental Animals (CICUAL N° 141021) and conducted according to the National Institutes of Health Guide for the Care and Use of Laboratory Animals of the National Research Council (National Academies, U.S.A., 8th Edition, 2011).

Drugs

Allopregnanolone (Sigma Chemical Co., St. Louis, MO, USA), Penicillin G Benzathine (Riched, Argentina), Ketamine HCL (Hollliday - Scott S.A, Buenos Aires, Argentina) and Xylazine (Koning Laboratories, Buenos Aires, Argentina) were used for experimental and surgical procedures. Stocks of ALLO were initially dissolved in propylene-glycol to a concentration of 0.6 mM. The dose of ALLO used in the experiments (6 μM) was obtained by dilutions in Krebs Ringer bicarbonate glucose buffer (KREBS) at pH 7.4. Bouin solution (Biopur Diagnostics, Santa Fe, Argentina) and Canada Balsam Synthetic (Biopack, Buenos Aires, Argentina) were purchased for histological procedures. Anti-cleaved caspase 3 (CASP3) (Biocare Medical, #CP229C, California, USA) raised in rabbit, anti-proliferating cell nuclear antigen (PCNA) raised in rabbit (Santa Cruz Biotechnology, sc-7907, USA), anti-α-actin raised in mouse (Santa Cruz Biotechnology, sc-56499, USA), polyclonal anti-Von Willebrand factor raised in rabbit (Dako Cytomation, A0082, USA), Anti-Rabbit HRP IgG (Sigma Aldrich, A4914, USA) , anti-mouse HRP IgG (R&D Systems HAF007, Minnesota, USA), and avidin-biotinylated HRP complex (Vectastain ABC system; Vector Laboratories, Burlingame, CA, USA) were used for immunohistochemistry technique.

Surgical Procedures

A stainless steel cannula was stereotaxically inserted into the right lateral ventricle under Ketamine/Xylazine anesthesia (50 mg/kg and 5 mg/kg body weight, respectively). The following coordinates were used: AP +0.4 mm, L +1.5 mm, and DV -4 mm [24]. At the end of the surgery, the cannula was sealed with a stainless steel wire to avoid obstruction. In order to prevent infections, each animal received a subcutaneous injection of 0.2 ml of 1.200.000 UI penicillin G Benzathine (1UI = 0.6 μg; 72 mg/rat). After the surgery, the animals were housed singly in plexiglas cages and maintained for a week undisturbed in order to recover the estrous cycle. At the end of the experiments, after decapitation, the location of the guide cannula was confirmed by the injection of blue ink. Only animals with confirmed microinjection

into right lateral ventricle were included in the experiments.

Experimental design

The rats were randomly assigned to either control or ALLO treated groups for each estrous cycle stage (n = 6/group, total of 48 animals) (Fig. 1). On the PE morning, the experimental groups received a single i.c.v. injection of ALLO: 6 μM, 1 μl, during 60 seconds to avoid reflux. A pharmacological dose of ALLO was administered as used in our previous reports of anxiety, memory and sexual behavior [17, 18, 21–23]. Control animals were injected with KREBS solution, containing propylene-glycol in equivalent concentrations to the used in ALLO groups. Six animals for each day of collection for experimental group were euthanized by decapitation 24 h (E), 48 h (D1), 72 h (D2) and 96 h (PE) after a unique injection of KREBS or ALLO. Serum samples were collected from each rat after blood centrifugation and stored at -20°C for RIA. From each rat, the right ovary and medial basal hypothalamus (MBH) were removed for 3β-HSD, 3α-HSOR and 20α-HSD enzymatic activity measurements. The left ovary was preserved for histological assays. One set of ovarian slides was stained with hematoxylin-eosin to quantify the number of structures at different stages of follicular development, and the other sections were used for immunohistochemistry.

Ovarian morphometry

The left ovaries from each rat were removed and immediately fixed in Bouin solution for 12 h. Then, dehydrated in a series of increasing concentration alcohols

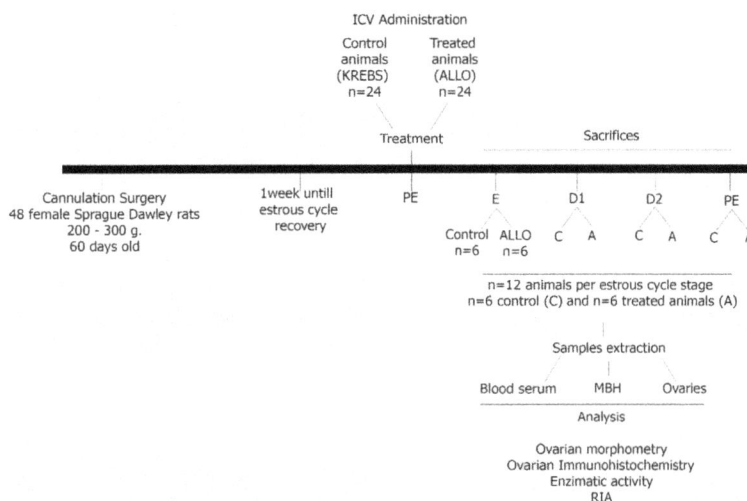

Fig. 1 Experimental design of the study. A: ALLO treated group, C: control, E: estrous, ICV: intracerebroventricular, D1: diestrous 1, D2: diestrous 2, MBH: medial basal hypothalamus, PE: proestrous, RIA: radioimmunoassay

and finally embedded in paraffin. Paraffin sections of 5 μm were taken every 50 μm and mounted onto microscope slides to prevent counting the same structure twice, according to the method described by Woodruff *et al.* (1990) [25]. Follicles were classified as primary (PF; a single layer of cuboidal granulosa cells, preantral (PAF; more than one layer of granulosa cells), early antral (EAF; three or more granulosa layers with an incipient antrum), antral (AF; more than three granulosa layers and a clearly defined antral space) and Graafian follicles (GF; polarized oocyte, defined cumulus granulosa layer and a cavity occupying most of the follicular volume) [26, 27]. *Corpora lutea* (CLs) were identified by the presence of large luteal cells and their characteristic cytoplasmic eosinophilia, surrounded by small lutein cells [28]. *Corpora albicans* were scarce, and they were not taken into account. Morphological characteristics of atretic follicles (ATF) include pyknotic *nuclei* (cell degeneration), detachment of the granulosa cell layer from the basal *laminae*, hypertrophy of external theca and oocyte degeneration [29]. Cysts can be subdivided into follicular and luteal cysts: follicular cysts are surrounded by a thin granulosa layer (≤ 3 mm) and contain a large antral cavity (the oocyte may be absent or present), while luteinized unruptured follicles (LUF) consist of an oocyte surrounded by luteinized granulosa cells and have a thicker wall (> 3 mm) [30–32]. The number of ovarian structures was determined in three ovarian sections from each ovary (three sections *per* ovary; n=6). Numbers of PF, PAF, EAF, AF, GF, CL, ATF and cysts (including LUFs) were determined for each left ovary/animal in each experimental group; then they were expressed as Mean ± S.E.M. of the number of structures in each ovary at each stage of the cycle.

The diameters of EAF, AF, GF and CL were measured using Image J software (Image Processing and Analysis in Java; National Institutes of Health, Bethesda, MD, USA). Results were expressed as mean diameter ± S.E.M.

Immunohistochemistry

Ovarian tissue sections were processed for *in situ* localization of CASP3, PCNA, α-actin and von Willebrand factor. Ovarian sections were deparaffinized in xylene and rehydrated in descending graduation ethanol washes. Endogenous peroxidase activity was blocked with 3% hydrogen peroxide in PBS and nonspecific binding was blocked with 2% BSA for 20 min at room temperature. Sections were incubated with the primary antibodies: CASP3 (1:300), PCNA (1:300), α-actin (1:100) and von Willebrand (1:100) overnight at 4°C in a humid chamber. After PBS washing, the slides were incubated with the corresponding secondary antibodies (anti-rabbit HRP-IgG 1:1000, anti-mouse HRP-

IgG 1:1000) for 2 h and then with avidin-biotinylated HRP complex (1:400) for 30 min. Protein expression was visualized using diaminobenzidine staining. The negative controls were obtained in the absence of primary antibodies. The reaction was stopped using distilled water, counterstained with hematoxylin and dehydrated before mounting. The images were digitized using a camera (Nikon, Melville, NY, USA) mounted on a conventional light microscope (Nikon).

Apoptosis and cellular proliferation were evaluated in EAF, AF, GF and CL by CASP3 and PCNA immunohistochemistry, respectively. EAF, AF and GF are the most sensitive ovarian structures to degeneration by atresia, since they have follicle-stimulating hormone (FSH) and LH receptors and are capable of sensing the balance between survival/apoptotic factors [33, 34]. Six ovaries from six different rats were used *per* experimental group (n=6, 48 ovaries in total). From each ovary, four follicles and four CL were selected and numbered to be analyzed. Within each follicle and each CL, four randomly selected fields were identified and numbered. In each ovary, thirty-two fields were analyzed in total: 16 fields for follicles and 16 fields for CL. Cell counting was performed using Image J software (NIH, Bethesda, MD). Proliferation or apoptotic index was calculated for each selected field as follows: CASP 3 or PCNA-positive cells divided by the total number of cells in the whole field. Results were expressed as mean ± S.E.M of positive immunostained cells for CASP3 or PCNA on the base of this raw data.

ALLO effects on ovarian angiogenesis were evaluated by immunohistochemistry for α-actin and von Willebrand at each stage of the estrous cycle. Six randomly selected fields were analyzed from each ovarian section (six sections *per* ovary; n=6). The percentage of endothelial cell area positively marked, either for α-actin or von Willebrand, with respect to the total area of the ovary was quantified using Image J software. The results obtained were expressed as mean ± S.E.M. of endothelial cell area positively marked.

RIA for LH, PRL, E2 and PG

Trunk blood was collected from each experimental group (n=6) in heparinized tubes and centrifuged during 15 min at 1500g (Beckman TJ-6RS). The plasma obtained was kept frozen (-20°C) until hormone assays were run. LH and PRL serum levels were determined by RIA using kits supplied by the National Hormone Pituitary Program, USA. The LH standard was NIDDK-rLH-RP-3 and the antibody NIDDK rLH-S-11. The PRL standard was NIDDK-rPRL-RP-3 and the antibody NIDDK-rPRL-S-9. The sensitivity of the assay was 0.5 ng/tube. The intra- and inter-assay coefficients of variation were 9 and 11%, respectively. The data were expressed in nanograms per milliliter (ng/ml) of serum in terms of NIDDK-rLH-RP-1 and NIDK-rPRL-RP-3 reference preparation. E2 serum concentration was determined by RIA using a commercial kit (Radim, Pomezia, Italy) based on competition between antigens labeled with iodine 125 (radioactive conjugate) and non-labeled antigens (calibrator sample) for specific binding sites in antiserum-coated tubes [22]. PG serum concentration was measured using a commercially obtained kit (Diagnostic Products Corporation, LA, CA, USA). The sensitivity of the assay was 0.02 ng/ml, and the inter- and intra-assay coefficients of variation were 5% and 6%, respectively. For each hormone analyzed, two measurements *per* animal *per* experimental group were obtained, and then the average between them was calculated. This final value was used to obtain mean ± S.E.M. for statistical analysis of LH, PRL, E2 and PG *per* experimental group.

Spectrophotometric measurements of enzymatic activity

The MBH and the ovaries were homogenized with a glass homogenizer at 0° C in a solution containing: 0.7 ml of 0.1 M Tris-HCl + 1 mM EDTA buffer (pH 8). The activities of 3β-HSD, 3α-HSOR and 20α-HSD were measured as described previously with minor modifications [21, 35, 36]. Lowry method was used for protein determination using bovine serum albumin (BSA) as standard. The homogenates were centrifuged at 105000g for 60 min, using a Beckman L T40.2 ultracentrifuge. The supernatants were used for determination of 20α-HSD activity. The precipitates were re-homogenized with 0.25 M sucrose and then centrifuged at 1200g for 5 min. The supernatants obtained were used as the enzyme solution to determine 3β-HSD activity. Then pregnenolone, the substrate for the reaction of 3α-HSOR, was added to the reaction mix. The latter contained Glycine-NaOH (pH 9. 4), BSA, NAD+ and a fraction of the enzyme solution. The enzymatic activities were determined spectrophotometrically using a Zeltec spectrophotometer. The assay of each enzyme measured the reduction of NAD+ or the oxidation rate of NADPH cofactor at 340 nm, respectively, as an increase in absorbance in 1 min at 37°C [35, 37, 38]. A fraction of the enzymatic solution was reserved for protein quantification. The values of enzymatic activity were expressed as mUI/mg protein/ min.

Statistical analysis

Raw data obtained were analyzed using Graph Pad Prism version 5.03 for Windows (Graph Pad Software, California, USA). Results were expressed as mean ± S.E.M. The aim of this work is to determine how certain parameters of the ovarian physiology are affected by two variables: treatment and stage of the estrous cycle. Therefore, ANOVA two-way was performed in all the experiments, followed by Bonferroni's posttest to determine the individual differences between control and ALLO groups at each stage of the cycle. D' Agostino-Pearson normality test was used prior to ANOVA two-way. Differences were considered significant at $p < 0.05$.

Results

Effect of ALLO on ovarian morphometry

Our results on E stage were published previously [22, 23] and they were included in this article in order to make comparisons easier. The results of the morphometric analysis are showed in Table 1. The number of PF decreased in D2 treated rats ($p < 0.01$). No significant differences were found in the number of PAF at any stage of the estrous cycle between control and ALLO groups. The number of EAF diminished significantly in treated rats at all stages of the cycle (E $p < 0.01$, D1 $p < 0.001$, D2 $p < 0.001$ and PE $p < 0.05$). AF decreased in treated rats of E ($p < 0.05$), D1 ($p < 0.001$) and D2 ($p < 0.01$). GF number decreased in ALLO treated rats at E stage ($p < 0.001$). There was a decrease in the number of CL in D2 ($p < 0.01$), but there were no significant differences in E, D1 and PE stages. ATF number increased substantially in ALLO treated ovaries from all stages of the estrous cycle (E $p < 0.001$, D1 $p < 0.01$, D2 $p < 0.001$ and PE $p < 0.01$). The number of cysts increased in E ($p < 0.001$), D1 ($p < 0.05$) and D2 ($p < 0.05$) treated groups; no cysts were found at PE stage, neither in control nor in ALLO groups. Finally, we found a decrease in EAF diameter at E and a decrease in CL diameter ($p < 0.01$) at D1 stage treated groups.

Effect of ALLO on ovarian apoptosis, proliferation and angiogenesis

Cleaved CASP3 expression was evaluated by immunohistochemistry in EAF, GF and CL from control and ALLO groups along the estrous cycle (Fig. 2). Cleaved CASP3 immunoreactivity was increased in granulosa cells at E and PE in ALLO treated groups, compared to control groups ($p < 0.001$). No differences were observed in the apoptotic index in follicles neither in D1 nor D2 stages between control and ALLO groups (Fig. 2a). In CL, cleaved CASP3 expression decreased in E, D1 and PE ALLO groups ($p < 0.001$, $p < 0.05$ and $p < 0.001$, respectively) (Fig. 2b).

PCNA immunoreactivity in granulosa cells decreased at all stages of the estrous cycle in ALLO treated groups, in comparison to control ones (E $p < 0.001$, D1 $p < 0.01$, D2 $p < 0.001$ and PE $p < 0.001$; Fig. 3a). On the contrary, PCNA immunoreactivity in CL increased in ALLO treated groups at all stages of the estrous cycle ($p < 0.001$; Fig. 3b).

In order to evaluate the effect of ALLO on endothelial cell density and stability, histological ovarian slides were

Table 1 Number and diameter of different ovarian structures in control and ALLO treated rats along the estrous cycle

Group (cyclic stage)	Control (E)	ALLO (E)	Control (D1)	ALLO (D1)	Control (D2)	ALLO (D2)	Control (PE)	ALLO (PE)
PF (n)	3.17 ± 0.75	2.83 ± 0.75	6.50 ± 0.65	5.75 ± 0.75	6.80 ± 1.74	5.00 ± 0.77**	3.50 ± 0.43	2.60 ± 0.40
PAF (n)	3.94 ± 0.56	2.77 ± 0.33	6.25 ± 1.32	7.75 ± 1.44	8.25 ± 1.32	7.40 ± 2.48	3.17 ± 0.65	1.80 ± 0.80
EAF (n)	4.83 ± 0.31	2.83 ± 0.31**	5.25 ± 0.85	2.50 ± 0.50***	9.20 ± 1.74	1.75 ± 2.08***	2.50 ± 0.34	0.80 ± 0.49*
AF (n)	2.67 ± 0.33	1.33 ± 0.33*	3.50 ± 0.65	0.50 ± 0.50***	4.40 ± 1.03	2.60 ± 1.08**	1.50 ± 0.56	1.00 ± 0.45
GF (n)	2.83 ± 0.31	0.67 ± 0.21***	0.75 ± 0.48	0.5 ± 0.5	0.08 ± 0.02	0.80 ± 0.58	0.67 ± 0.49	0.2 ± 0.2
CL (n)	7.65 ± 2.20	6.35 ± 1.10	7.25 ± 0.85	8.25 ± 1.18	13.50 ± 0.50	9.60 ± 0.93**	6.16 ± 1.08	8.40 ± 1.33
ATF (n)	2.75 ± 1.10	4.77 ± 0.90***	7.67 ± 1.20	11.75 ± 1.03**	5.00 ± 0.71	12.80±2.25***	9.33 ± 0.61	12.20 ± 0.97**
Cysts (n)	2.00 ± 0.55	6.00 ± 1.33***	0.01 ± 0.01	0.63 ± 0.26*	0.01 ± 0.01	0.63 ± 0.26*	0	0
EAF diameter (μm)	244.9 ± 19.84	208.70±14.14*	191.00 ± 21.48	189.30 ± 19.17	220.50 ± 31.65	212.80 ± 23.41	216.50 ± 25.55	234.30 ± 5.22
AF diameter (μm)	399.6 ± 26.25	413.15 ± 30.30	415.10 ± 37.51	420.80 ± 49.45	355.50 ± 37.82	378.70 ± 70.96	402.90 ± 12.97	375.00 ± 20.02
GF diameter (μm)	650.9 ± 34.03	603.62 ± 65.12	639.50 ± 20.01	646.10 ± 1.37	654.30 ± 55.29	614.30 ± 29.70	670.76 ± 32.98	689.87 ± 33.98
CL diameter (μm)	758 ± 65.01	836.30 ± 82.30	1019 ± 137.70	848 ±82.32**	946.60 ± 99.56	882.10 ± 97.88	1006 ± 66.93	999.89 ± 61.55

Number of ovarian structures (n) are expressed as Mean ± S.E.M. of primary (PF), preantral (PAF), early antral (EAF), antral (AF), Graafian (GF), atretic follicles (ATF), *corpora lutea* (CL) and cysts (follicular and luteal cysts). Mean diameter (μm) ± S.E.M of EAF, AF, GF and CL along the estrous cycle from control and ALLO treated rats. Two-way ANOVA followed by Bonferroni's *post hoc*, (n=6), ns $p>0.05$, *$p<0.05$, **$p<0.01$, ***$p<0.001$.

immunostained against α-actin and von Willebrand angiogenic factors. ALLO increased the vascular area labeled with α-actin at all stages of estrous cycle (E $p<0.001$, D1 $p<0.05$, D2 $p<0.001$ and PE $p<0.001$; Fig. 4). Similarly, ALLO augmented the vascular area labeled with von Willebrand factor at E ($p<0.001$), D2 ($p<0.05$) and PE ($p<0.001$) stages, with no significant differences at D1 (Fig. 4). Fig. 4c shows that cells

immunostained with von Willebrand factor in CL correspond to endothelial cells.

Effect of ALLO on LH, PRL, E2 and PG serum levels

Hormone serum levels from control and treated groups along the estrous cycle are presented in Fig. 5. ALLO injection induced a significant decrease in LH serum levels at E (control 0.22 ± 0.05 ng/ml vs.

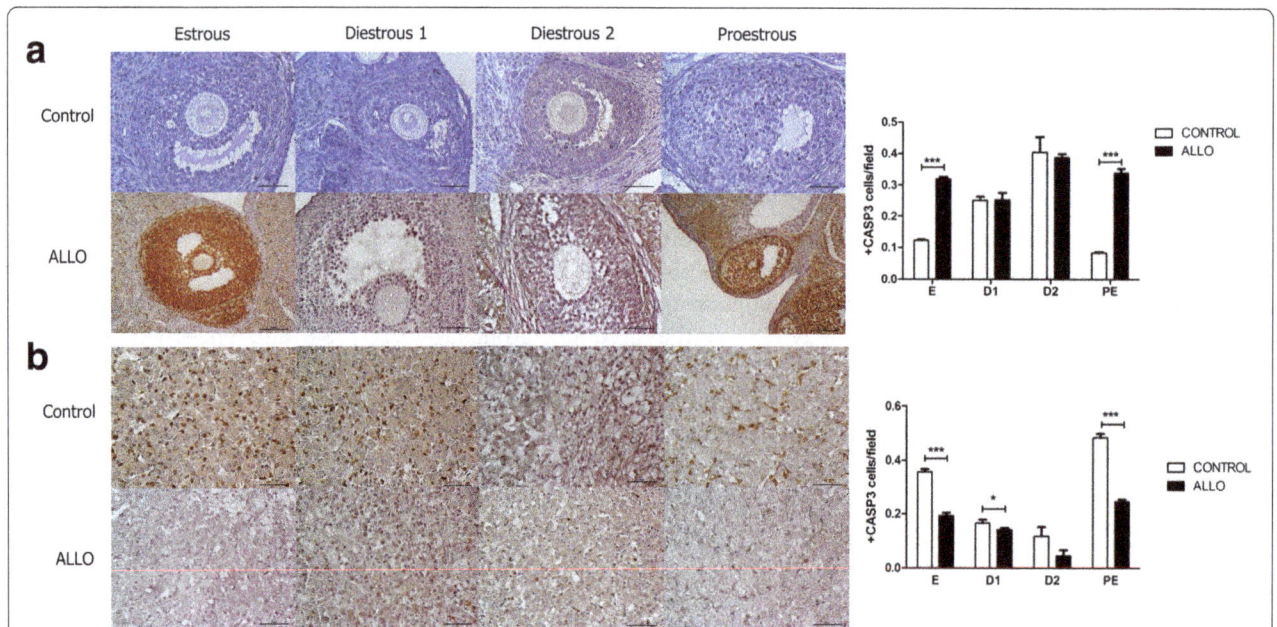

Fig. 2 Effect of ALLO on the apoptotic index (cleaved CASP3 positive immunostained cells over the total number of cells) in follicles (**a**) and *corpora lutea* (**b**). Control groups follicles (1A upper panel), ALLO treated follicles (1A lower panel), control groups CL (1B upper panel), ALLO treated groups CL (1B lower panel); E, D1, D2, PE from left to right. Representative photomicrographs of follicles and *corpora lutea* immunostained for cleaved CASP3 at each stage of the estrous cycle. Values are expressed as mean ± S.E.M. Two-way ANOVA followed by Bonferroni's post hoc, (n=6), *$p<0.05$, ***$p<0.001$. Magnification: follicles 200x, CL 400x

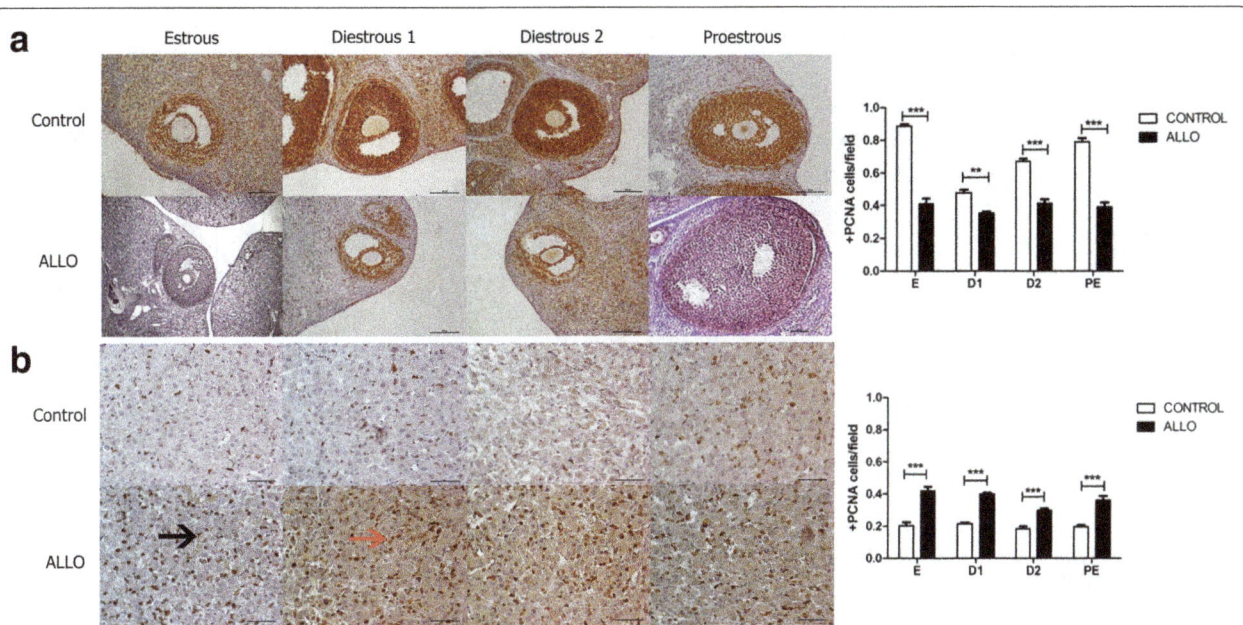

Fig. 3 Effect of ALLO on the proliferation index (PCNA positive immunostained cells over the total number of cells) in follicles (**a**) and *corpora lutea* (**b**). Control groups follicles (**a** upper panel), ALLO treated follicles (**a** lower panel), control groups CL (**b** upper panel), ALLO treated groups CL (**b** lower panel); E, D1, D2, PE from left to right. Representative photomicrographs of follicles and *corpora lutea* immunostained for PCNA at each stage of the estrous cycle. Black arrow indicate proliferating endothelial cells, red arrow indicate proliferating small luteal cells. Values are expressed as mean ± S.E.M. Two-way ANOVA followed by Bonferroni's post hoc, (n=6), *p<0.05, ***p<0.001. Magnification: follicles 200x, CL 400x

ALLO 0.098 ± 0.001 ng/ml, p<0.001) and PE stages (control 25.57 ± 3.37 ng/ml vs. ALLO 6.84 ± 2.07 ng/ml, p<0.001) (Fig. 5a, inset a). As regards PRL serum levels, ALLO induced an increase at E (control 2.10 ± 0.30 ng/ml vs. ALLO 9.60 ± 1.20 ng/ml, p<0.05) and a decrease at PE stage (control 65.56 ± 3.21 ng/ml vs. ALLO 18.37 ± 3.60 ng/ml, p<0.001) (Fig. 5b). E2 serum concentration decreased significantly in ALLO treated rats at PE (control 34.90 ± 8.09 pg/ml vs. ALLO 7.12 ± 2.01 pg/ml, p<0.01) (Fig. 5c). PG serum levels increased at D1 in ALLO treated rats (control 25.02 ± 13.22 ng/ml vs. ALLO 77 ± 12.44 ng/ml, p<0.01) (Fig. 5d).

Effect of ALLO on the enzymatic activities of 3β-HSD, 3α-HSOR and 20α-HSD in MBH and ovaries

3β-HSD enzymatic activity increased in treated ovaries at E (control 10 ± 1.2 mUI 3β-HSD/mg protein/min vs. ALLO 18 ± 2.1 mUI 3β-HSD/mg protein/min, p<0.001) (Fig. 6d). There was no effect of ALLO on 3α-HSOR (Fig. 6b and e) and 20α-HSD (Fig. 6c and f) enzymatic activity, neither in MBH nor in the ovaries.

Discussion

Allopregnanolone is the most active PG metabolite, and it has multiple functions, in addition to its role as neuromodulator in the nervous system. ALLO is also involved in the regulation of ovarian physiology [22, 23]. However,

the concrete correlation of ALLO with follicles and *corpora lutea* dynamics is still not well understood.

The data presented in this study showed, for the first time, how a single pharmacological dose of ALLO can alter the physiological dynamics of follicles and *corpora lutea* during the estrous cycle. Our research was conducted from different approaches: morphology of ovarian structures, molecular physiology (apoptosis, proliferation and angiogenesis) and steroidogenic process (hormone levels and enzymatic activity profiles).

In this work, the injection of ALLO decreased the number of EAF, AF and GF and increased ATF at several stages of the cycle; then, the processes of follicle maturation and selection have been impaired. On the other hand, the number of apoptotic granulosa cells increased and proliferating granulosa cells decreased at all stages in ALLO treated groups. These results suggest that ALLO promotes atresia of developing follicles by stimulating apoptosis on granulosa cells, and thus alters the apoptosis/proliferation balance in the whole follicle.

Granulosa cells are the most abundant cell population in ovarian follicles and the main source of E2 and PG in the ovary [39]. Since ALLO alters follicle maturation process, this neurosteroid might interfere with E2 secretion. The decline in E2 serum levels found in our experiments reflects the dysfunctionality of follicles as endocrine glands induced by ALLO. In a regular estrous cycle, once ovulation has occurred, E2 serum

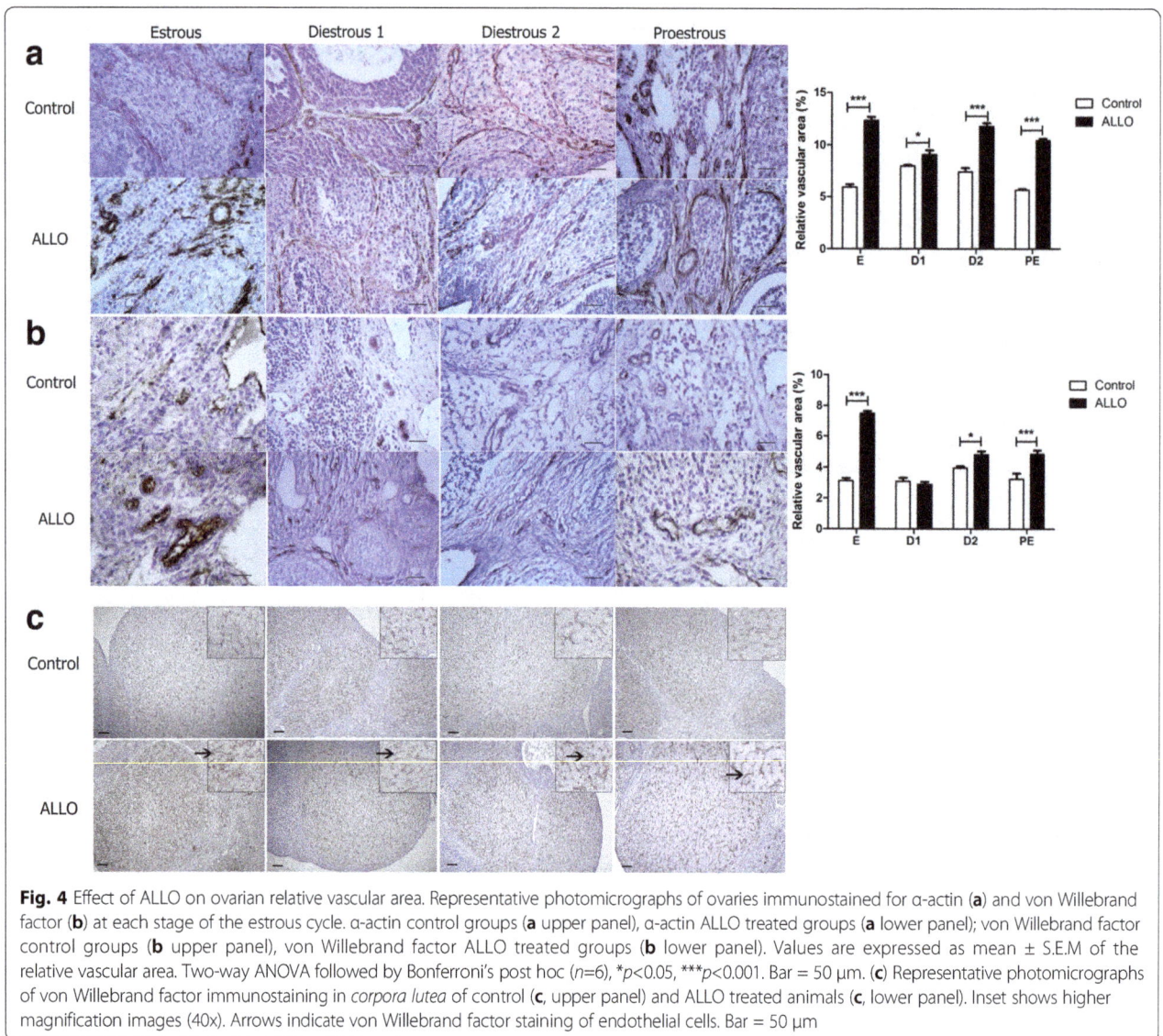

Fig. 4 Effect of ALLO on ovarian relative vascular area. Representative photomicrographs of ovaries immunostained for α-actin (**a**) and von Willebrand factor (**b**) at each stage of the estrous cycle. α-actin control groups (**a** upper panel), α-actin ALLO treated groups (**a** lower panel); von Willebrand factor control groups (**b** upper panel), von Willebrand factor ALLO treated groups (**b** lower panel). Values are expressed as mean ± S.E.M of the relative vascular area. Two-way ANOVA followed by Bonferroni's post hoc ($n=6$), $*p<0.05$, $***p<0.001$. Bar = 50 μm. (**c**) Representative photomicrographs of von Willebrand factor immunostaining in *corpora lutea* of control (**c**, upper panel) and ALLO treated animals (**c**, lower panel). Inset shows higher magnification images (40x). Arrows indicate von Willebrand factor staining of endothelial cells. Bar = 50 μm

concentration begins to increase to reach 40 pg/ml in PE [40]. However, our results showed that E2 serum levels were significantly reduced at the following PE (96 hs) after ALLO administration. This is not the first time that a correlation is established between follicular atresia and low E2 levels [41]. Although the activity of steroidogenic enzymes involved in E2 secretion was not affected, we assume that the low levels of E2 are related to ALLO effects on follicular atresia. In addition, the ovary is not the only sex steroid-producing gland; the adrenal gland of the rat secretes E2 at rates similar to the ovary and brain in minor concentrations, and the possible effect of ALLO on this gland and its secretion is still unknown [42]. It would be interesting to evaluate proliferation and apoptosis in granulosa and theca cells of cystic follicles, the expression of pro-apoptotic and anti-apoptotic regulatory proteins,

the balance between them (i.e.: BAX/BCL2) and the expression of steroid and gonadotropin receptors.

We have previously reported that ALLO caused a decrease in LH serum concentration of E rats [22], critical stage of the cycle in which LH induces ovulation. In the present research, we found that ALLO also decreased LH serum levels in PE rats as well. It has been shown that exogenous ALLO inhibits GnRH and LH secretion in rats through GABA action [21, 22]. These effects might be an outcome of the failure of the E2 negative feedback on GnRH [21, 43]. These results provide strong evidence that ALLO alters the cross-talk between the ovary and the hypothalamus, and thus ALLO causes the hypothalamus-hypophysis-ovarian (HHO) axis to dysregulate.

On the other hand, our results showed that ALLO injection increased the number of cystic structures. The

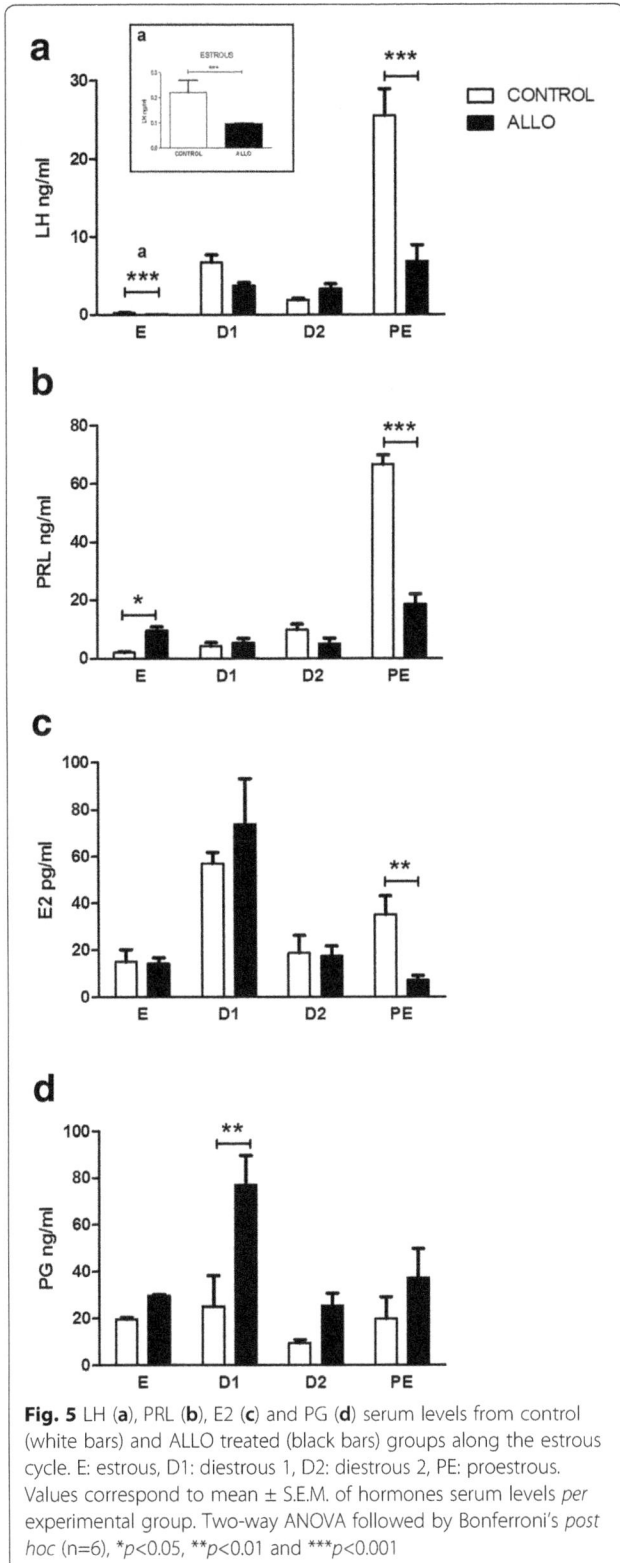

Fig. 5 LH (a), PRL (b), E2 (c) and PG (d) serum levels from control (white bars) and ALLO treated (black bars) groups along the estrous cycle. E: estrous, D1: diestrous 1, D2: diestrous 2, PE: proestrous. Values correspond to mean ± S.E.M. of hormones serum levels *per* experimental group. Two-way ANOVA followed by Bonferroni's *post hoc* (n=6), *$p<0.05$, **$p<0.01$ and ***$p<0.001$

and they are considered an abnormality in folliculogenesis [44]. Cystic ovarian follicles represent an ovarian disorder and an important cause of subfertility [30]. Although ALLO involvement in COD is still being investigated, it is well known that women with polycystic ovary have high levels of this PG metabolite. It is unknown whether elevated concentration and/or prolonged stimulation with ALLO in polycystic disease can cause the development of tolerance to it [45]. It has been shown that exposure of female rats to E2 induced a dysregulation of gonadal axis and a decreased brain and plasma ALLO [46]. Furthermore, GABA$_A$ receptors are involved in the pathophysiology of polycystic ovary syndrome [47, 48]. ALLO is able to alter GABA$_A$ receptor sensitivity [49]. Therefore, we conclude that the dysregulation of the HHO axis by ALLO injection contributes to the formation of cystic structures, probably by altering GABA$_A$ receptor sensibility to ALLO. It would be interesting to evaluate the expression of GABA receptors in the theca and granulosa cells of cystic structures.

The effects we have found could not only be related to the action of ALLO on GABA receptor but also they could be due to the action of ALLO over other ligands. ALLO affects brain function through actions at their cognate receptors (E2 receptor, PG receptor), or by modulating receptors whose primary transmitter is not a steroid (e.g. the GABA$_A$ receptor). Furthermore, previous works show that GABA$_A$ receptor is present not only in the CNS but also in the ovaries [50, 51]. Therefore, we assume that ALLO could exert its effects either at the brain or in the periphery (ovaries or adrenal gland). GABA$_A$ has different functions with respect to specific cell types in peripheral tissues as ovary [51]. GABA$_A$ receptor complex has been considered as the primary target of ALLO and majority of its inhibitory actions are mediated through GABA potentiation or direct activation of GABA currents [52]. However, GABA$_A$ receptor are highly expressed in endocrine tissues, particularly in the ovaries: the ovary express a total of 14 or 15 receptor subunit subtypes [53]. The high GABA content of these tissues supports the significant physiological role of GABA and GABA$_A$ receptors in ovaries. The results we present in the present article suggest that GABA receptors are involved in the regulation of follicular and luteal dynamics. We hypothesize that the action of ALLO might be mediated through GABA$_A$ receptor in the ovaries. Further research is needed to evaluate the possible mechanism of action of ALLO and the signaling pathways involved in the ovaries. The specific site of ALLO action (central or peripheral) still remains unclear; however, we assume there might be more than one tissue that responds to ALLO effects.

The angiogenic process is critical for the *corpus luteum* development and regression [28]. PG serum concentration

neuro-endocrine dysfunction of the HHO axis is closely associated with cystic ovarian disease pathogenesis (COD). As it is well known, cysts progression and persistence during the estrous cycle can lead to ovarian failure,

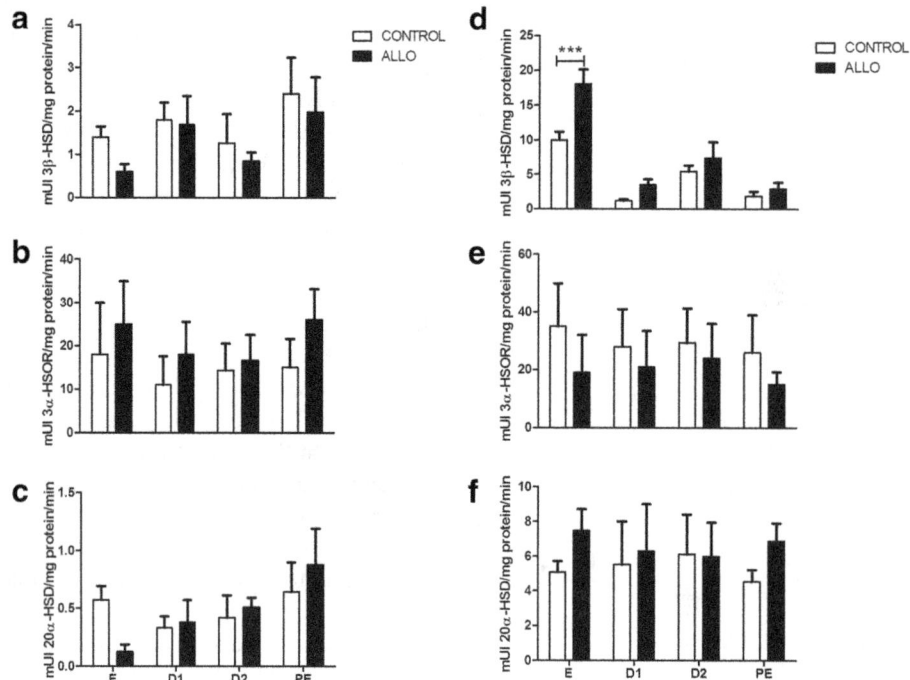

Fig. 6 Enzymatic activities of 3β-HSD (**a–d**), 3α-HSOR (**b–e**) and 20α-HSD (**c–f**) in the medial basal hypothalamus (MBH, left panel) and in the ovaries (right panel) at each stage of the estrous cycle. **e**: estrous, D1: diestrous 1, D2: diestrous 2, PE: proestrous. White bars correspond to control groups and black bars to ALLO treated groups. Values correspond to mean ± S.E.M. Two-way ANOVA followed by Bonferroni's *post hoc* ($n=6$), ***$p<0.001$

depends on the number and size of steroidogenic luteal cells (small and large), blood stream to the CL and on the ability of the steroidogenic tissue to synthesize PG. Mature CL receive most of blood ovarian irrigation and this could influence PG secretion [54]. Our results indicate that ALLO enhanced ovarian vascularization, increased ovarian 3β-HSD enzymatic activity in E (enzyme which converts pregnenolone in PG), and increased PG serum levels at D1. PCNA and von Willebrand staining pattern are similar, and they indicate that the cell type proliferating are endothelial cells. Moreover, PCNA staining in small luteal cells was increased in ALLO groups. It has been shown that PG interferes with luteal regression by a decrease in the number of apoptotic luteal cells and an increase in androstenedione levels [55]. Besides, it has been proved that PG maintains the functionality of CL through Notch pathway [45]. ALLO might be exerting a similar effect on CL in our experiments since PG levels and CL proliferation index are increased. In this work we found that ALLO increased proliferation and decreased apoptosis of luteal cells at all stages of the estrous cycle. Furthermore, we previously observed a decrease in the number of apoptotic *nuclei* in luteal cells from treated E rats [22]. Therefore, we could conclude that ALLO has a protective role on the function and survival of the CL. Further research is needed to distinguish CL cells types that undergo proliferation or apoptosis.

McCarthy et al., 1995 [56] showed that changes in serum ALLO concentration play an important role in the normal facilitation of estrous behavior in the rat; ALLO provoke this effect by acting at least in part through the PG receptor. In previous work, we found that ALLO inhibited lordosis behavior in rats through GABA action [18]. Micevych & Sinchak, 2008 [43] showed that circuits involved in controlling the LH surge and sexual behaviors were thought to be influenced by E2 and PG synthesized in the ovary and perhaps in the adrenal. It is now apparent that E2 of ovarian origin regulates the synthesis of neuroprogesterone (neuro-PG), and it is the locally produced neuro-PG that is involved in the initiation of the LH surge and subsequent ovulation. Moreover, E2 induces the transcription of PG receptors while stimulating synthesis of neuro-PG. Although the complete signaling cascade has not been elucidated, many of the features have been characterized.

Conclusion

The major findings of the present research article are that ALLO (1) interferes with follicular maturation affecting apoptosis/proliferation balance, (2) increases follicular atresia and cysts formation, (3) delays luteolysis by increasing serum PG and 3β-HSD enzymatic activity. ALLO has novel functions, which have not previously been identified in the rat ovary; thereby, these studies provide new insights about critical process for ovarian homeostasis (proliferation, apoptosis, angiogenesis and steroidogenesis). The effects of ALLO on these processes contribute to dysregulate the hypothalamus-hypophysis axis, and this results in inhibition of ovulation by neurosteroid action. On the basis of our discussion, the effects of ALLO strongly depend on the ovarian hormonal milieu that changes along the different stages of the estrous cycle. In order to comprehend the molecular mechanisms of ALLO action, a greater understanding of the role of hormonal milieu is strongly necessary.

Abbreviations
20α-HSD: 20α hydroxysteroid dehydrogenase; 3α-HSOR: 3α-hydroxysteroid oxidoreductase; 3β-HSD: 3β-hydroxysteroid dehydrogenase; AF: Antral follicle; ALLO: Allopregnanolone; ATF: Atretic follicles; CASP3: Caspase 3; CL: *Corpora lutea*; CNS: Central nervous system; D1: Diestrous 1; D2: Diestrous 2; E: Estrous; E2: 17β-estradiol; EAF: Early antral follicles; GF: Graafian follicles; LH: Luteinizing hormone; LUF: Luteinized unruptured follicles; MBH: Medial basal hypothalamus; neuroPG: Neuroprogesterone; PAF: Preantral follicles; PCNA: Proliferating cell nuclear antigen; PE: Proestrous; PF: Primary follicles; PG: Progesterone; PRL: Prolactin

Acknowledgements
Dr. Edgardo O. Álvarez for statistical advices, to Daniel Ibaceta (Veterinarian from Universidad Juan Agustín Maza) and Dr. Darío Cuello (IMBECU-CONICET) for assistance with histological experiments.

Funding
This study was supported by Universidad MAZA (Resolution N°562/17) and P-UE IMBECU, MINCyT-CONICET.

Authors' contributions
JAA and ARRC participated equally in this work. JAA, ARRC and MAS collected samples, performed laboratory work and data analysis; LTP, FP and MRL designed the project and drafted the manuscript. All authors read and approved the final manuscript.

Competing interests
The authors declare that they have no competing interests.

Author details
[1]Laboratorio de Fisiopatología Ovárica, Instituto de Medicina y Biología Experimental de Cuyo (IMBECU - CONICET), Mendoza, Argentina. [2]Facultad de Ciencias Veterinarias y Ambientales, Universidad Juan Agustín Maza, Mendoza, Argentina. [3]Laboratorio de Fisiopatología del Ovario, Instituto de Biología y Medicina Experimental (IByME - CONICET), Buenos Aires, Argentina. [4]Facultad de Ciencias Médicas, Universidad de Mendoza, Mendoza, Argentina.

References
1. Corpéchot C, Young J, Calvel M, Wehrey C, Veltz JN, Touyer G, Mouren M, Prasad VV, Banner C, Sjövall J, et al. Neurosteroids: 3 alpha-hydroxy-5 alpha-pregnan-20-one and its precursors in the brain, plasma, and steroidogenic glands of male and female rats. Endocrinology. 1993;133:1003–9.
2. Baulieu EE. Neurosteroids: Of the nervous system, by the nervous system, for the nervous system. Recent Prog Horm Res. 1997;52:1–32.
3. Zwain IH, Yen SS. Neurosteroidogenesis in astrocytes, oligodendrocytes, and neurons of cerebral cortex of rat brain. Endocrinology. 1999;140:3843–52.
4. Purdy RH, Morrow LA, Moore PH, Paul SM. Stress-induced elevations of γ-aminobutyric acid type A receptor-active steroids in the rat brain. PNAS. 1991;88:4553–7.
5. Paul SM, Purdy RH. Neuroactive steroids. FASEB J. 1992;6:2311–22.
6. Maguire J, Mody I. Neurosteroid synthesis-mediated regulation of GABA(A) receptors: relevance to the ovarian cycle and stress. J Neurosci. 2007;27(9):2155–62.
7. Micevych P, Sinchak K, Mills RH, Tao L, LaPolt P, Lu JK. The luteinizing hormone surge is preceded by an estrogen-induced increase of hypothalamic progesterone in ovariectomized and adrenalectomized rats. Neuroendocrinology. 2003;78(1):29–35.
8. Chappell PE, Lee J, Levine JE. Stimulation of gonadotropin-releasing hormone surges by estrogen. II. Role of cyclic adenosine 3'5'-monophosphate. Endocrinology. 2000;141(4):1486–92.
9. MacLusky NJ, McEwen BS. Oestrogen modulates progestin receptor concentrations in some rat brain regions but not in others. Nature. 1978;274(5668):276–8.
10. Soma KK, Sinchak K, Lakhter A, Schlinger BA, Micevych PE. Neurosteroids and female reproduction: estrogen increases 3beta-HSD mRNA and activity in rat hypothalamus. Endocrinology. 2005;146(10):4386–90.
11. Majewska MD. Neurosteroids: endogenous bimodal modulators of the GABAA receptor. Mechanism of action and physiological significance. Prog Neurobiol. 1992;38:379–95.
12. Guidotti A, Costa E. Can the antidysphoric and anxiolytic profiles of selective serotonin reuptake inhibitors be related to their ability to increase brain 3 alpha, 5 alpha tetrahydroprogesterone (Allopregnanolone) availability? Biol Psychiatry. 1998;44:865–73.
13. Smith SS, Gong QH, Moran MH, Bitran D, Frye CA, Hsu FC. Withdrawal from 3alpha-OH-5alpha-pregnan-20-one using a pseudopregnancy model alters the kinetics of hippocampal GABAA-gated current and increases the GABAA receptor alpha4 subunit in association with increased anxiety. J Neurosci. 1998;18:5275–84.
14. Frye CA, Duncan JE. Progesterone metabolites, effective at the GABAA receptor complex, attenuate pain sensitivity in rats. Brain Res. 1994;643:194–203.
15. Morrow AL, Devaud LL, Purdy RH, Paul SM. Neuroactive Steroid Modulators of the Stress Response. Ann N Y Acad Sci. 1995;771:257–72.
16. Wirth MM. Beyond the HPA axis: progesterone-derived neuroactive steroids in human stress and emotion. Front Endocrinol. 2011;2:1–14.
17. Laconi MR, Casteller G, Gargiulo P, Bregonzio C, Cabrera RJ. The anxiolytic effect of allopregnanolone is associated with gonadal hormonal status in female rats. Eur J Pharmacol. 2001;417:111–6.
18. Laconi MR, Cabrera RJ. Effect of centrally injected allopregnanolone on sexual receptivity, luteinizing hormone release, hypothalamic dopamine turnover and release in female rats. Endocrine. 2002;17:77–83.
19. Barbaccia ML, Roscetti G, Bolacchi F, Concas A, Mostallino MC, Purdy RH, Biggio G. Stress-Induced Increase in Brain Neuroactive Steroids: Antagonism by Abecarnil. Pharmacol Biochem Behav. 1996a;54:205–10.
20. Barbaccia ML, Roscetti G, Trabucchi M, Mostallino MC, Concas A, Purdy RH, Biggio G. Time-dependent changes in rat brain neuroactive steroid concentrations and GABAA receptor function after acute stress. Neuroendocrinology. 1996b;63:166–72.
21. Giuliani FA, Escudero C, Casas S, Bazzocchini V, Yunes R, Laconi MR, Cabrera R. Allopregnanolone and puberty: modulatory effect on glutamate and GABA release and expression of 3α-hydroxysteroid oxidoreductase in the hypothalamus of female rats. Neuroscience. 2013;243:64–75.
22. Laconi MR, Chavez C, Cavicchia JC, Fóscolo M, Sosa Z, Yunes RF, Cabrera RJ. Allopregnanolone alters the luteinizing hormone, prolactin, and progesterone serum levels interfering with the regression and apoptosis in rat corpus luteum. Horm Metab Res. 2012;44:1–17.

23. Pelegrina LT, Cáceres AR, Giuliani FA, Asensio JA, Parborell F, Laconi MR. A single dose of allopregnanolone affects the ovarian morphology and steroidogenesis. Reproduction. 2016;153:75–83.

24. Paxinos G, Watson C. The rat brain in stereotaxic coordinates. London: Academic Press; 2009.

25. Woodruff TK, Lyon RJ, Hansen SE, Rice GC, Mather JP. Inhibin and activin locally regulate rat ovarian folliculogenesis. Endocrinology. 1990;127: 3196–205.

26. Myers M, Britt KL, Wreford NGM, Ebling FJP, Kerr JB. Methods for quantifying follicular numbers within the mouse ovary. Reproduction. 2004;127:569–80.

27. Williams CJ, Erickson GF. 2012 Morphology and Physiology of the Ovary. Source Endotext [Internet]. South Dartmouth (MA): MDText.com, Inc.

28. Stocco C, Telleria C, Gibori G. The molecular control of corpus luteum formation, function, and regression. Endocr Rev. 2007;28:117–49.

29. Hsueh AJW, Billig H, Tsafriri A. Ovarian Follicle Atresia: A Hormonally Controlled Apoptotic Process. Endocr Rev. 1994;15:707–24.

30. Vanholder T, Opsomer G, de Kruif A. Aetiology and pathogenesis of cystic ovarian follicles in dairy cattle: a review. Reprod Nutr Dev. 2006;46:105–19.

31. Wang L, Qiao J, Liu P, Lian Y. Effect of luteinized unruptured follicle cycles on clinical outcomes of frozen thawed embryo transfer in Chinese women. J Assist Reprod Genet. 2008;25:229–33.

32. Fernandois D, Lara HE, Paredes AH. Blocking of β-adrenergic receptors during the subfertile period inhibits spontaneous ovarian cyst formation in rats. Horm Metab Res. 2012;44:682–7.

33. McGee EA, Hsueh AJ. Initial and cyclic recruitment of ovarian follicles. Endocr Rev. 2000;21:200–14.

34. Markstrom E, Svensson EC, Shao R, Svanverg B, Billig H. Survival factors regulating ovarian apoptosis - dependence on follicle differentiation. Reproduction. 2002;123:23–30.

35. Kawano T, Okamura H, Tajima C, Fukuma K, Katabuchi H. Effect of RU 486 on luteal function in the early pregnant rat. J Reprod Fertil. 1988;83:279–85.

36. Telleria CM, Deis RP. Effect of RU486 on ovarian progesterone production at proestrous and during pregnancy: a possible dual regulation of the biosynthesis of progesterone. J Reprod Fertil. 1994;102:379–84.

37. Takahashi M, Iwata N, Hara S, Mukai T, Takayama M, Endo T. Cyclic change in 3 alpha-hydroxysteroid dehydrogenase in rat ovary during the estrous cycle. Biol Reprod. 1995;53:1265–70.

38. Escudero C, Casas S, Giuliani F, Bazzocchini V, García S, Yunes R, Cabrera R. Allopregnanolone prevents memory impairment: effect on mRNA expression and enzymatic activity of hippocampal 3-alpha hydroxysteroid oxide-reductase. Brain Res Bull. 2012;87:280–5.

39. Amsterdam A, Dantes A, Hosokawa K, Schere-Levy CP, Kotsuji F, Aharoni D. Steroid regulation during apoptosis of ovarian follicular cells. Steroids. 1998; 63:314–8.

40. Levine JE. New concepts of the neuroendocrine regulation of gonadotropin surges in rats. Biol Reprod. 1997;56:293–302.

41. Uilenbrock JTJ, Woutersen PJA, van der Schoot P. Atresia of preovulatory follicles: gonadotropin binding and steroidogenic activity. Biol Reprod. 1980; 23:219–29.

42. Higashi S, Aizawa Y. Effect of ACTH on adrenal estrogens. Jpn J Pharmacol. 1980;30(3):273–8.

43. Micevych P, Sinchak K. The neurosteroid progesterone underlies estrogen positive feedback of the LH surge. Front Endocrinol. 2011;2:1–11.

44. Silvia WJ, Halter TB, Nugent AM, Laranja da Fonseca LF. Ovarian folicular cysts in dairy cows: an abnormality in folliculogenesis. Domest Anim Endocrinol. 2002;23:167–77.

45. Hedström H, Bäckström T, Bixo M, Nyberg S, Wang M, Gideonsson I, Turkmen S. Women with polycystic ovary syndrome have elevated serum concentrations of and altered GABAA receptor sensitivity to allopregnanolone. Clin Endocrinol. 2015;83(5):643–50.

46. Hedström H, Bäckström T, Bixo M, Nyberg S, Wang M, Gideonsson I, Turkmen S. Women with polycystic ovary syndrome have elevated serum concentrations of and altered GABAA receptor sensitivity to allopregnanolone. Clin Endocrinol. 2015;83:643–50.

47. Turkmen S, Andreen L, Cengiz Y. Effects of Roux-en-Y gastric bypass surgery on eating behaviour and allopregnanolone levels in obese women with polycystic ovary syndrome. Gynecol Endocrinol. 2015;31(4):301–5.

48. Zhu WJ, Wang JF, Krueger KE, Vicini S. Delta subunit inhibits neurosteroid modulation of GABAA receptors. J Neurosci. 1996;16(21):6648–56.

49. Hedblom E, Kirkness EF. A novel class of GABAA receptor subunit in tissues of the reproductive system. J Biol Chem. 1997;272(24):15346–50.

50. Huangguan D, Cuifang H, Xin H, Zhenteng L, Huaya L, Chang L. Different transcriptional levels of GABAA receptor subunits in mouse cumulus cells around oocytes at different mature stage. Gyn Endocrinol. 2016;32(12): 1009–13.

51. Faroni A, Magnaghi V. The Neurosteroid Allopregnanolone Modulates Specific Functions in Central and Peripheral Glial Cells. Front Endocrinol (Lausanne). 2011;2:103.

52. Akinci MK, Schofield PR. Widespread expression of GABAA receptor subunits in peripheral tissues. Neurosci Res. 1999;35:145–53.

53. Niswender GD, Juengel JL, Silva PJ, Rollyson MK, McIntush EW. Mechanisms controlling the function and life span of the corpus luteum. Physiol Revi. 2000;80:1–29.

54. Goyeneche AA, Deis RP, Gibori G, Telleria CM. Progesterone promotes survival of the rat corpus luteum in the absence of cognate receptors. Biol Reprod. 2003;68:151–8.

55. Acciliani P, Hernández SF, Bas D, Pazos MC, Irusta G, Abramovich D, Tesone M. A link between Notch and progesterone maintains the functionality of the rat corpus luteum. Reproduction. 2015;149:1–10.

56. McCarthy MM, Felzenberg E, Robbins A, Pfaff DW, Schwartz-Giblin S. Infusions of Diazepam and Allopregnanolone into the Midbrain Central Gray Facilitate Open-Field Behavior and Sexual Receptivity in Female Rats. Horm Behav. 1995;29(3):279–95.

17

Mild ovarian stimulation with letrozole plus fixed dose human menopausal gonadotropin prior to IVF/ICSI for infertile non-obese women with polycystic ovarian syndrome being pre-treated with metformin: a pilot study

Giuseppe D'Amato[1], Anna Maria Caringella[1], Antonio Stanziano[1], Clementina Cantatore[1], Simone Palini[1] and Ettore Caroppo[1,2]* ⓘ

Abstract

Background: Letrozole is widely employed as ovulation induction agent in women with PCOS, but its use in mild stimulation (MS) protocols for IVF is limited. Aim of the present study was to evaluate the feasibility of a MS protocol with letrozole plus hMG in non-obese PCOS women undergoing IVF after a metformin pre-treatment.

Methods: We retrospectively evaluated the data of 125 non-obese PCOS undergoing MS with letrozole plus hMG, 150 IU as starting dose, (group 1, $N = 80$) compared to those undergoing a conventional IVF stimulation protocols (CS) (group 2, $N = 45$) prior to IVF. All patients had received metformin extended release 1200–2000 mg daily for three to six months before IVF. GnRH antagonist was administered in both groups when the leading follicles reached 14 mm.

Results: Both groups were comparable for age, BMI and ovarian reserve markers. Both groups showed lower than expected AFC and AMH values as a consequence of metformin pre-treatment. Letrozole-treated patients required a significantly lower amount of gonadotropins units ($p < 0.0001$), and showed significantly lower day 5, day 8 and hCG day E2 levels compared to patients undergoing the CS protocol ($p < 0.0001$, $p < 0.0001$ and $p = 0.001$ respectively). The oocyte yield, in terms of total (6, IQR 3, vs 6, IQR 4 respectively,) and MII oocytes (5, IQR 3, vs 5, IQR 3, respectively) number, did not differ among groups; the number of total (3, IQR 2, vs 3, IQR 1 respectively) and good quality embryos (2, IQR1 vs 2, IQR 1,5 respectively) obtained was comparable as well in the two groups. The number of fresh transfers was significantly higher in group 1 compared to group 2 (80% vs 60%, $p = 0.016$). A trend for higher cumulative clinical pregnancy rate was found in women undergoing MS compared to CS (42.5%vs 24,4%, $p = 0.044$), but the study was not powered to detect this difference.

Conclusions: The present study suggests that the use of letrozole as adjuvant treatment to MS protocols for IVF may be an effective alternative to CS protocols for non-obese PCOS patients pre-treated with metformin, as it provides comparable IVF outcome without requiring high FSH dose, and avoiding supraphysiological estradiol levels.

Keywords: Letrozole, Human menopausal gonadotropin, Polycystic ovarian syndrome, Mild ovarian stimulation, IVF, Estradiol level, OHSS

---

* Correspondence: ecaroppo@teseo.it
[1]Asl Bari, Department of Maternal and Child Health, Reproductive and IVF Unit, Conversano, BA, Italy
[2]ASL Bari, PTA "F Jaia", Fisiopatologia della Riproduzione Umana e P.M.A, via de Amicis 30, 70014 Conversano, BA, Italy

Background

Mild ovarian stimulation (MS) for in vitro fertilization (IVF) consists in the administration of follicle stimulating hormone (FSH) or human menopausal gonadotropin (hMG) at lower dose and/or for a shorter duration, in a gonadotropin releasing hormone (GnRH)-antagonist co-treated cycle, with or without the concomitant use of oral compounds, antiestrogens or aromatase inhibitors (AI), with the aim of collecting fewer oocytes [1]. It is intended to offer a safer, cost-effective, patient-friendly protocol in which the risks of treatment are minimized [2], and in which the benefits are grossly comparable to those provided by conventional IVF stimulation protocols (CS). Relevant to this point, studies have demonstrated that increasing the FSH may not improve the IVF outcome, since there is no direct relationship between FSH dose and embryo quality [3], and the number of euploid embryos don't differ when MS or conventional ovarian stimulation protocols are employed [4].

Letrozole, together with clomiphene citrate, is one of the mostly used oral compounds in MS protocols, and is preferred to anastrazole due to its higher in vitro inhibitory effect on the enzyme aromatase and reduction of estrogen plasma levels [5]. Letrozole has been also utilized in ovulation induction cycles in clomiphene-resistant women with PCOS, without impacting the endometrial thickness despite the reduced total and per follicle estrogen levels on the day of hCG administration [6]; when compared to clomiphene citrate, it improves pregnancy and live birth rates in subfertile women with anovulatory PCOS [7].

Despite being promising as ovulation induction agent, letrozole has drawn limited attention as adjuvant treatment to MS protocols for IVF/ICSI cycles, as it doesn't appear to significantly improve pregnancy rates compared to the standard controlled ovarian stimulation protocols [8, 9]. As far as we could know, no study has been drawn to evaluate its use in infertile women with polycystic ovary syndrome undergoing IVF.

Aim of this pilot study was, therefore, to evaluate the feasibility of a MS protocol with letrozole plus hMG in non-obese infertile women with PCOS candidates to IVF/ICSI.

Methods

Patients

Among all infertile women with PCOS referred to our Reproductive Unit for couple infertility from January 2014 to December 2017, we retrospectively evaluated those who satisfied the following entry criteria: having received a MS protocol with letrozole plus hMG or a CS with hMG alone in a GnRH antagonist co-treated IVF/ICSI cycle, and having received metformin in the preceding three to six months (see below). Exclusion criteria were age > 40 years, BMI > 26 kg/cm^2, thyroid dysfunction, pituitary tumors,

congenital adrenal hyperplasia, adrenal tumors, Cushing syndrome, androgen-secreting tumors, moderate-to-severe endometriosis. Diagnosis of PCOS was based on the NIH 2012 extension of ESHRE/ASRM 2003 criteria [10].

12 patients in MS group (15%) and 6 (13,3%) in the CS group had an history of IUI cycles (1–3 cycles). None had a previous IVF cycle. Indication to IVF are displayed in Table 1. Since the IUI cycles were performed in other centers before metformin pre-treatment, we did not take into account the previous response to gonadotropin treatment when setting the FSH starting dose.

Before being enrolled for the IVF/ICSI program, all patients received a three to six months pre-treatment with metformin extended release (Glucophage Unidie, Bruno Farmaceutici Italy) 1200–2000 mg daily, in order to reduce the risk of ovarian hyperstimulation syndrome (OHSS) and to suppress the excessive ovarian production of androgens [11]. Obese patients were invited to lose weight by following a hypocaloric low glycemic index diet and exercise; patients whose BMI remained higher than 26 were excluded by the study.

In order to assess eligibility to IVF/ICSI, all patients underwent a careful physical examination, including height and weight measurement. Antral follicle count (AFC) was evaluated in the early follicular phase (day 2–5) by transvaginal ultrasound. Blood tests were performed on day 2 to assess basal FSH, LH, Estradiol (E2) and antimullerian hormone (AMH) serum levels. Endometrial thickness was evaluated by ultrasound.

Ovarian stimulation protocol and study design

125 patients that met the entry criteria were divided in two groups according to the received stimulation protocol: group 1 comprised 80 patients who received Letrozole (Ramates, Just Pharma, Rome, Italy) 2,5 mg daily starting from day 2 through day 6 of the menstrual cycle, plus hMG (Meropur, Ferring Italy) administered at a fixed-dose of 150 IU starting from day 3 to day 6 with further dose adjustments, while group 2 patients comprised 45 women who underwent an individualized, tailored hMG dose regimen starting from day 2 onwards, the starting dose being set according to a nomogram based on patients age, AFC and AMH [12]. The resulting mean ± SD starting dose was 182,22 IU/die ± 14,73 (range 100–300) IU/die. Allocation to treatment groups was determined by patients willingness to receive letrozole: some general practitioners dissuaded their patients from taking letrozole due to the recommendation against its use in premenopausal women provided in the drug label. All patients from group 1 gave written informed consent to the off-label use of letrozole in IVF.

In both groups a GnRH antagonist, Ganirelix acetate (Orgalutran, Merck Sharp & Dohme, UK), was started

Table 1 Comparison of clinical parameters in patients stratified in two groups according to stimulation protocol (letrozole plus HMG or HMG-only)

	Group 1 (Let-HMG)	Group 2 (HMG)	p-value*
N	80	45	/
Age (years)	34.5 (31–37) [24–40]	34 (31.5–36.5) [27–40]	0.959
Male factor infertility (%)	53.7	55.5	0.84
Endometriosis (%)	5	4.4	0.88
Tubal factor (%)	6	4	0.63
BMI (kg/cm^2)	21,9 (20–25) [16–31.5]	23 (20–24) [18–29]	0.736
Basal FSH (mIU/ml)	6.4 (5.3–7.4) [2–12]	6.4 (5.5–7.2) [4.5–9]	0.795
Basal LH (mIU/ml)	5.2 (4.15–6.7) [0.88–11]	4.7 (3.8–6.9) [2.55–11]	0.402
Basal E2 (pg/ml)	42.7 (30.2–59.9) [13–238]	43 (36–51) [13–91]	0.977
Antral follicle count (n)	12 (10–16) [7–27]	12 (10–14) [9–20]	0.316
AMH (ng/ml)	3.5 (2.4–4.9) [1.16–12.3]	4 (2.5–6.7) [1.2–10]	0.222

Data are displayed as median with upper and lower range in round parentheses and ranges in squared parentheses
*Two-tailed Mann-Whitney test

once the leading follicle(s) reached 14 mm in diameter. Serial ultrasound examination and evaluation of serum E2 levels were used to assess follicular maturation and endometrial thickness. Human chorionic gonadotropin (hCG) 7.500 to 10.000 IU s.c. was administered when at least two follicles reached a mean diameters of 18 mm. Progesterone level was assessed at hCG day.

IVF or ICSI was performed as clinically appropriate, with embryo transfer performed either in day 3 or in day 5, since no superiority of blastocyst compared to cleavage-state embryo transfer has been demonstrated [13]. Patients were eligible for frozen embryo transfer when serum progesterone (P) level was higher than 1.75 ng/ml [14] and/or E2 level was higher than 3500 pg/ml on hCG day. Luteal phase was supported by vaginal micronized progesterone 600 mg/day (Progeffik, Effik Italy).

Statistical analysis

Since the observed variables did not follow a normal distribution according to one-sample Kolmogorov-Smirnov test, the differences in clinical parameters and in IVF outcome in patients stratified in two groups according to the stimulation protocol were evaluated by two-sided Mann Whitney U test for continuous variables, by chi square for categorical variables, and by z-test for proportions.

Statistical significance was set at $p < 0.05$ for all analyses. All computations were performed using SPSS for Windows.

IRB approval

The present study was approved by the local IRB (IEC Azienda Ospedaliera Universitaria Policlinico di Bari, register number 4990, April 5, 2016).

Results

Patients clinical parameters are summarized in Table 1. Both groups were comparable for age, BMI and ovarian reserve markers.

Table 2 display the stimulation and IVF outcome variables obtained to both group of patients. Group 1 patients required a significantly lower amount of gonadotropins units, and showed significantly lower day 5, day 8 and hCG day E2 levels compared to group 2 (Fig. 1). This difference in E2 level, however, did not affect the number of maturing follicles (Table 3), which were comparable among groups.

The use of letrozole did not impact on progesterone levels (at hCG day) and on endometrial thickness, both resulting comparable among groups; on the other hand, MS with letrozole resulted in an higher percentage of fresh cycles compared to the CS protocol (80 vs 60%, $p = 0.016$). In the MS group, the freeze-all policy was applied to 16 patients (20%): in 9 cases for elevated E2 levels, in 5 cases for P rise, in 2 patients for both factors. In the CS group, the freeze-all strategy was applied to 18 patients (40%): 11 cases for high E2 levels, in 4 cases for P rise, in 3 cases for both reasons. 6 patients (7%) in MS group and 12 (26,6%) in the CS group (p-value = 0.0036) received a GnRH agonist trigger (0,3 mg of triptorelin) to prevent OHSS. No patient from both groups needed hospitalization for OHSS.

The oocyte yield, in terms of total and MII oocytes number, did not differ among groups; the number of total and good quality embryos obtained was comparable as well in the two groups.

The clinical pregnancy rate (CPR) in fresh transfers did not differ among groups; only a trend for higher cumulative CPR was observed in group 1 compared to group 2 (critical z 1.9599640, 1-β 0.55).

Table 2 Stimulation and IVF outcome variables of PCOS patients under letrozole plus HMG or HMG-only stimulation protocol

	Group 1 (Let-HMG)	Group 2 (HMG)	p-value
Days of stimulation (N)	11 (10–12) [8–15]	10 (10–12) [9–15]	0.246*
HMG dose (units)	1350 (1200–1500) [626–2475]	1800 (1337–3110) [1050–5325]	< 0.0001*ᵖ
E2 day 5 (pg/ml)	103 (73–182) [14–495]	525 (284–703) [82–1328]	< 0.0001*ᵖ
E2 day 8 (pg/ml)	502 (322–826) [39–1639]	1056 (829–1439) [147–4244]	< 0.0001*ᵖ
E2 hcg day (pg/ml)	1538 (1043–2391) [300–7845]	2561 (1600–3238) [482–7793]	0.001*
Progesterone at hCG day (ng/ml)	0.8 (0.6–1.1) [0.17–2.5]	0.86 (0.6–1.37) [0.2–4.9]	0.183*
Endometrial thickness (mm)	9.5 (8.6–10.7) [6.7–13]	10 (8.7–10.9) [7.3–15.3]	0.25*
N. oocytes retrieved	6 (5–8) [3–17]	6 (5–9) [3–17]	0.361*
N. MII oocytes	5 (4–7) [2–12]	5 (4–7) [2–14]	0.593*
hCG day E2/follicles > 16 mm ratio	193 (128–292) [28–569]	320 (219–434) [87–974]	< 0.0001ᵖ
hCG day E2/total oocyte ratio	233 (169–329([53–590]	372 (309–660) [116–1025]	0.001ᵖ
hCG E2/MII oocytes ratio	313 (221–430) [60–1077]	473 (309–660) [120–1025]	0.001ᵖ
N. embryos	3 (2–4) [1–12]	3 (2–3) [1–9]	0.895*
N. good quality embryos	2 (2–3) [0–8]	2 (1.5–3) [0–5]	0.864*
N. transferred embryos	2 (2–3) [1–3]	2 (2–3) [0–3]	0.605*
N. good quality embryos transferred	2 (1–2) [0–3]	2 (1–2) [0–3]	0.815*
N. fresh cycles (%)	80	60	0.016#
Fertilization rate (%)	78.9	79.9	0.941#
Pregnancy rate in fresh cycles N (%)	33/64 (51)	10/36 (27.7)	0.021§
Clinical pregnancy rate in fresh cycles N (%)	30/64 (46.8)	10/36 (27.7)	0.061§
Cumulative pregnancy rates (fresh + cryo) N (%)	36/80 (48.7)	12/45 (26.6)	0.016§ᵖ
Cumulative clinical pregnancy rate N(%)	34/80 (42.5)	11/45 (24.4)	0.044§

Data are displayed as median with upper and lower range in round parentheses and ranges in squared parentheses, or as count with percentages in parentheses
*Two-tailed Mann-Whitney test
#2-sided Pearson Chi-square test
§Z-test for two independent proportions
ᵖthe study is powered to detect this difference

No side effects were reported by patients who received Letrozole.

Discussion

The results of this pilot study suggest that a mild stimulation protocol with Letrozole may represent an effective alternative to standard IVF stimulation protocols for non-obese PCOS women pre-treated with metformin, as it provides a comparable IVF outcome to the standard GnRH antagonist protocol, with the advantage of reducing the FSH dose, lowering the estradiol levels under stimulation, and reducing the need of embryo cryopreservation to prevent OHSS.

It has been proposed that the major advantage of using MS protocols is to allow the development of the healthier follicles with more competent eggs, given that higher gonadotropins dose may disrupt the physiologic hormonal milieu inside the follicles [15]. Indeed, earlier studies suggest that CS protocols may have a negative impact on the developmental and implantation potential of human embryos [reviewed in 2]. These results were challenged by other studies demonstrating that the degree of exposure to exogenous gonadotropins did not significantly modify the likelihood of blastocyst aneuploidy in patients with a normal ovarian response to stimulation [16]; relevantly, those earlier results were obtained from the analysis of cleavage stage embryos, so that the embryos aneuploidy rates were artificially increased by the inclusion of mosaic embryos with likely innate abilities to self-correct downstream beyond blastocyst stage (reviewed in [17]).

It has to be highlighted that the patients enrolled in the present study displayed lower than expected AFC and AMH values. The median AFC found in our patients was comparable, while the median AMH was slightly higher, than that of an age-matched cohort of 5705 women comprising poor, normal and hyperresponders, [18]. It has to be pointed out, however, that AMH and AFC values were obtained at the end of metformin treatment and before the start of the stimulation protocols: since metformin has been found to significantly reduce both AMH and AFC in PCOS patients [19] we

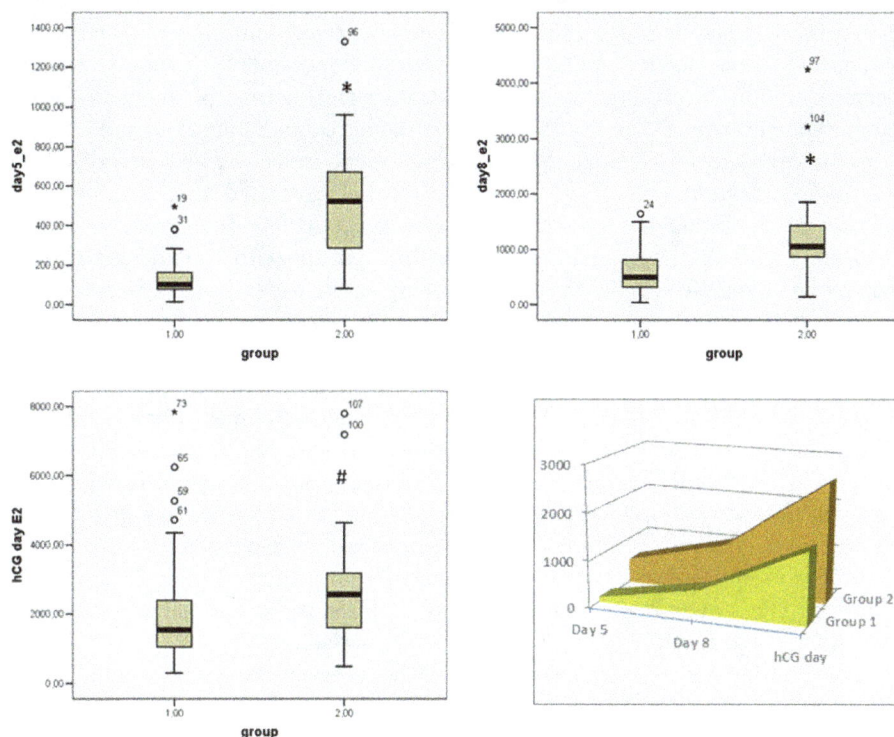

Fig. 1 Serum estradiol levels during ovarian stimulation protocol in patients with PCOS receiving letrozole plus fixed-dose hMG (Group 1) or tailored dose hMG (Group 2). A – C: Box plot displaying the estradiol levels in stimulation day 5 (A), 8 (B) and at hCG day (C). D: area graph displaying the dynamic of estradiol levels rise during ovarian stimulation in the two groups of patients. * = $p < 0.0001$

hypothesize that the resulting AFC and AMH values are the consequence of metformin treatment. The mechanism trough which metformin reduces AFC and AMH hasn't been fully clarified to date, although the demonstrated effect on metformin in reducing the number of primary, preantral and atretic follicles while increasing that of antral follicles by angiogenic factors levels restoration [20] could explain this finding. Also the low number of oocytes obtained in both groups may be explained by the lower AFC and AMH values than expected in PCOS patients. Still the number of MII oocytes was extremely variable in both groups, ranging from 2 to 12 and from 2 to 14 in both groups respectively (Table 2),

this variability being probably due to the wide age range of patients enrolled in the study (24–40 and 27–40 respectively, Table 1).

MS protocols may also improve/optimize the endometrial receptivity by lowering the estradiol levels [15]. It has been demonstrated that supraphysiologic estradiol levels may impact on the endometrial receptivity [21, 22]. Recent large-sample studies has even found that supraphysiologic estradiol levels may expose the offspring to an higher risk of low birth weight [23–25].

Although MS cannot be used as first line protocol for every patient [8, 17], the present study is suggestive for its preferable employment in non-obese PCOS patients

Table 3 Ovarian follicles behavior under letrozole plus HMG or HMG-only stimulation protocol

Parameter	GROUP 1 (LET-HMG)	GROUP 2 (HMG)	p-value*
Day 5 follicles < 10 mm	9 (5.5–11) [0–21]	9 (8–13) [4–20]	0.097
Day 8 follicles < 10 mm	4 (2–7) [0–13]	5 (4–8) [2–18]	0.031[P]
hCG day follicles < 10 mm	3 (0–4) [0–11]	4 (2–4.7) [0–13]	0.024[P]
Day 5 follicles > 11 mm	3 (1–5.5) [0–20]	2 (1–4) [0–8]	0.131
Day 8 follicles > 13 mm	6 (5–8) [0–23]	5 (2–7) [1–20]	0.009[P]
hCG day follicles > 16 mm	7 (6–9) [3–25]	7 (6–9) [3–15]	0.836

Data are displayed as median with upper and lower range in round parentheses and ranges in squared parentheses
*Two-tailed Mann-Whitney test
[P]the study is powered to detect this difference

pretreated with metformin, as it provided a comparable IVF outcome to CS despite significantly lower estradiol-to-follicles and estradiol-to-MII oocytes ratios (Table 2), suggesting that higher estradiol levels are unneeded when letrozole is employed. The reason for this finding could be explained by the dynamics of androgen secretion following letrozole administration.

Letrozole plays its role by inhibiting the cytochrome P450 isoenzymes 2A6 and 2C19 of the aromatase enzyme complex, resulting in a release of the hypothalamic–pituitary axis from estrogenic negative feedback and, consequently, in stronger GnRH pulses and FSH secretion rise, with the consequential stimulating effect on the growth of ovarian follicles [26]. In addition, the increase of intra-ovarian androgens, secondary to aromatase inhibition, augments the follicular sensitivity to FSH and enhances the early follicular growth. Several studies have demonstrated a direct relationship between androgen receptor (AR) mRNA and FSH receptor (FSHr) in granulosa cells, as well as the priming effect of androgens on FSHr expression modulated by the enhanced AR expression (reviewed in [27]). The relationship between AR and FSHr in granulosa cells is amplified in PCOS patients [28]. Moreover, androgens have been found to attenuate follicular atresia through nuclear and extranuclear signaling pathway by enhancing the expression of the microRNA miR-125b [29]. When Letrozole is administered in the early follicular phase, an increased expression of FSHrs together with an higher FSH release from the pituitary is expected, resulting in increased androgen pool which prevent follicular atresia. High androgen levels could, therefore, promote follicular growth in the early follicular phase in a way that could be independent, to a certain extent, from estradiol level. Indeed, at that stage the estradiol levels were very low in letrozole-treated patients compared to controls (Table 2). Interestingly, it has been demonstrated that lower estradiol levels in the early follicular phase don't affect the follicular development [30]. Conversely, when follicles growth proceeds, the role of androgens in follicular growth begins negligible; indeed, a lower expression of the AR gene in human GC in the large pre-ovulatory follicles compared to small ones have been reported [28, 31].

Another potentially beneficial effect of using the present MS protocol for IVF in non-obese PCOS women is the lower need to proceed with embryo cryopreservation to prevent OHSS compared to controls. It has been suggested that reducing the need of frozen embryo transfer could have a beneficial impact on the perinatal outcome of IVF singletons [32, 33], as embryo cryopreservation may promote alteration of DNA methylation reprogramming enzymes [34].

Letrozole is still contraindicated in premenopausal women due to the results of a follow up study, presented at the 2005 ASRM meeting but never published on a peer reviewed journal, on 150 babies born to women who took letrozole for ovulation induction, showing that cardiac and locomotor anomalies were overrepresented in the letrozole babies compared with the control group of normal fertile women Indeed, a further multicentre study demonstrated that the major malformation rate was lower in letrozole group compared to clomiphene citrate group, with the incidence of cardiac anomalies being seven times lower compared to clomiphene [35]. Recently, letrozole has been even found to significantly decrease the risk of miscarriage, without increasing the risk of major congenital anomalies or adverse pregnancy or neonatal outcomes, when compared with natural cycles in patients undergoing ART [36]. Still, as no therapeutic indication has been listed for ovulation induction or IVF in the letrozole package information, and the recommendation against its use in premenopausal women persists, obtaining IRB approvals for clinical trials aiming at evaluating the use of letrozole in MS-IVF protocols remains challenging.

The present study has some limitations. Data have been retrospectively evaluated, however since all data were stored in a database management system being in use to the IVF unit, no data was missed. The study sample size, although large enough to reject the null hypothesis in some comparisons (see Tables 2-3), is too small to allow generalization of our findings with regards to the IVF outcome. It has to be highlighted, furthermore, that the results of the present study may apply only to non-obese PCOS women pre-treated with metformin for at least three months, in view of the lower than expected AFC and AMH values observed in our patients.

Conclusions

In conclusion, the present study suggests that the use of letrozole as adjuvant treatment to mild stimulation protocols for IVF may be a safe and cost-effective an effective alternative to standard ovarian stimulation protocols for non-obese PCOS patients undergoing metformin pre-treatment, as it provides comparable IVF outcome without requiring high FSH dose, and avoids supraphysiological estradiol levels, which may be detrimental to the developmental and implantation potential of embryos.

Abbreviations
AFC: Antral follicle count; AMH: Anti mullerian hormone; CS: Conventional IVF stimulation protocols; E2: Estradiol; GnRH: Gonadotropin releasing hormone; hCG: Human chorionic gonadotropin; HMG: Human menopausal gonadotropin; ICSI: Intracytoplasmic sperm injection; IVF: In vitro fertilization; MII: Metaphase II; MS: Mild stimulation; OHSS: Ovarian hyperstimulation syndrome; PCOS: Polycystic ovarian syndrome

Acknowledgements
We grateful acknowledge the Reviewers for their thoughtful and detailed comments that significantly helped us in improving the manuscript quality.

Authors' contributions

GD: conception and design of the study. AMC: performed the research and acquired the data. AS: performed the research. CC: performed the research. SP: collected all the embryological data. EC: study design, data analysis and interpretation, manuscript drafting. Each Author gave final approval of the version to be published.

Competing interests

The authors declare that they have no competing interests.

References

1. Nargund G, Fauser BC, Macklon NS, Ombelet W, Nygren K, Frydman R. Rotterdam ISMAAR consensus group on terminology for ovarian stimulation for IVF. The ISMAAR proposal on terminology for ovarian stimulation for IVF. Hum Reprod. 2007;22:2801–4.
2. Verberg MFG, Macklon NS, Nargund G, Frydman R, Devroey P, Broekmans FJ, Fauser BCJM. Mild ovarian stimulation for IVF. Hum Reprod Update. 2009;15:13–29.
3. Arce JC, Andersen AN, Fernández-Sánchez M, Visnova H, Bosch E, García-Velasco JA, Barri P, de Sutter P, Klein BM, Fauser BC. Ovarian response to recombinant human follicle-stimulating hormone: a randomized, antimüllerian hormone-stratified, dose-response trial in women undergoing in vitro fertilization/intracytoplasmic sperm injection. Fertil Steril. 2014;102:1633–40.
4. Baart EB, Martini E, Eijkemans MJ, Van Opstal D, Beckers NG, Verhoeff A, Macklon NS, Fauser BC. Milder ovarian stimulation for in-vitro fertilization reduces aneuploidy in the human preimplantation embryo: a randomized controlled trial. Hum Reprod. 2007;22(4):980–8.
5. Bhatnagar AS, Hausler A, Schieweck K, Lang M, Bowman R. Highly selective inhibition of estrogen biosynthesis by CGS 20267, a new non-steroidal aromatase inhibitor. J Steroid Biochem Mol Biol. 1990;37:1021–7.
6. Mitwally MFM, Casper RF. Use of an aromatase inhibitor for induction of ovulation in patients with an inadequate response to clomiphene citrate. Fertil Steril. 2000;75:305–9.
7. Franik S, Kremer JAM, Nelen WLDM, Farquhar C. Aromatase inhibitors for subfertile women with polycystic ovary syndrome. Cochrane Database Syst Rev. 2014;2:CD010287.
8. Papanikolaou EG, Polyzos NP, Humaidan P, Pados G, Bosch E, Tournaye H, Tarlatzis B. Aromatase inhibitors in stimulated IVF cycles. Reprod Biol Endocrinol. 2011;9:85.
9. Haas J, Casper RF. In vitro fertilization with the use of clomiphene citrate or letrozole. Fertil Steril. 2017;108:568–71.
10. National Institutes of Health. Evidence-based methodology workshop on polycystic ovary syndrome, December 3–5, 2012. Executive summary. Available at: https://prevention.nih.gov/docs/programs/pcos/FinalReport.pdf
11. Tso LO, Costello MF, Albuquerque LE, Andriolo RB, Macedo CR. Metformin treatment before and during IVF or ICSI in women with polycystic ovary syndrome. Cochrane Database Syst Rev. 2014;11:CD006105.
12. La Marca A, Sunkara SK. Individualization of controlled ovarian stimulation in IVF using ovarian reserve markers: from theory to practice. Hum Reprod Update. 2014;20:124–40.
13. Martins WP, Nastri CO, Rienzi L, van der Poel SZ, Gracia C, Racowsky C. Blastocyst vs cleavage-state embryo transfer: systematic review and meta-analysis of reproductive outcomes. Ultrasound Obstet Gynecol. 2017;49:583–91.
14. Venetis CA, Kolibianakis EM, Bosdou JK, Tarlatzis BC. Progesterone elevation and probability of pregnancy after IVF: a systematic review and meta-analysis of over 60 000 cycles. Hum Reprod Update. 2013;19:433–57.
15. Nargund G, Kumar Datta A, Fauser BCJM. Mild stimulation for in vitro fertilization. Fertil Steril. 2017;108:558–67.
16. Sekhon L, Shaia K, Santistevan A, Cohn KH, Lee JA, Beim PY, Copperman AB. The cumulative dose of gonadotropins used for controlled ovarian stimulation does not influence the odds of embryonic aneuploidy in patients with normal ovarian response. J Assist Reprod Genet. 2017;34:749–58.
17. Orvieto R, Vanni VS, Gleicher N. The myths surrounding mild stimulation in vitro fertilization (IVF). Reprod Biol Endocrinol. 2017;15:48.
18. Broer SL, van Disseldorp J, Broeze KA, Dolleman M, Opmeer BC, Bossuyt P, Eijkemans MJ, Mol BW, Broekmans FJ. IMPORT study group. Added value of ovarian reserve testing on patient characteristics in the prediction of ovarian response and ongoing pregnancy: an individual patient data approach. Hum Reprod Update. 2013;19:26–36.
19. Piltonen T, Morin-Papunen L, Koivunen R, Perheentupa A, Ruokonen A, Tapanainen JS. Serum anti-Müllerian hormone levels remain high until late reproductive age and decrease during metformin therapy in women with polycystic ovary syndrome. Hum Reprod. 2005;20:1820–6.
20. Di Pietro M, Parborell F, Irusta G, Pascuali N, Bas D, Bianchi MS, Tesone M, Abramovich D. Metformin regulates ovarian angiogenesis and follicular development in a female polycystic ovary syndrome rat model. Endocrinology. 2015;156:1453–63.
21. Haouzi D, Assou S, Dechanet C, Anahory T, Dechaud H, De Vos J, et al. Controlled ovarian hyperstimulation for in vitro fertilization alters endometrial receptivity in humans: protocol effects. Biol Reprod. 2010;82:679–86.
22. Zhang Y, Chen Q, Zhang H, Wang Q, Li R, Jin Y, Wang H, Ma T, Qiao J, Duan E. Aquaporin-dependent excessive intrauterine fluid accumulation is a major contributor in hyper-estrogen induced aberrant embryo implantation. Cell Res. 2015;25:139–42.
23. Pereira N, Elias RT, Christos PJ, Petrini AC, Hancock K, Lekvich JP, Rosenwaks Z. Supraphysiologic estradiol is an independent predictor of low birth weight in full-term singletons born after fresh embryo transfer. Hum Reprod. 2017;13:1–8.
24. Liu S, Kuang Y, Wu Y, Feng Y, Lyu Q, Wang L, Sun Y, Sun X. High oestradiol concentration after ovarian stimulation is associated with lower maternal serum beta-hCG concentration and neonatal birth weight. Reprod BioMed Online. 2017;35:189–96.
25. Imudia A, Awonuga AO, Doyle JO, Kaimal AJ, Wright DL, Toth TL, Styer AK. Peak serum estradiol level during controlled ovarian hyperstimulation is associated with increased risk of small for gestational age and preeclampsia in singleton pregnancies after in vitro fertilization. Fertil Steril. 2012;97:1374–9.
26. Casper RF, Mitwally MFM. Review: aromatase inhibitors for ovulation induction. J Clin Endocrinol Metab. 2006;91:760–71.
27. Dewailly D, Robin G, Peigne M, Decanter C, Pigny P, Catteau-Jonard S. Interactions between androgens, FSH, anti-Müllerian hormone and estradiol during folliculogenesis in the human normal and polycystic ovary. Hum Reprod Update. 2016;22:709–24.
28. Catteau-Jonard S, Jamin SP, Leclerc A, Gonzales J, Dewailly D, di Clemente N. Anti-Mullerian hormone, its receptor, FSH receptor, and androgen receptor genes are overexpressed by granulosa cells from stimulated follicles in women with polycystic ovary syndrome. J Clin Endocrinol Metab. 2008;93:4456–61.
29. Sen A, Prizant H, Light A, Biswas A, Hayes E, Lee H-J, Barad D, Gleicher N, Hammes SR. Androgens regulate ovarian follicular development by increasing follicle stimulating hormone receptor and microRNA-125b expression. Proc Natl Acad Sci U S A. 2014;111:3008–13.
30. Kolibianakis EM, Albano C, Camus M, Tournaye H, Van Steirteghem AC, Devroey P. Initiation of gonadotropin-releasing hormone antagonist on day 1 as compared to day 6 of stimulation: effect on hormonal levels and follicular development in in vitro fertilization cycles. J Clin Endocrinol Metab. 2003;88:5632–7.
31. Prizant H, Gleicher N, Sen A. Androgen actions in the ovary: balance is key. J Endocrinol. 2014;222:R141–51.
32. Nelissen EC, Van Montfoort AP, Coonen E, Derhaag JG, Geraedts JP, Smiths LJ, Land JA, Evers JL, Dumoulin JC. Further evidence that culture media

affect perinatal outcome: findings after transfer of fresh and cryopreserved embryos. Hum Reprod. 2012;27:1966–7.

33. Korosec S, Frangez HB, Steblovnik L, Verdenik I, Bokal EV. Independent factors influencing large-for-gestation birth weight in singletons born after in vitro fertilization. J Assist Reprod Genet. 2016;33:9–17.

34. Petrussa L, Van de Velde H, De Rycke M. Dynamic regulation of DNA methyltransferases in human oocytes and preimplantation embryos after assisted reproductive technologies. Mol Hum Reprod. 2014;20:861–74.

35. Tulandi T, Martin J, Al-Fadhli R, Kabli N, Forman R, Hitkari J, Librach C, Greenblatt E, Casper RF. Congenital malformations among 911 newborns conceived after infertility treatment with letrozole or clomiphene citrate. Fertil Steril. 2006;85:1761–5.

36. Tatsumi T, Jwa SC, Kuwahara A, Irahara M, Kubota T, Saito H. No increased risk of major congenital anomalies or adverse pregnancy or neonatal outcomes following letrozole use in assisted reproductive technology. Hum Reprod. 2017;32:125–32.

18

Body mass index and basal androstenedione are independent risk factors for miscarriage in polycystic ovary syndrome

Wan Yang[1], Rui Yang[1], Mingmei Lin[1], Yan Yang[1], Xueling Song[1], Jiajia Zhang[1], Shuo Yang[1], Ying Song[1], Jia Li[1], Tianshu Pang[1], Feng Deng[1], Hua Zhang[2], Ying Wang[1*], Rong Li[1] and Jie Jiao[1]

Abstract

Background: There is limited literature investigating the effects of body mass index (BMI) and androgen level on in vitro fertilization (IVF) outcomes with a gonadotropin-releasing hormone (GnRH)-antagonist protocol in polycystic ovary syndrome (PCOS). Androgen-related variation in the effect of body mass index (BMI) on IVF outcomes remains unknown.

Methods: In this retrospective study, 583 infertile women with PCOS who underwent IVF using the conventional GnRH-antagonist protocol were included. Patients were divided into four groups according to BMI and androgen level: overweight- hyperandrogenism(HA) group, $n = 96$, overweight-non-HA group, $n = 117$, non-overweight-HA group, $n = 152$, and non-overweight-non-HA group, $n = 218$.

Results: A significantly higher number of oocytes were retrieved, and the total Gn consumption as well Gn consumption per day was significantly lower, in the non-overweight groups than in the overweight groups. The number of available embryos was significantly higher in the HA groups than in the non-HA groups. Clinical pregnancy rate was of no significant difference among four groups. Live-birth rates in the overweight groups were significantly lower than those in non-overweight-non-HA group (23.9, 28.4% vs. 42.5%, $P<0.05$). The miscarriage rate in overweight-HA group was significantly higher than that in non-overweight-non-HA group (45.2% vs. 14.5%, $P<0.05$). Multivariate logistic regression analysis revealed that BMI and basal androstenedione (AND) both acted as significantly influent factors on miscarriage rate. The area under the curve (AUC) in receiver operating characteristic (ROC) analysis for BMI and basal AND on miscarriage rate were 0.607 ($P = 0.029$) and 0.657 ($P = 0.001$), respectively, and the cut-off values of BMI and basal AND were 25.335 kg/m^2 and 10.95 nmol/L, respectively.

Conclusions: In IVF cycles with GnRH-antagonist protocol, economic benefits were seen in non-overweight patients with PCOS, with less Gn cost and more retrieved oocytes. BMI and basal AND were both significantly influential factors with moderate predictive ability on the miscarriage rate. The predictive value of basal AND on miscarriage was slightly stronger than BMI.

Keywords: Gonadotropin-releasing hormone antagonist, Polycystic ovary syndrome, Hyperandrogenism, Body mass index, In vitro fertilization

* Correspondence: wang_163ying@163.com
[1]Center for Reproductive Medicine, Department of Obstetrics and Gynecology, Peking University Third Hospital, 49 N Garden Rd, Haidian District, Beijing 100191, China
Full list of author information is available at the end of the article

Introduction

For infertile women with polycystic ovary syndrome (PCOS) who fail lifestyle intervention and ovulation induction therapy or who have additional infertility factors, in vitro fertilization (IVF) can be used. Moderate evidence suggests that a gonadotropin (Gn)-releasing hormone (GnRH)-antagonist protocol can significantly reduce the incidence of ovarian hyperstimulation syndrome (OHSS) [1–3], and the use of a GnRH-antagonist protocol is gradually being adopted by clinicians. Phenotypic expressions of PCOS include oligo-ovulation/anovulation, hyperandrogenism (HA), polycystic ovaries, overweight/ obesity, and insulin resistance/metabolic syndrome [4]. There is limited literature investigating the clinical phenotype of patients with PCOS who can benefit the most from a GnRH-antagonist protocol during IVF.

In China, 34.63% of patients with PCOS have a body mass index (BMI) above 23 kg/m^2 [5]. There are different opinions about the role of BMI in IVF outcomes. In 2016, Provost et al. [6] analyzed a total of 239,127 fresh IVF cycles and demonstrated a progressive and statistically significant worsening of outcomes in groups with higher BMIs, including cycles performed specifically for PCOS or male-factor infertility. Bailey et al. [7] also indicated that obese women with PCOS had lower odds of clinical pregnancy and live birth than lean women with PCOS, while there was a trend toward decreased OHSS incidence with increasing BMI among women with PCOS. However, Dechaud et al. [8] showed that obese patients required a higher recombinant follicle-stimulating hormone (r-FSH) dose, but it did not have any adverse impact on IVF, including the cancellation rate, implantation rate, and pregnancy rate. Metwally et al. [9] found that obesity adversely affected embryo quality in young women undergoing IVF/intracytoplasmic sperm injection, while the oocyte quality was not affected.

The prevalence of biochemical HA in patients with PCOS is 78.2% [10]. Studies on the role of HA in IVF outcomes are limited. A recent study reported that HA in women with PCOS did not compromise IVF results, in contrast, facilitated the retrieval of a significantly higher number of oocytes [11]. In our recent study, HA also had a positive effect on the number of retrieved oocytes, where it is associated with miscarriage rate as well [12]. Conversely, another study inferred that the combination of HA and chronic anovulation was associated with a negative impact on the clinical pregnancy rate in patients with PCOS [13]. Endocrine disturbances are complicated in patients with PCOS. HA and obesity interact with each other and promote the progression of PCOS. However, few studies to date have investigated BMI and androgen level together. Therefore, the present study was designed to evaluate whether the effect of BMI on IVF outcomes vary with the level of androgen in PCOS with a GnRH-antagonist protocol.

Materials and methods

Between January 2013 and December 2015, a total of 583 infertile patients with PCOS treated with the conventional GnRH-antagonist protocol at the Center for Reproductive Medicine of Peking University Third Hospital were screened and enrolled in the study. Patients with PCOS between 20 and 35 years of age who were undergoing their first IVF cycle were included. Exclusion criteria included endometriosis, previous ovarian surgical history, hydrosalpinx, severe oligoasthenospermia or azoospermia, and systemic diseases such as diabetes mellitus and hypo- or hyperthyroidism. This retrospective cohort study was approved by the Institutional Review Board of the Department of Obstetrics and Gynecology, Peking University Third Hospital of Beijing, China.

In all cases, PCOS was diagnosed according to the Rotterdam 2003 criteria [14]. BMI was calculated by the following formula: $BMI = weight/height^2 \text{ (kg/m}^2)$. HA was diagnosed by a testosterone level $\geq 2.2 \text{ nmol/L}$ or AND level $\geq 12 \text{ nmol/L}$. Testosterone and AND levels were obtained from basal sex hormone assessments. This cohort study included four groups of patients with PCOS: $BMI \geq 25 \text{ kg/m}^2$ with HA (overweight-HA group, $n = 96$), $BMI \geq 25 \text{ kg/m}^2$ with normal androgen (overweight-non-HA group, $n = 117$), $BMI < 25 \text{ kg/m}^2$ with HA (non-overweight-HA group, $n = 152$), and $BMI < 25 \text{ kg/m}^2$ with normal androgen (non-overweight-non-HA group, $n = 218$).

All patients were stimulated with a combination of a GnRH antagonist (cetrorelix; SeronoMunich, Germany) and an r-FSH drug (Gonal-f; Merck Serono, Munich, Germany) to develop multiple follicles. Controlled ovarian hyperstimulation was started from 2nd day of the menstrual period when no follicle > 10 mm in diameter was detected by ultrasound, and serum estradiol levels were < 50 pg/mL. The Gn dose was modified in accordance with the ovarian response. Highly purified human menopausal gonadotropin (menogon; Ferring, Kiel, Germany) was occasionally added. A GnRH antagonist was injected subcutaneously at a daily dose of 0.25 mg when follicles with a mean diameter $\geq 14 \text{ mm}$ were detected. The criterion for administration of recombinant human chorionic gonadotropin (hCG) (250 µg) was the observation of at least two follicles with a mean diameter $\geq 18 \text{ mm}$. Thirty-six hours after the trigger, oocyte retrieval was performed with ultrasound guidance, using a 16-G double-lumen aspiration needle. Conventional fertilization and embryo culture were performed. In cases where the number of retrieved oocytes was ≥ 20 or estradiol levels were above 15,000 pmol/L on the day of hCG administration, all available embryos were cryopreserved by the vitrification method for future transfer to prevent OHSS. Two embryos were transferred three days after oocyte retrieval. Supportive therapy with progesterone was administered vaginally (90 mg daily), starting on the day of oocyte collection, and was continued until 10 weeks of gestation.

Primary outcome measures were rate of clinical pregnancy, miscarriage rate, and rate of live birth. Secondary outcome measures were Gn dosage, number of oocytes collected, and number of available embryos.

Data were analyzed with SPSS 20.0 (Chicago, IL). The chi-square test was used for categorical variables, and analysis of variance was used for continuous variables. Logistic regression analysis was performed using these binary variables in a forward stepwise method. The optimal cut-off values were calculated by receiver operating characteristic (ROC) analysis using the Youden index. A P value of < 0.05 was considered statistically significant for all analyses.

Results

Baseline characteristics of patients are shown in Table 1. There were no significant differences in age, basal FSH, and antral follicle count between the groups. The duration of infertility was significantly higher in the overweight groups than in the non-overweight groups. The basal luteinizing hormone (LH) levels were significantly higher in the HA groups than in the non-HA groups.

Characteristics of ovarian responses among the four patient groups are shown in Table 2. The number of oocytes retrieved and the estradiol levels on the day of hCG administration were significantly higher in the non-overweight groups than in the overweight groups, although the total Gn consumption, as well as Gn consumption per day, was significantly lower in the non-overweight groups. Despite the effect of BMI, Gn consumption per kilogram was significantly lower in the HA groups. As with the number of oocytes retrieved, the cancellation rates of embryo transfer to prevent OHSS were significantly higher in the non-overweight groups than in the overweight

groups. Unlike the basal LH levels that were related to basal androgen levels, LH levels on the day of hCG administration were significantly lower in the non-overweight groups than in the overweight groups. The number of available embryos was higher in non-overweight-HA group than in overweight-non-HA group. The level of progesterone (P4) and the endometrial thickness on the day of hCG administration were not different among the four groups. Similarly, the fertilization rate and the cleavage rate were comparable among the four groups.

Pregnancy outcomes are presented in Table 3. The miscarriage rate was significantly higher in overweight-HA group than in non-overweight-non-HA group. The live-birth rates were significantly lower in the overweight groups than in non-overweight-non-HA group. There were no ectopic pregnancies in HA groups. There were no differences in the rates of clinical pregnancy, preterm pregnancy, twin pregnancy, or caesarean section among the study groups.

Multivariate logistic regression analyses and ROC analysis were performed to define the predictive factors of miscarriage rate. Parameters that could have adverse effects on miscarriage rate were age, BMI, basal testosterone, basal AND, Gn consumption/kg/day, and number of oocytes retrieved. These parameters, as well as LH levels (both basal LH and LH on the day of hCG administration), were chosen for multivariate logistic regression analyses. After adjusting the effects of other parameters, BMI and basal AND showed independently significant differences in predicting the miscarriage rate (Table 4). A ROC analysis was performed to define the optimal cut-off values of BMI and basal AND (Fig. 1). The areas under the curve (AUCs) for the BMI and basal AND were 0.607 ($P = 0.029$) and 0.657 ($P = 0.001$), respectively (Table 5). These two parameters were demonstrated to have moderate predictive ability on miscarriage, with a sensitivity of 0.511–0.723 and a specificity of 0.584–0.737.

Table 1 Baseline characteristics of patients

Parameter	Non-overweight		Overweight		P value
	Non-HA ($n = 218$)	HA ($n = 152$)	Non-HA ($n = 117$)	HA ($n = 96$)	
Age (y)	29.2 ± 3.6	29.0 ± 3.4	29.8 ± 3.2	29.1 ± 3.2	NS
BMI (kg/m²)	21.5 ± 2.1 [a]	21.6 ± 2.2 [a]	28.5 ± 2.3 [b]	28.7 ± 3.1 [b]	<0.001
Infertile duration (y)	3.7 ± 2.5 [a]	3.7 ± 2.1 [a]	4.6 ± 2.7 [b]	4.4 ± 2.8 [b]	<0.001
Basal FSH (IU/L)	6.1 ± 1.5	6.3 ± 1.8	5.9 ± 1.8	6.1 ± 1.7	NS
Basal LH (IU/L)	5.7 ± 3.8 [a]	9.7 ± 5.9 [b]	5.5 ± 3.8 [a]	8.9 ± 4.6 [b]	<0.001
Basal T(ng/ml)	0.8 ± 0.3 [a]	1.4 ± 1.0 [b]	0.9 ± 0.3 [a]	2.0 ± 3.0 [c]	<0.001
Basal AND (nmol/L)	8.0 ± 2.5 [a]	17.3 ± 6.0 [b]	8.6 ± 2.3 [a]	19.2 ± 7.3 [c]	<0.001
Total AFC (n)	19.0 ± 6	19.8 ± 5	19.1 ± 6	20.8 ± 7	NS

Data are presented as mean ± standard deviation unless otherwise specified

NS not significant; *HA* hyperandrogenism; *AFC* antral follicle count; *BMI* body mass index; *FSH* follicle-stimulating hormone; *LH* luteinizing hormone; *T* testosterone; *AND* androstenedione

[a] Significantly different from [b] or [c] groups

Table 2 Characteristics of ovarian responses

Parameter	Non-overweight		Overweight		P value
	Non-HA (n = 218)	HA (n = 152)	Non-HA (n = 117)	HA (n = 96)	
Gn stimulation days	10.5 ± 2.1[a]	9.8 ± 1.8[b]	11.3 ± 2.6[c]	10.5 ± 2.4[a]	<0.001
Total Gn dosage (IU)	1588 ± 659[a]	1420 ± 595[a]	2081 ± 885[b]	1828 ± 750[c]	<0.001
Gn dosage /day (IU)	148 ± 40[a]	141 ± 35[a]	180 ± 49[b]	170 ± 40[c]	<0.001
Gn consumption/kg (IU)	28.3 ± 12[a]	25.1 ± 10[b]	27.6 ± 11	24.9 ± 10[b]	<0.05
Gn consumption/ kg/day	2.6 ± 0.7[a]	2.5 ± 0.6	2.4 ± 0.6	2.3 ± 0.5[b]	<0.001
E2 on HCG day (pmol/L)	12,708 ± 7621[a]	13,663 ± 8165 [a]	9219 ± 6685[b]	11,143 ± 7556	<0.001
LH on HCG day (mIU/mL)	2.4 ± 2.2[a]	2.4 ± 2.3[a]	3.0 ± 3.6	3.2 ± 2.6[b]	<0.001
P4 on HCG day (nmol/L)	2.4 ± 1.4	2.4 ± 1.4	2.2 ± 1.3	2.5 ± 1.5	NS
Endometrial thickness	10.7 ± 1.7	10.4 ± 1.7	10.7 ± 1.8	10.2 ± 1.9	NS
Oocyte retrieved (n)	16.7 ± 8.4[a]	18.2 ± 9.9[a]	12.1 ± 6.9[b]	13.8 ± 8.5[b]	<0.001
ET cancellation rate[d]	26.6%[a]	35.5%[a]	14.5%[b]	18.8%[b]	<0.05
Fertilization rate (%)	78.0 ± 19	76.5 ± 19	76.2 ± 24	75.1 ± 21	NS
Cleavage rate (%)	96.7 ± 11	98.9 ± 03	98.6 ± 05	97.6 ± 08	NS
Available embryos	7.75 ± 5.6	8.91 ± 6.9[a]	5.34 ± 4.7 [b]	6.68 ± 6.0	<0.001

Data are presented as mean ± standard deviation unless otherwise specified
NS not significant; BMI body mass index; HA hyperandrogenemia; PCOS polycystic ovary syndrome; Gn gonadotropin; E2 estradiol; LH luteinizing hormone; P4 progesterone; hCG human chorionic gonadotropin; ET embryo transfer
[a] Significantly different from [b] or [c] groups
[d]The cancellation rate of embryo transfer to prevent ovarian hyperstimulation syndrome

Cut-off values were as follows: BMI, 25.335 kg/m^2; and basal AND, 10.95 nmol/L.

Discussion

Nearly 70–80% of anovulatory infertility cases are caused by PCOS [15]. As a therapy, IVF can be safely used in infertile women with PCOS, especially with a GnRH-antagonist protocol. There is few studies to date have investigated the parameters of BMI and androgen together with the use of GnRH antagonists. In this study, the aim was to assess Androgen-related variation in the effect of body mass index (BMI) on IVF outcomes.

In this study, the duration of infertility was significantly higher in the overweight groups than in the non-overweight groups, indicating that body weight may contribute to a longer duration of infertility. The number of oocytes retrieved was significantly higher in the non-overweight groups than in the overweight groups, although the total Gn consumption as well as Gn consumption per day was significantly lower. There is an economic benefit of using a GnRH-antagonist protocol in non-overweight patients with PCOS, because of less cost and larger number of retrieved oocytes. Despite the effect of BMI, Gn consumption per kilogram was significantly

Table 3 Pregnancy outcomes

Parameter	Non-overweight		Overweight		P value
	Non-HA (n = 218)	HA (n = 152)	Non-HA (n = 117)	HA (n = 96)	
Clinical PR	49.7% (76/153)	43.6% (41/94)	40.9% (36/88)	43.7% (31/71)	NS
Miscarriage rate	14.5% (11/76)[a]	26.8% (11/41)	30.6% (11/36)	45.2% (14/31)[b]	<0.05
Live-birth rate	42.5% (65/153)[a]	31.9% (30/94)	28.4% (25/88)[b]	23.9% (17/71)[b]	<0.05
Ectopic PR	3.3% (5/153)	0% (0/94)[a]	5.7% (5/88)[b]	0% (0/71)	<0.05
Singleton PR	60.5%(46/76)	56.1%(23/41)	58.3% (21/36)	58.1% (18/31)	NS
Twin PR	39.5%(30/76)	43.9%(18/41)	41.7% (15/36)	41.9% (13/31)	NS
Preterm rate	22.4%(17/76)	19.5%(8/41)	19.4% (7/36)	12.9% (4/31)	NS
Full term rate	63.2%(48/76)	53.7%(22/41)	50.0%(18/36)	41.9% (13/31)	NS
CS rate	72.3% (47/65)	70.0% (21/30)	84.0% (21/25)	94.1% (16/17)	NS

HA hyperandrogenemia; PCOS polycystic ovary syndrome; BMI body mass index; NS not significant; PR pregnancy rate; CS caesarean section
[a] Significantly different from [b] groups

Table 4 Multivariate logistic regression analysis for predictive factors of miscarriage rate

Parameter	β	P value	Odds ratio	CI(95%)
Age (y)	0.040	0.502	1.040	0.927–1.168
BMI (kg/m²)[a]	0.093	0.049	1.097	1.000–1.204
Basal LH (IU/L)	0.030	0.379	1.031	0.963–1.103
Basal T(ng/ml)	0.095	0.684	1.100	0.695–1.742
Basal AND (nmol/L)[a]	0.069	0.034	1.071	1.005–1.141
Gn consumption/kg/day	0.579	0.061	1.785	0.974–3.273
LH on HCG day (mIU/mL)	0.061	0.258	1.063	0.957–1.180
Oocyte retrieved (n)	0.022	0.533	1.023	0.953–1.098
Constant	−7.630	0.001	0.000	

BMI body mass index; *LH* luteinizing hormone; *T* testosterone; *AND* androstenedione; *CI* confidence interval; *Gn* gonadotropin; *hCG* human chorionic gonadotropin
[a]Significant difference

Table 5 ROC analysis of BMI and AND on prediction of miscarriage rate

Parameter	Cut-off value	AUC	P value	Sensitivity	Specificity
BMI (kg/m²)	25.335	0.607	0.029	0.511	0.737
Basal AND (nmol/L)	10.95	0.657	0.001	0.723	0.584

BMI body mass index; *AND* androstenedione; *ROC* receiver operating characteristic; *AUC* area under the curve

lower in the HA groups, indicating that when over-weight PCOS patients lose weight, patients with HA gain economic benefits. The number of available embryos was higher in non-overweight-HA group than in overweight-non-HA group, indicating that a non-over-weight build and over-secretion of androgen may be protective factors for good-quality embryos. The miscarriage rate was significantly higher in overweight-HA group than in non-overweight-non-HA group, indicating that being overweight and having HA may play an important role in higher miscarriage rates. It appeared that being over-weight was a risk factor for both low-quality embryos and miscarriage. However, HA was a positively influential factor for good-quality embryos but a risk factor for miscarriage. Meanwhile, in multivariate logistic regression analyses, BMI and basal AND showed independently significant differences on prediction of miscarriage, after considering the effects of other parameters that may cause miscarriage. ROC analysis showed that the optimal cut-off values of BMI and basal AND were 25.335 kg/m² and 10.95 nmol/L, respectively. Although the predictive abilities of both BMI and basal AND on miscarriage were moderate, with a sensitivity of 0.511–0.723 and a spe-cificity of 0.584–0.737, they may still provide predict-ive values in clinical treatment since the AUCs for BMI and basal AND level were significantly different ($P = 0.029$ and $P = 0.001$, respectively). In addition, the predictive value of basal AND on miscarriage was slightly stronger than that of BMI.

PCOS is closely related to miscarriages. The molecular mechanisms underlying PCOS-associated miscarriages are controversial. Obesity and HA are factors that may contribute to miscarriage [13], which was confirmed by our previous study. By observational analysis of the developmental kinetics and metabolic activity of oocytes,

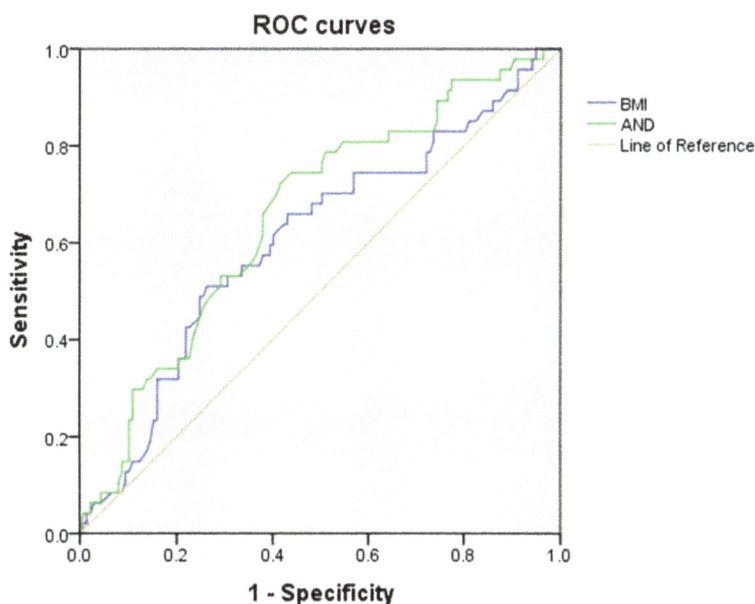

Fig. 1 Receiver operating characteristic (ROC) curves analysis of body mass index (BMI) and androstenedione (AND) on prediction of miscarriage rate. The green line and blue lines represent AND and BMI, respectively, and the beige line is the reference

some researchers have observed that oocytes from women who are overweight or obese are smaller than those from women of healthy weight (BMI < 25 kg/m^2), yet post-fertilization they reach the morula stage faster and, as blastocysts, show reduced glucose consumption and elevated endogenous triglyceride levels [16]. The data indicate that a high BMI in women is associated with distinct phenotypic changes in the embryo, which may reduce the quality of embryos and cause miscarriage. Valckx et al. showed that metabolic alterations in the serum were reflected in the follicular fluid, and that some of these alterations may have affected oocyte quality; however, there were poor BMI-related associations [17]. As for HA-related miscarriages, there are several potential mechanisms. First, the basal LH levels are related to basal androgen levels, as shown in our study. HA contributes to the secretion of excessive amounts of LH that may cause oocyte maturation disturbances and miscarriage. Second, HA may have an adverse effect on ovarian folliculogenesis and granulosa cell function. Follicular atresia is potentiated by androgens in the immature rat, and granulose cell apoptosis in rats is inducible by androgens [18]. Increased expression of AKT1 and AKT2 may be a possible mechanism linking HA to granulosa cell dysfunction in patients with HA PCOS [19]. Finally, testosterone may impact the endometrium. Testosterone was reported to have a dose-dependent negative effect on the proliferation of decidualized endometrial stromal cells [20] and to suppress the expression of HOXA10, which is essential to endometrial receptivity [21]. In patients with PCOS, HA and obesity interact with each other and promote the progression of PCOS.

One limitation of our study is its retrospective design. The effects of BMI and HA are assessed in the cohort study with logistic regression analysis and ROC analysis, showing the optimal cut-off values of BMI and basal AND. Although AUCs in ROC analysis are significantly different, the predictive ability of both parameters on miscarriage is moderate, due to the relatively limited sample size. Prospective studies with a larger sample size are needed in the future, along with studies investigating the effects of hyperinsulinemia.

Conclusions

In conclusion, being overweight was a risk factor for both low-quality embryos and miscarriage. However, HA was a positively influential factor for good-quality embryos but a risk factor for miscarriage. Multivariate logistic regression analyses show that BMI and basal AND were both significantly influential factors on miscarriage rate, with moderate predictive ability. The predictive value of basal AND on miscarriage was slightly stronger than BMI.

Acknowledgments

The authors thank the Research Center of Clinical Epidemiology, Peking University Third Hospital, for support in statistical analyses. The authors thank Rozella, an experienced editor whose first language is English, for carefully reviewing the article.

Funding

This work was supported by the National Natural Science Foundation of China [81550022].

Authors' contributions

WY designed research. WY, RY, MML, SY, JJZ, YY, SLS, YS and TSP collected data. WY, FD, JL, HZ analyzed data. WY, YW, RL and JQ wrote and revised the manuscript. All authors read and approved the final manuscript.

Competing interests

The authors declare that they have no competing interests.

Author details

[1]Center for Reproductive Medicine, Department of Obstetrics and Gynecology, Peking University Third Hospital, 49 N Garden Rd, Haidian District, Beijing 100191, China. [2]Research Center of Clinical Epidemiology, Peking University Third Hospital, Beijing, China.

References

1. Balen AH, Morley LC, Misso M, et al. The management of anovulatory infertility in women with polycystic ovary syndrome: an analysis of the evidence to support the development of global WHO guidance. Hum Reprod Update. 2016;22(6):687–708.
2. Kollmann M, Martins WP, Lima ML, et al. Strategies for improving outcome of assisted reproduction in women with polycystic ovary syndrome: systematic review and meta-analysis. Ultrasound Obstet Gynecol. 2016;48(6):709–18.
3. Xiao J, Chen S, Zhang C, et al. Effectiveness of GnRH antagonist in the treatment of patients with polycystic ovary syndrome undergoing IVF: a systematic review and meta-analysis. Gynecol Endocrinol. 2013;29(3):187–91.
4. Fauser BC, Tarlatzis BC, Rebar RW, et al. Consensus on women's health aspects of polycystic ovary syndrome (PCOS): the Amsterdam ESHRE/ASRM-sponsored 3rd PCOS consensus workshop group. Fertil Steril. 2012;97(1):28–38.
5. Chen X, Ni R, Mo Y, et al. Appropriate BMI levels for PCOS patients in southern China. Hum Reprod. 2010;25(5):1295–302.
6. Provost MP, Acharya KS, Acharya CR, et al. Pregnancy outcomes decline with increasing body mass index: analysis of 239,127 fresh autologous in vitro fertilization cycles from the 2008-2010 Society for Assisted Reproductive Technology registry. Fertil Steril. 2016;105(3):663–9.
7. Bailey AP, Hawkins LK, Missmer SA, et al. Effect of body mass index on in vitro fertilization outcomes in women with polycystic ovary syndrome. Am J Obstet Gynecol. 2014;211(2):163–e1.

8. Dechaud H, Anahory T, Reyftmann L, et al. Obesity does not adversely affect results in patients who are undergoing in vitro fertilization and embryo transfer. Eur J Obstet Gynecol Reprod Biol. 2006;127(1):88–93.

9. Metwally M, Cutting R, Tipton A, et al. Effect of increased body mass index on oocyte and embryo quality in IVF patients. Reprod BioMed Online. 2007; 15(5):532–8.

10. Alexiou E, Hatziagelaki E, Pergialiotis V, et al. Hyperandrogenemia in women with polycystic ovary syndrome: prevalence, characteristics and association with body mass index. Horm Mol Biol Clin Investig. 2017;29(3):105–11.

11. Gaddas M, Chaouache N, Ajina M, et al. Does hyperandrogenic statute in the polycystic ovary syndrome constitutes an obstacle to the success of in vitro fertilization? J Gynecol Obstet Biol Reprod. 2016;45(9):1091–8.

12. Yang W, Yang R, Yang S, et al. Infertile polycystic ovary syndrome patients undergoing in vitro fertilization with the gonadotropin-releasing hormone-antagonist protocol: role of hyperandrogenism. Gynecol Endocrinol. 2018 Aug;34(8):715–8.

13. Ramezanali F, Ashrafi M, Hemat M, et al. Assisted reproductive outcomes in women with different polycystic ovary syndrome phenotypes: the predictive value of anti-Mullerian hormone. Reprod BioMed Online. 2016; 32(5):503–12.

14. Rotterdam ESHRE/ASRM-Sponsored PCOS consensus workshop group. Revised 2003 consensus on diagnostic criteria and long-term health risks related to polycystic ovary syndrome (PCOS). Hum Reprod. 2004;19(1):41–7.

15. Brassard M, AinMelk Y, Baillargeon JP. Basic infertility including polycystic ovary syndrome. Med Clin North Am. 2008;92(5):1163–92.

16. Leary C, Leese HG, Sturmey RG. Human embryos from overweight and obese women display phenotypic and metabolic abnormalities. Hum Reprod. 2015;30(1):122–32.

17. Valckx SD, De Pauw I, De Neubourg D, et al. BMI-related metabolic composition of the follicular fluid of women undergoing assisted reproductive treatment and the consequences for oocyte and embryo quality. Hum Reprod. 2012;27(12):3531–9.

18. Kimura S, Matsumoto T, Matsuyama R, et al. Androgen receptor function in folliculogenesis and its clinical implication in premature ovarian failure. Trends Endocrinol Metab. 2007;18(5):183–9.

19. Nekoonam S, Naji M, Nashtaei MS, et al. Expression of AKT1 along with AKT2 in granulosa-lutein cells of hyperandrogenic PCOS patients. Arch Gynecol Obstet. 2017;295:1041–50.

20. Freis A, Renke T, Kammerer U, et al. Effects of a hyperandrogenaemic state on the proliferation and decidualization potential in human endometrial stromal cells. Arch Gynecol Obstet. 2017;295:1005–13.

21. Cermik D, Selam B, Taylor HS. Regulation of HOXA-10 expression by testosterone in vitro and in the endometrium of patients with polycystic ovary syndrome. J Clin Endocrinol Metab. 2003;88:238–43.

19

Effect of levothyroxine supplementation on pregnancy outcomes in women with subclinical hypothyroidism and thyroid autoimmuneity undergoing in vitro fertilization/intracytoplasmic sperm injection: an updated meta-analysis of randomized controlled trials

Meng Rao[1], Zhengyan Zeng[2], Shuhua Zhao[1] and Li Tang[1]* 📵

Abstract

Background: Evidence suggests that subclinical hypothyroidism (SCH) and thyroid autoimmunity (TAI) are associated with adverse pregnancy outcomes. This systematic review and meta-analysis was conducted to determine whether levothyroxine (LT4) supplementation would improve pregnancy outcomes among infertile women with SCH and/or TAI who underwent in vitro fertilization (IVF) or intracytoplastic sperm injection (ICSI).

Methods: We searched databases of PubMed, EMBASE, Web of Science, Cochrane Controlled Trials Register databases, and Clinicaltrials.gov up to April 2018 to identify eligible studies. Studies that focused on the treatment effect of LT4 on pregnancy outcomes of women with SCH and/or TAI who underwent IVF/ICSI were included in the data synthesis. We only included randomized controlled trials (RCTs). Relative risks (RR) and 95% confidence intervals (CI) were calculated using a random-effects model to assess the results of pregnancy outcomes, including clinical pregnancy rate, miscarriage rate, live birth rate and preterm birth rate.

Results: Four published RCTs including 787 infertile couples undergoing IVF/ICSI were included in this meta-analysis. Notably, the study observed no significant associations of LT4 treatment with the clinical pregnancy rate (RR = 1.46, 95% CI: 0.86–2.48), live birth rate (RR = 2.05, 95% CI: 0.96–4.36), or preterm birth rate (RR = 1.13, 95% CI: 0.65–1.96). However, patients receiving LT4 supplementation had a significantly decreased miscarriage rate relative to those receiving a placebo or no treatment (RR = 0.51, 95% CI: 0.32–0.82). A further sub-group analysis showed that LT4 supplementation did not improve the miscarriage rates among patients with SCH (RR = 0.67, 95% CI: 0.39–1.15) or TAI (RR = 0.28, 95% CI: 0.07–1.06).

Conclusions: Given its potential to reduce the miscarriage rate, LT4 supplementation is recommended for infertile women with SCH and/or TAI who are undergoing IVF/ICSI. However, additional population-based RCTs are needed to confirm this recommendation.

Keywords: Subclinical hypothyroidism, Thyroid autoimmunity, Levothyroxine, Pregnancy outcome, IVF/ICSI

---

* Correspondence: tanglikm@163.com
[1]Department of Reproduction and Genetics, the First Affiliated Hospital of Kunming Medical University, No. 295 Xi Chang road, Kunming 650032, China
Full list of author information is available at the end of the article

Background

Subclinical hypothyroidism (SCH) is a common mild thyroid disorder among women of childbearing age, with a prevalence of 3–8% [1, 2]. SCH is defined as an elevated serum thyrotropin (TSH) level and normal serum thyroxine (T4) level. Thyroid autoimmunity (TAI), defined as the presence of thyroid autoantibodies, antithyroperoxidase antibody (TPO-Ab), or antithyroglobulin antibody (Tg-Ab), is the most common cause of hypothyroidism among women of childbearing age [3].

Many studies have established the association between SCH and/or TAI and adverse pregnancy outcomes, including preeclampsia, placental abruption, miscarriage, preterm birth and neonatal mortality, in both spontaneous pregnancies and those achieved using assisted reproductive technologies (ART) [2, 4–6]. Subsequently, several meta-analyses have further confirmed these associations [7–9]. Theoretically, levothyroxine (LT4) supplementation may therefore attenuate the risks of adverse pregnancy outcomes.

One retrospective study showed that TAI-positive infertile female patients who were undergoing IVF did not receive benefits from LT4 treatment in terms of pregnancy outcomes [10]. In a randomized controlled trial (RCT) of TPO-Ab positive women undergoing IVF/ICSI, Negro et al. reported no differences in the pregnancy rates, live birth rates and miscarriage rates between the LT4-treated and placebo groups [11]. Nevertheless, a RCT conducted by Rahman et al. [12] showed that LT4 supplementation enhanced the fertilization rate, clinical pregnancy rate and live birth rate, while decreasing the miscarriage rate. The conclusion by Rahman and colleagues was supported by another RCT [13], which showed improved embryo implantation rate and live birth rate and a decreased miscarriage rate with LT4 treatment, although no effects on the clinical pregnancy rate were observed. In 2013, Velkeniers et al. systematically reviewed the above-listed RCTs and conducted a meta-analysis to determine whether LT4 treatment attenuated adverse pregnancy outcomes in patients with SCH and/or TAI [14]. The authors concluded that LT4 supplementation could improve the live birth rate and decrease the miscarriage rate but had no obvious effect on the clinical pregnancy rate. Therefore LT4 supplementation should be recommended as a means of improving clinical pregnancy outcomes in women with SCH and/or TAI who were undergoing ART.

It is worth noting that all previously published RCTs regarding the treatment effect of LT4 on pregnancy outcomes after IVF/ICSI involved small patient samples [11–13]. In 2017, however, a Chinese research group conducted a population-based RCT to reevaluate whether TPO-Ab-positive infertile women with normal thyroid function would benefit from LT4 supplementation with

respect to pregnancy outcomes following IVF/ICSI [15]. However, these authors observed no differences in the clinical pregnancy, live birth and miscarriage rates between the LT4-treated and untreated groups, in contrast to the previous meta-analysis. Therefore, this report aims to conduct a necessary re-summarization of the evidence from RCTs that addressed the topic of "treatment effect of LT4 on pregnancy outcomes of infertile women with SCH and/or TAI undergoing IVF/ICSI", with the intent to provide updated information for clinicians and patients.

Methods

Literature search

A systematic literature review of the PubMed, EMBASE, Web of Science, Cochrane Controlled Trials Register databases, other electronic databases, and Clinicaltrials.gov was performed to identify all relevant published studies up to April 2018. The search was limited to human studies published in English, and the following search terms were applied: (subclinical hypothyroidism OR thyroid autoimmunity OR thyroperoxidase antibody (TPO-Ab) OR thyroglobulin antibody (Tg-Ab)) AND (assisted reproductive technology (ART) OR in vitro fertilization (IVF) OR intracytoplasmic sperm injection (ICSI) OR ovarian stimulation) AND (levothyroxine OR euthyrox) AND (pregnancy outcome OR delivery OR live birth OR miscarriage OR preterm birth). The reference lists of the relevant publications were also manually searched for related studies. Two researchers independently completed the literature search and identified eligible studies. Conflicting decisions were resolved through consensus with a third researcher.

Study selection

Studies were included if they satisfied the following criteria: 1) subjects were infertile couples treated with ART, 2) women were diagnosed with SCH and/or TAI prior to ART cycles; 3) pregnancy outcomes were compared between levothyroxine-treated and placebo-treated or untreated women and 4) an RCT design. Studies were excluded for the following reasons: 1) publication as an abstract, letter to editor, case report or review and 2) a failure to provide sufficient data for analysis. Generally, clinical pregnancy was diagnosed via ultrasonography 4 weeks after embryo transfer. The miscarriage rate was defined as the number of miscarriages during the first 28 weeks of gestation per clinical pregnancy. The live birth rate was defined as the number of deliveries that resulted in at least 1 live-born baby per initiated cycle beyond 28 weeks of gestation. Preterm birth was defined as the delivery of a live neonate before 37 weeks of gestation.

Data extraction

Two reviewers independently extracted the following types of data from the included articles: first author, year of publication, country, patient characteristics, details of ART, causes of infertility, age, body mass index (BMI), reference values for thyroid status, patients' thyroid status and thyroid hormone values and interventions. Data related to pregnancy outcomes, including clinical pregnancy, live birth, miscarriage and preterm delivery, were collected and expressed as numbers of events in the LT4-treated and control groups. The corresponding author was contacted for more information if the data presented in the article were inadequate for the analysis.

Quality assessment of included studies

We included only RCT studies in this review. Accordingly, we used the Jadad quality assessment scale [16] and the PEDro scoring systems (available at http://www.pedro.org.au/english/downloads/pedro-scale/. accessed April 28, 2018) for the quality assessment.

Quality of evidence

For all outcomes, the quality of the evidence was assessed using the criteria of the Grading of Recommendations Assessment, Development and Evaluation (GRADE) system (study limitations, consistency of effect, imprecision, indirectness, and publication bias), which specifies four levels of evidence: high, moderate, low and very low quality [17, 18]. Serious or very serious deficiencies in these criteria could lead to a downgrading of the quality of evidence by one or two levels.

Statistical analysis

All analyses were conducted using Review Manager version 5.2 software (The Cochrane Collaboration). A standard meta-analytical method was used to compare the studies included in this analysis, and the effect size and corresponding 95% confidence interval (CI) were applied to express the combined results. We used the relative risk (RR) to describe the effect sizes. We additionally used a random-effects model. The degree of heterogeneity was also measured using the I^2 statistic, where values of < 25%, 25–50, and > 50% indicated low, moderate and high heterogeneity, respectively [19]. Inter-study variance was evaluated by calculating Tau^2, which represents the estimated standard deviation of the underlying effects across studies. Potential publication bias was evaluated using funnel plots. A subgroup analysis was also conducted to further analyze the effects of LT4 treatment on pregnancy outcomes among patients characterized by a positive TPO-Ab level or SCH diagnosis. The level of statistical significance was set at a P value < 0.05.

Results

Literature search

The literature search yielded 538 articles for review. After removing duplicate studies and reviewing the titles and abstracts, 16 full-text articles were screened further and assessed for eligibility. Thereafter, another 12 articles were excluded because of non-RCT design ($n = 4$), not focusing on infertile couples undergoing IVF/ICSI ($n = 3$), results not compared between LT4 treated and placebo-treated/no treated patients (n = 3), failure to provide data on the pregnancy rate, miscarriage rate or live birth rate ($n = 2$). Finally, 4 full-text RCTs comprising 787 infertile couples were included in the meta-analysis, as shown in Fig. 1.

Characteristics of included RCTs

The four included studies were published between 2005 and 2017, and the patients were from Italy [11], Egypt [12], South Korea [13] and China [15]. The study by Rahman and colleagues [12] did not provide BMI values; otherwise the ages and BMI values of patients in the LT4-treated and control groups were all comparable. In two studies, thyroid disorders were diagnosed based on the presence of TPO-Abs [11, 15], whereas an increased TSH value with a cut-off level of 4.0 or 4.5 mIU/L was used for diagnosis in the other two studies [12, 13]. The causes of infertility and controlled ovarian stimulation protocols were comparable among the trials, although the studies by Negro et al. [11] and Kim et al. [13] did not include male factor infertility or ovarian dysfunction, respectively, while the trial conducted by Wang et al. [15] included patients with uterine malformation and

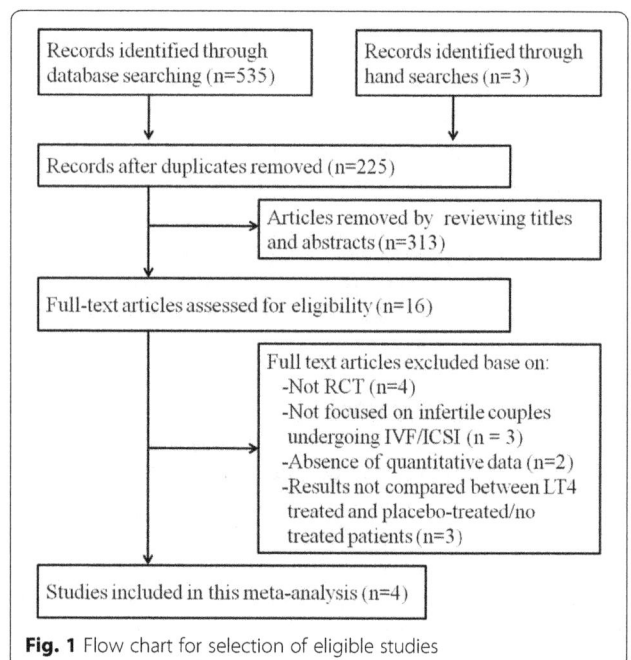

Fig. 1 Flow chart for selection of eligible studies

intrauterine insemination failure. However, the ratios of infertility causes were similar in each trial (Table 1).

In all trials, LT4 treatment was maintained throughout a diagnosed clinical pregnancy. Nevertheless, the starting time and dosing of LT4 supplementation varied among the trials. Patients in 3 trials [11, 12, 15] began LT4 supplementation 1 month before controlled ovarian stimulation (COS), whereas patients in the fourth trial [13] began supplementation on the first day of COS. In two trials, the LT4 doses were fixed [12, 13], while individually adjusted doses were provided in the other two trials [11, 15]. In the trial by Wang et al. [15], 282 of 300 patients in the treatment group, and 285 of 300 patients in the control group were enrolled in the last data analysis, whereas no patients dropped out of the other three trials [11–13]. Detailed information about the trial characteristics is presented in Table 1.

Quality assessment
As shown in Additional file 1: Table S1, the Jadad scores of the enrolled RCTs ranged from 3 to 5 (maximum total score = 5). The studies by Negro [11] and Rahman [12] were categorized as "excellent," whereas the studies by Kim [13] and Wang [15] were categorized as "good" because double-blinding had not been applied. Additionally, the enrolled studies received PEDro quality scores ranging from 8 to 10. The deducted items were all related to the blinding of subjects, therapists or assessors.

Clinical pregnancy rate
All four included studies reported clinical pregnancy rates. Of these, one study showed a significant improvement in the clinical pregnancy rate [12], whereas the other three studies [11, 13, 15] failed to find any difference between the LT4-treated and untreated patients. The meta-analysis found no significant association of LT4 treatment with the clinical pregnancy rate (RR = 1.46, 95% CI: 0.86–2.48, n = 787, I^2 = 86%, moderate quality evidence) (Fig. 2a). The high and statistically significant heterogeneity was mainly attributed to the study by Rahman [12], as the I^2 decreased to 12% without a significant change in the combined effect when this study was removed from the meta-analysis. LT4 supplementation was initiated a month prior to cycle start in three of the included studies [11, 12, 15], whereas at the cycle start in the other study by Kim et al. [13]. When excluding this study, the combined results also showed no significant association of LT4 treatment with the clinical pregnancy rate (RR = 1.49, 95% CI: 0.75–2.94, n = 723, I^2 = 90%) (Table 2).

Live birth rate
Two studies reported increased live birth rates among women receiving LT4 treatment [12, 13], whereas the other two did not [11, 15]. The combined results of all four studies indicated no significant effect of LT4 treatment on the live birth rate, with a pooled RR of 2.05 (95% CI: 0.96–4.36, n = 787, I^2 = 84%, moderate quality evidence) (Fig. 2b). However, the pooled result changed when the study by Wang et al. [15] was removed from the meta-analysis (RR = 2.80, 95% CI: 1.16–6.75, n = 220, I^2 = 73%). When excluding the study by Kim et al. [13], the combined results also showed no significant effect of LT4 treatment on the live birth rate (RR = 2.11, 95% CI: 0.76–5.84, n = 723, I^2 = 88%) (Table 2).

Miscarriage rate
Only one study [12] reported a significant decrease in the miscarriage rate for patients treated with LT4, whereas the other three studies [11, 13, 15] showed no significant effect. The combined results suggested a significantly lower miscarriage rate among LT4-treated patients relative to placebo-treated/untreated patients, with an RR of 0.51 (95% CI: 0.32–0.82, n = 787, I^2 = 15%, moderate quality evidence) (Fig. 2C). The pooled result changed when the study by Rahman et al. [12] was removed from the meta-analysis (RR = 0.61, 95% CI: 0.34–1.10, n = 787, I^2 = 10%). When excluding the study by Kim et al. [13], the combined results also suggested a significantly lower miscarriage rate among LT4-treated patients relative to placebo-treated/untreated patients (RR = 0.53, 95% CI: 0.35–0.82, n = 723, I^2 = 0) (Table 2).

Preterm birth rate
Preterm birth data were only reported by Wang et al. [15]. Specifically, the results showed that LT4 supplementation had no effect on the preterm birth rate, with an RR of 1.13 (95% CI: 0.65–1.96, I^2 not applicable) (Fig. 2D).

Publication bias
We evaluated the publication bias in each outcome and found the funnel plot virtually symmetrical, this indicated that there was little publication bias (Data not shown).

Discussion
The effects of SCH and/or TAI on clinical pregnancy have long been investigated. Most studies observed strong associations of SCH and/or TAI with adverse clinical outcomes [2, 5–7], especially miscarriage [8, 9]. However, a consensus has not been reached regarding whether LT4 supplementation could attenuate these risks. In this RCT-based meta-analysis, LT4 supplementation versus placebo/no treatment yielded a significant decrease in miscarriage rate but had no effects on the clinical pregnancy, live birth and preterm birth rates.

Several recently published meta-analyses have emphasized the adverse effects of SCH or TAI on clinical outcomes following either spontaneous pregnancies or those

Table 1 Summary of included studies

Study	Country	Study population	ART details	Causes of infertility	Patients age	Patients BMI
Negro 2005	Italy	86 TPO-Abs-positive infertile women undergoing ART	The first cycle of IVF/ICSI	In treated group: 11, 10, 7 and 8 patients were due to ovarian dysfunction, tubal factors, endometriosis and idiopathic causes, respectively; In control group: the number was 13, 9, 9 and 5, respectively.	Treated group:29.2 ± 4; Placebo: 30.1 ± 5	Unclear
Rahman 2010	Egypt	70 infertile women with subclinical hypothyroidism undergoing ART	All patients underwent ICSI	In treated group: 13, 9, 7 and 6 patients were due to ovarian dysfunction, tubal factors, endometriosis and idiopathic causes, respectively; In control group: the number was 12, 11, 5 and 7, respectively.	Treated group:31.2 ± 4.7; Placebo: 30 ± 4.3	Unclear
Kim 2011	South Korea	64 infertile patients with subclinical hypothyroidism undergoing ART	In both treated and control group: 18 and 14 patients underwent IVF and ICSI, respectively.	In treated group: 10, 6, 13 and 3 patients were due to tubal factors, endometriosis, male factors and idiopathic causes, respectively; In control group: the number was 9, 7, 13 and 3, respectively.	Treated group:36.0 ± 2.4; Placebo: 36.1 ± 2.2	Treated group:21.5 ± 1.9; Placebo: 21.7 ± 2.1
Wang 2017	China	600 TPO-Abs-positive infertile women undergoing ART	The first or second fresh IVF cycle	In treated group: 140, 37, 10, 15, 37, 128 and 21 patients were due to tubal factors, PCOS, endometriosis, Uterine malformation, Intrauterine insemination failure, male factors and idiopathic causes, respectively; In control group: the number was 142, 35, 14, 22, 27, 110 and 12, respectively.	Treated group: 31.3 ± 3.9; Placebo: 31.7 ± 3.8	Treated group: 22.7 ± 3.3; Placebo: 22.8 ± 3.2

Study	Reference values for thyroid status	Thyroid status and thyroid hormone values in patients	Intervention	Pregnancy outcomes
Negro 2005	TSH 0.27–4.2 mIU/L fT4 9.3–18.0 ng/L (12–33.5 pmol/L) TPO-Ab 0–100 kIU/L	For all patients:TPO-Ab (+). TSH and fT4 within normal range. Treated group: TSH 1.9 ± 0.7 mIU/L before treatment, fT4 11.2 ± 1.8 ng/L before treatment; TSH 1.1 ± 0.3 mIU/L after treatment, fT4 14.1 ± 2.5 ng/L after treatment; Conttrol group:TSH 1.7 ± 0.7 mIU/L, fT4 11.7 ± 2.1 ng/L	Patients in treated group underwent LT4 1 μg/kg/day treatment, one month before ART, this treatment was maintained throughout pregnancy	CPR, LBR, MR
Rahman 2010	TSH 0.27–4.2 mIU/L, fT3 2.56–4.4 pg/mL, fT4 0.9–2.59 ng/dL	For all patients:TSH > 4 mUI/L, fT4 within normal range. Treated group: TSH 4.7 ± 0.5 mIU/L before treatment, fT3 2.85 ± 0.7 ng/L before treatment, fT4 1 ± 0.4 before treatment; Conttrol group:TSH 4.8 ± 0.7 mIU/L, fT3 2.79 ± 0.8 ng/L, fT4 1.04 ± 0.49 ng/L	Patients in treated group underwent LT4 50–100 μg/day, one month before ART, this treatment was maintained throughout pregnancy	CPR, LBR, MR
Kim 2011	TSH 0.27–4.0 mIU/L fT4 0.9–2.59 ng/dL	For all patients:TSH>4.5 mUI/L, fT4 within normal range. Treated group: TSH 6.6 ± 1.7 mIU/L before treatment, fT4 1.2 ± 0.2 before treatment; Conttrol group:TSH 6.7 ± 1.8 mIU/L, fT4 1.2 ± 0.2 ng/L	Patients in treated group underwent LT4 50 μg/day, from the first day of controlled ovarian stimulation, this treatment was maintained throughout pregnancy	CPR, LBR, MR
Wang 2017	TSH 0.5–4.78 mIU/L TPO-Ab 0–60 IU/mL	For all patients:TPO-Ab (+). TSH and fT4 within normal range. Treated group: TSH (mean (interquartile range)), 2.94 (2.04–3.74) mIU/L before treatment, fT4 (mean ± SD), 1.16 ± 0.13 before treatment; Conttrol group: TSH 2.12 (1.5–2.8) mIU/L, ft 4 1.19 ± 0.14 ng/L	LT4 was supplemented between 2 and 4 weeks before the COS and continued through the end of pregnancy. For individuals with a TSH level ≥ 2.5 mIU/L, the starting dose was 50 μg/d; for those with a TSH level < 2.5 mIU/L, the starting dose was 25 μg/d. For individuals with body weight < 50 kg, the starting dose was decreased by 50%. The LT4 dose was titrated to keep the TSH level within 0.1 to 2.5 mIU/L in the first trimester, 0.2 to 3.0 mIU/L in the second trimester, and 0.3 to 3.0mIU/L in the third trimester.	CPR, LBR, MR, PBR

TPO-Ab thyroperoxidase antibody; *TSH* thyrotropin; *LT4* levothyroxine; *CPR* clinical pregnancy rate; *LBR* live birth rate; *MR* miscarriage rate; *PBR* preterm birth rate; *COS* controlled ovarian stimulation

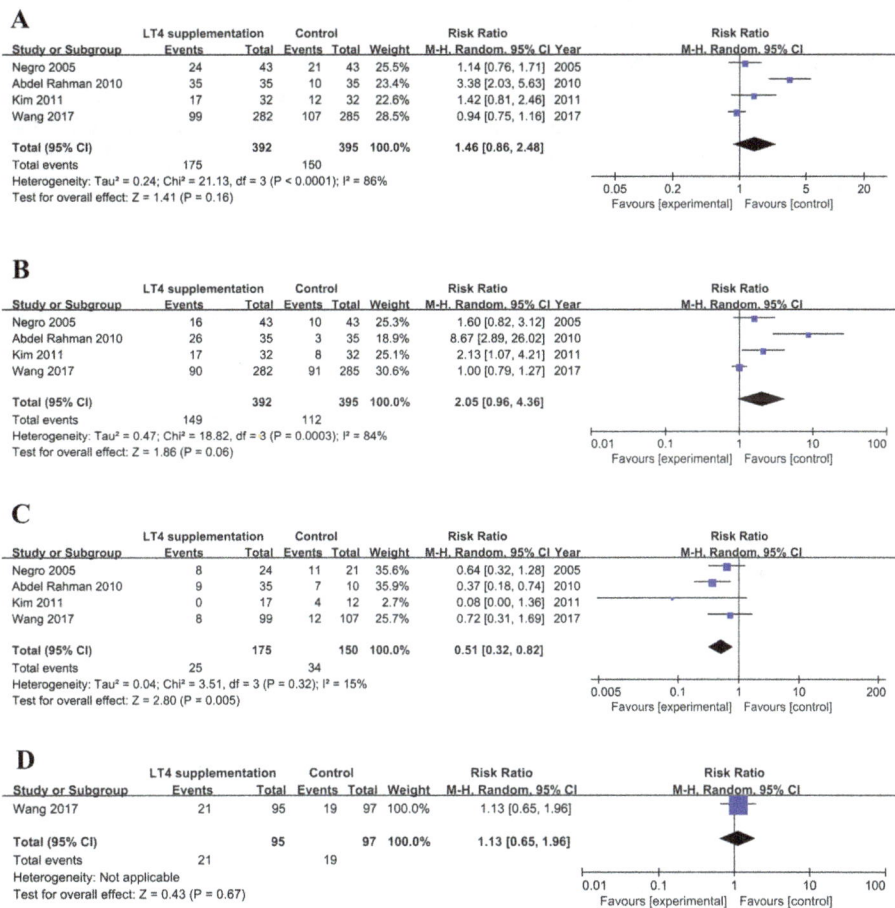

Fig. 2 Forest plot (random-effects model) of LT4 supplementation and pregnancy outcome following IVF/ICSI cycles. (**a**), clinical pregnancy rate; (**b**), live birth rate; (**c**), miscarriage rate and (**d**), preterm birth rate

achieved by ART [2, 8, 9]. A meta-analysis by Boogaard et al. [9] indicated that pregnant women with SCH or TAI have an increased risk of complications, especially pre-eclampsia, perinatal mortality and (recurrent) miscarriage. In a meta-analysis of 31 studies on miscarriage and 5 studies on preterm birth, Thangaratinam observed a significant difference in the miscarriage rate between patients with and without TAI [odds ratio (OR) = 3.90, 95% CI: 2.48–6.12 for cohort studies and OR = 1.80, 95% CI: 1.25–2.60 for case-control studies] [8]. The authors also observed a 2.07-fold higher risk of preterm birth among women

positive for thyroid autoantibodies (95% CI: 1.17–3.68). In 2016, Maraka et al. [2] published a meta-analysis focused on adverse pregnancy and neonatal outcomes in pregnant women with SCH. These authors also identified a 2.01-fold increased risk of pregnancy loss in women with SCH, but no association of this factor with preterm birth.

Notably, the above studies were all based on patients with spontaneous pregnancies or a mixture of those with spontaneous and ART pregnancies. By contrast, a very recent meta-analysis focused on the association of TAI and IVF/ICSI outcomes. Here, the results suggested that

Table 2 LT4 supplementation and pregnancy outcomes following IVF/ICSI, in women with SCH and/or TAI, without combining the study by Kim et al.

Subgroup	Number of studies	Number of patients	Statistical method	Effect size	I^2 (%)
Clinical pregnancy	3	723	RR (Random, 95% CI)	1.49 (0.75, 2.94)	90
Live birth	3	723	RR (Random, 95% CI)	2.11 (0.76, 5.84)	88
Miscarriage	3	723	RR (Random, 95% CI)	0.53 (0.35, 0.82)	0
Preterm birth	1	567	RR (Random, 95% CI)	1.13 (0.65, 1.96)	N/A

SCH subclinical hypothyroidism; *TAI* thyroid autoimmunity; *RR* risk ratio; *CI* confidence interval; *N/A* not available

women with TAI had a significantly increased rate of miscarriage (OR = 1.44, 95% CI: 1.06–1.09) and decreased rate (OR = 0.73, 95% CI: 0.54–0.99) of live birth, whereas the fertilization and implantation rates appeared to be unaltered [7]. These studies all concluded that SCH or TAI lead to adverse pregnancy outcomes and that LT4 supplementation could theoretically attenuate this risk.

This study, which is an update of a previously published 2013 meta-analysis [14], enrolled an additional population-based RCT conducted in China [15] in which the results were inconsistent with the conclusions of the earlier meta-analysis. In the previous meta-analysis, LT4 treatment was found to significantly increase the live birth rate relative to placebo/no treatment (RR = 2.76, 95% CI: 1.20–6.44), with no effect on the clinical pregnancy rate (RR = 1.46, 95% CI: 0.86–2.48). However, our updated meta-analysis found no significant improvements in the live birth and clinical pregnancy rates among women receiving LT4 supplementation. This result was consistent with another prospective study that showed no difference in the live birth and clinical pregnancy rates between women with SCH who had TSH levels controlled to < 2.5 mIU/L or 2.5–4.2 mIU/L before IVF [20]. These negative results suggest that LT4 intervention is a weakly influential factor, as clinical pregnancy and live birth are considered the most important benefits for infertile patients. However, both this and the previous meta-analysis suggested that the LT4 intervention reduced miscarriage rates, consistent with the findings of many other studies focused on spontaneous pregnancies and those achieved by ART [21, 22]. Even though no significant improvement was observed in clinical pregnancy and live birth rates in women supplemented with LT4, we still emphasize the importance of LT4 intervention for patients with SCH and/or TAI due to its potential in decreasing the risk of miscarriage. We hypothesize that significant improvement of clinical pregnancy and live birth would be possible when more RCTs would be enrolled into the meta-analysis in the future. Considering that the initial tome of LT4 supplementation in the study by Kim et al. [13] was different from the other three studies [11, 12, 15], the combined results of these three studies were consistent with the precious analysis in which all studies were enrolled. This may indicate that the initial time of LT4 supplementation may not significantly affect pregnancy outcomes, as long as LT4 is supplemented prior to IVF/ICSI cycle start.

In an earlier study, Blumenthal et al. observed no differences in adverse pregnancy outcomes between women treated for SCH and euthyroid women [23], which suggests the beneficial effects of LT4 for the former group. Infertile patients always undergo thyroid function screening before pregnancy, whereas pregnant women do not usually undergo an initial screening until the first trimester. A series of studies reported no effects of LT4 treatment on miscarriage among women with SCH and/or TAI who received LT4 supplementation when screened and diagnosed after becoming pregnant. [24–26]. These inconsistent conclusions may be attributable to the different time windows in which thyroid function testing was conducted and LT4 supplementation was initiated [27].

The molecular mechanism underlying the association between adverse pregnancy outcomes and SCH and/or TAI is not fully understood. However, several hypotheses based on current studies may explain this issue. Firstly, human granulosa cells express TSH and thyroid hormone receptors, and both tri-iodothyronine (T3) and thyroxine (T4) are found in the follicular fluid. Therefore, alterations in TSH levels may negatively influence oocyte quality and function in patients with (sub)clinical hypothyroidism [3, 28]. Secondly, TPO and Tg are also expressed in the endometrium, where they may be responsible for local thyroxine production [29]. Accordingly, the endometrium is susceptible to the actions of anti-TPO and anti-Tg autoantibodies. Finally, TAI may be considered an expression of general autoimmunity, and adverse fertility outcomes such as spontaneous miscarriage may be attributable to the presence of anticardiolipin antibodies [30]. However, this meta-analysis only provides findings to support the beneficial effects of LT4 on miscarriage, but not on clinical pregnancy, live birth or preterm birth. In patients with SCH and/or TAI, LT4 supplementation may decrease the risk of miscarriage mainly by driving the balance away from thyroid dysfunction. A recent meta-analysis by Thangaratinam indicated strong associations of the presence of maternal thyroid autoantibodies with miscarriage and preterm delivery [8]. Furthermore, a very recent RCT conducted by Nazarpour et al. [25] found that LT4 supplementation could precisely decrease the preterm birth rate among pregnant women with SCH diagnosed using a TSH cutoff of ≥4.0 mIU/L. However, our meta-analysis only observed a decreased risk of miscarriage, but not preterm birth (only one enrolled study), with LT4 supplementation. More well-designed studies are needed to confirm this preliminary conclusion.

We observed a high level of heterogeneity among studies of the clinical outcomes of clinical pregnancy and live birth. The following aspects may have affected the combined results. First, the enrolled studies differed in terms of the methodology and normal ranges of thyroid function test results, as listed in Table 1. Second, the studies differed in terms of LT4 dose, as shown in Table 1. In addition, other factors, such as controlled ovarian hyperstimulation protocols and IVF or ICSI cycles, might also affect the combined effects and degree of heterogeneity.

The strength of this meta-analysis is that we focused on the effect of LT4 on SCH and/or TAI, a very common mild thyroid disorder among women of childbearing age, and the conclusion is very critical when providing consultation to infertile couples. Additionally, we only enrolled RCTs, this enhanced the evidence of the pooled results. There are also some limitations in this meta-analysis. Firstly, there were only 4 eligible studies enrolled in data analysis. Secondly, the number of patients in 3 of the 4 included studies was limited. Third, patients characterized by TPO-positivity and increased TSH levels were mixed in data synthesis. Future meta-analysis regarding the effect of LT4 supplementation on women with only SCH or TAI is necessary to better clarify this issue, when more RCTs would have been conducted.

In conclusion, this current RCT-based meta-analysis confirmed the beneficial effects of LT4 supplementation in terms of decreasing the risk of miscarriage among female patients with TAI and SCH who are undergoing IVF/ICSI. However, LT4 treatment did not improve the rates of clinical pregnancy, live birth and preterm birth. Further studies are needed to determine whether LT4 intervention can also improve long-term complications such as neurodevelopmental delays in women with SCH and/or TAI.

Abbreviations
ART: Assisted reproductive technology; BMI: body mass index; CI: confidence interval; ICSI: Intracytoplasmic sperm injection; IVF: in vitro fertilization; LT4: levothyroxine; RCT: randomized controlled trial; RR: relative risks; SCH: subclinical hypothyroidism (SCH); TAI: thyroid autoimmunity; Tg-Ab: antithyroglobulin antibody; TPO-Ab: antithyroperoxidase antibody

Acknowledgements
We acknowledge the professional manuscript editing services of Armstrong-Hilton Ltd. Ethics approval and consent to participate
Not applicable.

Funding
This study was supported by the scientific funding from the first affiliated hospital of Kunming medical university (No. 2017BS008).

Authors' contributions
MR and LT participated in the conception and design of the study. MR and ZZ searched and collected the data, performed the analysis and wrote the manuscript. LT and SZ revised the manuscript and gave final approval of this manuscript. All authors read and approved the final manuscript.

Competing interest
The authors declare that they have no competing interests.

Author details
[1]Department of Reproduction and Genetics, the First Affiliated Hospital of Kunming Medical University, No. 295 Xi Chang road, Kunming 650032, China. [2]Department of Neurology, the First Affiliated Hospital of Kunming Medical University, Kunming 650032, China.

References
1. Karmisholt J, Andersen S, Laurberg P. Variation in thyroid function tests in patients with stable untreated subclinical hypothyroidism. Thyroid. 2008;18: 303–8.
2. Maraka S, Ospina NM, O'Keeffe DT, Espinosa De Ycaza AE, Gionfriddo MR, Erwin PJ, Coddington CC, 3rd, Stan MN, Murad MH, Montori VM. Subclinical hypothyroidism in pregnancy: a systematic review and meta-analysis. Thyroid. 2016;26:580–590.
3. Vissenberg R, Manders VD, Mastenbroek S, Fliers E, Afink GB, Ris-Stalpers C, Goddijn M, Bisschop PH. Pathophysiological aspects of thyroid hormone disorders/thyroid peroxidase autoantibodies and reproduction. Hum Reprod Update. 2015;21:378–s87.
4. Sen A, Kushnir VA, Barad DH, Gleicher N. Endocrine autoimmune diseases and female infertility. Nat Rev Endocrinol. 2014;10:37–50.
5. Haddow JE, Cleary-Goldman J, McClain MR, Palomaki GE, Neveux LM, Lambert-Messerlian G, Canick JA, Malone FD, Porter TF, Nyberg DA, Bernstein PS, D'Alton ME. First, second-trimester risk of aneuploidy research C. Thyroperoxidase and thyroglobulin antibodies in early pregnancy and preterm delivery. Obstet Gynecol. 2010;116:58–62.
6. Rushworth FH, Backos M, Rai R, Chilcott IT, Baxter N, Regan L. Prospective pregnancy outcome in untreated recurrent miscarriers with thyroid autoantibodies. Hum Reprod. 2000;15:1637–9.
7. Busnelli A, Paffoni A, Fedele L, Somigliana E. The impact of thyroid autoimmunity on IVF/ICSI outcome: a systematic review and meta-analysis. Hum Reprod Update. 2016;22:775–90.
8. Thangaratinam S, Tan A, Knox E, Kilby MD, Franklyn J, Coomarasamy A. Association between thyroid autoantibodies and miscarriage and preterm birth: meta-analysis of evidence. BMJ. 2011;342:d2616.
9. van den Boogaard E, Vissenberg R, Land JA, van Wely M, van der Post JA, Goddijn M, Bisschop PH. Significance of (sub)clinical thyroid dysfunction and thyroid autoimmunity before conception and in early pregnancy: a systematic review. Hum Reprod Update. 2011;17:605–19.
10. Revelli A, Casano S, Piane LD, Grassi G, Gennarelli G, Guidetti D, Massobrio M. A retrospective study on IVF outcome in euthyroid patients with anti-thyroid antibodies: effects of levothyroxine, acetyl-salicylic acid and prednisolone adjuvant treatments. Reprod Biol Endocrinol. 2009;7:137.
11. Negro R, Mangieri T, Coppola L, Presicce G, Casavola EC, Gismondi R, Locorotondo G, Caroli P, Pezzarossa A, Dazzi D, Hassan H. Levothyroxine treatment in thyroid peroxidase antibody-positive women undergoing assisted reproduction technologies: a prospective study. Hum Reprod. 2005; 20:1529–33.
12. Abdel Rahman AH, Aly Abbassy H, Abbassy AA. Improved in vitro fertilization outcomes after treatment of subclinical hypothyroidism in infertile women. Endocr Pract. 2010;16:792–7.
13. Kim CH, Ahn JW, Kang SP, Kim SH, Chae HD, Kang BM. Effect of levothyroxine treatment on in vitro fertilization and pregnancy outcome in infertile women with subclinical hypothyroidism undergoing in vitro fertilization/intracytoplasmic sperm injection. Fertil Steril. 2011;95:1650–4.
14. Velkeniers B, Van Meerhaeghe A, Poppe K, Unuane D, Tournaye H, Haentjens P. Levothyroxine treatment and pregnancy outcome in women with subclinical hypothyroidism undergoing assisted reproduction

technologies: systematic review and meta-analysis of RCTs. Hum Reprod Update. 2013;19:251–8.

15. Wang H, Gao H, Chi H, Zeng L, Xiao W, Wang Y, Li R, Liu P, Wang C, Tian Q, Zhou Z, Yang J, Liu Y, Wei R, Mol BWJ, Hong T, Qiao J. Effect of levothyroxine on miscarriage among women with Normal thyroid function and thyroid autoimmunity undergoing in vitro fertilization and embryo transfer: a randomized clinical trial. JAMA. 2017;318:2190–8.

16. Jadad AR, Moore RA, Carroll D, Jenkinson C, Reynolds DJ, Gavaghan DJ, McQuay HJ. Assessing the quality of reports of randomized clinical trials: is blinding necessary? Control Clin Trials. 1996;17:1–12.

17. Atkins D, Best D, Briss PA, Eccles M, Falck-Ytter Y, Flottorp S, Guyatt GH, Harbour RT, Haugh MC, Henry D, Hill S, Jaeschke R, Leng G, Liberati A, Magrini N, Mason J, Middleton P, Mrukowicz J, O'Connell D, Oxman AD, Phillips B, Schunemann HJ, Edejer T, Varonen H, Vist GE, Williams JW Jr, Zaza S, Group GW. Grading quality of evidence and strength of recommendations. BMJ. 2004;328:1490.

18. Guyatt G, Oxman AD, Akl EA, Kunz R, Vist G, Brozek J, Norris S, Falck-Ytter Y, Glasziou P, DeBeer H, Jaeschke R, Rind D, Meerpohl J, Dahm P, Schunemann HJ. GRADE guidelines: 1. Introduction-GRADE evidence profiles and summary of findings tables. J Clin Epidemiol. 2011;64:383–94.

19. Higgins JPT, Cochrane GS. Cochrane handbook for systematic reviews of interventions. Version 5.1.0 [updated march 2011]. Oxford: The Cochrane Collaboration; 2011.

20. Cai Y, Zhong L, Guan J, Guo R, Niu B, Ma Y, Su H. Outcome of in vitro fertilization in women with subclinical hypothyroidism. Reprod Biol Endocrinol. 2017;15:39.

21. Ma L, Qi H, Chai X, Jiang F, Mao S, Liu J, Zhang S, Lian X, Sun X, Wang D, Ren J, Yan Q. The effects of screening and intervention of subclinical hypothyroidism on pregnancy outcomes: a prospective multicenter single-blind, randomized, controlled study of thyroid function screening test during pregnancy. J Matern Fetal Neonatal Med. 2016;29:1391–4.

22. Negro R, Formoso G, Mangieri T, Pezzarossa A, Dazzi D, Hassan H. Levothyroxine treatment in euthyroid pregnant women with autoimmune thyroid disease: effects on obstetrical complications. J Clin Endocrinol Metab. 2006;91:2587–91.

23. Blumenthal NJ, Eastman CJ. Beneficial effects on pregnancy outcomes of thyroid hormone replacement for subclinical hypothyroidism. J Thyroid Res 2017;2017:4601365.

24. Maraka S, Singh Ospina NM, O'Keeffe DT, Rodriguez-Gutierrez R, Espinosa De Ycaza AE, Wi CI, Juhn YJ, Coddington CC, 3rd, Montori VM, Stan MN. Effects of levothyroxine therapy on pregnancy outcomes in women with subclinical hypothyroidism. Thyroid 2016;26:980–986.

25. Nazarpour S, Ramezani Tehrani F, Simbar M, Tohidi M, Alavi Majd H, Azizi F. Effects of levothyroxine treatment on pregnancy outcomes in pregnant women with autoimmune thyroid disease. Eur J Endocrinol. 2017;176:253–65.

26. Negro R, Schwartz A, Stagnaro-Green A. Impact of levothyroxine in miscarriage and preterm delivery rates in first trimester thyroid antibody-positive women with TSH less than 2.5 mIU/L. J Clin Endocrinol Metab. 2016;101:3685–90.

27. Busnelli A, Vannucchi G, Paffoni A, Faulisi S, Fugazzola L, Fedele L, Somigliana E. Levothyroxine dose adjustment in hypothyroid women achieving pregnancy through IVF. Eur J Endocrinol. 2015;173:417–24.

28. Aghajanova L, Stavreus-Evers A, Lindeberg M, Landgren BM, Sparre LS, Hovatta O. Thyroid-stimulating hormone receptor and thyroid hormone receptors are involved in human endometrial physiology. Fertil Steril. 2011; 95:230–7 7 e1–2.

29. Catalano RD, Critchley HO, Heikinheimo O, Baird DT, Hapangama D, Sherwin JR, Charnock-Jones DS, Smith SK, Sharkey AM. Mifepristone induced progesterone withdrawal reveals novel regulatory pathways in human endometrium. Mol Hum Reprod. 2007;13:641–54.

30. Toulis KA, Goulis DG, Venetis CA, Kolibianakis EM, Negro R, Tarlatzis BC, Papadimas I. Risk of spontaneous miscarriage in euthyroid women with thyroid autoimmunity undergoing IVF: a meta-analysis. Eur J Endocrinol. 2010;162:643–52.

20

The effects of vitamin D supplementation on metabolic profiles and gene expression of insulin and lipid metabolism in infertile polycystic ovary syndrome candidates for in vitro fertilization

Majid Dastorani[1], Esmat Aghadavod[1*], Naghmeh Mirhosseini[2], Fatemeh Foroozanfard[3], Shahrzad Zadeh Modarres[4], Mehrnush Amiri Siavashani[5] and Zatollah Asemi[1*]

Abstract

Background: Vitamin D deficiency in women diagnosed with polycystic ovary syndrome (PCOS) remarkably decreases the chance of pregnancy, which might be related to its impact on metabolic abnormalities in these patients. It is hypothesized that vitamin D supplementation influences metabolic profile of these patients and indirectly might affect fertility and the outcomes. Therefore, this study was conducted to determine the effects of vitamin D supplementation on the levels of anti-Müllerian hormone (AMH), metabolic profiles, and gene expression of insulin and lipid metabolism in infertile women with PCOS who were candidate for in vitro fertilization (IVF).

Methods: This study was a randomized, double-blinded, placebo-controlled trial conducted among 40 infertile women, aged 18–40 years, diagnosed with PCOS and was candidate for IVF. Participants were randomly assigned into two intervention groups for receiving either 50,000 IU vitamin D or placebo ($n = 20$ each group) every other week for 8 weeks. Gene expression for insulin and lipid metabolism was conducted using peripheral blood mononuclear cells (PBMCs) of women with PCOS, via RT-PCR method.

Results: Vitamin D supplementation led to a significant reduction in serum AMH ($- 0.7 \pm 1.2$ vs. $- 0.1 \pm 0.5$ ng/mL, $P = 0.02$), insulin levels ($- 1.4 \pm 1.6$ vs. -0.3 ± 0.9 μIU/mL, $P = 0.007$), homeostatic model of assessment for insulin resistance ($- 0.3 \pm 0.3$ vs. -0.1 ± 0.2, $P = 0.008$), and a significant increase in quantitative insulin sensitivity check index ($+ 0.009 \pm 0.01$ vs. $+ 0.001 \pm 0.004$, $P = 0.04$), compared with the placebo. Moreover, following vitamin D supplementation there was a significant decrease in serum total- ($- 5.1 \pm 12.6$ vs. $+ 2.9 \pm 10.9$ mg/dL, $P = 0.03$) and LDL-cholesterol levels ($- 4.5 \pm 10.3$ vs. $+ 2.5 \pm 10.6$ mg/dL, $P = 0.04$) compared with the placebo.

Conclusion: Overall, the findings of this trial supported that 50,000 IU vitamin D supplementation every other week for 8 weeks had beneficial effects on insulin metabolism, and lipid profile of infertile women with PCOS who are candidate for IVF. These benefits might not be evident upon having sufficient vitamin D levels.

Keywords: Vitamin D supplementation, Glycemic control, Cardio-metabolic, In vitro fertilization

* Correspondence: aghadavod_m@yahoo.com; asemi_r@yahoo.com; asemi_z@Kaums.ac.ir
[1]Research Center for Biochemistry and Nutrition in Metabolic Diseases, Kashan University of Medical Sciences, Kashan, I.R, Iran
Full list of author information is available at the end of the article

Background

Polycystic ovary syndrome (PCOS) is one of the most common endocrine disorders among women affecting 4% to 12% of women in reproductive age [1]. It is a multifactorial syndrome presented with obesity, insulin resistance, dyslipidemia and other metabolic abnormalities. Obesity leads to more than 70% insulin resistance in these patients [2]. Insulin resistance, occurs in patients with PCOS, is significantly associated with different metabolic abnormalities including elevated aromatase activity, increased androgen production, and impaired progesterone synthesis in granulosa cells [2]. Current evidence has reported a high risk of metabolic disorders predisposing individuals to cardiovascular disease (CVD) in in vitro fertilization (IVF) pregnancies [3, 4] and animal models [5, 6]. However, the independent role of insulin resistance in in vitro fertilization (IVF) outcomes is less defined in the literature [7].

There is a significant association between serum vitamin D levels and reproductive function, already reported in murine models [8]. Further, studies investigating the role of vitamin D receptor (VDR) in reproductive tissues have supported a positive correlation between vitamin D status and reproduction [9]. VDR is located in different reproductive tissues including ovary (particularly granulosa cells), uterus, placenta and testis [10]. Diverse expression of VDR suggests a potential role of vitamin D in female reproductive function [11]. Moreover, in PCOS, ovarian physiology is influenced by the metabolic disorders observed in these patients; therefore, a beneficial effect of vitamin D on metabolic abnormalities might translate into an ideal ovarian physiology [12, 13]. Vitamin D supplementation is recommended as a potential therapeutic adjunct for the ovulatory dysfunction and metabolic disorders observed in women with PCOS [14, 15]. Evidence evaluating the impact of vitamin D deficiency on the success rate of reproduction following IVF in humans is limited [16, 17]. Moreover, vitamin D deficiency is correlated with poor ovarian stimulation in PCOS but not unexplained infertility [18]. Likewise, vitamin D has been shown to be involved in a minor pathway related to metabolic and hormonal dysregulation in women with PCOS [19]. Therefore, the beneficial effects of vitamin D on the metabolic disorders in PCOS might translate into an improvement in ovarian physiology. The majority of current studies investigating the effects of vitamin D supplementation on metabolic status in patients with PCOS have not specifically looked into IVF. And to our best knowledge, this trial is the first study assessing the effects of vitamin D supplementation on glycemic control, markers of cardiometabolic risk and gene expression of insulin and lipid metabolism in infertile women diagnosed with PCOS who were candidate for IVF. In a study conducted by Seyyed Abootorabi et al. [20] vitamin D supplementation at a dosage of 50,000 IU/week for 8 weeks reduced fasting glucose and increased adiponectin levels in women diagnosed with PCOS who were vitamin D deficient. Further, in a meta-analysis performed by Xue et al. [21], vitamin D administration to patients with PCOS significantly decreased triglycerides levels, while did not change insulin metabolism and other markers of lipid profiles. On the other hand, recently there are concerns about the risks associated to uncontrolled vitamin D supplementation [22].

Current evidence and the physiological role of vitamin D in reproductive activity might support the significance of vitamin D supplementation while doing IVF in infertile women with PCOS F. So, this study was aimed to determine the effects of vitamin D supplementation on glycemic control, markers of cardiometabolic abnormalities and gene expression of insulin and lipid metabolism in infertile women diagnosed with PCOS and candidate for IVF.

Methods

Trial design and participants' characteristics

This study was a randomized, double-blinded, placebo-controlled trial conducted on 40 infertile women, aged 18 to 40 years old, with PCOS, diagnosed using Rotterdam criteria [23], who were candidate for IVF. The study was registered in the Iranian website for clinical trials registration (http://www.irct.ir: IRCT20170513033941N2 7). Recruited participants were referred patients at Research and Clinical Center for Infertility and Naghavi Clinic, Kashan, Iran, from December 2017 through March 2018. Any case of metabolic disorders, including thyroid disorder, diabetes or impaired glucose tolerance was excluded at screening phase. This study was performed following Declaration of Helsinki and was approved by the research ethics committee of Kashan University of Medical Sciences (KAUMS). Written informed consent was signed by all subjects prior to the intervention.

Intervention

Participants were randomly assigned into two intervention groups to receive either 50,000 IU vitamin D ($n = 20$) or placebo (n = 20) every other week for 8 weeks. Vitamin D and placebo (paraffin) capsules were similarly matched in color, shape, size and packaging, and were manufactured by Zahravi (Tabriz, Iran) and Barij Essence (Kashan, Iran), respectively. Random number table was used for randomization by one of the researchers not involved in other processes of trial. Randomization and allocation were concealed from the investigators and study participants until the completion of analyses. Compliance rate was assessed through measuring serum 25(OH)D levels and asking patients to return back the medication containers. To increase the compliance, all subjects were received a short message on their cell phones every day, throughout the trial, to take the supplements.

Assessment of outcomes

Insulin metabolism was considered as the primary outcome. Lipid profiles and gene expression of insulin and lipid metabolism were defined as the secondary outcomes. Fifteen milliliter fasting blood was collected at the beginning and end of the trial at Naghavi Clinic laboratory, Kashan, Iran. Fasting plasma glucose (FPG) concentrations were measured on the day of blood collection, using enzymatic kits with the coefficient variances (CVs) of less than 5%. Serum 25-hydroxyvitamin D (25 (OH) D) concentrations were determined by an ELISA kit (IDS, Boldon, UK) with inter- and intra-assay CVs of lower than 7%. Serum AMH levels were measured using an ELISA kit (Bioactiva, Homburg, Germany) with CVs of lower than 6%. Serum insulin concentrations were measured by an ELISA kit (DiaMetra, Milano, Italy) with inter- and intra-assay CVs of 3.5 and 5.0%, respectively. The homeostasis model of assessment-insulin resistance (HOMA-IR) and the quantitative insulin sensitivity check index (QUICKI) were determined according to the published formula [24]. Enzymatic kits (Pars Azmun, Tehran, Iran) were applied to measure serum lipid profiles with inter- and intra-assay of less than 5%.

Isolation of lymphocyte cells

Blood samples were used to extract lymphocyte cells, using 50% percoll (Sigma-Aldrich, Dorset, UK). Cell count and viability test were performed using trypan blue, RNA and DNA extraction [25].

RNA extraction and real-time PCR (RT-PCR)

RNA was extracted from blood samples using RNX-plus kit (Cinnacolon, Tehran, Iran). RNA suspension was frozen at – 20 °C until cDNA was derived. RNA quantification was conducted using UV spectrophotometer and total RNAs were extracted from each sample. Each sample OD 260/280 ratio was considered to range from 1.7 to 2.1, representing no contamination with either protein or DNA [25].

The isolated RNA was reverse transcribed to cDNA library, using moloney murine leukemia virus reverse transcriptase (RT). Gene expressions of peroxisome proliferator-activated receptor gamma (PPAR-γ), glucose transporter 1 (GLUT-1) and low-density lipoprotein receptor (LDLR) were done using peripheral blood mononuclear cells (PBMCs) via SYBR green detection and Amplicon Kit, applying quantitative RT-PCR and Light Cycler technology (Roche Diagnostics, Rotkreuz, Switzerland) (Table 1). Glyceraldehyde-3-phosphate

dehydrogenase (GAPDH) primers were used as a housekeeping gene. Primers were designed using Primer Express Software (Applied Biosystems, Foster City, USA) and Beacon designer software (Takaposizt, Tehran, Iran). Relative transcription levels were calculated using Pffafi or $2^{-\Delta\Delta CT}$ methods [25].

Sample size

Clinical trial sample size formula was used to calculate sample size considering a type one error (α) of 0.05 and type two error (β) of 0.20 with the power of 80%. Mean difference (d) of HOMA-IR equal to 0.8 and SD of 0.8 were used for the calculation [26]. Sample size was defined as 16 participants in each group. Considering 4 probable dropouts in each group, the final sample size was determined to be 20 participants in each group.

Statistical methods

Kolmogorov-Smirnov test was used to assess the normal distribution of variables. Analyses were replicated using intention-to-treat (ITT) approach. To determine the differences in anthropometric measures and gene expression of insulin and lipid metabolism between the intervention groups, we used independent samples t-test. The effects of vitamin D supplementation on glycemic control and markers of cardiometabolic risk were assessed using repeated measures ANOVA test. The P-values of < 0.05 were considered statistically significant. Statistical analyses were conducted using the Statistical Package for Social Science version 18 (SPSS Inc., Chicago, Illinois, USA).

Results

We had three dropouts in each intervention group due to personal reasons, and 34 participants [infertile women with PCOS candidate for IVF receiving vitamin D (n = 17) and placebo (n = 17)] completed the study (Fig. 1). Using ITT protocol, all 40 participants (20 in each group) were included in the final analysis. Compliance rate in this trial ranged 90% to100% in both groups. No side effects were reported following vitamin D supplementation in infertile women with PCOS who were candidate for IVF throughout the study. Mean age, height, weight and BMI were not statistically different between the intervention groups throughout the trial (Table 2).

After 8-week intervention, vitamin D supplementation led to a significant reduction in serum AMH (– 0.7 ± 1.2 vs. -0.1 ± 0.5 ng/mL, P = 0.02) and insulin levels (– 1.4 ± 1.6 vs. -0.3 ± 0.9 μIU/mL, P = 0.007), HOMA-IR (– 0.3 ± 0.3 vs. -0.1 ± 0.2, P = 0.008), as well as a significant increase in QUICKI (+ 0.009 ± 0.01 vs. + 0.001 ± 0.004, P = 0.04) compared with placebo (Table 3). Further, taking vitamin D supplements significantly decreased serum total- (– 5.1 ± 12.6 vs. + 2.9 ± 10.9 mg/dL, P = 0.03) and

Table 1 Specific primers used for real-time quantitative PCR

Gene	Primer	Product size (bp)	Annealing temperature ©
GAPDH	F: AAGCTCATTTCCTGGTATGACAACG	126	61.3
	R: TCTTCCTCTTGTGCTCTTGCTGG		
PPAR-γ	F: ATGACAGACCTCAGACAGATTG	210	54
	R: AATGTTGGCAGTGGCTCAG		
GLUT-1	F: TATCTGAGCATCGTGGCCAT	238	62.1
	R: AAGACGTAGGGACCACACAG		
LDLR	F: ACTTACGGACAGACAGACAG	223	57
	R: GGCCACACATCCCATGATTC		

GAPDH glyceraldehyde-3-Phosphate dehydrogenase, *GLUT-1* glucose transporter 1, *LDLR* low-density lipoprotein receptor, *PPAR-γ* peroxisome proliferator-activated receptor gamma

LDL-cholesterol levels (-4.5 ± 10.3 vs. $+2.5 \pm 10.6$ mg/dL, $P = 0.04$) compared with the placebo. There was no significant effect of vitamin D supplementation on fasting glucose and other parameters of lipid profiles.

RT-PCR quantitative tests showed a significant upregulation of gene expression of PPAR-γ ($P = 0.01$), GLUT-1 ($P = 0.009$) and LDLR ($P = 0.03$) in PBMCs of infertile women diagnosed with PCOS who were candidate for IVF following vitamin D supplementation rather than placebo (Fig. 2).

Discussion

The results of this trial demonstrated the beneficial effects of 50,000 IU vitamin D supplementation every other week for 8 weeks on improving insulin metabolism and some of the markers of lipid profile among infertile women diagnosed with PCOS who were candidate for IVF. These benefits might not be evident upon having sufficient vitamin D levels. To our best knowledge, this study has reported the effects of vitamin D supplementation on AMH, glycemic control, lipid profiles and gene expression of insulin and lipid metabolism in infertile women for the first time.

Polycystic ovary syndrome predisposes patients to different metabolic abnormalities, such as insulin resistance and dyslipidemia [27, 28]. This study demonstrated that 50,000 IU vitamin D supplementation every other week for 8 weeks resulted in significant decreases in serum AMH, insulin levels and HOMA-IR score, and a significant increase in QUICKI in infertile women with PCOS who were

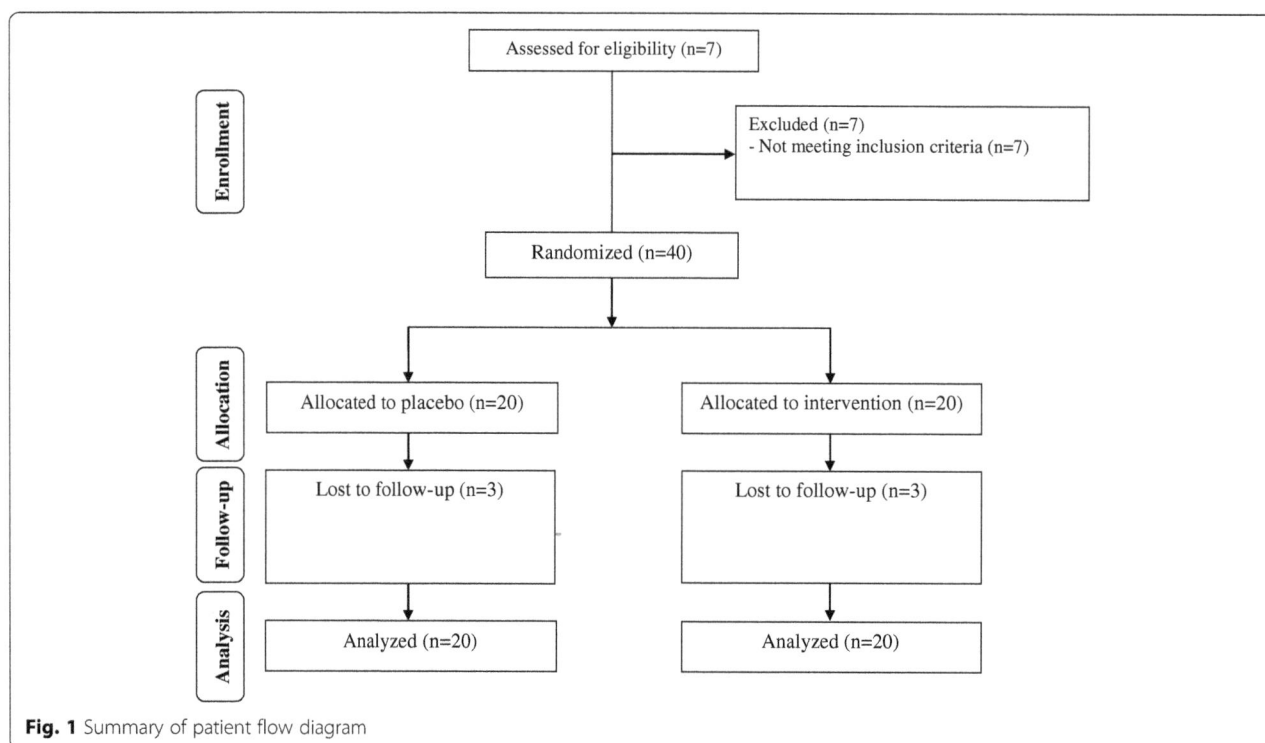

Fig. 1 Summary of patient flow diagram

Table 2 General characteristics of study participants

	Placebo group (n = 20)	Vitamin D group (n = 20)	P[a]
Age (y)	30.1 ± 3.4	29.9 ± 4.4	0.87
Height (cm)	159.2 ± 2.0	160.4 ± 3.3	0.16
Weight at study baseline (kg)	72.0 ± 6.9	71.3 ± 9.9	0.77
Weight at end-of-trial (kg)	72.2 ± 6.8	71.5 ± 9.6	0.79
Weight change (kg)	0.1 ± 0.8	0.2 ± 0.9	0.70
BMI at study baseline (kg/m^2)	28.4 ± 2.6	27.7 ± 3.9	0.49
BMI at end-of-trial (kg/m^2)	28.5 ± 2.6	27.8 ± 3.7	0.50
BMI change (kg/m^2)	0.1 ± 0.3	0.1 ± 0.3	0.68

Data are means± SDs
[a] Obtained from independent t-test

candidate for IVF. Further, vitamin D supplementation significantly increased gene expression levels of PPAR-γ and GLUT-1. In the agreement with our study, Gupta et al. [29] demonstrated that vitamin D supplementation at a dosage of 60,000 IU weekly for 12 weeks significantly reduced insulin levels and HOMA-IR, and significantly increased QUICKI in vitamin D-deficient women with PCOS. In another study, taking vitamin D supplements at a dosage of 20,000 IU per week for 24 weeks by women with PCOS, having serum calcium levels < 2.65 mmol/L and uncertain serum 25 (OH) D status at baseline, improved glucose metabolism and menstrual frequency [30]. However, there are also studies with discrepant findings. Garg et al. [31], showed that vitamin D supplementation at a dose of 4000 IU/day for 6 months to vitamin D-deficient women with PCOS did not have any significant effect on insulin resistance and insulin secretion. Insulin resistance is associated with increased synthesis of vasoconstriction factors, which might be the reason for vascular stiffness in women

diagnosed with PCOS [32]. Therefore, improved insulin metabolism by vitamin D supplementation may decrease the risk of metabolic complications subsequent to insulin resistance in these patients. The mechanisms involved in the impact of vitamin D on insulin metabolism could be direct and indirect effects of vitamin D on stimulating insulin release through improved vitamin D receptor expression, enhancing insulin sensitivity for glucose transportation and suppressing the release of pro-inflammatory cytokines [33].

We found that 50,000 IU vitamin D supplementation every other week for 8 weeks significantly decreased total- and LDL-cholesterol levels in infertile women with PCOS who were candidate for IVF, compared with the placebo, though other lipid profiles parameters remained unchanged. Moreover, vitamin D supplementation significantly increased gene expression levels of LDLR. Similar to our findings, vitamin D supplementation at a dosage of 4000 IU/day for 12 weeks significantly decreased total cholesterol

Table 3 Glycemic control, markers of cardio-metabolic risk and oxidative stress at baseline and after the 8-week intervention in infertile polycystic ovary syndrome women candidate for in vitro fertilization that received either vitamin D supplements or placebo

	Placebo group (n = 20)			Vitamin D group (n = 20)			P[a]
	Baseline	End-of-trial	Change	Baseline	End-of-trial	Change	
Vitamin D (ng/mL)	11.0 ± 2.4	10.9 ± 2.1	-0.1 ± 0.6	10.5 ± 2.5	21.7 ± 5.9	11.2 ± 5.0	< 0.001
AMH (ng/mL)	8.7 ± 2.7	8.6 ± 2.5	-0.1 ± 0.5	7.7 ± 3.4	7.0 ± 3.1	−0.7 ± 1.2	0.02
FPG (mg/dL)	92.9 ± 5.5	93.5 ± 5.6	0.5 ± 3.0	90.3 ± 10.5	89.4 ± 10.6	−0.9 ± 7.4	0.42
Insulin (μIU/mL)	11.4 ± 1.9	11.1 ± 2.0	−0.3 ± 0.9	11.2 ± 2.2	9.8 ± 2.7	−1.4 ± 1.6	0.007
HOMA-IR	2.6 ± 0.5	2.5 ± 0.4	−0.1 ± 0.2	2.5 ± 0.7	2.2 ± 0.7	−0.3 ± 0.3	0.008
QUICKI	0.33 ± 0.008	0.33 ± 0.009	0.001 ± 0.004	0.33 ± 0.01	0.34 ± 0.02	0.009 ± 0.01	0.04
Triglycerides (mg/dL)	111.5 ± 35.5	117.4 ± 34.8	5.9 ± 13.2	105.3 ± 33.5	107.5 ± 38.1	2.1 ± 17.4	0.44
VLDL-cholesterol (mg/dL)	22.3 ± 7.1	23.5 ± 6.9	1.2 ± 2.6	21.1 ± 6.7	21.5 ± 7.6	0.4 ± 3.5	0.44
Total cholesterol (mg/dL)	197.1 ± 36.3	200.0 ± 36.5	2.9 ± 10.9	203.6 ± 26.6	198.5 ± 24.7	−5.1 ± 12.6	0.03
LDL-cholesterol (mg/dL)	124.9 ± 35.9	127.4 ± 35.3	2.5 ± 10.6	133.1 ± 21.1	128.7 ± 20.8	−4.5 ± 10.3	0.04
HDL-cholesterol (mg/dL)	49.9 ± 7.5	49.1 ± 8.2	−0.8 ± 3.9	49.4 ± 5.7	48.4 ± 5.4	−1.0 ± 2.8	0.81

Data are means± SDs
[a] Obtained from repeated measures ANOVA test
AMH anti-Müllerian hormone, *FPG* fasting plasma glucose, *HOMA-IR* homeostasis model of assessment-estimated insulin resistance, *QUICKI* quantitative insulin sensitivity check index

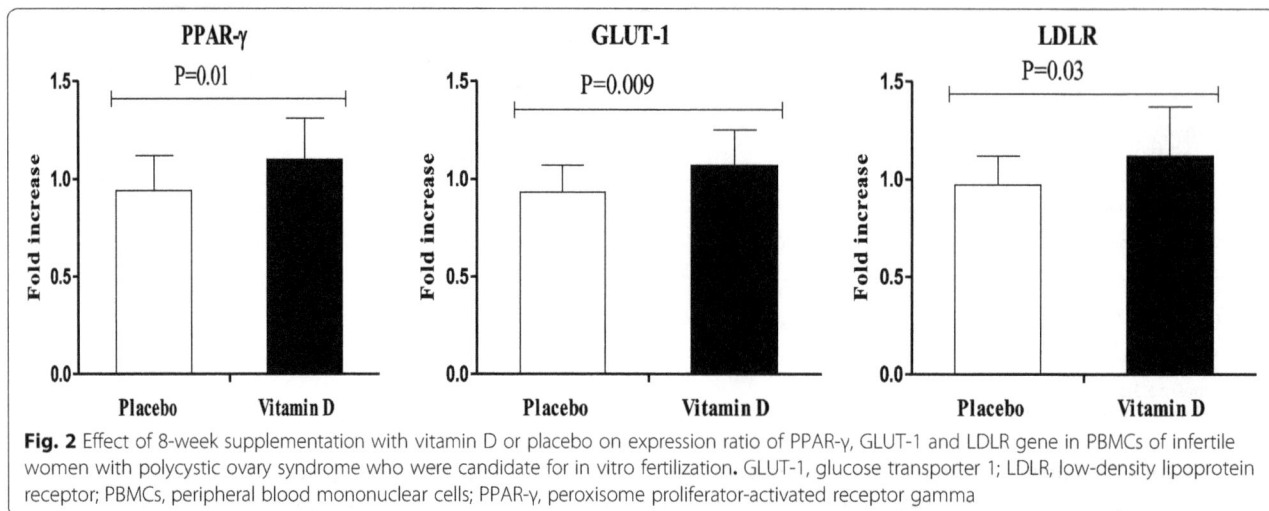

Fig. 2 Effect of 8-week supplementation with vitamin D or placebo on expression ratio of PPAR-γ, GLUT-1 and LDLR gene in PBMCs of infertile women with polycystic ovary syndrome who were candidate for in vitro fertilization. GLUT-1, glucose transporter 1; LDLR, low-density lipoprotein receptor; PBMCs, peripheral blood mononuclear cells; PPAR-γ, peroxisome proliferator-activated receptor gamma

concentrations in vitamin D deficient HIV-infected patients [34]. In a meta-analysis conducted by Akbari et al. [35], vitamin D supplementation significantly decreased LDL-cholesterol levels in gestational diabetes patients, though other lipid profiles parameters did not change. There are also contrary studies demonstrating that vitamin D supplementation (100,000 IU loading dose, followed by 20,000 IU/week) did not improve CVD risk factors including blood pressure, lipid profiles and glucose metabolism parameters in vitamin D insufficient population [36]. Current evidence suggested that increased insulin and androgens levels may negatively influence lipid profiles in women with PCOS [37]. Fatty acids byproducts have an important role in inflammation and reproduction [37]. Improved insulin sensitivity and decreased production of PTH by vitamin D might decrease total- and LDL-cholesterol [38]. Further, insulin reduces biosynthesis of cholesterol via increased 3-hydroxy-3-methylglutaryl CoA (HMG-CoA) reductase activity [39], which in turn decreases total- and LDL-cholesterol levels.

There are a few limitations in this study. First, the evaluation of insulin resistance in the current study, was only based on HOMA-IR. We did not assess any direct dynamic test, such as glucose tolerance test or hyperinsulinemic euglycemic clamp. Second, some of the insignificant results might be related to the short duration of intervention. So, further studies are required with longer duration and higher sample size to confirm our findings. In addition, all the participants were vitamin D deficient, so the observed effects might be correlated with the correction of vitamin D deficiency, rather than the supplementation per se. This should be considered in the interpretation of our finding.

Conclusions

Overall, the findings of this trial supported that 50,000 IU vitamin D supplementation every other week

for 8 weeks had beneficial effects on insulin metabolism, and some parameters of lipid profiles among infertile women with PCOS who were candidate for IVF. These benefits might not be evident upon having sufficient vitamin D levels.

Abbreviations

25 (OH) D: 25-hydroxyvitamin D; AMH: anti-Müllerian hormone; FPG: fasting plasma glucose; GAPDH: glyceraldehyde-3-phosphate dehydrogenase; HOMA-IR: homeostasis model of assessment-estimated insulin resistance; HMG-CoA: 3-hydroxy-3-methylglutaryl CoA; ITT: intention-to-treat; QUICKI: quantitative insulin sensitivity check index; GLUT-1: glucose transporter 1; LDLR: low-density lipoprotein receptor; PBMCs: peripheral blood mononuclear cells; PPAR-γ: peroxisome proliferator-activated receptor gamma

Acknowledgements

Research reported in this publication was supported by Kashan University of Medical Sciences, Kashan, Iran.

Funding

This study was founded by a grant from the Vice-chancellor for Research, Kashan University of Medical Sciences, Kashan, Iran.

Authors' contributions

ZA and EA contributed in conception, design, statistical analysis and drafting of the manuscript. MD, NM, FF, SZ-M and MA-S contributed in data collection and manuscript drafting. All authors approved the final version for submission.

Competing interests

The authors declare that they have no competing interests.

Author details

[1]Research Center for Biochemistry and Nutrition in Metabolic Diseases, Kashan University of Medical Sciences, Kashan, I.R. Iran. [2]School of Public Health, University of Saskatchewan, Saskatoon, SK, Canada. [3]Department of Gynecology and Obstetrics, School of Medicine, Kashan University of Medical Sciences, Kashan, I.R. Iran. [4]Laser Application in Medical Science Research Center, Shahid Beheshti University of Medical Sciences, Tehran, Iran. [5]Taleghani Educational Hospital, IVF Center, Shahid Beheshti University of Medical Sciences, Tehran, Iran.

References

1. Sheehan MT. Polycystic ovarian syndrome: diagnosis and management. Clin Med Res. 2004;2:13–27.

2. Fica S, Albu A, Constantin M, Dobri GA. Insulin resistance and fertility in polycystic ovary syndrome. J Med Life. 2008;1:415–22.

3. Ceelen M, van Weissenbruch MM, Roos JC, Vermeiden JP, van Leeuwen FE. Delemarre-van de Waal HA. Body composition in children and adolescents born after in vitro fertilization or spontaneous conception. J Clin Endocrinol Metab. 2007;92:3417–23.

4. Ceelen M, van Weissenbruch MM, Vermeiden JP, van Leeuwen FE. Delemarre-van de Waal HA. Cardiometabolic differences in children born after in vitro fertilization: follow-up study. J Clin Endocrinol Metab. 2008;93: 1682–8.

5. Rexhaj E, Paoloni-Giacobino A, Rimoldi SF, Fuster DG, Anderegg M, Somm E, et al. Mice generated by in vitro fertilization exhibit vascular dysfunction and shortened life span. J Clin Invest. 2013;123:5052–60.

6. Scott KA, Yamazaki Y, Yamamoto M, Lin Y, Melhorn SJ, Krause EG, et al. Glucose parameters are altered in mouse offspring produced by assisted reproductive technologies and somatic cell nuclear transfer. Biol Reprod. 2010;83:220–7.

7. Vlaisavljevic V, Kovac V, Sajko MC. Impact of insulin resistance on the developmental potential of immature oocytes retrieved from human chorionic gonadotropin-primed women with polycystic ovary syndrome undergoing in vitro maturation. Fertil Steril. 2009;91:957–9.

8. Halloran BP, DeLuca HF. Effect of vitamin D deficiency on fertility and reproductive capacity in the female rat. J Nutr. 1980;110:1573–80.

9. Daftary GS, Taylor HS. Endocrine regulation of HOX genes. Endocr Rev. 2006; 27:331–55.

10. Kinuta K, Tanaka H, Moriwake T, Aya K, Kato S, Seino Y. Vitamin D is an important factor in estrogen biosynthesis of both female and male gonads. Endocrinology. 2000;141:1317–24.

11. Johnson LE, DeLuca HF. Vitamin D receptor null mutant mice fed high levels of calcium are fertile. J Nutr. 2001;131:1787–91.

12. Wehr E, Pilz S, Schweighofer N, Giuliani A, Kopera D, Pieber TR, et al. Association of hypovitaminosis D with metabolic disturbances in polycystic ovary syndrome. Eur J Endocrinol. 2009;161:575–82.

13. Yildizhan R, Kurdoglu M, Adali E, Kolusari A, Yildizhan B, Sahin HG, et al. Serum 25-hydroxyvitamin D concentrations in obese and non-obese women with polycystic ovary syndrome. Arch Gynecol Obstet. 2009;280:559–63.

14. Turer CB, Lin H, Flores G. Prevalence of vitamin D deficiency among overweight and obese US children. Pediatrics. 2013;131:e152–61.

15. Zadeh-Vakili A, Ramezani Tehrani F, Daneshpour MS, Zarkesh M, Saadat N, Azizi F. Genetic polymorphism of vitamin D receptor gene affects the phenotype of PCOS. Gene. 2013;515:193–6.

16. Aleyasin A, Hosseini MA, Mahdavi A, Safdarian L, Fallahi P, Mohajeri MR, et al. Predictive value of the level of vitamin D in follicular fluid on the outcome of assisted reproductive technology. Eur J Obstet Gynecol Reprod Biol. 2011;159:132–7.

17. Anifandis GM, Dafopoulos K, Messini CI, Chalvatzas N, Liakos N, Pournaras S, et al. Prognostic value of follicular fluid 25-OH vitamin D and glucose levels in the IVF outcome. Reprod Biol Endocrinol. 2010;8:91.

18. Butts SF, Seifer DB, Koelper N, Senapati S, Sammel MD, Hoofnagle AN, et al. Vitamin D deficiency is associated with poor ovarian stimulation outcome in pcos but not unexplained infertility. J Clin Endocrinol Metab. 2018. https://doi.org/10.1210/jc.2018-00750.

19. He C, Lin Z, Robb SW, Ezeamama AE. Serum vitamin D levels and polycystic ovary syndrome: a systematic review and meta-analysis. Nutrients. 2015;7: 4555–77.

20. Seyyed Abootorabi M, Ayremlou P, Behroozi-Lak T, Nourisaeidlou S. The effect of vitamin D supplementation on insulin resistance, visceral fat and adiponectin in vitamin D deficient women with polycystic ovary syndrome: a randomized placebo-controlled trial. Gynecol Endocrinol. 2018;34:489–94.

21. Xue Y, Xu P, Xue K, Duan X, Cao J, Luan T, et al. Effect of vitamin D on biochemical parameters in polycystic ovary syndrome women: a meta-analysis. Arch Gynecol Obstet. 2017;295:487–96.

22. Taylor PN, Davies JS. A review of the growing risk of vitamin D toxicity from inappropriate practice. Br J Clin Pharmacol. 2018;84:1121–7.

23. Rotterdam ESHRE/ASRM-Sponsored PCOS Consensus Workshop Group. Revised 2003 consensus on diagnostic criteria and long-term health risks related to polycystic ovary syndrome. Fertil Steril. 2004;81:19–25.

24. Pisprasert V, Ingram KH, Lopez-Davila MF, Munoz AJ, Garvey WT. Limitations in the use of indices using glucose and insulin levels to predict insulin sensitivity: impact of race and gender and superiority of the indices derived from oral glucose tolerance test in African Americans. Diabetes Care. 2013; 36:845–53.

25. Dunkley PR, Jarvie PE, Robinson PJ. A rapid Percoll gradient procedure for preparation of synaptosomes. Nat Protoc. 2008;3:1718–28.

26. Maktabi M, Chamani M, Asemi Z. The effects of vitamin D supplementation on metabolic status of patients with polycystic ovary syndrome: a randomized, double-blind, placebo-controlled trial. Horm Metab Res. 2017; 49:493–8.

27. Asemi Z, Foroozanfard F, Hashemi T, Bahmani F, Jamilian M, Esmaillzadeh A. Calcium plus vitamin D supplementation affects glucose metabolism and lipid concentrations in overweight and obese vitamin D deficient women with polycystic ovary syndrome. Clin Nutr. 2015;34:586–92.

28. Foroozanfard F, Jamilian M, Bahmani F, Talaee R, Talaee N, Hashemi T, et al. Calcium plus vitamin D supplementation influences biomarkers of inflammation and oxidative stress in overweight and vitamin D-deficient women with polycystic ovary syndrome: a randomized double-blind placebo-controlled clinical trial. Clin Endocrinol. 2015;83:888–94.

29. Gupta T, Rawat M, Gupta N, Arora S. Study of effect of vitamin D supplementation on the clinical, hormonal and metabolic profile of the PCOS women. J Obstet Gynaecol India. 2017;67:349–55.

30. Wehr E, Pieber TR, Obermayer-Pietsch B. Effect of vitamin D3 treatment on glucose metabolism and menstrual frequency in polycystic ovary syndrome women: a pilot study. J Endocrinol Investig. 2011;34:757–63.

31. Garg G, Kachhawa G, Ramot R, Khadgawat R, Tandon N, Sreenivas V, et al. Effect of vitamin D supplementation on insulin kinetics and cardiovascular risk factors in polycystic ovarian syndrome: a pilot study. Endocr Connect. 2015;4:108–16.

32. Kelly CJ, Speirs A, Gould GW, Petrie JR, Lyall H, Connell JM. Altered vascular function in young women with polycystic ovary syndrome. J Clin Endocrinol Metab. 2002;87:742–6.

33. Alvarez JA, Ashraf A. Role of vitamin d in insulin secretion and insulin sensitivity for glucose homeostasis. Int J Endocrinol. 2010;2010:351385.

34. Longenecker CT, Hileman CO, Carman TL, Ross AC, Seydafkan S, Brown TT, et al. Vitamin D supplementation and endothelial function in vitamin D deficient HIV-infected patients: a randomized placebo-controlled trial. Antivir Ther. 2012;17:613–21.

35. Akbari M, Mosazadeh M, Lankarani KB, Tabrizi R, Samimi M, Karamali M, et al. The effects of vitamin D supplementation on glucose metabolism and lipid profiles in patients with gestational diabetes: a systematic review and meta-analysis of randomized controlled trials. Horm Metab Res. 2017;49:647–53.

36. Kubiak JM, Thorsby PM, Kamycheva E, Jorde R. Vitamin D supplementation does not improve CVD risk factors in vitamin D insufficient subjects. Endocr Connect. 2018;7:840–9.

37. Li S, Chu Q, Ma J, Sun Y, Tao T, Huang R, et al. Discovery of novel lipid profiles in PCOS: do insulin and androgen oppositely regulate bioactive lipid production? J Clin Endocrinol Metab. 2017;102:810–21.

38. Wang H, Xia N, Yang Y, Peng DQ. Influence of vitamin D supplementation on plasma lipid profiles: a meta-analysis of randomized controlled trials. Lipids Health Dis. 2012;11:42. https://doi.org/10.1186/1476-511X-11-42.

39. Kaplan M, Kerry R, Aviram M, Hayek T. High glucose concentration increases macrophage cholesterol biosynthesis in diabetes through activation of the sterol regulatory element binding. Protein 1 (SREBP1): inhibitory effect of insulin. J Cardiovasc Pharmacol. 2008;52:324–32.

21

Spatio-temporal expression profile of matrix metalloproteinase (Mmp) modulators Reck and Sparc during the rat ovarian dynamics

Gabriel Levin[1†], Tatiane Maldonado Coelho[1,2†], Nathali Guimarães Nóbrega[1], Marina Trombetta-Lima[1,2], Mari Cleide Sogayar[1,2] and Ana Claudia Oliveira Carreira[1,2,3*] [ID]

Abstract

Background: Matrix metalloproteinases (Mmps) and their tissue inhibitors (Timps) are widely recognized as crucial factors for extracellular matrix remodeling in the ovary and are involved in follicular growth, ovulation, luteinization, and luteolysis during the estrous cycle. Recently, several genes have been associated to the modulation of Mmps activity, including *Basigin (Bsg)*, which induces the expression of Mmps in rat ovaries; *Sparc*, a TGF-β modulator that is related to increased expression of Mmps in cancer; and *Reck*, which is associated with Mmps inhibition. However, the expression pattern of Mmp modulators in ovary dynamics is still largely uncharacterized.

Methods: To characterize the expression pattern of Mmps network members in ovary dynamics, we analyzed the spatio-temporal expression pattern of Reck and Sparc, as well as of Mmp2, Mmp9 and Mmp14 proteins, by immunohistochemistry (IHC), in pre-pubertal rat ovaries obtained from an artificial cycle induced by eCG/hCG, in the different phases of the hormone-induced estrous cycle. We also determined the gene expression profiles of *Mmps (2, 9, 13 14)*, *Timps (1, 2, 3)*, *Sparc*, *Bsg*, and *Reck* to complement this panel.

Results: IHC analysis revealed that Mmp protein expression peaks at the early stages of folliculogenesis and ovulation, decreases during ovulation-luteogenesis transition and luteogenesis, increasing again during *corpus luteum* maintenance and luteolysis. The protein expression patterns of these metalloproteinases and Sparc were inverse relative to the pattern displayed by Reck. We observed that the gene expression peaks of Mmps inhibitors *Reck* and *Timp2* were closely paraleled by *Mmp2* and *Mmp9* suppression. The opposite was also true: increased *Mmp2* and *Mmp9* expression was concomitant to reduced *Reck* and *Timp2* levels.

Conclusion: Therefore, our results generate a spatio-temporal expression profile panel of Mmps and their regulators, suggesting that Reck and Sparc seem to play a role during ovarian dynamics: Reck as a possible inhibitor and Sparc as an inducer of Mmps.

Keywords: Folliculogenesis, Ovary remodeling, Mmps system, Extracellular matrix, Reck, Sparc

* Correspondence: ancoc@iq.usp.br; ancoc@iq.usp.br;
anaclaudiaoli@gmail.com
†Gabriel Levin and Tatiane Maldonado Coelho contributed equally to this work.
[1]NUCEL (Cell and Molecular Therapy Center), Internal Medicine Department, Medical School, University of São Paulo, Rua Pangaré, 100, Cidade Universitária, São Paulo, SP 05360-130, Brazil
[2]Chemistry Institute, Biochemistry Department, University of São Paulo, São Paulo, SP 05508-000, Brazil
Full list of author information is available at the end of the article

Background

The ovarian dynamics comprehended by different phases of the estrous cycle involves extensive tissue remodeling [1], and major extracellular matrix (ECM) reorganization is a key part of this process. This tissue remodeling is dependent upon cyclic hormonal variation, proteins and peptide growth factors and is a pre-requisite for expansion of the growing ovulatory follicle, breakdown of follicular walls during ovulation, luteinization of the postovulatory follicles, and regression of the *corpus luteum* (CL) [2, 3]. Matrix metalloproteinases (Mmps), a large family of zinc-dependent proteases, and their also numerous inhibitors (Timps) play a major role in ovarian ECM reorganization [2–5]. Together, Mmps and Timps form a network that regulates tissue remodelling and is modulated not only by gonadotropins and steroid hormones, but, also, by the expression of other factors, such as TNF-α, IGF-1 [5–9], and Bsg, which is an inducer of Mmps during the luteinization process [10]. A complete map of the components of this network, as well as a precise characterization of their expression pattern, may allow us to better understand this tight regulation involved in ovarian tissue remodelling that occur during the estrous cycle.

It is already known from the literature that Mmp2, Mmp9, Mmp14 (Mt1-Mmp), and Mmp19 expression and activity in granulosa and/or theca cells are extensively linked to the disruption of ovarian ECM in rats, which is rich in collagen, laminin, and fibronectin, leading to follicular growth and release of the oocyte during the ovulatory process [11]. MMP1, MMP2 e MMP9 have been detected in cultures of luteinized granulosa cells [12–14].

The expression and activity of Mmps have been known to be upregulated by gonadotropins during these phases [15–19]. However, hCG also was shown to reduce the expression of MMP2 and MMP9 [12, 13]. Following ovulation, the ruptured follicle is transformed into a CL by extensive cellular reorganization, migration, and neovascularization [20–22], which is associated with notable gelatinolytic activity, whereas the regression and absorption of CL is marked by an increase in Mmp13 levels and activity [23, 24].

Tissue inhibitors of metalloproteinases (Timps) have also been extensively studied in ovaries during the estrous cycle. Timp1 is upregulated by gonadotropins during folliculogenesis and ovulation in rats [25–27], providing proteolytic homeostasis to the ECM, through inhibition of metalloproteinases in the corpus luteum, while Timp3 levels decrease slightly [28].

Timp1 mRNA levels increase during luteal formation and regression [24, 29], while *Timp3* levels are elevated during luteal maintenance [29]. TIMP-2 has a role in the local regulation of MMP1 and MMP2 in the corpus luteum [30]. Moreover, in addition to these inhibitors, there are also proteins, which have already been described as being responsible for inducing the expression of Mmps and ensuring system homeostasis in the ovary. In this context, it is worth mentioning Basigin (Bsg), a protein associated with Mmps induction and also with tumor progression and endometriosis, being expressed in granulosa and theca cells of pre-ovulatory follicles, and also in CL [10, 31]. However, the expression pattern of Mmp modulators in ovary dynamics is still largely uncharacterized, and there is evidence that members of the network are still to be identified. In particular, two proteins implied in tumor aggressiveness and invasive potential, through modulation of ECM integrity, namely, Sparc and Reck, may have an important role in ovarian tissue remodeling, since they are expressed in ovarian cells and are involved in the regulation of the Mmp system in other tissues [32–36].

Sparc (secreted protein acid and rich in cysteine), also known as Osteonectin, a 43 K protein, and basement-membrane protein 40 (BM-40), is a calcium-binding matrix cellular protein that plays a role in matrix mineralization [37], modulates TGF-β [34], and is expressed in the internal theca and follicular basal lamina of ovine follicles and theca-derived small luteal cells [35]. Even though SPARC is highly expressed in several tumors, it may be able to inhibit tumorigenesis or tumor progression in human ovarian cancer [38] and its expression is reduced in ovarian cancer cell lines [38]. Additionally, Sparc is implicated in indirect Mmp modulation and turnover of many physiological processes, but it has not yet been described in whole ovary dynamics. Despite the fact that Bagavandoss et al. described Sparc in the ovary of the late stages of estrous cycle, its expression in the initial phases (folliculogenesis, ovulation and ovulation-luteinization transition) of this process is still unknown [32]. On the other hand, RECK (REversion-inducing-Cystein-rich protein with Kazal motifs) is a key regulator of extracellular matrix integrity and angiogenesis that is linked to the cell membrane by a GPI-anchor [36] and inhibits the activity of MMP2, MMP9, and MMP14 at different steps of their activation cascades in humans [36, 39]. *Reck* gene is expressed in several mouse tissues during development, including the uterus and ovaries, but at lower levels in most tissues, when compared to those of Timps 1, 2, 3, and 4 [33]. Reck expression is inhibited by estrogen within the mouse uterus, but this inhibition is partially blocked by progesterone [40]. To date, no information is available regarding the expression profile and function of Reck in rat ovaries development and maturation.

To analyse the ovarian extracellular matrix remodeling, we analyzed an artificial estral cycle, with a combination of equine chorionic gonadotropin (eCG) and human CG (hCG) in pre-pubertal rats [41], that have not yet started their estrous cycle, to induce multiple follicular development and ovulation. The rats only start their estrus cycles after the vaginal orifice opens, which tends to occur between postnatal 32 and 36 days [41]. The literature describes that the administration of 10UI eCG stimulates the folliculogenesis and after 48 h the injection of 10UI of hCG can induce ovulation [42, 43]. In sequence, it is observed formation of corpus luteum, and 24 and 48 h post-hCG injection, the luteal formation in the ovaries. After 4 and 8 days, a peak of progesterone production is maximal resulting in the luteal maintenance, and corpus luteum regression can be analyzed at 14 days.

Therefore, understanding Reck and Sparc expression during the estrous cycle is essential to understand which role, if any, they play in the regulation of ovarian tissue remodeling, which allows all of the complex physiological processes that take place in the ovary. In this context, our hypothesis is that the Mmps regulators Reck and Sparc are modulated in ovarian dynamics possibly controlling the expression of Mmps, Reck being a possible inhibitor and Sparc a possible inducer of Mmps in this process.

To address these questions, we characterized the spatio-temporal expression pattern of Reck and Sparc proteins, as well as of Mmp2, Mmp9 and Mmp14 by immunohistochemistry in pre-pubertal rat ovaries during different phases of the hCG/eCG induced estrous cycle. To complement these data, we used qRT-PCR to investigate *Mmps 2, 9, 13, 14, and 19, Timps 1, 2, and 3, Reck, Sparc, and Bsg* mRNA levels and generate a complete expression profile panel of these targets during induced folliculogenesis, ovulation, luteogenesis, and luteolysis in prepubertal rat ovaries.

Methods
Animal model
All animal experimentation was approved by the Ethics Committee for Animal Use of the Chemistry Institute (CEUA) on 08/28/2010, University of São Paulo, São Paulo, Brazil, in accordance with the National Council for the Control of Animal Experimentation (CONCEA).

To create an artificial estral cycle, we carried out the protocol to induce multiple follicular development and ovulation described by Jo and Curry and Ying and Meyer [42, 43]. First, 21 day-old pre-pubertal Sprague-Dawley female rats were induced by subcutaneous injection of 10 IU of equine chorionic gonadotropin (eCG) (Folligon, MSD Saúde Animal, São Paulo, SP, Brazil), resulting in animals in folliculogenesis phase. In sequence, ovulation and CL formation were induced by subcutaneous injection of 10 IU of human chorionic gonadotropin (hCG) (Choragon, Ferring

GmbH, Kiel, Alemanha) 48 h after eCG injection. To analyze the relative expression pattern of the genes of interest throughout the hormonally induced estrous cycle, 10 experimental groups were established and different hormonal treatments were adopted to recreate the various stages of the estrous cycle. Treatment groups varied depending on the hormones applied (eCG only or both eCG and hCG) and induction and euthanasia periods of time. Animals were euthanized at 0, 24, or 48 h after eCG administration or 12, 24, or 48 h or 4, 8, or 14 days after hCG administration (Table 1). Two independent experiments were carried out, using three animals per experimental group. Animals injected with phosphate-buffered saline (PBS [137 mM NaCl, 2.7 mM KCl, 8 mM anhydrous Na_2HPO_4, and 1.4 mM KH_2PO_4; pH = 7.2]) were used as controls.

Tissue samples
Both ovaries were collected from each animal. One ovary was stored in RNAholder solution (BioAgency Laboratories, São Paulo, SP, Brazil) at – 80 °C for total RNA extraction and the contralateral ovary was fixed in 4% paraformaldehyde solution (Sigma-Aldrich, St. Louis, MO, USA), stored at 4 °C, and subsequently included in paraffin for immunohistochemical analysis.

Immunohistochemistry
The paraffin-embedded tissues were sectioned into 4 μm-thick sections using a microtome (Leica Biosystems, Wetzlar, HE, Germany) and placed onto polylysine-treated slides. The sections were then dewaxed in xylene (Synth, São Paulo, SP, Brazil), incubated with decreasing concentrations of ethanol (Synth), and rehydrated in PBS-T (0.1% Triton X-100 in PBS [123 mM NaCl, 9.7 mM Na_2HPO_4, and 51.1 mM KH_2PO_4; pH = 7.4]). Next, tissue antigens were retrieved using phosphate-citrate buffer (pH = 6.0; Sigma-Aldrich) at 98 °C for 20 min, slowly cooled down to room temperature, and

Table 1 Experimental groups and treatments

GROUP	10 IU eCG	10 IU hCG	PHASE
G1	0 h	–	Control
G2	24 h	–	Folliculogenesis
G3	48 h	–	
G4	48 h	12 h	Ovulation
G5	48 h	24 h	Transition: ovulation-luteinization
G6	48 h	48 h	Transition: ovulation-luteinization, *corpus luteum* formation
G7	48 h	4 days	*Corpus luteum* maintenance
G8	48 h	8 days	
G9	48 h	14 days	*Corpus luteum* regression

washed in PBS-T. To block endogenous peroxidase, the tissues were incubated with 3% hydrogen peroxide at room temperature for 45 min, washed in PBS-T, and incubated for 20 min in 3% nonfat milk solution in PBS for blocking of non-specific sites. The tissues were individually incubated overnight with rabbit polyclonal antibodies against Mmp2 (1:1000 dilution, product no. ab79781; Abcam, Inc., Cambridge, MA, USA), Mmp9 (1:100 dilution, product no. ab38898; Abcam, Inc.), and Sparc (1:100 dilution, product no. #5420; Cell Signaling Technology, Danvers, MA, USA) or rabbit monoclonal antibodies anti-Mmp14 (1:100 dilution, product no. ab51074; Abcam, Inc.) and anti-Reck (1:200 dilution, product no. #3433; Cell Signaling Technology) at 4 °C. Information on the antibodies and dilutions used in the IHC experiments are summarized in Additional file 1: Table S1. Antibody dilutions were made in PBS with 0.1% bovine serum albumin (BSA). The signal was amplified using the labeled streptavidin-biotin (LSAB) method with the Universal Dako LSAB + peroxidase kit (Dako North America, Inc., Via Real Carpinteria, CA, USA). Tissues were incubated for 30 min with the biotinylated link, washed twice with PBS-T, and incubated with streptavidin conjugated to horseradish peroxidase. For the IHC-negative control, the primary antibody was omitted. Tissues were revealed using the DAB kit (Dako North America) and counterstained with Harris hematoxylin (Easypath, São Paulo, SP, Brazil). Lastly, the sections were dehydrated, xylene embedded, and assembled with VectaMount permanent mounting medium (Vector

Laboratories, Burlingame, CA, USA). Immunohistochemically stained sections were scanned using the Pannoramic P250 Flash II Slide Scanner (3DHISTECH, Budapest, Hungary), and the images were selected using the Case-Viewer software (3DHISTECH, version 2.0). Representative areas of the tissue were selected for each condition to compose Fig. 1 and IHC scores were generated after analysis by three independent researchers (Table 2). IHC kits were provided by Dako North America.

RNA isolation, cDNA synthesis, and reverse transcriptase PCR

Total RNA was isolated using the TRIzol (Invitrogen, Carlsbad, CA, USA) protocol. RNA quality was evaluated by the spectrophotometric absorbance ratios at 280/260 nm and 230/260 nm (Nanodrop, Thermo Scientific, Waltham, MA, USA). Equal amounts of RNA treated with DNaseI (Thermo Scientific) from each of the three ovaries were mixed into a single pool for reverse transcription. Complementary DNA was synthetized from 2µg of total RNA pool using ImProm-II Reverse Transcriptase (Promega, Madison, WI, USA) according to the manufacturer's instructions.

qRT-PCR

The relative mRNA expressions of the target genes were assessed using the Maxima SYBR Green/ROX qPCR Master Mix (Thermo Scientific) in a GeneAmp 7300

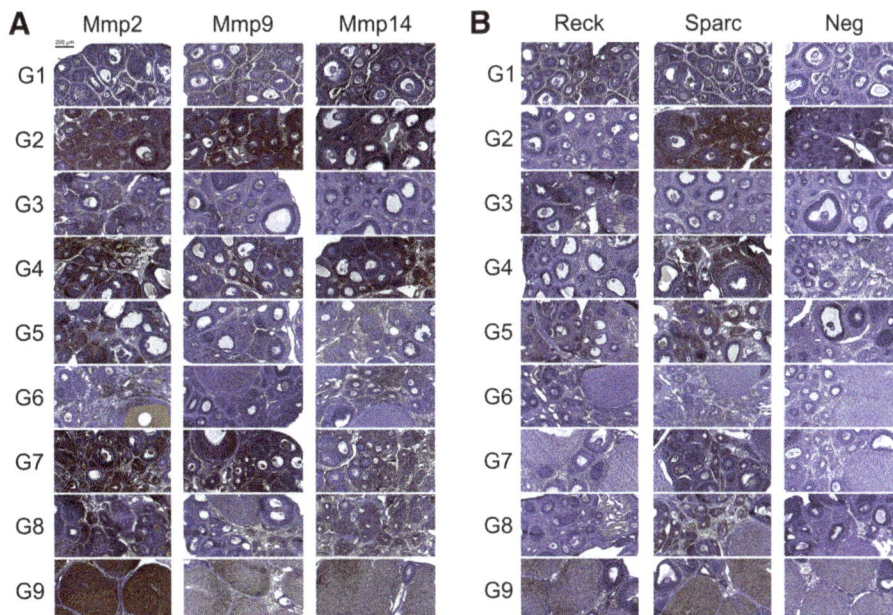

Fig. 1 Immunohistochemistry (IHC) analysis of target proteins Mmp2, 9, 14, Reck, and Sparc during ovary dynamics across hormone-induced estrous cycle in rats. Brown staining indicates the presence of the protein. **a** Mmp2, Mmp9 and Mmp14; **b** Reck, Sparc and negative control (Neg)

Table 2 Intensity and localization of target proteins in ovarian tissue during hormone-induced estrous cycle

GROUP	PHASE	Mmp2	Mmp9	Mmp14	Reck	Sparc
PBS	Vehicle control	(4) G^a/T/E/O	(2) E	(2) E	(2) T/E	(2) T/E/O
			(3) O			
G1	Control	(2) T/O	(3) T/E/O	(3) T/E	(3) T/E	(2) T/E/O
G2	Folliculogenesis	(4) G^a/T/E/O	(5) G^a/T/E/O	(4) T/E	0	(4) G^a/T/E/O
G3		(3) T/E/O	(2) E	0	(2) T/E	0
			(3) O			
G4	Ovulation	(5) T/E/O	(4) G^a/T/E/O	(5) G^a/T/E	0	(4) T/E/O
G5	Transition: ovulation-luteinization	(4) T/E/O	(2) T/E/O	(2) E	(3) T/E	(3) T/E/O
G6	Transition: ovulation-luteinization, luteinization	(3) CL/T/E/O	(2) CL/E/O	(2) E	(1) CL	(2) CL/E/O
G7	CL maintenance	(5) CL/G^a/T/E/O	(5) CL	(3) T/E	(1) CL/T/E	(3) CL/T/E/O
			(4) G^a/T/E/O			
G8		(4) CL/T/E/O	(2) CL	(2) E	(2) T/E	(3) CL/T/E/O
			(3) G^a/T/E/O			
G9	Luteolysis	(6)	(3) CL/O	(4) CL	(3) CL/T/E	(4) CL
		CL/G^a/T/E/O		(3) T/E		(2) T/E/O

Localization is identified as: CL: *corpus luteum*; T: theca; G: granulosa; E: stroma; O: oocyte. Staining intensity (0–6): unstained (0), low staining (1–2), moderate staining (3–4), and strong staining (5–6)
^{a}Expression unevenly detected across the tissue

Sequence Detection System (Applied Biosystems, Foster City, CA, USA), according to the manufacturer's instructions. The primers used to amplify the *Mmps* (*2, 9, 13, 14,* and *19*), *Timps* (*1, 2,* and *3*), *Sparc, Bsg,* and *Reck* genes are listed in Additional file 1: Table S2. A dissociation cycle was performed after each run to check for non-specific amplification. Relative mRNA expression levels were estimated using the method described in [44], which generates a normalization value in geNorm Software using *β-Actin* and *Hprt* as housekeeping genes.

Statistical analysis

Relative mRNA expression levels across treatment groups were normalized relative to the average expression of control animals treated with saline solution and compared using One-way analysis of variance (ANOVA), followed by Dunnett's post hoc comparison test. Spearman correlations were calculated for each gene pair (Additional file 1: Table S3). All analyses were carried out using the SPSS Software (IBM SPSS Statistics; version 20). A p value of $p < 0.05$ was considered significant (* $p < 0.05$, ** $p < 0.01$, and *** $p < 0.001$).

Results

Expression profile of Mmps during ovary ECM remodeling across hormone-induced estrous cycle

We studied the spatio-temporal patterns of expression of Mmps 2, 9, and 14 proteins within the ovarian tissue using immunohistochemistry. Figure 1a shows representative images for each condition, with the target staining intensities and respective localizations being summarized in Table 2. All Mmps analyzed were mainly restricted

to the theca and stromal cells, except during the late stages of the estrous cycle (G7 and G8), when expression was also detected in the *corpus luteum*. Oocytes and granulosa cells were immune-reactive to gelatinases only. Ovaries showed a global increase in Mmp protein expression during the early stages of folliculogenesis (G2), followed by another expression peak during ovulation (G4). Nevertheless, the expression levels of gelatinases were lower during the ovulation-luteogenesis transition and CL formation and increased during CL maintenance, more specifically, at luteolysis.

Figure 2 shows the relative expression pattern of *Mmps*, at the mRNA level, by qRT-PCR. *Mmp2* mRNA levels were significantly lower in ovaries from the control group, when compared to the early folliculogenesis ovaries (G2), displaying a peak at the ovulation-luteogenesis transition phase (G5) followed by a sharp decrease (Fig. 2a). Similarly, *Mmp9* rapidly increased, peaked at G5 and decreased after G6 (Fig. 2b). Meanwhile, *Mmp13* peaked at late stages of the G8-G9 protocol (Fig. 2c). *Mmp14* (Fig. 2d) and *Mmp19* were not modulated during the process (data not shown).

Expression profile of the Mmps' modulators Reck, Bsg and Sparc during ovary ECM remodeling across hormone-induced estrous cycle

Figure 3 presents the mRNA expression profile of different Mmps modulators during the hormone-induced estrous cycle, the inhibitors *Timps* (*Timp1, Timp2,* and *Timp3*) (Fig. 3a, B, and C, respectively) and *Reck* (Fig. 3d) and the *Mmps* inducers *Bsg* and *Sparc* (Fig. 3e and f,

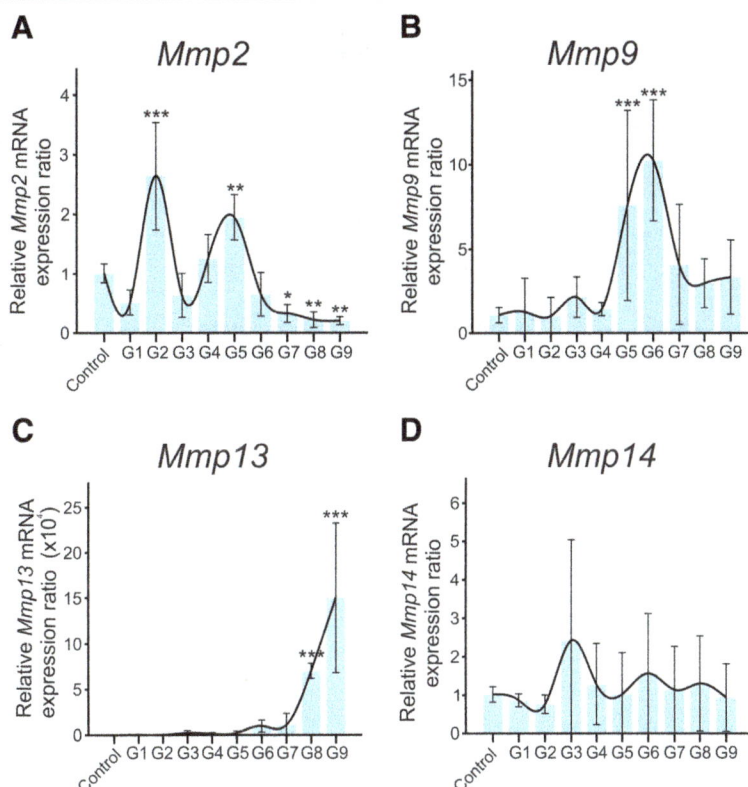

Fig. 2 mRNA expression profile of matrix metalloproteinases (*Mmps*) during ovary dynamics across hormone-induced estrous cycle in rats. (**a**) *Mmp2*, (**b**) *Mmp9*, (**c**) *Mmp13* and (**d**) *Mmp14*. Expression levels were normalized to the average expression of control animals treated with saline solution. The statistical significances were relative to control group. * *Mmp2* expression level was lower in the *corpus luteum* (G7) ($p < 0.05$). ** *Mmp2* levels were significantly higher at the ovulation-luteogenesis transition phase (G5) and lower at late stages of the CL maintenance and luteolysis G8-G9 ($p < 0.01$). *** *Mmp2* levels were significantly higher in early folliculogenesis ovaries (G2) than in ovaries from the control group; *Mmp9* levels were higher at ovulation-luteinization Transition (G5) and luteinization (G6); *Mmp13* were levels higher at late stages of the CL maintenance and luteolysis (G8-G9) ($p < 0.001$)

respectively) in whole ovarian RNA extracts. *Timp1* mRNA showed a clear expression peak during ovulation (G4 and G5, Fig. 3a), while *Timp2* and *Timp3* apparently are not significantly modulated in this model (Fig. 3b and c). Expression levels were normalized relative to the average expression of control animals treated with saline solution.

As may be observed in Fig. 1b and Table 2, the Reck protein, the only Mmp inhibitor which is anchored to the membrane by a glycosyl phosphatidyl anchor, was expressed in theca cells, ovarian stroma, and CL, but the protein expression pattern was opposite to that of Mmps, namely: no Reck protein expression was detected during early folliculogenesis and ovulation, while the highest Reck levels occurred immediately following eCG administration (G1) and during ovulation-luteogenesis transition (G5). The only exception was luteolysis (G9), during which Reck protein and the Mmps were both detected at high levels. Additionally, *Reck* mRNA was upregulated at the early stages of the estrous cycle during folliculogenesis, with an expression peak at G2 (Fig. 3d). Furthermore, its gene

expression negatively correlated with *Mmp13* collagenase expression (Additional file 1: Table S2). Conversely, the Mmp inducer *Bsg* displayed an mRNA expression peak during the late stage of CL maintenance (G8) (Fig. 3e).

The ovarian tissue expressed the Sparc protein in theca, granulosa and stromal cells, in oocytes and CL. The Sparc modulation pattern across the estrous cycle was similar to that of Mmps, with protein expression peaks during early folliculogenesis (G2), ovulation (G4), and luteolysis (G9), and lower expression levels between these phases (Fig. 1b, Table 2). High *Sparc* mRNA expression was observed at late folliculogenesis (G3) and from ovulation-luteogenesis transition to CL maintenance (G5 and G6, Fig. 3f).

Discussion

In this study, we evaluated the spatio-temporal expression pattern of several Mmps and their regulating proteins in whole ovaries at several stages of the estrous cycle using immunohistochemistry to generate a panel

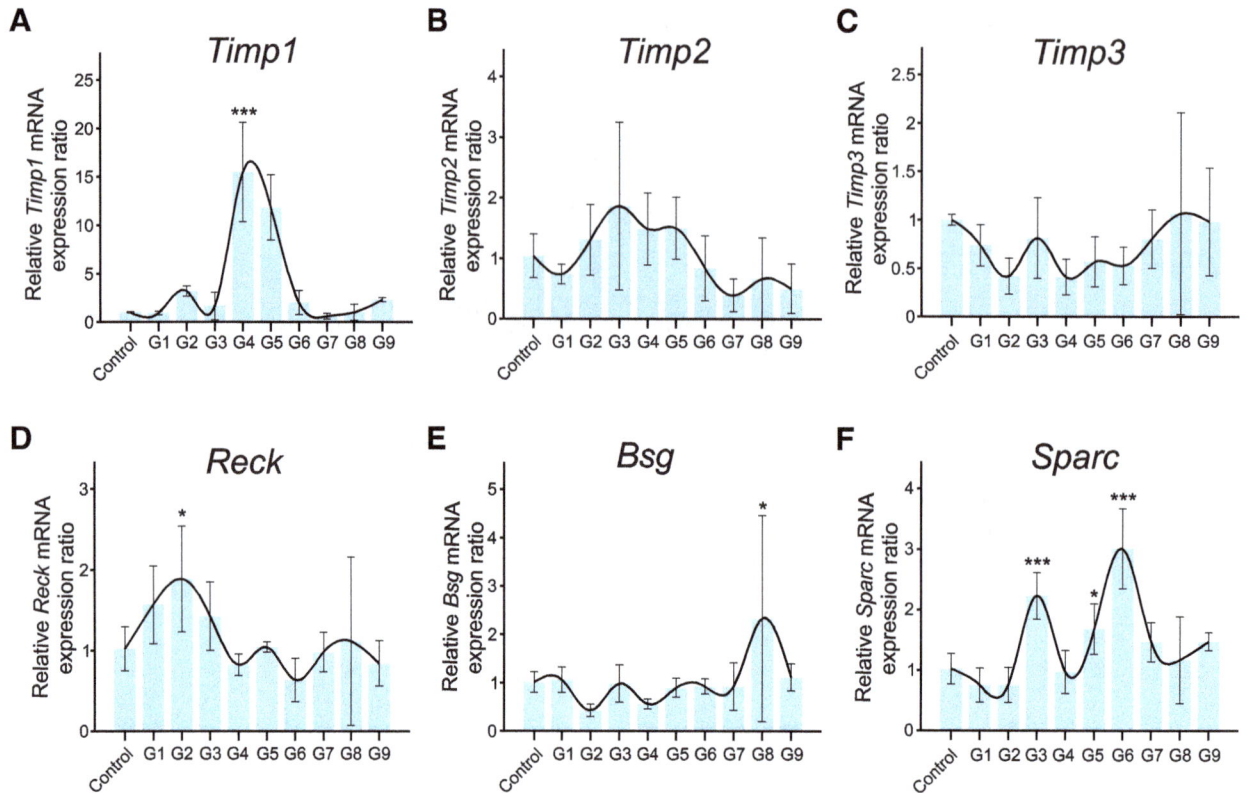

Fig. 3 Mmps modulators mRNA expression profile of matrix metalloproteinase (*Mmp*) modulators during ovary dynamics across hormone-induced estrous cycle in rats. Mmp inhibitors: (**a**) *Timp1*, (**b**) *Timp2*, (**c**) *Timp3*, (**d**) *Reck*; Mmp inducers: (**e**) *Bsg* and (**f**) *Sparc*. Expression levels were normalized to the average expression of control animals treated with saline solution. The statistical significances were relative to control group. * Reck level was significantly higher at folliculogenesis phase (G2); *Bsg* level was significantly higher during the late stage of *corpus luteum* maintenance (G8); *Sparc* levels were significantly higher at late folliculogenesis (G3) and at ovulation-luteogenesis transition to *corpus luteum* maintenance (G6) ($p < 0.05$). *** *Timp1* level was significantly higher during ovulation (G4 and G5); *Sparc* levels were higher at late folliculogenesis (G3) and at ovulation-luteogenesis transition to *corpus luteum* maintenance (G5 and G6) ($p < 0.001$)

of these players in rat ovarian dynamics. In addition, we also quantitatively assessed the mRNA expression of *Mmps* and their regulators at those same estrous cycle stages. Interestingly, some of the analyzed genes (*Mmp9*, *Reck* and *Sparc*) displayed a discrepancy between the observed mRNA and protein levels at specific phases of the induced estrous cycle. A poor correlation between mRNA and protein levels has been extensively reported highlighting the importance of an integrative approach [45–47] or the development of a gene specific RNA-to-protein conversion factor [48]. Particularly, MMPs and their inhibitors have been shown to display discrepancies in their mRNA to protein correspondence in human prostate tissue and in skeletal muscle cancer in cachexia-associated matrix remodeling [49, 50] and further studies are necessary to identify the mechanisms that lead to this disparity for this particular targets.

Analysis of Mmp spatial and temporal protein distribution, through immunohistochemistry, revealed that the Mmp2 and Mmp9 gelatinases display an overall

higher expression during the rat estrous cycle, when compared to the Mmp14 collagenase. Gelatinases had a widespread spatial distribution in the ovaries, being detected in the theca, stromal, and granulosa cells, oocytes and CL. Mmp14 protein expression, on the other hand, was mainly restricted to theca and stromal cells, but at late stages of the estrous cycle, during luteolysis (G9), being also detected at the CL. The *Mmp14* transcript levels apparently did not vary across ovulation and CL lifespan, similarly to what has been described in the literature [24, 51]. Nevertheless, high Mmp14 protein levels were detected in CL during its regression, indicating a possible contribution of this MMP to local tissue remodeling.

Mmp2 mRNA levels displayed a 2.8-fold increase during early folliculogenesis (G2), followed by a reduction (G3) and displayed a peak during the ovulation-luteogenesis transition phase (G5). At this same stage (G5), 24 h after hCG injection, *Mmp9* expression displayed an increase, peaking at luteinization (G6). Furthermore, both gelatinases displayed a reduced mRNA expression during CL maintenance (G7-G8) and regression (G9). Our results support previously published gene expression data from other groups, corroborating the increased gelatinolytic and collagenolytic activity during folliculogenesis and *Mmp2* and *Mmp9* expression 24 h post-hCG injection (luteogenesis, G5) in other studies [16, 23, 24, 51], indicating a role for this enzyme in the tissue remodeling associated with luteolysis.

We observed an increase in *Mmp13* mRNA expression during the hormone-induced estrous cycle, which reached a peak of 150,000-fold 14 days after hCG injection (G9), suggesting that this gene is strongly correlated with luteal regression. These data are supported by others: Nothnick et al. [23] observed a 15-fold increase in *Mmp13* mRNA expression 12 days after hCG and Liu et al. [24], using an adult pseudo-pregnant rat model, also showed an increase in *Mmp13* expression during luteal regression [24].

Our data suggest that Mmp expression is tightly related to the main biological events taking place during the estrous cycle, supporting previously published data and adding evidence to the importance of proteolytic tissue-degradation for ovulation in primates and rodents [52]. Equally important as determining Mmps expression during the estrous cycle is to evaluate the expression of their inhibitors and inducers, since the balance between all of these proteins is what determines the extent and nature of ECM remodeling.

Timp1 was the only member of the Timp family to show significant mRNA modulation in this work, presenting a sharp increase in mRNA levels during ovulation (G4), 12 h after hGC administration. Conversely, for an Mmp inhibitor, its expression positively correlates with *Mmp2* gene expression. Li and Curry [53] reported that the expression of both *Timp1* and *Timp3* mRNAs was induced upon treatment with hCG in pre-ovulatory rat granulosa cells in an epidermal growth factor receptor tyrosine kinase and mitogen-activated protein kinase (MAPK) pathway-dependent fashion [53]. This differential regulation is of extreme interest because Timps are multifunction proteins, whose Mmp-inhibition independent functions might have an important role in this model.

Takahashi and colleagues observed that the RECK MMP inhibitor has a privileged peri-cellular localization in human cells, due to its anchoring to the cell membrane by GPI [36]. Although *RECK* gene is widely expressed in normal organs [36], no description is available to date about its expression pattern in ovaries, despite the intense MMP-directed ECM remodeling that occurs in these organs. Our analysis of Reck expression in rat ovarian dynamics, by immunohistochemistry, showed no detectable Reck protein expression in early folliculogenesis (G2) and ovulation (G4), while Mmps 2, 9 and 14 levels were elevated. Following the same

pattern, Reck protein is expressed at detectable levels in theca and stromal cells at the end of folliculogenesis (G3) whereas expression of Mmps is lower. In addition, during the ovulation-luteogenesis transition phase (G5), an increase in Reck protein expression in theca and stromal cells was observed in parallel to a decrease in Mmp9 expression, but not of Mmp2, in the same cells. Also, at late stages of ovarian remodeling, Reck was expressed in the *corpus luteum*, during luteogenesis, CL maintenance and regression (G6-G9). Moreover, *Reck* mRNA reached a significant expression peak during the late stages of folliculogenesis (G3), 48 h post-eCG stimulus, opposite to the reduction observed in gelatinases mRNA levels at this point. This orchestrated modulation of Reck and Mmps expression suggests that Reck may be involved in Mmps modulation in this model. In support of this hypothesis, the literature describes that RECK controls MMPs 2, 9, and 14 activities through several mechanisms, including inhibition of their proteolytic activity and activation cascade, as well as their sequestration [36, 39, 54].

Regarding Mmp inducers, our gene expression analysis shows that *Bsg* mRNA levels peak at CL manteinance (G8). In agreement, other authors used a rat hormone-induced estrous cycle model to determine a *Bsg* mRNA expression panel, observing that this gene displayed increased expression during luteinization, which persisted until CL regression [10]. Sparc, another Mmp inducer, was also investigated, revealing a spatio-temporal pattern modulation in rat ovaries during the estrous cycle. Spatial and temporal expression of Sparc protein was widespread, similarly to the pattern observed for Mmps. The Sparc protein profile was the similar to that of Mmps and opposite to the one displayed by Reck. According to Bagavandoss and collaborators, Sparc protein has been detected in theca and interstitial cells and its expression has been shown to increase in rat granulosa cells following hCG administration, during the final phases of ovarian development [32]. However, in the current study, we also detected Sparc protein expression in theca, stromal, granulosa cells and oocytes in the whole hormone-induced estrous cycle, except at late folliculogenesis. It is important to note that this is the first time that Sparc protein was observed in oocytes and in the initial stages of the ovarian remodeling, namely folliculogenesis, ovulation and ovulation-luteinization transition in rat model. In addition, gene expression analyses indicate high levels of relative *Sparc* mRNA expression during late folliculogenesis (G3) and ovulation-luteogenesis transition (G5, G6). Taken together, these results suggest that the Sparc transcript and protein may also play a role in the estrous cycle. In this same direction, Smith et al., using an ovine model, suggested that *SPARC* gene is an important modulator of ovarian development and dynamics which is involved in tissue reconstruction during pregnancy [35].

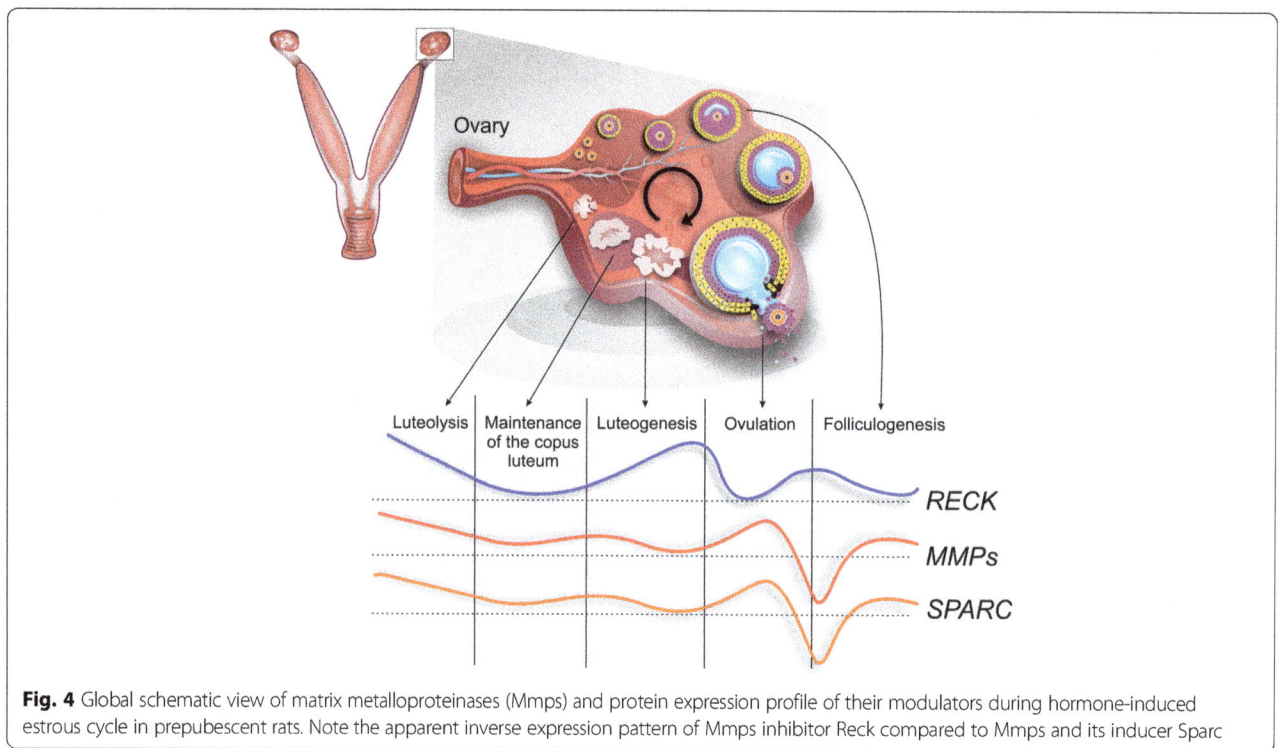

Fig. 4 Global schematic view of matrix metalloproteinases (Mmps) and protein expression profile of their modulators during hormone-induced estrous cycle in prepubescent rats. Note the apparent inverse expression pattern of Mmps inhibitor Reck compared to Mmps and its inducer Sparc

Therefore, our results generate an expression profile panel of Mmps and their regulators, suggesting that Reck and Sparc seem to play an important role at specific steps of the process, being part of a larger picture in rat ovarian dynamics.

Conclusions

Here we present a global view of Mmps and their regulators during a hormone-induced estrous cycle in pre-pubertal rats (Fig. 4). Our results show that both Reck and Sparc are differentially expressed in the rat ovary model, suggesting that these proteins may play important roles in ovary ECM remodeling. For the first time, a spatio-temporal profile of Reck and Sparc was described, evidencing an opposite regulation pattern between these Mmps regulators, with Reck as a possible inhibitor and Sparc as an inducer of Mmps, during ovarian dynamics.

metalloproteinases; PBS: Phosphate-buffered saline; PBS-T: 0.1% Triton X-100 in Phosphate-buffered saline; Reck: Reversion-inducing-Cystein-rich protein with Kazal motifs; Sparc: Secreted protein acid and rich in cysteine; Timps: Tissue inhibitors of metalloproteinases

Acknowledgements

We are grateful to Zizi de Mendonça, Debora Cristina da Costa, Ingrid da Silva Cunha, Raquel Santana and Amanda Cordeiro de Mello Pereira for their excellent technical support, to MSc. Marluce da Cunha Mantovani, MSc. Mateus Contar Adolfi, and Dr. Gustavo Gross Belchior for experimental support and advice, and to Carlos DeOcesano Pereira for help with the figures.

Funding

The following Brazilian Federal and State research agencies provided financial support for this study: São Paulo Research Foundation (FAPESP) [grant number 2013/18842–8], National Bank for Economical and Social Development (BNDES), National Council for Scientific and Technological Development (CNPq), Coordination for the Improvement of Higher Education Personnel (CAPES), National Financier of Research and Projects (FINEP), Ministry of Science, Technology and Innovation (MCTI), and Ministry of Health of Brazil/Department of Science and Technology (MS-DECIT).

Abbreviations

Bsg: Basigin; CL: Corpus Luteum; eCG: Equine chorionic gonadotropin; ECM: Extracellular matrix; hCG: Human chorionic gonadotropin; IHC: Immunohistochemistry; IU: International unit; Mmps: Matrix

Authors' contributions

GL and TC wrote the manuscript, performed the experiments and contributed to the design of the study. NN performed some of the experiments. ML helped with the data and statistical analysis and wrote part of the manuscript. MS and AC contributed to the design of the study, manuscript writing and editorial revisions. All authors approved the final submitted version of the article.

Competing interests

The authors declare that they have no competing interests.

Author details

[1]NUCEL (Cell and Molecular Therapy Center), Internal Medicine Department, Medical School, University of São Paulo, Rua Pangaré, 100, Cidade Universitária, São Paulo, SP 05360-130, Brazil. [2]Chemistry Institute, Biochemistry Department, University of São Paulo, São Paulo, SP 05508-000, Brazil. [3]Department of Surgery, School of Veterinary Medicine and Animal Science, University of São Paulo, São Paulo, SP 05508-270, Brazil.

References

1. Irving-Rodgers HF, Roger J, Luck MR, Rodgers RJ. Extracellular matrix of the corpus luteum. Semin Reprod Med. 2006;24:242–50.
2. Curry TE, Osteen KG. Cyclic changes in the matrix metalloproteinase system in the ovary and uterus. Biol Reprod. 2001;64:1285–96.
3. Curry TE, Osteen KG. The matrix metalloproteinase system: changes, regulation, and impact throughout the ovarian and uterine reproductive cycle. Endocr Rev. 2003;24:428–65.
4. McCawley LJ, Matrisian LM. Matrix metalloproteinases: they're not just for matrix anymore! Curr Opin Cell Biol. 2001;13:534–40.
5. Portela VM, Veiga A, Price CA. Regulation of MMP2 and MMP9 metalloproteinases by FSH and growth factors in bovine granulosa cells. Genet Mol Biol. 2009;32:516–20.
6. Kleiner DE, Stetler-Stevenson WG. Structural biochemistry and activation of matrix metalloproteases. Curr Opin Cell Biol. 1993;5:891–7.
7. Gomez DE, Alonso DF, Yoshiji H, Thorgeirsson UP. Tissue inhibitors of metalloproteinases: structure, regulation and biological functions. Eur J Cell Biol. 1997;74:111–22.
8. Brew K, Dinakarpandian D, Nagase H. Tissue inhibitors of metalloproteinases: evolution, structure and function. Biochim Biophys Acta. 2000;1477:267–83.
9. Gaddy-Kurten D, Hickey GJ, Fey GH, Gauldie J, Richards JS. Hormonal regulation and tissue-specific localization of alpha 2-macroglobulin in rat ovarian follicles and corpora lutea. Endocrinology. 1989;125:2985–95.
10. Smedts AM, Curry TE. Expression of basigin, an inducer of matrix metalloproteinases, in the rat ovary. Biol Reprod. 2005;73:80–7.
11. Huet C, Monget P, Pisselet C, Hennequet C, Locatelli A, Monniaux D. Chronology of events accompanying follicular atresia in hypophysectomized ewes. Changes in levels of steroidogenic enzymes, connexin 43, insulin-like growth factor II/mannose 6 phosphate receptor, extracellular matrix components, and matrix metalloproteinases. Biol Reprod. 1998;58:175–85.
12. Aston KE, Stamouli A, Thomas EJ, Vyas S, Iredale JP, Arthur MJ, Richardson MC. Effect of gonadotrophin on cell and matrix retention and expression of metalloproteinases and their inhibitor in cultured human granulosa cells modelling corpus luteum function. Mol Hum Reprod. 1996;2:26–30.
13. Stamouli A, O'Sullivan MJ, Frankel S, Thomas EJ, Richardson MC. Suppression of matrix metalloproteinase production by hCG in cultures of human luteinized granulosa cells as a model for gonadotrophin-induced luteal rescue. J Reprod Fertil. 1996;107:235–9.
14. Nothnick WB, Soloway P, Curry TE Jr. Assessment of the role of tissue inhibitor of metalloproteinase-1 (TIMP-1) during the periovulatory period in female mice lacking a functional TIMP-1 gene. Biol Reprod. 1997;56:1181–8.
15. Bagavandoss P. Differential distribution of gelatinases and tissue inhibitor of metalloproteinase-1 in the rat ovary. J Endocrinol. 1998;158:221–8.
16. Cooke RG, Nothnick WB, Komar C, Burns P, Curry TE. Collagenase and gelatinase messenger ribonucleic acid expression and activity during follicular development in the rat ovary. Biol Reprod. 1999;61:1309–16.
17. Robker RL, Russell DL, Espey LL, Lydon JP, O'Malley BW, Richards JS. Progesterone-regulated genes in the ovulation process: ADAMTS-1 and cathepsin L proteases. Proc Natl Acad Sci U S A. 2000;97:4689–94.
18. Liu K, Wahlberg P, Ny T. Coordinated and cell-specific regulation of membrane type matrix metalloproteinase 1 (MT1-MMP) and its substrate matrix metalloproteinase 2 (MMP-2) by physiological signals during follicular development and ovulation. Endocrinology. 1998;139:4735–8.
19. Hägglund AC, Ny A, Leonardsson G, Ny T. Regulation and localization of matrix metalloproteinases and tissue inhibitors of metalloproteinases in the mouse ovary during gonadotropin-induced ovulation. Endocrinology. 1999;140:4351–8.
20. Rothchild I. The regulation of the mammalian corpus luteum. Recent Prog Horm Res. 1981;37:183–298.
21. Smith MF, McIntush EW, Smith GW. Mechanisms associated with corpus luteum development. J Anim Sci. 1994;72:1857–72.
22. Niswender GD, Juengel JL, Silva PJ, Rollyson MK, McIntush EW. Mechanisms controlling the function and life span of the corpus luteum. Physiol Rev. 2000;80:1–29.
23. Nothnick WB, Keeble SC, Curry TE. Collagenase, gelatinase, and proteoglycanase messenger ribonucleic acid expression and activity during luteal development, maintenance, and regression in the pseudopregnant rat ovary. Biol Reprod. 1996;54:616–24.
24. Liu K, Olofsson JI, Wahlberg P, Ny T. Distinct expression of gelatinase a [matrix metalloproteinase (MMP)-2], collagenase-3 (MMP-13), membrane type MMP 1 (MMP-14), and tissue inhibitor of MMPs type 1 mediated by physiological signals during formation and regression of the rat corpus luteum. Endocrinology. 1999;140:5330–8.
25. Reich R, Daphna-Iken D, Chun SY, Popliker M, Slager R, Adelmann-Grill BC, Tsafriri A. Preovulatory changes in ovarian expression of collagenases and tissue metalloproteinase inhibitor messenger ribonucleic acid: role of eicosanoids. Endocrinology. 1991;129:1869–75.
26. Mann JS, Kindy MS, Edwards DR, Curry TE. Hormonal regulation of matrix metalloproteinase inhibitors in rat granulosa cells and ovaries. Endocrinology. 1991;128:1825–32.
27. Murray SC, Keeble SC, Muse KN, Curry TE. Regulation of granulosa cell-derived ovarian metalloproteinase inhibitor(s) by prolactin. J Reprod Fertil. 1996;107:103–8.
28. Kennedy JL, Muse KN, Keeble SC, Curry TE. Hormonal regulation of tissue inhibitors of metalloproteinases during follicular development in the rat ovary. Endocrine. 1996;5:299–305.
29. Nothnick WB, Edwards DR, Leco KJ, Curry TE. Expression and activity of ovarian tissue inhibitors of metalloproteinases during pseudopregnancy in the rat. Biol Reprod. 1995;53:684–91.
30. Duncan WC, McNeilly AS, Illingworth PJ. The effect of luteal "rescue" on the expression and localization of matrix metalloproteinases and their tissue inhibitors in the human corpus luteum. J Clin Endocrinol Metab. 1998;83:2470–8.
31. Smedts AM, Lele SM, Modesitt SC, Curry TE. Expression of an extracellular matrix metalloproteinase inducer (basigin) in the human ovary and ovarian endometriosis. Fertil Steril. 2006;86:535–42.
32. Bagavandoss P, Sage EH, Vernon RB. Secreted protein, acidic and rich in cysteine (SPARC) and thrombospondin in the developing follicle and corpus luteum of the rat. J Histochem Cytochem. 1998;46:1043–9.
33. Nuttall RK, Sampieri CL, Pennington CJ, Gill SE, Schultz GA, Edwards DR. Expression analysis of the entire MMP and TIMP gene families during mouse tissue development. FEBS Lett. 2004;563:129–34.
34. Podhajcer OL, Benedetti LG, Girotti MR, Prada F, Salvatierra E, Llera AS. The role of the matricellular protein SPARC in the dynamic interaction between the tumor and the host. Cancer Metastasis Rev. 2008;27:691–705.
35. Smith GW, Gentry PC, Long DK, Smith MF, Roberts RM. Differential gene expression within the ovine corpus luteum: identification of secreted protein acidic and rich in cysteine as a major secretory product of small but not large luteal cells. Endocrinology. 1996;137:755–62.
36. Takahashi C, Sheng Z, Horan TP, Kitayama H, Maki M, Hitomi K, Kitaura Y, Takai S, Sasahara RM, Horimoto A, et al. Regulation of matrix metalloproteinase-9 and inhibition of tumor invasion by the membrane-anchored glycoprotein RECK. Proc Natl Acad Sci U S A. 1998;95:13221–6.
37. Bornstein P, Sage EH. Matricellular proteins: extracellular modulators of cell function. Curr Opin Cell Biol. 2002;14:608–16.
38. Yiu GK, Chan WY, Ng SW, Chan PS, Cheung KK, Berkowitz RS, Mok SC. SPARC (secreted protein acidic and rich in cysteine) induces apoptosis in ovarian cancer cells. Am J Pathol. 2001;159:609–22.

39. Oh J, Takahashi R, Kondo S, Mizoguchi A, Adachi E, Sasahara RM, Nishimura S, Imamura Y, Kitayama H, Alexander DB, et al. The membrane-anchored MMP inhibitor RECK is a key regulator of extracellular matrix integrity and angiogenesis. Cell. 2001;107:789–800.

40. Zhang X, Healy C, Nothnick WB. Estrogen suppresses expression of the matrix metalloproteinase inhibitor reversion-inducing cysteine-rich protein with Kazal motifs (RECK) within the mouse uterus. Endocrine. 2012;42:97–106.

41. Zarrow MX, Quinn DL. Superovulation in the immature rat following treatment with PMS alone and inhibition of PMS-induced ovulation. J Endocrinol. 1963;26:181–8.

42. Jo M, Curry TE. Regulation of matrix metalloproteinase-19 messenger RNA expression in the rat ovary. Biol Reprod. 2004;71:1796–806.

43. Ying SY, Meyer RK. Ovulation induced by PMS and HCG in hypophysectomized immature rats. Proc Soc Exp Biol Med. 1972;139:1231–3.

44. Pfaffl MW. A new mathematical model for relative quantification in real-time RT-PCR. Nucleic Acids Res. 2001;29:e45.

45. Tian Q, Stepaniants SB, Mao M, Weng L, Feetham MC, Doyle MJ, Yi EC, Dai H, Thorsson V, Eng J, et al. Integrated genomic and proteomic analyses of gene expression in mammalian cells. Mol Cell Proteomics. 2004;3:960–9.

46. Maier T, Guell M, Serrano L. Correlation of mRNA and protein in complex biological samples. FEBS Lett. 2009;583:3966–73.

47. Liu Y, Beyer A, Aebersold R. On the dependency of cellular protein levels on mRNA abundance. Cell. 2016;165:535–50.

48. Edfors F, Danielsson F, Hallstrom BM, Kall L, Lundberg E, Ponten F, Forsstrom B, Uhlen M. Gene-specific correlation of RNA and protein levels in human cells and tissues. Mol Syst Biol. 2016;12:883.

49. Lichtinghagen R, Musholt PB, Lein M, Romer A, Rudolph B, Kristiansen G, Hauptmann S, Schnorr D, Loening SA, Jung K. Different mRNA and protein expression of matrix metalloproteinases 2 and 9 and tissue inhibitor of metalloproteinases 1 in benign and malignant prostate tissue. Eur Urol. 2002;42:398–406.

50. Devine RD, Bicer S, Reiser PJ, Velten M, Wold LE. Metalloproteinase expression is altered in cardiac and skeletal muscle in cancer cachexia. Am J Physiol Heart Circ Physiol. 2015;309:H685–91.

51. Jo M, Thomas LE, Wheeler SE, Curry TE. Membrane type 1-matrix metalloproteinase (MMP)-associated MMP-2 activation increases in the rat ovary in response to an ovulatory dose of human chorionic gonadotropin. Biol Reprod. 2004;70:1024–32.

52. Chaffin CL, Vandevoort CA. Follicle growth, ovulation, and luteal formation in primates and rodents: a comparative perspective. Exp Biol Med (Maywood). 2013;238:539–48.

53. Li F, Curry TE. Regulation and function of tissue inhibitor of metalloproteinase (TIMP) 1 and TIMP3 in periovulatory rat granulosa cells. Endocrinology. 2009;150:3903–12.

54. Welm B, Mott J, Werb Z. Developmental biology: vasculogenesis is a wreck without RECK. Curr Biol. 2002;12:R209–11.

22

Dehydroepiandrosterone (DHEA) supplementation improves in vitro fertilization outcomes of poor ovarian responders, especially in women with low serum concentration of DHEA-S: a retrospective cohort study

Chyi-Uei Chern[1], Kuan-Hao Tsui[1,2,3], Salvatore Giovanni Vitale[4], San-Nung Chen[1], Peng-Hui Wang[2,5,6], Antonio Cianci[4], Hsiao-Wen Tsai[1,2], Zhi-Hong Wen[7] and Li-Te Lin[1,2,8*] (iD)

Abstract

Background: Dehydroepiandrosterone (DHEA) is now widely used as an adjuvant for in vitro fertilization (IVF) cycles in poor ovarian responders (PORs). Several studies showed that DHEA supplementation could improve IVF outcomes of PORs. However, most of the PORs do not respond to DHEA clinically. Therefore, the aim of this study is to confirm the beneficial effects of DHEA on IVF outcomes of PORs and to investigate which subgroups of PORs can best benefit from DHEA supplementation.

Methods: This retrospective cohort study was performed between January 2015 and December 2017. A total of 151 PORs who fulfilled the Bologna criteria and underwent IVF cycles with the gonadotropin-releasing hormone antagonist protocol were identified. The study group ($n = 67$) received 90 mg of DHEA daily for an average of 3 months before the IVF cycles. The control group ($n = 84$) underwent the IVF cycles without DHEA pretreatment. The basic and cycle characteristics and IVF outcomes between the two groups were compared using independent t-tests, Chi-Square tests and binary logistic regression.

Results: The study and control groups did not show significant differences in terms of basic characteristics. The study group demonstrated a significantly greater number of retrieved oocytes, metaphase II oocytes, fertilized oocytes, day 3 embryos and top-quality embryos at day 3 and a higher clinical pregnancy rate, ongoing pregnancy rate and live birth rate than those measures in the control group. The multivariate analysis revealed that DHEA supplementation was positively associated with clinical pregnancy rate (OR = 4.93, 95% CI 1.68–14.43, $p = 0.004$). Additionally, in the study group, the multivariate analysis showed that serum dehydroepiandrosterone-sulfate (DHEA-S) levels < 180 μg/dl were significantly associated with a rate of retrieved oocytes > 3 (OR = 5.92, 95% CI 1.48–23.26, $p = 0.012$).

(Continued on next page)

* Correspondence: litelin1982@gmail.com
[1]Department of Obstetrics and Gynecology, Kaohsiung Veterans General Hospital, No.386, Dazhong 1st Rd., Zuoying Dist, Kaohsiung City 81362, Taiwan
[2]Department of Obstetrics and Gynecology, National Yang-Ming University School of Medicine, No. 155, Sec. 2, Li-Nong Street, Pei-Tou, Taipei 112, Taiwan
Full list of author information is available at the end of the article

(Continued from previous page)

Conclusions: DHEA supplementation improves IVF outcomes of PORs. In PORs with DHEA pretreatment, women with lower DHEA-S level may have greater possibility of attaining more than 3 oocytes.

Keywords: Dehydroepiandrosterone, DHEA, Diminished ovarian reserve, In vitro fertilization, Poor ovarian responders

Background

Poor ovarian responders (PORs) are the women who respond suboptimally to ovarian stimulation with gonadotropins. While a variety of definitions exist for POR [1], the ESHRE consensus group standardized the definition of POR and established the Bologna criteria in 2011 [2]. It is a great challenge for PORs to reach live birth in in vitro fertilization (IVF) cycles [3, 4]. No certain protocol or single intervention is accepted as an effective method to overcome the poor prognosis of PORs [5]. Therefore, multiple strategies, including various IVF protocols [6], the use of adjuvant supplements [7, 8] and accumulation of vitrified oocytes or embryos [9] have been attempted for PORs undergoing IVF cycles. However, the optimal management for PORs remains an unsolved problem.

Regarding adjuvant supplements, dehydroepiandrosterone (DHEA) is currently widely used worldwide and is considered a potential agent to ameliorate the IVF outcomes of PORs. DHEA is an endogenous steroid generated by the adrenal glands and ovarian theca cells, and acts as a precursor for testosterone [10], which was reported to be engaged in early follicular development [11]. DHEA was first used in PORs in 2000 by Casson et al. who demonstrated that DHEA treatment could enhance response to ovarian stimulation [12]. Later, several studies showed the beneficial effects of DHEA on ovarian reserve [13], oocytes and embryo quality [14, 15] and pregnancy outcomes [16, 17] in PORs. Recent meta-analyses also revealed that DHEA supplementation could improve ongoing pregnancy or live birth in PORs undergoing IVF cycles [18, 19]. However, there is a lack of large-scale, well-designed randomized controlled trials to verify the beneficial effects of DHEA in PORs.

In clinical practice, some PORs saw improvement in IVF outcomes after DHEA supplementation; however, others failed to respond to DHEA treatment. It is believed that there are certain subgroups of PORs who could benefit more from DHEA supplementation than others. Therefore, the aim of this study is to confirm the beneficial effects of DHEA on IVF outcomes and to identify the subgroups of PORs that may benefit more from DHEA supplementation.

Methods

Study design

This is a retrospective cohort study. Patients were treated at the Reproductive Center of the Kaohsiung Veterans General Hospital between January 2015 and December 2017. The study conformed with the "Declaration of Helsinki for Medical Research involving Human Subjects." Additionally, approval was obtained from the institutional review board at Kaohsiung Veterans General Hospital, with the identifier VGHKS18-CT6–09. The study was performed in accordance with approved guidelines.

Study participants

A total of 1658 IVF cycles were performed during the study period. Among these cycles, women who met the Bologna criteria were defined as PORs. Bologna criteria [2] included at least two of the three following features: (1) advanced maternal age ($\geq$ 40 years) or any other risk factor for POR, (2) a previous poor ovarian response ($\leq$ 3 oocytes with a conventional stimulation protocol), and (3) an abnormal ovarian reserve test. An abnormal ovarian reserve test was defined as antral follicle count (AFC) < 5 or anti-Müllerian hormone (AMH) < 1 ng/mL in this study. Additionally, two episodes of a previous POR after maximal stimulation alone would be sufficient to define a patient as a POR. The exclusion criteria were as follows: (1) patients who did not undergo gonadotropin-releasing hormone (GnRH) antagonist protocol, (2) patients who underwent fresh embryo transfer, (3) patients who underwent oophorectomy, and (4) patients who took herbal drugs or other supplementation (e.g., growth hormone). PORs identified in this study were then divided into POR and POR/DHEA groups. In the POR group, patients directly underwent an IVF cycle without DHEA pretreatment. In the POR/DHEA group, patients received daily DHEA supplementation (CPH; Formulation Technology, Oakdale, CA, USA) of 90 mg for an average of 3 months before entry into an IVF cycle. DHEA supplementation or not was decided based on patients' consideration and preference after full consultation provided by a doctor. The study flow chart is shown in Fig. 1.

Treatment protocol

The efficacy of IVF protocols, especially between GnRH agonist and antagonist regimens, is still controversial [20, 21]. However, the GnRH antagonist protocol was the most popular one for PORs in a worldwide survey [22]. Therefore, a GnRH antagonist protocol was routinely used for PORs in our reproductive center. Controlled ovarian stimulation was conducted within 5 days of the menstrual cycle, with 300 IU of recombinant FSH

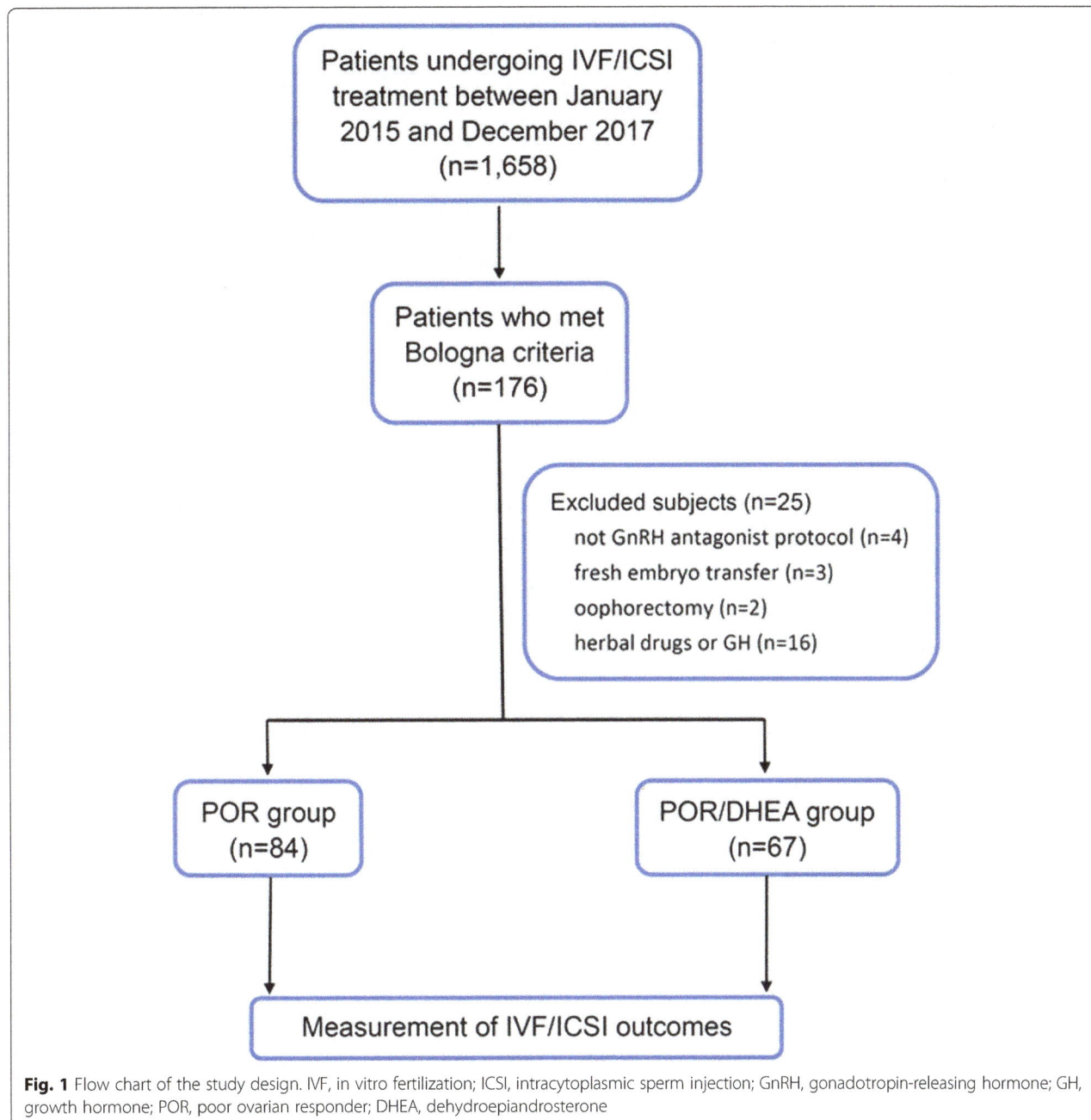

Fig. 1 Flow chart of the study design. IVF, in vitro fertilization; ICSI, intracytoplasmic sperm injection; GnRH, gonadotropin-releasing hormone; GH, growth hormone; POR, poor ovarian responder; DHEA, dehydroepiandrosterone

(Gonal-F, Merck KGaA, Darmstadt, Germany) or recombinant FSH + LH (Pergovaris, Merck Serono, Aubonne, Switzerland or Merional, Institut Biochimique SA, Lamone, Switzerland). Daily injections of a GnRH antagonist (Cetrotide 0.25 mg, Merck Serono, Idron, France) were given from the day the leading follicle reached 12–14 mm in diameter until the day of oocyte trigger. Dual trigger, combined recombinant hCG (Ovidrel 250 µg, Merck Serono, Modugno, Italy) and GnRH agonist (Lupro 2 mg, Nang Kuang Pharmaceutical Co, Ltd., Tainan, Taiwan), were administered when at least one dominant follicle reached a mean diameter of 17 mm. Oocytes were retrieved 34–36 h after oocyte trigger under the guidance of transvaginal ultrasound. Intracytoplasmic sperm injection (ICSI) was performed in all patients to diminish the potential of fertilization failure. Embryos were evaluated and graded according to the criteria established by the Istanbul consensus workshop [23]. All embryos were cryopreserved by vitrification on the third day after oocyte retrieval for subsequent frozen embryo transfer (FET) cycles. An artificial cycle was used for endometrial preparation of FET, as previously described [24]. Embryo transfer was done under transabdominal sonographic guidance. Regarding luteal phase support, daily progesterone, including

Crinone 8% gel (Merck Serono, Hertfordshire, UK) and Duphaston 40 mg (Abbott, Olst, the Netherlands) were given. A pregnancy test was carried out 15 days after embryo transfer. Once a positive pregnancy test was observed, progesterone was continued until 8–10 weeks of gestation.

Main measurement and outcomes

The primary outcome measures were the number of retrieved oocytes and clinical pregnancy rate. Clinical pregnancy was confirmed if a visible fetal heart beat was found in an intrauterine gestational sac by transvaginal ultrasound. The secondary outcome measures included number of mature oocytes, fertilized oocytes, day 3 embryos, top-quality day 3 embryos, ongoing pregnancy rate and live birth rate. Ongoing pregnancy was defined as the presence of a fetal heart beat beyond 20 weeks of gestation. Live birth was determined by delivery of a live fetus after 20 completed weeks of gestation. Cycle cancellation was defined as incomplete cycles due to no response to gonadotropins or no retrieved oocyte.

Statistical analysis

Normality of quantitative variables was revealed by Kolmogorov-Smirnov test. Independent t-tests were used to compare quantitative variables. The categorical variables were compared using Chi-Square tests. In addition, binary logistic regression was used to assess odds ratios (ORs) and 95% confidence intervals (CIs) of clinical pregnancy and the number of retrieved oocytes > 3 after adjusting for confounders. All analyses were performed using the Statistical Package for Social Sciences (SPSS) version 20.0 (Chicago, IL, USA). Comparisons with a p-value less than 0.05 were considered significant.

Results

A total of 176 cycles met the Bologna criteria (10.6%). Among these cycles, there were 4 cycles that did not receive GnRH antagonist protocol, 3 cycles that received fresh embryo transfer, 2 cycles that underwent oophorectomy, and 16 cycles that received herbal drugs or growth hormone and were excluded from the study. Ultimately, 151 cycles were identified in this study and divided into the POR group ($n = 84$) and the POR/DHEA group ($n = 67$). There were no differences between the two groups regarding age, body mass index, infertility duration, previous IVF attempts, primary or secondary infertility, basal follicle stimulation hormone (FSH), dehydroepiandrosterone-sulfate (DHEA-S) concentration, AFC, AMH and Bologna criteria category (Table 1).

The cycle characteristics and IVF outcomes between the two groups are presented in Table 2. There were no significant differences in terms of stimulation duration or gonadotropin dose. The POR/DHEA group had a greater number of retrieved oocytes (3.3 ± 2.5 vs. 2.0 ± 1.5, $p < 0.001$), metaphase II oocytes (1.9 ± 1.5 vs. 1.0 ± 1.1, $p < 0.001$), fertilized oocytes (2.3 ± 1.7 vs. 1.4 ± 1.2, $p < 0.001$), day 3 embryos (2.1 ± 1.6 vs. 1.3 ± 1.2, $p = 0.001$) and top-quality embryos at day 3 (1.0 ± 1.1 vs. 0.4 ± 0.8, $p = 0.001$) than did the POR group. Furthermore, the rate of retrieved oocytes > 3 (34.3% vs. 14.3%, $p = 0.004$), the clinical pregnancy rate (23.9% vs. 7.1%, $p = 0.004$), ongoing pregnancy rate (17.9% vs. 6.0%, $p = 0.021$) and live birth rate (16.4% vs. 6.0%, $p = 0.038$) were significantly higher in the POR/DHEA group than in the POR group. Cycle cancellation rate was similar between the two groups.

As shown in Table 3, the multivariate analysis revealed that DHEA supplementation was significantly associated with clinical pregnancy rate (OR = 4.93, 95% CI 1.68–14.53, $p = 0.004$). In addition, in the POR/DHEA group, multivariate analysis (Table 4) showed POR with serum concentration of DHEA-S less than 180 μg/dl was significantly associated with the possibility to retrieve more than 3 oocytes (OR = 5.92, 95% CI 1.48–23.26, $p = 0.012$).

Discussion

In this retrospective cohort study, the incidence rate of POR based on Bologna criteria was 10.6% (176/1658) and was compatible with that of previous study [25]. Additionally, the poor prognosis of Bologna PORs undergoing IVF/ICSI cycles without DHEA supplementation in this study was also consistent with previous study [3]. However, after DHEA pretreatment, the present study demonstrated that number of retrieved oocytes, metaphase II oocytes, fertilized oocytes, day 3 embryos, top-quality embryos at day 3 as well as clinical pregnancy rate, ongoing pregnancy rate and live birth rate significantly improved. Furthermore, the multivariate analysis displayed that PORs with DHEA supplementation exhibited a 4.93-fold increase in the clinical pregnancy rate (95% CI 1.68–14.53, $p = 0.004$) compared to those without DHEA supplementation (Table 3). Numerous studies [15, 17, 26–28] and some meta-analyses [18, 19, 29] also support the beneficial effects of DHEA on PORs undergoing IVF/ICSI cycles. The systematic review and meta-analysis conducted by Zhang et al. showed that DHEA supplementation increased the clinical pregnancy rate, live birth rate and ovarian reserve in patients with poor ovarian response [18]. However, few randomized controlled trials with limited cases were analyzed, and the inclusive criteria for PORs were heterogeneous. Moreover, the Cochrane Review included only randomized controlled trials and concluded that pretreatment with DHEA may be associated with improved live birth rate in patients undergoing IVF/ICSI cycles [19]. Nevertheless, the Cochrane Review also included the studies of pretreatment with testosterone and the patients who were not identified as PORs. An updated randomized controlled trial performed by Kotb and colleagues, enrolled PORs according to the

Table 1 Basic characteristics of poor ovarian responders with or without DHEA

Parameters	POR (n = 84)	POR with DHEA (n = 67)	p value
Age (years)	39.8 ± 3.7	39.1 ± 3.3	0.208
Body mass index (kg/m2)	21.8 ± 3.8	21.9 ± 2.9	0.857
Infertility duration (year)	5.3 ± 4.5	5.6 ± 4.2	0.712
Previous IVF attempts(n)	2.3 ± 2.2	2.6 ± 2.2	0.480
Types of infertility n (%)			0.548
Primary infertility	41/84 (48.8%)	36/67 (53.7%)	
Secondary infertility	43/84 (51.2%)	31/67 (46.3%)	
Basal FSH (IU/l)	6.3 ± 4.6	7.1 ± 4.2	0.305
DHEA-S (µg/dl)	212.9 ± 85.9	199.2 ± 65.0	0.316
Antral follicle counts (n)	3.3 ± 1.4	3.3 ± 1.3	0.921
Anti-Müllerian hormone(ng/ml)	0.7 ± 0.4	0.7 ± 0.5	0.932
[a]Bologna criteria category n (%)			0.170
1 + 2	16/84 (19.0%)	5/67 (7.5%)	
1 + 3	16/84 (19.0%)	19/67 (28.4%)	
2 + 3	21/84 (25.0%)	17/67 (25.4%)	
1 + 2 + 3	31/84 (36.9%)	26/67 (38.8%)	

Data are presented as mean ± standard deviation and n (%)

POR poor ovarian responder, *DHEA* dehydroepiandrosterone, *IVF* in vitro fertilization, *FSH* follicle stimulation hormone, *DHEA-S* dehydroepiandrosterone-sulfate

[a]PORs meet the Bologna criteria, having at least two of the three following features: (1) advanced maternal age (≥ 40 years) or any other risk factor for POR; (2) a previous POR (≤ 3 oocytes with a conventional stimulation protocol); (3) an abnormal ovarian reserve test. Abnormal ovarian reserve test was defined as antral follicle count (AFC) < 5 or anti-Müllerian hormone (AMH) < 1 ng/mL in this study

Bologna criteria and revealed that DHEA supplementation significantly increased the number of oocytes, fertilization rate, fertilized oocytes, clinical pregnancy rate and ongoing pregnancy rate [26]. Similarly, the small sample size was also a limitation of the study. Therefore, taken together, based on current evidence and our retrospective cohort study, DHEA supplementation seems to improve IVF/ICSI outcomes and ovarian reserve in PORs. However, additional large-scale, well-designed randomized controlled trials are necessary to confirm the beneficial role of DHEA in PORs. Furthermore, although we used a GnRH antagonist protocol in this study, we believed that other protocols, especially a non-suppressive stimulation protocol, like microcode agonist protocol could also reach better results

Table 2 Cycle characteristics and pregnancy outcome of poor ovarian responders with or without DHEA

Parameters	POR (n = 84)	POR with DHEA (n = 67)	p value
Stimulation duration (days)	10.1 ± 2.2	10.5 ± 1.9	0.310
Gonadotropin dosage (IU)	2884.4 ± 872.5	2975.4 ± 649.4	0.126
No. of oocytes retrieved (n)	2.0 ± 1.5	3.3 ± 2.5	< 0.001
Oocytes retrieved > 3, % (n)	14.3 (12/84)	34.3 (23/67)	0.004
No. of metaphase II oocytes (n)	1.0 ± 1.1	1.9 ± 1.5	< 0.001
Maturation rate (%)	35.5 ± 36.2	56.2 ± 33.9	< 0.001
No. of fertilized oocytes (n)	1.4 ± 1.2	2.3 ± 1.7	< 0.001
Fertilization rate (%)	58.0 ± 42.5	67.9 ± 32.7	0.108
No. of Day 3 embryos (n)	1.3 ± 1.2	2.1 ± 1.6	0.001
No. of top-quality Day 3 embryos (n)	0.4 ± 0.8	1.0 ± 1.1	0.001
Clinical pregnancy rate, % (n)	7.1 (6/84)	23.9 (16/67)	0.004
Ongoing pregnancy rate, % (n)	6.0 (5/84)	17.9 (12/67)	0.021
Live birth rate, % (n)	6.0 (5/84)	16.4 (11/67)	0.038
Cancellation rate, % (n)	16.7 (14/84)	10.4 (7/67)	0.273

Data are presented as mean ± standard deviation and % (n)

POR poor ovarian responder, *DHEA* dehydroepiandrosterone

Table 3 Analyses of factors affecting clinical pregnancy rate in poor ovarian responders

	Univariate analysis		Multivariate analysis	
	OR (95% CI)	p value	Adjusted OR (95% CI)	p value
DHEA				
Yes vs. No	4.08(1.50–11.11)	0.006	4.93(1.68–14.53)	0.004
Age (years)	0.91(0.81–1.02)	0.114	0.95(0.84–1.09)	0.466
BMI (kg/m2)	1.05(0.93–1.20)	0.397		
Infertility duration	0.90(0.79–1.03)	0.120	0.88(0.76–1.03)	0.106
Previous IVF attempts (n)	0.95(0.77–1.20)	0.670		
Types of infertility				
Primary vs. Secondary	1.05(0.42–2.59)	0.920		
Basal FSH (IU/l)	1.04(0.94–1.15)	0.435		
AFC (n)	1.56(1.11–2.21)	0.011	1.62(1.11–2.37)	0.012
AMH (ng/ml)	1.44(0.52–4.00)	0.484		
[a]Bologna criteria category				
(1 + 3) vs. (1 + 2)	4.14(0.46–37.06)	0.204		
(2 + 3) vs. (1 + 2)	5.33(0.62–46.00)	0.128		
(1 + 2 + 3) vs. (1 + 2)	2.80(0.32–24.24)	0.350		

OR odd ratio, CI confidence interval, DHEA dehydroepiandrosterone, BMI body mass index, IVF in vitro fertilization, FSH follicle stimulation hormone, AFC antral follicle counts, AMH anti-Müllerian hormone

[a]Poor ovarian responders (PORs) meet the Bologna criteria, having at least two of the three following features: (1) advanced maternal age (≥ 40 years) or any other risk factor for POR; (2) a previous POR (≤ 3 oocytes with a conventional stimulation protocol); (3) an abnormal ovarian reserve test. Abnormal ovarian reserve test was defined as antral follicle count (AFC) < 5 or anti-Müllerian hormone (AMH) < 1 ng/mL in this study

after DHEA supplementation. However, further studies are needed to prove this concept.

The major mechanism of DHEA on the improvement of reproductive outcomes is associated with increased androgen after DHEA supplementation. DHEA, a precursor of estradiol and testosterone, serves as a prohormone of follicular fluid testosterone during ovarian induction [30].

Androgen receptors (ARs) have been identified in the granulosa cells (GCs) at any follicular stage, especially preantral and antral follicles [31, 32]. In GC-specific AR knockout mice, mice were subfertile with longer estrous cycles, fewer ovulated oocytes, reduced follicle progression and increased follicle atresia [33, 34]. GC-specific ARs seemed to be pivotal regulators of follicular development

Table 4 Analyses of factors affecting retrieved oocytes > 3 in poor ovarian responders with DHEA supplementation

	Univariate analysis		Multivariate analysis	
	OR (95% CI)	p value	Adjusted OR (95% CI)	p value
DHEA-S, μg/dl				
< 180 vs. ≥ 180	6.62(1.90–22.73)	0.003	5.92(1.48–23.26)	0.012
Age, years	0.94(0.80–1.09)	0.404		
BMI, kg/m2	1.00(0.84–1.20)	0.986		
Infertility duration	1.03(0.92–1.16)	0.620		
Previous IVF attempts, n	1.07(0.86–1.34)	0.541		
Types of infertility				
Primary vs. Secondary	1.81(0.65–5.02)	0.258		
[a]Bologna criteria category				
(1 + 3) vs. (1 + 2)	0.09(0.01–1.00)	0.050	0.22(0.02–2.92)	0.253
(2 + 3) vs. (1 + 2)	0.18(0.02–1.92)	0.154	0.43(0.03–6.05)	0.530
(1 + 2 + 3) vs. (1 + 2)	0.09(0.01–0.97)	0.047	0.17(0.01–2.05)	0.164

DHEA dehydroepiandrosterone, OR odd ratio, CI confidence interval, DHEA-S dehydroepiandrosterone-sulfate, BMI body mass index, IVF in vitro fertilization

[a]Poor ovarian responders (PORs) meet the Bologna criteria, having at least two of the three following features: (1) advanced maternal age (≥ 40 years) or any other risk factor for POR; (2) a previous POR (≤ 3 oocytes with a conventional stimulation protocol); (3) an abnormal ovarian reserve test. Abnormal ovarian reserve test was defined as antral follicle count (AFC) < 5 or anti-Müllerian hormone (AMH) < 1 ng/mL in this study

and fertility. Indeed, androgen has been reported to play roles in recruitment and initiation of primordial follicles [35, 36], promotion of follicular growth by increasing FSH receptor expression [37, 38], and prevention of follicular atresia by reducing apoptosis [37]. Moreover, DHEA administration increases serum concentration of insulin-like growth factor-1 (IGF-1) [39], which has been reported to be correlated with oocyte quality and embryo development [40, 41]. Therefore, indirect action of DHEA was mainly presented. However, direct action of DHEA on the target organs has been proposed [42, 43] but is still inconclusive. Regarding the molecular mechanism, our previous studies revealed that DHEA supplementation could improve mitochondrial function and reduce apoptosis in the cumulus cells [44] and human granulosa cell line [45].

Returning to clinical practice, however, not all PORs benefit from the DHEA pretreatment. Thus, we attempted to investigate which subgroups of PORs with DHEA supplementation benefit most from such pretreatment. The current study found that PORs with lower DHEA-S concentration (< 180 μg/dl) exhibited a 5.92-fold increase in the rate of retrieved oocytes > 3 (95% CI 1.48–23.26, $p = 0.012$) compared to those with higher DHEA-S concentration (≥ 180 μg/dl) (Table 4). Hypoandrogenism has been reported to be in association with diminished ovarian reserve [46]. Low androgen levels can be of ovarian and/or adrenal etiology. Since DHEA-S is almost exclusively produced by adrenals, it is generally accepted that low DHEA-S reflects an adrenal cause for low androgen levels. Therefore, our finding would suggest that DHEA supplementation was especially effective if androgen deficiency was of adrenal origin. Gleicher et al. demonstrated that patients with secondary ovarian insufficiency induced by adrenal hypoandrogenism dramatically improved in ovarian function after DHEA supplementation [47]. Another study conducted by Gleicher and colleagues showed that in women with high-AMH/low-testosterone phenotype associated with adrenal insufficiency, DHEA supplementation equalizes low to normal testosterone and normalizes IVF cycle outcomes [48]. Taken together, patients with low DHEA-S levels, implying adrenal hypoandrogenism, could obtain greater improvement from DHEA supplementation. In addition, in developed countries, most cases of primary adrenal insufficiency are caused by autoimmunity, frequently coexisting with other autoimmune abnormalities [49]. Therefore, further survey for autoimmunity in these patients may be needed.

The strength of this study lies in its strict exclusion criteria and subgroup analysis. However, there were some limitations in this study. First, this is a retrospective study with relatively small sample size. Second, the patients identified based on the Bologna criteria may be heterogeneous. Moreover, serum DHEA-S levels were checked not at the time when patients were included in the study, but within 6 months before DHEA supplementation or IVF cycles. We believed that the serum DHEA-S levels of this study were representative. However, potential bias could not be excluded.

Conclusion

In conclusion, the IVF outcomes of PORs could potentially benefit from pretreatment with DHEA. In PORs who received DHEA supplementation, women with lower DHEA-S levels could achieve higher possibility of retrieving more than 3 oocytes.

Abbreviations
AFC: Antral follicle count; AMH: Anti-Müllerian hormone; AR: Androgen receptor; BMI: Body mass index; CI: Confidence interval; DHEA: Dehydroepiandrosterone; DHEA-S: Dehydroepiandrosterone-sulfate; FET: Frozen embryo transfer; FSH: Follicle stimulation hormone; GC: Granulosa cell; GnRH: Gonadotropin-releasing hormone; ICSI: Intracytoplasmic sperm injection; IGF-1: Insulin-like growth factor-1; IVF: In vitro fertilization; OR: Odd ratio; POR: Poor ovarian responder

Acknowledgements
This work was generously supported by grants VGHKS18-CT6-09 from Kaohsiung Veterans General Hospital.

Authors' contributions
CUC and LTL are responsible for drafting the article. PHW, ZHW and AC are responsible for design of the study. SGV, SNC and HWT are responsible for analysis and interpretation of data. KHT and LTL are responsible for supervising the research and revising the manuscript. All authors read and approved the final manuscript.

Competing interests
The authors declare that they have no competing interests.

Author details
[1] Department of Obstetrics and Gynecology, Kaohsiung Veterans General Hospital, No.386, Dazhong 1st Rd., Zuoying Dist, Kaohsiung City 81362, Taiwan. [2] Department of Obstetrics and Gynecology, National Yang-Ming University School of Medicine, No. 155, Sec. 2, Li-Nong Street, Pei-Tou, Taipei 112, Taiwan. [3] Department of Pharmacy and Master Program, College of Pharmacy and Health Care, Tajen University, No.20, Weixin Rd, Yanpu, Township, Pingtung County 90741, Taiwan. [4] Department of General Surgery and Medical Surgical Specialties, University of Catania, 95123 Catania, Italy. [5] Department of Obstetrics and Gynecology, Taipei Veterans General Hospital, No. 201, Section 2, Shih-Pai Road, Taipei 112, Taiwan. [6] Department of Medical Research, China Medical University Hospital, No. 2, Yude Road, North District, Taichung City 40447, Taiwan. [7] Department of Marine Biotechnology and Resources, National Sun Yat-sen University, 70 Lienhai Rd, Kaohsiung

City 80424, Taiwan. [8]Department of Biological Science, National Sun Yat-Sen University, 70 Lienhai Rd, Kaohsiung City 80424, Taiwan.

References

1. Polyzos NP, Devroey P. A systematic review of randomized trials for the treatment of poor ovarian responders: is there any light at the end of the tunnel? Fertil Steril. 2011;96(5):1058–61.e7.

2. Ferraretti AP, La Marca A, Fauser BC, Tarlatzis B, Nargund G, Gianaroli L. ESHRE consensus on the definition of 'poor response' to ovarian stimulation for in vitro fertilization: the Bologna criteria. Hum Reprod. 2011;26(7):1616–24.

3. Polyzos NP, Nwoye M, Corona R, Blockeel C, Stoop D, Haentjens P, et al. Live birth rates in Bologna poor responders treated with ovarian stimulation for IVF/ICSI. Reprod BioMed Online. 2014;28(4):469–74.

4. Xu B, Chen Y, Geerts D, Yue J, Li Z, Zhu G, et al. Cumulative live birth rates in more than 3,000 patients with poor ovarian response: a 15-year survey of final in vitro fertilization outcome. Fertil Steril. 2018;109(6):1051–9.

5. Pandian Z, McTavish AR, Aucott L, Hamilton MP, Bhattacharya S. Interventions for 'poor responders' to controlled ovarian hyper stimulation (COH) in in-vitro fertilisation (IVF). Cochrane Database Syst Rev. 2010;(1):Cd004379.

6. Sunkara SK, Coomarasamy A, Faris R, Braude P, Khalaf Y. Long gonadotropin-releasing hormone agonist versus short agonist versus antagonist regimens in poor responders undergoing in vitro fertilization: a randomized controlled trial. Fertil Steril. 2014;101(1):147–53.

7. Bosdou JK, Venetis CA, Kolibianakis EM, Toulis KA, Goulis DG, Zepiridis L, et al. The use of androgens or androgen-modulating agents in poor responders undergoing in vitro fertilization: a systematic review and meta-analysis. Hum Reprod Update. 2012;18(2):127–45.

8. Li XL, Wang L, Lv F, Huang XM, Wang LP, Pan Y, et al. The influence of different growth hormone addition protocols to poor ovarian responders on clinical outcomes in controlled ovary stimulation cycles: a systematic review and meta-analysis. Medicine (Baltimore). 2017;96(12):e6443.

9. Chamayou S, Sicali M, Alecci C, Ragolia C, Liprino A, Nibali D, et al. The accumulation of vitrified oocytes is a strategy to increase the number of euploid available blastocysts for transfer after preimplantation genetic testing. J Assist Reprod Genet. 2017;34(4):479–86.

10. Burger HG. Androgen production in women. Fertil Steril. 2002;77(Suppl 4):S3–5.

11. Prizant H, Gleicher N, Sen A. Androgen actions in the ovary: balance is key. J Endocrinol. 2014;222(3):R141–R51.

12. Casson PR, Lindsay MS, Pisarska MD, Carson SA, Buster JE. Dehydroepiandrosterone supplementation augments ovarian stimulation in poor responders: a case series. Hum Reprod. 2000;15(10):2129–32.

13. Singh N, Zangmo R, Kumar S, Roy KK, Sharma JB, Malhotra N, et al. A prospective study on role of dehydroepiandrosterone (DHEA) on improving the ovarian reserve markers in infertile patients with poor ovarian reserve. Gynecol Endocrinol. 2013;29(11):989–92.

14. Barad D, Gleicher N. Effect of dehydroepiandrosterone on oocyte and embryo yields, embryo grade and cell number in IVF. Hum Reprod. 2006; 21(11):2845–9.

15. Zangmo R, Singh N, Kumar S, Vanamail P, Tiwari A. Role of dehydroepiandrosterone in improving oocyte and embryo quality in IVF cycles. Reprod BioMed Online. 2014;28(6):743–7.

16. Barad D, Brill H, Gleicher N. Update on the use of dehydroepiandrosterone supplementation among women with diminished ovarian function. J Assist Reprod Genet. 2007;24(12):629–34.

17. Wiser A, Gonen O, Ghetler Y, Shavit T, Berkovitz A, Shulman A. Addition of dehydroepiandrosterone (DHEA) for poor-responder patients before and during IVF treatment improves the pregnancy rate: a randomized prospective study. Hum Reprod. 2010;25(10):2496–500.

18. Zhang M, Niu W, Wang Y, Xu J, Bao X, Wang L, et al. Dehydroepiandrosterone treatment in women with poor ovarian response undergoing IVF or ICSI: a systematic review and meta-analysis. J Assist Reprod Genet. 2016;33(8):981–91.

19. Nagels HE, Rishworth JR, Siristatidis CS, Kroon B. Androgens (dehydroepiandrosterone or testosterone) for women undergoing assisted reproduction. Cochrane Database Syst Rev. 2015;11:Cd009749.

20. Orvieto R, Patrizio P. GnRH agonist versus GnRH antagonist in ovarian stimulation: an ongoing debate. Reprod BioMed Online. 2013;26(1):4–8.

21. Lambalk CB, Banga FR, Huirne JA, Toftager M, Pinborg A, Homburg R, et al. GnRH antagonist versus long agonist protocols in IVF: a systematic review and meta-analysis accounting for patient type. Hum Reprod Update. 2017; 23(5):560–79.

22. Patrizio P, Vaiarelli A, Levi Setti PE, Tobler KJ, Shoham G, Leong M, et al. How to define, diagnose and treat poor responders? Responses from a worldwide survey of IVF clinics. Reprod BioMed Online. 2015;30(6):581–92.

23. Alpha Scientists in Reproductive Medicine and ESHRE Special Interest Group of Embryology. The Istanbul consensus workshop on embryo assessment: proceedings of an expert meeting. Hum Reprod. 2011;26(6):1270–83.

24. Zheng Y, Dong X, Huang B, Zhang H, Ai J. The artificial cycle method improves the pregnancy outcome in frozen-thawed embryo transfer: a retrospective cohort study. Gynecol Endocrinol. 2015;31(1):70–4.

25. Yang S, Chen X, Zhen X, Wang H, Ma C, Li R, et al. The prognosis of IVF in poor responders depending on the Bologna criteria: a large sample retrospective study from China. Biomed Res Int. 2015;2015:296173.

26. Kotb MM, Hassan AM, AwadAllah AM. Does dehydroepiandrosterone improve pregnancy rate in women undergoing IVF/ICSI with expected poor ovarian response according to the Bologna criteria? A randomized controlled trial. Eur J Obstet Gynecol Reprod Biol. 2016;200:11–5.

27. Xu B, Li Z, Yue J, Jin L, Li Y, Ai J, et al. Effect of dehydroepiandrosterone administration in patients with poor ovarian response according to the Bologna criteria. PLoS One. 2014;9(6):e99858.

28. Jirge PR, Chougule SM, Gavali VG, Bhomkar DA. Impact of dehydroepiandrosterone on clinical outcome in poor responders: a pilot study in women undergoing in vitro fertilization, using bologna criteria. J Hum Reprod Sci. 2014;7(3):175–80.

29. Li J, Yuan H, Chen Y, Wu H, Wu H, Li L. A meta-analysis of dehydroepiandrosterone supplementation among women with diminished ovarian reserve undergoing in vitro fertilization or intracytoplasmic sperm injection. Int J Gynaecol Obstet. 2015;131(3):240–5.

30. Haning RV,J, Hackett RJ, Flood CA, Loughlin JS, Zhao QY, Longcope C. Plasma dehydroepiandrosterone sulfate serves as a prehormone for 48% of follicular fluid testosterone during treatment with menotropins. J Clin Endocrinol Metab. 1993;76(5):1301–7.

31. Hillier SG, Tetsuka M, Fraser HM. Location and developmental regulation of androgen receptor in primate ovary. Hum Reprod. 1997;12(1):107–11.

32. Slomczynska M, Tabarowski Z. Localization of androgen receptor and cytochrome P450 aromatase in the follicle and corpus luteum of the porcine ovary. Anim Reprod Sci. 2001;65(1–2):127–34.

33. Sen A, Hammes SR. Granulosa cell-specific androgen receptors are critical regulators of ovarian development and function. Mol Endocrinol. 2010;24(7): 1393–403.

34. Walters KA, Middleton LJ, Joseph SR, Hazra R, Jimenez M, Simanainen U, et al. Targeted loss of androgen receptor signaling in murine granulosa cells of preantral and antral follicles causes female subfertility. Biol Reprod. 2012; 87(6):151.

35. Smith P, Steckler TL, Veiga-Lopez A, Padmanabhan V. Developmental programming: differential effects of prenatal testosterone and dihydrotestosterone on follicular recruitment, depletion of follicular reserve, and ovarian morphology in sheep. Biol Reprod. 2009;80(4):726–36.

36. Magamage MPS, Zengyo M, Moniruzzaman M, Miyano T. Testosterone induces activation of porcine primordial follicles in vitro. Reprod Med Biol. 2011;10(1):21–30.

37. Sen A, Prizant H, Light A, Biswas A, Hayes E, Lee HJ, et al. Androgens regulate ovarian follicular development by increasing follicle stimulating hormone receptor and microRNA-125b expression. Proc Natl Acad Sci U S A. 2014;111(8):3008–13.

38. Laird M, Thomson K, Fenwick M, Mora J, Franks S, Hardy K. Androgen stimulates growth of mouse Preantral follicles in vitro: interaction with follicle-stimulating hormone and with growth factors of the TGFbeta superfamily. Endocrinology. 2017;158(4):920–35.

39. Genazzani AD, Stomati M, Strucchi C, Puccetti S, Luisi S, Genazzani AR. Oral dehydroepiandrosterone supplementation modulates spontaneous and growth hormone-releasing hormone-induced growth hormone and insulin-like growth factor-1 secretion in early and late postmenopausal women. Fertil Steril. 2001;76(2):241–8.

40. Fried G, Remaeus K, Harlin J, Krog E, Csemiczky G, Aanesen A, et al. Inhibin B predicts oocyte number and the ratio IGF-I/IGFBP-1 may indicate oocyte

quality during ovarian hyperstimulation for in vitro fertilization. J Assist Reprod Genet. 2003;20(5):167–76.

41. Liu HC, He ZY, Mele CA, Veeck LL, Davis O, Rosenwaks Z. Human endometrial stromal cells improve embryo quality by enhancing the expression of insulin-like growth factors and their receptors in cocultured human preimplantation embryos. Fertil Steril. 1999;71(2):361–7.

42. Alexaki VI, Charalampopoulos I, Panayotopoulou M, Kampa M, Gravanis A, Castanas E. Dehydroepiandrosterone protects human keratinocytes against apoptosis through membrane binding sites. Exp Cell Res. 2009; 315(13):2275–83.

43. Liu D, Si H, Reynolds KA, Zhen W, Jia Z, Dillon JS. Dehydroepiandrosterone protects vascular endothelial cells against apoptosis through a Galphai protein-dependent activation of phosphatidylinositol 3-kinase/Akt and regulation of antiapoptotic Bcl-2 expression. Endocrinology. 2007;148(7):3068–76.

44. Lin LT, Wang PH, Wen ZH, Li CJ, Chen SN, Tsai EM, et al. The application of Dehydroepiandrosterone on improving mitochondrial function and reducing apoptosis of cumulus cells in poor ovarian responders. Int J Med Sci. 2017;14(6):585–94.

45. Tsui KH, Wang PH, Lin LT, Li CJ. DHEA protects mitochondria against dual modes of apoptosis and necroptosis in human granulosa HO23 cells. Reproduction. 2017;154(2):101–10.

46. Gleicher N, Kim A, Weghofer A, Kushnir VA, Shohat-Tal A, Lazzaroni E, et al. Hypoandrogenism in association with diminished functional ovarian reserve. Hum Reprod. 2013;28(4):1084–91.

47. Gleicher N, Kushnir VA, Weghofer A, Barad DH. The importance of adrenal hypoandrogenism in infertile women with low functional ovarian reserve: a case study of associated adrenal insufficiency. Reprod Biol Endocrinol. 2016;14:23.

48. Gleicher N, Kushnir VA, Darmon SK, Wang Q, Zhang L, Albertini DF, et al. New PCOS-like phenotype in older infertile women of likely autoimmune adrenal etiology with high AMH but low androgens. J Steroid Biochem Mol Biol. 2017;167:144–52.

49. Charmandari E, Nicolaides NC, Chrousos GP. Adrenal insufficiency. Lancet. 2014;383(9935):2152–67.

23

The ovarian estrogen synthesis function was impaired in Y123F mouse and partly restored by exogenous FSH supplement

Xiaoyu Tu[1,2], Miao Liu[1], Jianan Tang[1], Yu Zhang[1], Yan Shi[1], Lin Yu[1] and Zhaogui Sun[1,3*]

Abstract

Background: LepR tyrosine site mutation mice (Y123F) exhibit decreased serum E2 levels, immature reproductive organs, infertility as well as metabolic abnormalities. Although the actions of leptin and lepR in the control of reproductive function are thought to be exerted mainly via the hypothalamic-pituitary-gonadal axis, relatively less is known regarding their local effects on the peripheral ovary, especially on steroid hormone synthesis. Meanwhile, whether the decreased fertility of Y123F mouse could be restored by gonadotropin has not been clear yet.

Methods: The serum levels of E2, P4, FSH, LH, T and leptin of Y123F and WT mice at the age of 12 weeks were measured by enzyme-linked immunosorbent assay. Immunohistochemistry was used to compare the distribution of hormone synthases (STAR, CYP11A1, CYP19A1, HSD17B7) and FSHR in adult mouse ovaries of two genotypes. Western blot and real-time PCR were used to detect the expression levels of four ovarian hormone synthases and JAK2-STAT3 / STAT5 signaling pathway in 4 and 12 weeks old mice, as well as the effects of exogenous hFSH stimulation on hormone synthases and FSHR.

Results: Compared with WT mice, the serum levels of FSH, LH and E2 in 12-week-old Y123F mice were significantly decreased; T and leptin levels were significantly increased; but there was no significant difference of serum P4 levels. STAR, CYP11A1, HSD17B7 expression levels and the phosphorylation levels of JAK2 and STAT3 were significantly decreased in adult Y123F mice, while the expression of CYP19A1 and phospho-STAT5 were significantly increased. No significant differences were found between 4-week-old Y123F and WT mice. After exogenous hFSH stimulation, E2 levels and expression of CYP19A1 and HSD17B7 were significantly higher than that in the non-stimulated state, but significant differences still existed between Y123F and WT genotype mice under the same condition.

Conclusions: Abnormal sex hormone levels of Y123F mice were due to not only decreased gonadotropin levels in the central nervous system, but also ovarian hormone synthase abnormalities in the peripheral gonads. Both FSH signaling pathway and JAK2-STAT3/STAT5 signaling pathway were involved in regulation of ovarian hormone synthases expression. Exogenous FSH just partly improved the blood E2 levels and ovarian hormone synthase expression.

Keywords: Leptin receptor, Tyrosine site mutations, Infertility, Ovarian steroid hormone synthases

* Correspondence: sunzgbio@126.com
[1]Key Lab of Reproduction Regulation of NPFPC, SIPPR, IRD, Fudan University, Xietu Road 2140, Xuhui District, Shanghai 200032, China
[3]Key Laboratory of Contraceptive Drugs & Devices of NPFPC, Shanghai Institution of Planned Parenthood Research, Xietu Road 2140, Xuhui District, Shanghai 200032, China
Full list of author information is available at the end of the article

Background

Obesity has been one of the most important health problems within the world's population; the prevalence of overweight and obesity is increasing in reproductive-aged women [1]. It has detrimental impact on female reproductive health, including ovulatory disorders [2], decreased rates of conception, infertility [3], early pregnancy loss etc. [2]. Therefore, it is of great clinical significance to study the molecular mechanisms of impaired fertility in association with obesity.

Leptin, as an important adipokine, is encoded by ob gene and secreted by adipose tissue. Leptin receptor (lepR), with multiple isoforms (lepR a, b, c, d, e, and f), was encoded by db gene [4–6]. After ligand binding, lepR activates intracellular signal transduction pathways mainly including JAK2-STAT3/STAT5 through three tyrosine residues tyr985, tyr1077 and tyr1138 [7]. Previous studies reported leptin and lepR-deficient mice, such as ob/ob or db/db mice, all displayed metabolic abnormalities and reproductive disorders [6, 8]. These fully illustrated that, in addition to controlling energy balance and body weight, leptin also served as a necessary signal to regulate female reproduction. Y123F mice are transgenic mice that are expressed mutant leptin receptors with phenylalanine (F) substitution for all three tyrosine (Y) residues [9]. Our previous study showed that Y123F female mice were infertile similar with db/db mice, including no estrous cycle, anovulation and a significant decrease in serum estradiol (E2) levels [10]. But Y123F mice's symptoms of obesity, hyperphagia, hyperinsulinemia and impairment in glucose tolerance are less severe than db/db mice due to the remaining tyrosine-independent mechanisms. Also, Y123F mice have a longer life span than db/db mice [9]. Therefore, Y123F mice are more suitable to be a new animal model to investigate the role of leptin and lepR in reproduction, especially in obesity-related infertility.

The expression of lepR has been documented not only in the central nervous system such as hypothalamus or pituitary, but also in the peripheral gonads such as ovary granulosa or embryonic cells of several species [5, 7, 11]. However, the actions of leptin and lepR in the control of reproductive function are thought to be exerted mainly via the hypothalamic-pituitary-gonadal (HPG) axis, relatively less is known regarding their local effects on the peripheral ovary [12], especially on ovarian hormone synthesis. Therefore, in this study, we decided to observe effects of leptin and lepR on ovary itself, particularly on its steroid hormone synthesis with Y123F mouse model.

During ovarian steroidogenesis, the first step takes place within mitochondria where steroidogenic acute regulatory protein (STAR) is to facilitate the movement of cholesterol from outer mitochondrial membrane to the inner mitochondrial membrane [13]. Then, the cholesterol side-chain cleavage enzyme (P450scc or CYP11A1) converts cholesterol to pregnenolone to initiate steroidogenesis, which is a rate-limiting and quantitative regulation step. Next, most enzymes can be divided into two groups to mediate qualitative regulation determining the type of steroid to be produced: cytochrome P450 enzymes and hydroxysteroid dehydrogenases. Among them, CYP19 (P450arom) catalyzes the conversion of the C19 androgen, androstenedione and testosterone, to the C18 estrogen, estrone and estradiol respectively. HSD17B7 primarily activates estrone to estradiol, especially in the luteal phase of the rodent ovarian cycle, which is responsible for the final step in estradiol synthesis [13, 14]. In our previous study, we verified an elevated expression of site-mutated lepR in Y123F mouse ovaries and showed some accompanied gene profiling changes, particularly including steroid hormone biosynthesis enzyme genes such as Hsd17b7 or Star [10]. So far there has been no study regarding the relation between lepR and steroidogenic enzymes as well as involved mechanism. Accordingly, in this study, we evaluate sex hormone levels in adult Y123F female mice compared with WT mice; then we focus on Y123F mice ovaries to investigate changes of steroidogenic enzymes and JAK2-STAT3/STAT5 signaling pathway. Finally, we explore whether the decreased fertility of Y123F mouse could be restored by exogenous hFSH supplement.

Methods

Transgenic mice

Y123F mice, a knock-in line of mice that expressed mutant leptin receptors with phenylalanine substitution for all three tyrosines, were generated by Liu Yong, et al. [9]. Heterozygous Y123F mice were kindly provided by Dr. Shi Huijuan at Shanghai Institute of Planned Parenthood Research, Shanghai, China. They were backcrossed to C57BL/6 mice (purchased from Shanghai Laboratory Animal Research Center, Shanghai, China) for at least three generations to yield heterozygous Y123F mice in the C57BL/6 background, then heterozygous Y123F mice inbred to produce homozygous Y123F mice and WT littermates as described previously [10]. The mice were genotyped by PCR analysis of tail-tip DNA at 4 weeks of age with primers: F: CTA CTG GAA TGG AAC CTT GAG GCT TC; R: CAT TTT TCC TTT TAT CAG ACC AGC AAC C. All mice were housed in standard plastic rodent cages and maintained in a temperature- and light-controlled room (22–24 °C with 55–65% relative humidity and a 12/12 h light/dark cycle) with ad libitum feed and water. The study was approved by the Animal Ethics Committee at Shanghai Institute of Planned Parenthood Research. Animals were cared for in accordance with the guidelines of Experimental Animals.

Sample collection and hormone test

At the 4th week and 12th week after birth, mice were euthanized by cervical dislocation, ovaries were excised, cleaned of fat, weighed, and frozen at -80 °C. At 12 weeks of age, blood samples were collected and centrifuged, and the serum was stored at -20 °C for further analysis. 12-week-old female mice were divided into homozygous Y123F group and WT group. Mice in each group were randomly administered an intraperitoneal injection of 10 IU human follicle stimulating hormone (hFSH, gonal-f, Merck Serono Co., Ltd.) or equal does of phosphate buffer solution (PBS). After 48 h, they were sacrificed to collect ovaries and serum as above. All WT mice that were chosen as the control were at the stage of metestrus or diestrus. Serum hormone levels of progesterone (P4) and E2 were determined with Roche Cobas e601 electrochemical luminescence immunity analyzer (Roche, Switzerland) and were carried out in the Clinical Laboratory of ShangHai Institute of Planned Parenthood Research Hospital. Leptin, follicle stimulating hormone (FSH) and luteinizing hormone (LH) were measured by commercial ELISA kits (Elabscience Biotechnology Co., Ltd., Wuhan, China) according to the manufacturer's instructions. Testosterone (T) was measured by commercial ELISA kit (R&D, USA) according to the manufacturer's instructions. Intra-assay and inter-assay coefficients of variation were both < 10%.

Immunohistochemistry

To determine the cellular localization of steroidogenic enzymes and related receptors in the ovary, immunohistochemistry (IHC) were performed as described previously [10, 15]. Mouse ovaries were randomly collected from 12-week-old female mice of WT and Y123F groups (WT mice, n = 3; Y123F mice, n = 3). In brief, ovarian tissue was embedded by paraffin. Sections of paraffin-embedded ovaries (5 μm) were collected on glass slides, then deparaffinized and hydrated. Antigen retrieval was achieved by microwaving the slides in 0.01 M sodium citrate solution (pH 6.0) for 15 min, cooling to room temperature and washing three times in phosphate buffered saline (PBS) each for 5 min. After washing, the slides were blocked with 3% hydrogen peroxide in PBS for 10 min to quench endogenous peroxidase activity. The nonspecific background was eliminated by blocking with 10% lamb serum in PBS for 1 h at room temperature. The slides were then incubated with the primary antibody at 4 °C overnight. The primary antibodies included STAR (1:100 dilution, Proteintech Group, USA), CYP11A1 (1:100 dilution, Proteintech Group, USA), CYP19A1 (1:100 dilution, Proteintech Group, USA), HSD17B7 (1:100 dilution, Proteintech Group, USA), and FSHR (1:200 dilution, Abways, China). The next day, after washing with PBS, the slides

were incubated for 1 h at room temperature with biotinylated goat anti-rabbit IgG secondary antibody (1:200 dilution, Invitrogen, USA). The antibody dilution buffer was 10% lamb serum in PBS. Immunoreactive signals were detected using streptavidin-HRP and VECTOR Nova RED Peroxidase (HRP) Substrate Kit (Vectorlabs, Burlingame, USA) at room temperature. Slides were counterstained with hematoxylin. A negative control was performed without the primary antibody incubation step. Immunostaining was observed using a Nikon Eclipse 50i microscope (Nikon, Tokyo, Japan) and captured by NIS-Element F Software. Every antibody was repeated in slides from three separate ovaries with identical genotype.

Protein extraction and western blot

Total protein was extracted from mixed ovaries (WT mice, n = 5; Y123F mice, n = 5) as described earlier [10]. In brief, ovary tissues were harvested and lysed in lysis buffer adding with 1 mM phenylmethylsulphonyl fluoride on ice (Beyotime, Shanghai, China). Lysates were homogenized using a homogenizer and centrifuged at 12000 g for 15 min at 4 °C and the protein concentrations were measured using a BCA Protein Assay Kit (CWBIO, Beijing, China). A total of 30 μg protein was boiled in 1× loading buffer to denature, then added to each lane and separated by 10% SDS-PAGE for 1.5 h. The bands were transferred to a 0.45-μm nitrocellulose membrane (ImmobilonTM-NC Millipore Corporation, USA) for 1.5~ 2 h. The membranes were then blocked with 7% nonfat dry milk powder (NFDMP) in Tris-buffered saline (TBS: 2 mM Tris-HCl, 15 mM NaCl, pH 7.4), containing 0.1% Tween-20 (TBST) for 2 h at room temperature. Then they were incubated with the primary antibody at 4 °C overnight. The primary antibodies included STAR, CYP11A1, CYP19A1, HSD17B7 (1:1000 dilution, Proteintech Group, USA), JAK2, Phospho-JAK2 (Tyr1007/1008) (1:1000 dilution, Cell Signaling Technology, USA), STAT3, Phospho-STAT3 (Tyr705), STAT5A/B, Phospho-STAT5A (Tyr694) and FSHR (1:1000 dilution, Abways, China). Beta Actin antibody (1:5000 dilution, Proteintech Group, USA) was used as the internal control. These antibodies were diluted in TBST with 3.5% NFDMP. The next day, the membranes were washed three times in TBST each for 5 min and further incubated with HRP conjugated anti-rabbit or anti-mouse secondary antibodies (1:5000 dilution, Proteintech Group, USA) for 1 h at room temperature. After washing again in TBST, the signal was detected by Tanon™ High-sig ECL Western Blotting Substrate (Tanon, China) and analyzed using the FluorChem Gel documentation system (Tanon, China). The results were obtained from three independent repeated experiments with three pools of mixed ovary protein.

RNA extraction and quantitative real-time PCR (qPCR)

QPCR was performed to quantify the expressions of *Star, Cyp19A1, Cyp11A1, Hsd17b7, Fshr, Jak2, Stat3* and *Stat5* in the ovary. Expression levels were normalized against *Gapdh* expression. The primer sets are shown in Table 1. Total RNA was extracted from mixed ovaries (WT mice, $n = 3$; Y123F mice, $n = 3$) using Trizol (Invitrogen, USA) according to the manufacturer's instructions. RNA quantity and purity was confirmed by NanoDrop ASP-3700 spectrophotometer (ACTGene, Piscataway, NJ, USA), OD 260/280 nm ratios between 1.8 and 2.0 were obtained for all RNA samples. Total RNA from each sample was reverse transcribed into cDNA using a standard oligo-dT RT protocol with a ReverTra Ace qPCR RT Master Mix with gDNA Remover Kit (Toyobo, Osaka, Japan) according to the manufacturer's instructions. QPCR reactions were performed on an Illumina-Eco System (Illumina, USA) in a 10μl reaction volume with SYBR Green I Master Mix reagent (Toyobo, Osaka, Japan) and 5 pmol of the specific primer pairs shown in Table 1. The PCR thermal cycling conditions were 95 °C for 10 min for polymerase activation and the initial denaturation step, followed by 40 cycles with denaturation at 95 °C for 30s, annealing at 60 °C for 30s and extension at 72 °C for 30s. A melting curve analysis was recorded at the end of the amplification to evaluate the absence of contaminants or primer dimers. Each set of qPCR reactions was repeated three times, and the levels of gene expression were expressed in the form of $2^{-\Delta\Delta Ct}$. The results were repeated in three pools of total RNA from mixed ovaries.

Table 1 Primers used in quantitative real-time PCR

Gene	Accession number	Primer sequences (5′–3′)
Star	NM_011485.4	Upstream: CGGGTCTTGGGTCCTGGATTGT
		Downstream: GCTGCCCTCGCTCACCTTAAG
Cyp19a1	NM_007810.3	Upstream: TCGTCGCAGAGTATCCAGAGGT
		Downstream: CGCATGACCAAGTCCACAACAG
Cyp11a1	NM_019779.3	Upstream: GCTCAACCTGCCTCCAGACTTC
		Downstream: CCTCCTGCCAGCATCTCGGTAA
Hsd17b7	NM_010476.3	Upstream: CTGTGACACCGTACAACGGA
		Downstream: GCTCGGGTGATCCGATTTCT
Jak2	NM_008413.3	Upstream: AGATGGGAAGGGAAGGGTGTGG
		Downstream: AAGAGGGAGCAGCACGAAGGAT
Stat3	NM_213659.3	Upstream: TCGGTTGGAGGTGTGAGGTAGG
		Downstream: GTGGGAAAGGAAGGCAGGTTGA
Stat5	NM_001164062.1	Upstream: CAGAGTCGGTGACGGAGGAGAA
		Downstream: GCACGGTGGCAGTAGCATTGT
Gapdh	NM_001289726.1	Upstream: GTGAAGGTCGGTGTGAACGGATT
		Downstream: GGTCTCGCTCCTGGAAGATGGT

Statistical analysis

All data are presented as Mean ± SD or Mean ± SEM as indicated. The statistical analyses and data graphing were conducted using the GraphPad Prism 5 software. WB band intensities were analyzed by Image J software. The statistical analyses were performed with unpaired two-tailed Student's t test; a p-value < 0.05 was considered statistically significant.

Results

Y123F mice exhibited disordered sex hormone secretion

In view of the uncertainty of mouse breeding, the difficulty of blood collection, the estrous cycle of WT mice and the limited volume of blood samples, the final sample size of each indicator in both groups is not necessarily equal. The results showed that serum FSH of Y123F mice ($n = 9$) were lower than that of WT mice ($n = 8$) ($p < 0.05$) (Fig. 1a). Serum LH levels of Y123F mice ($n = 9$) were lower than that of WT mice ($n = 7$) ($p < 0.05$) (Fig. 1b). T levels were significantly higher in Y123F mice ($n = 5$) ($p < 0.01$) than that of WT mice ($n = 5$) ($p < 0.01$) (Fig. 1c). Leptin levels were significantly higher in Y123F mice ($n = 9$) than that of WT mice ($n = 7$) ($p < 0.01$) (Fig. 1d).

Steroidogenic enzymes changed in adult Y123F mouse ovaries compared with WT mouse ovaries

According to cDNA Microarray results of Y123F ovaries in our previous research [10], we decided to investigate the expression of four ovary steroidogenic enzymes in 12-week-old Y123F ovaries: STAR, CYP11A1, CYP19A1, HSD17B7. WB results showed that STAR, CYP11A1 and HSD17B7 expressions were significantly decreased ($p < 0.05$); while CYP19A1 expressions were increased ($p < 0.01$) in adult Y123F mouse ovaries compared with WT ovaries (Fig. 2a, c). Meanwhile, relative mRNA expression levels of these genes were all dramatically decreased in adult Y123F mouse ovaries ($p < 0.05$) (Fig. 2e). However, comparing these steroidogenic enzymes expression changes of immature mouse ovaries (4-week-old) in both groups, only relative mRNA expression levels of CYP11A1 were higher in Y123F mouse ovaries than that of WT ovaries ($p < 0.01$). Apart from that, there was nearly no difference of four steroidogenic enzyme expressions between two groups through WB and qRT-PCR tests ($p > 0.05$) (Fig. 2b, d, f). The contradictory results of CYP19A1 protein and mRNA levels in Y123F mouse ovaries gave the impetus for us to examine these enzymes distribution and expression in ovaries through IHC. The IHC results showed that CYP19A1 mainly located in cumulus granulosa cells of tertiary follicles in Y123F mouse ovaries while in the granulosa cells of secondary follicle and corpus luteum in WT mouse ovaries (Fig. 3c, C1). Meanwhile, STAR widely

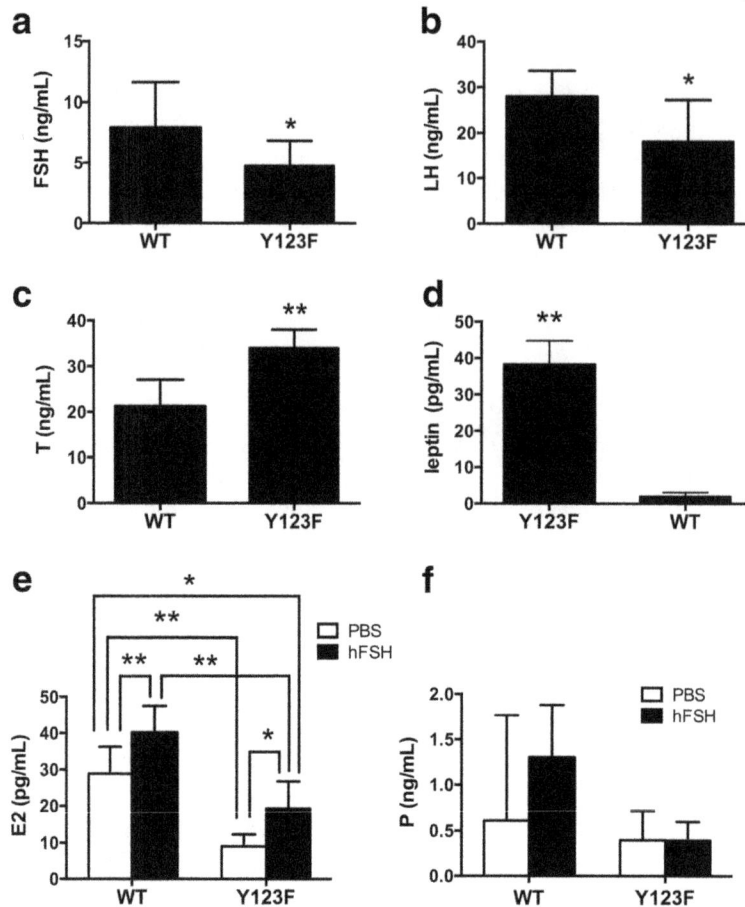

Fig. 1 The hormone determination in wild type (WT) and Y123F homozygous (Y123F) mice. The FSH, LH, T, E2, P and leptin levels in wild type and Y123F homozygous mouse blood were determined. **a** The blood FSH levels in WT ($n = 8$) were significantly higher than Y123F ($n = 9$) mice ($p < 0.05$). **b** The blood LH levels in WT ($n = 7$) were significantly higher than Y123F ($n = 9$) mice ($p < 0.05$). **c** The blood T levels in WT ($n = 5$) were significantly lower than Y123F ($n = 5$) mice ($p < 0.01$). **d** The blood leptin levels in WT ($n = 7$) were significantly lower than Y123F ($n = 9$) mice ($p < 0.01$). **e** The blood E2 levels in WT ($n = 9/13$) and Y123F ($n = 7/6$) mice after an intraperitoneal injection of 10 IU hFSH or PBS. **f** The blood P levels in WT ($n = 5/8$) and Y123F ($n = 9/6$) mice after an intraperitoneal injection of 10 IU hFSH or PBS. Data are expressed as the mean $\pm$ SD, $*p < 0.05$, $**p < 0.01$ indicate a significant difference between the WT and Y123F groups

distributed in the whole WT ovaries but only in some granulosa cells of Y123F ovaries (Fig. 3a, A1). CYP11A1 had the similar distribution with CYP19A1 in mouse ovaries of both groups (Fig. 3b, B1). HSD17B7 demonstrated fewer expressions in the whole Y123F mouse ovary than WT ovary where most of the corpora lutea were positive (Fig. 3d, D1). As a whole, these results indicated that lepR deficiency had a negative influence on steroidogenic enzymes production in adult Y123F mouse ovaries.

LepR deficiency affected JAK2-STAT3/STAT5 signaling pathway in ovaries

As a lepR tyrosine site mutations transgenic mouse model, whether the JAK2-STAT3/STAT5 signaling pathway changed in local ovaries of Y123F mice needed to be determined. So we compared the levels of phospho-

JAK2, JAK2, phospho-STAT3, STAT3, phospho-STAT5, STAT5 between Y123F and WT mouse ovaries. All determinations were performed in 4-week-old and 12-week-old mice respectively, and we found no significant differences in WB and qRT-PCR results at the age of 4 weeks ($p > 0.05$) (Fig. 4b, d, f). However, in 12-week-old ovaries, WB and qRT-PCR results showed that phosphorylation of JAK2 and STAT3 markedly decreased while phosphorylation of STAT5 dramatically increased in Y123F ovaries ($p < 0.05$) (Fig. 4a, c, e).

Exogenous hFSH partly restored serum E2 levels and ovary steroidogenic enzymes expression of Y123F mouse

Since serum E2 and FSH levels were decreased in Y123F mice, we considered whether supplement of exogenous hFSH could improve ovary function. With PBS as a control, we found that E2 levels were increased after hFSH

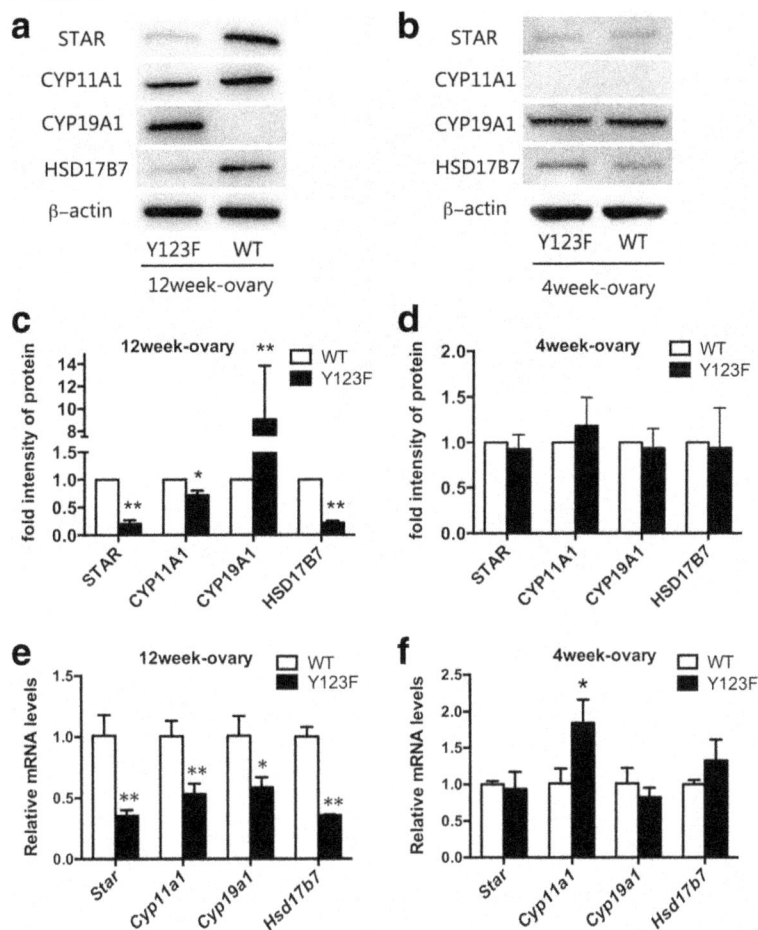

Fig. 2 Comparison of ovary steroidogenic enzyme protein and mRNA levels of WT and Y123F mouse ovaries at the age of 4 weeks and 12 weeks. **a** Western blotting analysis of ovary steroidogenic enzyme expressions in WT and Y123F mouse ovaries at the age of 12 weeks. **c** Densitometric analysis of Western blotting detection of ovary steroidogenic enzyme expressions in WT and Y123F mouse ovaries at the age of 12 weeks. **e** QPCR analysis of ovary steroidogenic enzyme relative mRNA expressions levels in WT and Y123F mouse ovaries at the age of 12 weeks. **b** Western blotting analysis of ovary steroidogenic enzyme expressions in WT and Y123F mouse ovaries at the age of 4 weeks. **d** Densitometric analysis of Western blotting detection of ovary steroidogenic enzyme expressions in WT and Y123F mouse ovaries at the age of 4 weeks. **f** QPCR analysis of ovary steroidogenic enzyme relative mRNA expressions levels in WT and Y123F mouse ovaries at the age of 4 weeks. Data of WB results are expressed as the mean ± SD of three independent experiments. Data of QPCR results are expressed as the mean ± SEM of three independent experiments, *$p < 0.05$, **$p < 0.01$ indicate a significant difference between the WT and Y123F groups

stimulation in both genotypes, for Y123F mice ($p < 0.05$), but for WT mice ($p < 0.01$). When comparing between genotypes, for PBS injection mice, E2 levels were higher in WT mice ($n = 13$) than Y123F mice ($n = 6$) ($p < 0.01$); for hFSH injection mice, E2 levels were higher in WT mice ($n = 9$) than Y123F mice ($n = 7$) ($p < 0.01$). E2 levels in Y123F mice with hFSH injection ($n = 7$) were still lower than that in WT mice with PBS injection ($n = 13$) ($p < 0.05$) (Fig. 1e). However, there was no significant difference of serum P4 levels after hFSH injection in both genotypes ($p > 0.05$) (Fig. 1f). At the same time, we found that only CYP19A1 increased responding to hFSH induction in Y123F ovaries, which was consistent with that in WT mice ($p < 0.05$) (Fig. 5b, e). HSD17B7 just had a slight increase in Y123F ovaries after hFSH

injection ($p < 0.05$) (Fig. 5c, f). Surprisingly, Y123F mouse ovaries had higher expression of FSHR than WT ovaries, but FSHR in Y123F ovaries showed no significant changes after stimulation (Fig. 5a, d). So we further detected FSHR distribution in ovaries of both groups and found that positive FSHR staining mostly located in follicular cavities and rarely in corpus luteum by IHC (Fig. 3e, E1), which contributed to the raised expression in Y123F mouse ovaries detected by WB.

Discussion

Observational studies from humans or animal models with leptin or leptin-receptor deficiency have fully indicated that leptin-lepR system are involved in maintaining normal reproductive function [6, 16–18]. Although

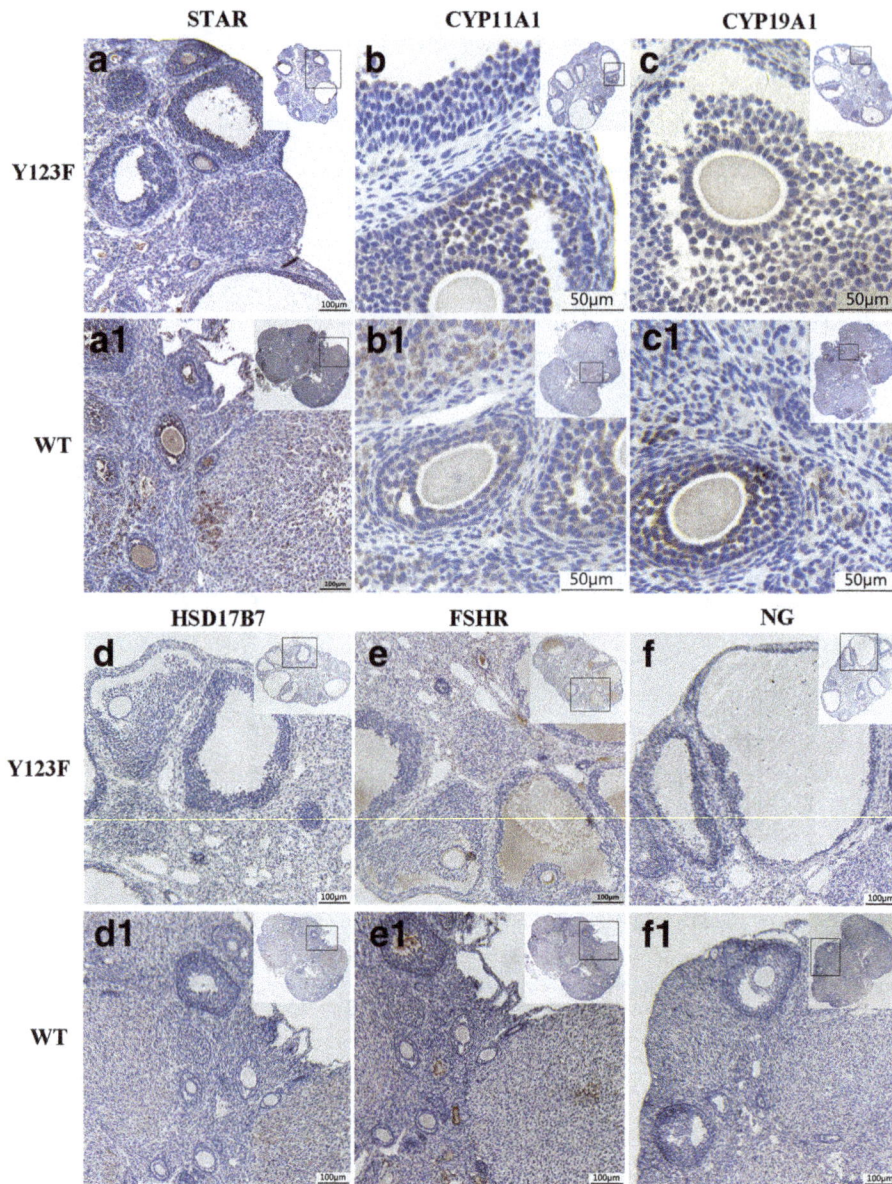

Fig. 3 Immunohistochemical detection of ovary steroidogenic enzyme expressions in 12-week-old Y123F and WT mouse ovaries. (A-A1) The 10 × 10 magnification immunocytochemistry images of STAR expression as indicated by the dotted squares in Y123F mouse ovaries (**a**) and WT mouse ovaries (A1). (B-B1) The 40 × 10 magnification immunocytochemistry images of CYP11A1 expression as indicated by the dotted squares in Y123F mouse ovaries (**b**) and WT mouse ovaries (B1). (C-C1) The 40 × 10 magnification immunocytochemistry images of CYP19A1 expression as indicated by the dotted squares in Y123F mouse ovaries (**c**) and WT mouse ovaries (C1). (D-D1) The 10 × 10 magnification immunocytochemistry images of HSD17B7 expression as indicated by the dotted squares in Y123F mouse ovaries (**d**) and WT mouse ovaries (D1). (E-E1) The 10 × 10 magnification immunocytochemistry images of FSHR expression as indicated by the dotted squares in Y123F mouse ovaries (**e**) and WT mouse ovaries (E1). (F-F1) The 10 × 10 magnification immunocytochemistry images of negative control as indicated by the dotted squares in Y123F mouse ovaries (**f**) and WT mouse ovaries (F1)

the central effects of leptin on hypothalamic and pituitary function have been examined extensively [19, 20], the contribution of direct leptin actions on the ovary in obesity-related infertility/subfertility remains incompletely understood. In this study, using the Y123F mouse model, we mainly explored the effects of lepR tyrosine site mutations on serum estrogen levels and local ovary steroidogenic enzymes changes. The novel finding of

direct actions of leptin on the ovary may account for some adverse effects of obesity on ovarian function.

Firstly, according to our previous study that Y123F mice had low E2 level, no estrous cycle and anovulation [10], we fully tested sex hormone levels of Y123F mice at the age of 12 weeks and found that the hypothalamic hypogonadism existed. In accordance with this result, previous studies demonstrated that leptin null (ob/ob)

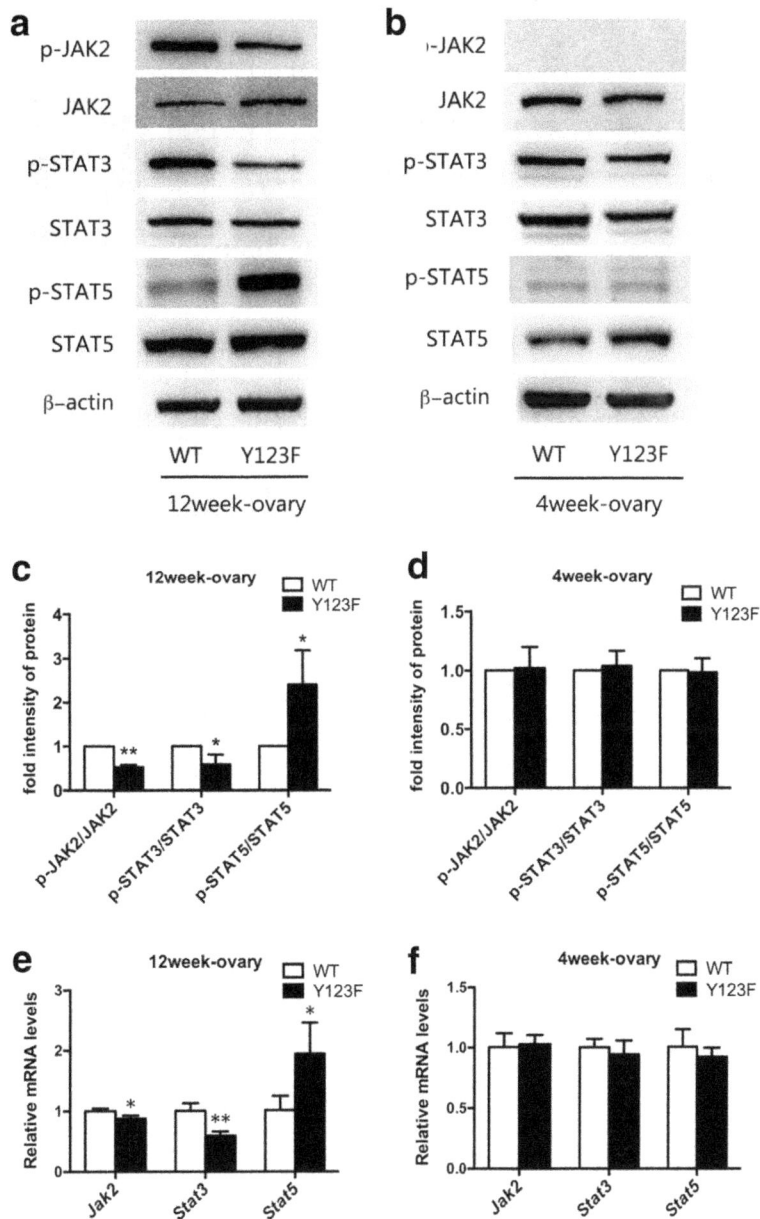

Fig. 4 Detections of JAK2-STAT3/STAT5 signaling pathway of WT and Y123F mouse ovaries at the age of 4 weeks and 12 weeks. **a** Western blotting analysis of phospho-JAK2, JAK2, phospho-STAT3, STAT3, phospho-STAT5, STAT5 expressions in WT and Y123F mouse ovaries at the age of 12 weeks. **c** Densitometric analysis of Western blotting detection of phospho-JAK2, phospho-STAT3 and phospho-STAT5 levels in WT and Y123F mouse ovaries at the age of 12 weeks. **e** QPCR analysis of *Jak2, Stat3* and *Stat5* relative mRNA expressions levels in WT and Y123F mouse ovaries at the age of 12 weeks. **b** Western blotting analysis of phospho-JAK2, JAK2, phospho-STAT3, STAT3, phospho-STAT5, STAT5 expressions in WT and Y123F mouse ovaries at the age of 4 weeks. **d** Densitometric analysis of Western blotting detection of phospho-JAK2, phospho-STAT3 and phospho-STAT5 levels in WT and Y123F mouse ovaries at the age of 4 weeks. **f** QPCR analysis of *Jak2, Stat3* and *Stat5* relative mRNA expressions levels in WT and Y123F mouse ovaries at the age of 4 weeks. Data of WB results are expressed as the mean ± SD of three independent experiments. Data of QPCR results are expressed as the mean ± SEM of three independent experiments, *$p < 0.05$, **$p < 0.01$ indicate a significant difference between the WT and Y123F groups

and leptin receptor null (db/db) mice exhibited low gonadotrophin concentrations, immature reproductive organs, and impaired sexual maturation [21]. Also, leptin and leptin receptor gene defects result in human obesity and delayed puberty, oligo-anovulation, or subfertility in most human populations [22]. Since leptin receptor is expressed abundantly within the hypothalamus and pituitary [7, 23, 24], Watanobe, et al. showed that leptin acted within the hypothalamus of animals to stimulate the release of GnRH within the median eminence-arcuate

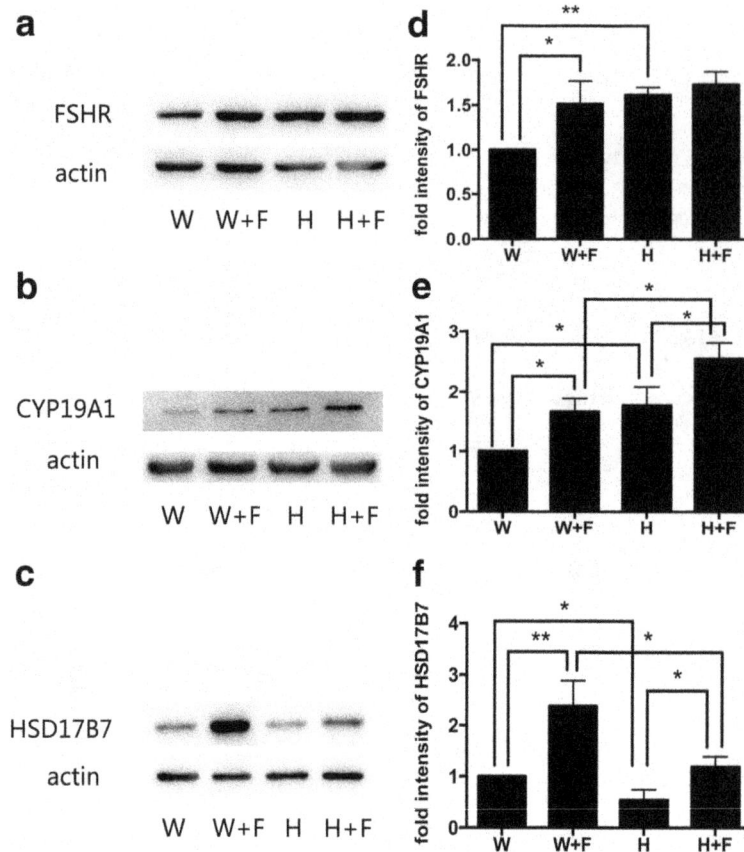

Fig. 5 Detections of FSHR, CYP19A1, HSD17B7 expression changes in WT and Y123F mouse ovaries after injection of hFSH or PBS at the age of 12 weeks. **a** FSHR expression changes in WT mouse ovaries after injection of PBS (W) or hFSH (W + F) and in Y123F mouse ovaries after injection of PBS (H) or hFSH (H + F). **b** CYP19A1 expression changes in WT mouse ovaries after injection of PBS (W) or hFSH (W + F) and in Y123F mouse ovaries after injection of PBS (H) or hFSH (H + F). **c** HSD17B7 expression changes in WT mouse ovaries after injection of PBS (W) or hFSH (W + F) and in Y123F mouse ovaries after injection of PBS (H) or hFSH (H + F). **d-f** Densitometric analysis of Western blotting detection of FSHR (**d**), CYP19A1 (**e**) and HSD17B7 (**f**) expression changes in WT and Y123F mouse ovaries after injection of hFSH or PBS. Data are expressed as the mean ± SD of three independent experiments, *$p < 0.05$, **$p < 0.01$ indicate a significant difference between the WT and Y123F groups

nucleus in fasted animals [25]. Nicole Bellefontaine, et al. reported that leptin plays a central role in regulating the HPG axis to increase circulating LH levels in vivo through the activation of neuronal NO synthase in neurons of the preoptic region [26], in addition to through neuropeptides such as NPY [27] or kisspeptin [28]. Wen H. Yu, et al. also confirmed that, in vitro pituitary tissue culture; leptin induces a dose-related increase in LH, FSH, and prolactin release [20] via nitric oxide synthase activation in the gonadotropes [29]. Female fertility relies on the regulation of sex hormones and positive/ negative feedback exists in HPG axis [30, 31]. Due to the direct stimulatory effects of leptin on the HPG axis, thus for Y123F mice, abnormal lepR in central nervous systems resulted in low gonadotropin secretion, subsequently contributing to the low E2 levels.

Considering clinical patients undergoing assisted reproductive technology (ART), classic controlled ovarian hyperstimulation was performed using GnRH-agonist long protocol with exogenous recombinant FSH to stimulate oocyte development as well as increase E2 levels [2, 32]. We tried to elevate E2 levels in Y123F mice by supplementing exogenous hFSH. Surprisingly, low serum E2 levels were only partly restored due to the active response of the ovary to FSH, still remained a significant lower level compared with WT mice. So we hypothesized that low E2 levels of Y123F mouse were not only due to low gonadotropin levels, but also probably due to the local factors in the ovary directly relating to leptin and lepR, such as steroidogenisis disorder,

It is well established that a series of ovary steroidogenic enzymes modulate hormone biosynthesis, which subsequently regulates reproductive functions such as follicle development and ovulation [13]. Here, we found that ovary steroidogenic enzymes changed in 12-week-old Y123F mice, with a remarkable decrease of STAR, CYP11A1, HSD17B7, as well as an increase of CYP19A1, fully confirmed our hypothesis. Several studies have reported direct local leptin effects on ovarian functions. Zachow RJ, et al. indicated that leptin antagonizes the stimulatory effects of transforming growth factor-β and insulin-like growth factor-I on FSH-dependent estrogen production by a mechanism involving the leptin-induced attenuation of P450arom activity and mRNA expression in rat ovarian granulosa cells (GC) in vitro [33, 34]. Ghizzoni L, et al. found that 30% decrease in E2 production was caused by the certain Leptin concentration; while P4 levels were not influenced in the culture media of human granulosa-lutein cells obtained from follicular fluid of women undergoing in vitro fertilization. They concluded that leptin suppresses E2 secretion by interfering with either the translational or post-translational steps of the baseline CYP17 and/or aromatase synthesis and/or the activation of the enzymes [35]. In other species, such as sheep or bovine, leptin also inflicted a negative effect on ovarian steroidogenesis in vitro and in vivo experiments, which were corresponding with our results [36, 37]. However, some studies showed stimulatory effects of leptin on the ovary [38, 39]. These discrepancies may stem from differences in the doses of leptin and species as well as experiment design. In our study, ovary steroidogenic enzymes expressed abnormally in local ovary of lepR-deficient Y123F mice, even if to supplement exogenous hFSH, the expression defects of ovary steroidogenic enzymes were just partly recovered. But WB results showed that FSHR had higher expression in Y123F mice than WT mice, which had no significant increase after hFSH stimulation. By means of IHC, we found that higher expression of FSHR overall in Y123F mouse ovaries dectected by WB was due to more antral follicles in Y123F ovaries than in WT ovaries. But its feedback regulation may be up to saturation, leading to limited improvement of ovary steroidgenesis via hFSH supplement. Overall, our results fully illustrated that leptin and lepR in the Y123F mouse ovary had a negative effect on local ovarian steroidogenesis, independently of its central actions in the hypothalamus and pituitary.

Apart from previous studies above, Clark BJ and Lin D, et al. confirmed that overexpression of mouse STAR in mouse leydig MA-10 cells increased their basal steroidogenic rate [40], and co-transfection of expression vectors for both StAR and the P450scc system in nonsteroidogenic COS-1 cells augmented pregnenolone synthesis more than that obtained with the P450scc system alone [41]. Thus, in this study, the insufficiency of STAR, CYP11A1 and HSD17B7 can directly disrupt estradiol biosynthesis, leading to the low E2 levels of Y123F mice. It's worth mentioning that Y123F mouse ovaries had higher expression of CYP19A1 and higher level of testosterone. As the substrate of estrogen biosynthesis, we considered that testosterone induced a compensatory response of higher expression of CYP19A1 to facilitate

more conversion from testosterone to estradiol [13]. But IHC showed that CYP19A1 mainly distributed in cumulus granulosa cells of tertiary follicles of Y123F mouse ovaries; and while mostly in the granulosa cells of secondary follicle and corpora lutea of WT mouse ovaries. So we supposed that estradiol produced in granulosa cells of Y123F mouse ovaries could be less available to get into the blood circulation due to the lack of corpus luteum that had enriching blood vessels, ultimately resulting in low blood E2 levels.

Intriguingly, there was no significant difference in all 4-week-old mice. These findings suggested that lepR tyrosine site mutations led to ovary steroidogenic enzymes changes only in adult mice, which had correlations with metabolic abnormalities due to fatness. Before 4 weeks, on one hand, mice did not reach up to sexual maturity and most of steroidogenic enzymes remained inactive; on the other hand, Y123F mice still maintained regular body weight due to complete compensation for lepR deficiency by other signal pathway [9]. Corresponding with our finding, Luba Sominsky and colleagues have shown that neonatal overfeeding increased circulating levels of leptin and reduced the number of ovarian follicles, specifically, the primordial follicle pool in adult rats. The adult rats had increased levels of ovarian leptin and its receptor, but diminished release of pituitary gonadotropins at ovulation and altered expression of ovarian markers, such as GDF9, important for follicular recruitment and survival [42]. So our results also confirmed the negative effects of leptin/lepR related obesity on reproduction.

In view of the local effects of leptin on ovary, although estradiol production is mainly regulated by FSH acting via the cAMP-dependent protein kinase (PKA) pathway in ovary granulosa cells [43, 44], lepR mediated JAK2-STAT3/STAT5 signaling pathway in local ovary was worthy of being determined. Leptin has been shown to primarily activate the JAK2-STAT3/STAT5 signaling pathway through three tyrosine sites on long isoform leptin receptor [45–47]. The long isoform LepR, which contains an intact intracellular domain with necessary protein motifs, can activate the JAK2, further stimulating the phosphorylation of multiple residues (Tyrosine 985, Tyrosine 1138, and Tyrosine 1077) on the intracellular domain of LEPR [48]. Phosphorylation of tyrosine residue 1138 mainly recruits STAT3 and it has been reported that hypothalamic leptin control to reproduction is regulated by signals independent of STAT3 signaling [49]. Meanwhile, Tyrosine 1077, the major phosphorylation site mediating leptin's effects on reproduction, promotes the recruitment and transcriptional activation of STAT5 [50] and is required for ongoing appropriate function of the female reproductive function [51]. As expected, we found that in 12-week-old ovaries, phosphorylation of

JAK2, STAT3 and STAT5 changed in Y123F ovaries, but no significant differences in 4-week-old ovaries between two genotypes.

Previously, Ding, et al. found that sileptin treatment decreased the secretion of E2 and the cell proliferation, but increased the secretion of progesterone and cell apoptosis in human ovarian granulosa cells in vitro. They confirmed that impaired activation of lepR mediating JAK2/STAT3 signal pathway contributed to ovarian granulosa cell apoptosis [52]. Therefore, our results indicated that LepR was involved in adult ovary steroidogenesis by mediating JAK2-STAT3/STAT5 signaling pathway in local ovaries.

Conclusion

In conclusion, lepR tyrosine site mutations of Y123F mice not only decreased gonadotropin levels through the central nervous system, but also impaired steroidogenic enzymes expression of local ovary through JAK2-STAT3/STAT5 signaling pathways. Both effects led to abnormal sex hormones levels and infertility of Y123F mice. Owing to the local ovarian factors, exogenous hFSH supplement just partly restored the defects in serum E2 levels and ovary steroidogenic enzymes expression. Since obesity and obesity-related infertility/subfertility are growing problems in human beings, our finding that direct effects of leptin and lepR on ovary were involved in infertility of Y123F mice, suggested a new viewpoint on the relationship between obesity and reproduction. Accordingly, clinicians can try to improve their ovarian hormone synthesis function in obese patients with impaired fertility via supplement exogenous hFSH or hMG. Meanwhile, the founding that is, the feedback of gonadotropin action of Y123F mouse still existed, provides animal experimental basis for follow-up therapy with assisted reproductive technology on obesity-related infertility.

Abbreviations

CYP11A1: P450scc, cholesterol side-chain cleavage enzyme; CYP19A1: Aromatase; E2: Estradiol; ELISA: Enzyme-linked immunosorbent assay; F: Phenylalanine; FSH: Follicle stimulating hormone; FSHR: Follicle stimulating hormone receptor; HPG: Hypothalamic-pituitary-gonadal; HSD17B7: Hydroxysterold Dehydrogenase 17B7; IHC: Immunohistochemistry; JAK2: Janus kinase 2; LepR: Leptin receptor; LH: Luteinizing hormone; P: Progesterone; QPCR: Real-time quantitative PCR; STAR: Steroidogenic acute regulatory protein; STAT3: Signal transducer and activator of transcription 3; STAT5: Signal transducer and activator of transcription 5; T: Testosterone; WB: Western blot; WT: Wild type; Y: Tyrosine; Y123F: LepR tyrosine site mutation mice

Acknowledgements

The authors would like to thank Shunheng Yao for his assistance with the animal experiments.

Funding

This work was supported by the National Natural Science Foundation of China (No.81370682).

Authors' contributions

ZS conceived and designed the experiments. XT and ZS wrote the manuscript. XT, ML and JT performed the experiments. XT and YZ analyzed the data. YS and LY contributed to experimental reagents, materials and analysis tools. All authors approved the final submitted version of the article.

Competing interests

The authors declare that they have no competing interests.

Author details

[1]Key Lab of Reproduction Regulation of NPFPC, SIPPR, IRD, Fudan University, Xietu Road 2140, Xuhui District, Shanghai 200032, China. [2]Women's Hospital, School of Medicine, Zhejiang University, Hangzhou, China. [3]Key Laboratory of Contraceptive Drugs & Devices of NPFPC, Shanghai Institution of Planned Parenthood Research, Xietu Road 2140, Xuhui District, Shanghai 200032, China.

References

1. Ng M, Fleming T, Robinson M, Thomson B, Graetz N, Margono C, Mullany EC, Biryukov S, Abbafati C, Abera SF. Global, regional, and national prevalence of overweight and obesity in children and adults during 1980-2013: a systematic analysis for the global burden of disease study 2013. Lancet. 2014;384:766–81.
2. Lin XH, Wang H, Wu DD, Ullah K, Yu TT, Ur Rahman T, Huang HF. High leptin level attenuates embryo development in overweight/obese infertile women by inhibiting proliferation and promotes apoptosis in granule cell. Horm Metab Res. 2017;49:534–41.
3. Medicine PCoASfR. Obesity and reproduction: an educational bulletin. Fertil Steril. 2008;90:21–9.
4. Barash IA, Cheung CC, Weigle DS, Ren H, Kabigting EB, Kuijper JL, Clifton DK, Steiner RA. Leptin is a metabolic signal to the reproductive system. Endocrinology. 1996;137:3144–7.
5. Fei H, Okano HJ, Li C, Lee GH, Zhao C, Darnell R, Friedman JM. Anatomic localization of alternatively spliced leptin receptors (Ob-R) in mouse brain and other tissues. Proc Natl Acad Sci U S A. 1997;94:7001–5.
6. Zhang Y, Proenca R, Maffei M, Barone M, Leopold L, Friedman JM. Positional cloning of the mouse obese gene and its human homologue. Nature. 1994; 372:425–32.
7. Zhou Y, Rui L. Leptin signaling and leptin resistance. Front Med. 2013;7: 207–22.
8. Moschos S, Chan JL, Mantzoros CS. Leptin and reproduction: a review. Fertil Steril. 2002;77:433–44.
9. Jiang L, You J, Yu X, Gonzalez L, Yu Y, Wang Q, Yang G, Li W, Li C, Liu Y. Tyrosine-dependent and -independent actions of leptin receptor in control of energy balance and glucose homeostasis. Proc Natl Acad Sci U S A. 2008; 105:18619–24.
10. Tu X, Kuang Z, Gong X, Shi Y, Yu L, Shi H, Wang J, Sun Z. The influence of LepR tyrosine site mutations on mouse ovary development and related gene expression changes. PLoS One. 2015;10:e0141800.
11. Archanco M, Muruzabal FJ, Llopiz D, Garayoa M, Gomez-Ambrosi J, Fruhbeck G, Burrell MA. Leptin expression in the rat ovary depends on estrous cycle. J Histochem Cytochem. 2003;51:1269–77.
12. Ksinanova M, Cikos S, Babel'ova J, Sefcikova Z, Spirkova A, Koppel J, Fabian D. The responses of mouse preimplantation embryos to leptin in vitro in a transgenerational model for obesity. Front Endocrinol (Lausanne). 2017;8:233.

13. Payne AH, Hales DB. Overview of steroidogenic enzymes in the pathway from cholesterol to active steroid hormones. Endocr Rev. 2004;25:947–70.

14. Miller WL, Auchus RJ. The molecular biology, biochemistry, and physiology of human steroidogenesis and its disorders. Endocr Rev. 2011;32:81–151.

15. Li J, Ye Y, Zhang R, Zhang L, Hu X, Han D, Chen J, He X, Wang G, Yang X, Wang L. Robo1/2 regulate follicle atresia through manipulating granulosa cell apoptosis in mice. Sci Rep. 2015;5:9720.

16. Clement K, Vaisse C, Lahlou N, Cabrol S, Pelloux V, Cassuto D, Gourmelen M, Dina C, Chambaz J, Lacorte JM, et al. A mutation in the human leptin receptor gene causes obesity and pituitary dysfunction. Nature. 1998;392: 398–401.

17. Strobel A, Issad T, Camoin L, Ozata M, Strosberg AD. A leptin missense mutation associated with hypogonadism and morbid obesity. Nat Genet. 1998;18:213–5.

18. Tartaglia LA, Dembski M, Weng X, Deng N, Culpepper J, Devos R, Richards GJ, Campfield LA, Clark FT, Deeds J, et al. Identification and expression cloning of a leptin receptor, OB-R. Cell. 1995;83:1263–71.

19. Jin L, Burguera BG, Couce ME, Scheithauer BW, Lamsan J, Eberhardt NL, Kulig E, Lloyd RV. Leptin and leptin receptor expression in normal and neoplastic human pituitary: evidence of a regulatory role for leptin on pituitary cell proliferation. J Clin Endocrinol Metab. 1999;84:2903–11.

20. Yu WH, Kimura M, Walczewska A, Karanth S, McCann SM. Role of leptin in hypothalamic-pituitary function. Proc Natl Acad Sci U S A. 1997;94:1023–8.

21. Chehab FF, Qiu J, Mounzih K, Ewart-Toland A, Ogus S. Leptin and reproduction. Nutr Rev. 2002;60:S39–46. discussion S68-84, 85-37

22. Dubern B, Clement K. Leptin and leptin receptor-related monogenic obesity. Biochimie. 2012;94:2111–5.

23. Mercer JG, Hoggard N, Williams LM, Lawrence CB, Hannah LT, Trayhurn P. Localization of leptin receptor mRNA and the long form splice variant (Ob-Rb) in mouse hypothalamus and adjacent brain regions by in situ hybridization. FEBS Lett. 1996;387:113–6.

24. Iqbal J, Pompolo S, Considine RV, Clarke IJ. Localization of leptin receptor-like immunoreactivity in the corticotropes, somatotropes, and gonadotropes in the ovine anterior pituitary. Endocrinology. 2000;141:1515–20.

25. Watanobe H. Leptin directly acts within the hypothalamus to stimulate gonadotropin-releasing hormone secretion in vivo in rats. J Physiol. 2002; 545:255–68.

26. Bellefontaine N, Chachlaki K, Parkash J, Vanacker C, Colledge W, d'Anglemont de Tassigny X, Garthwaite J, Bouret SG, Prevot V. Leptin-dependent neuronal NO signaling in the preoptic hypothalamus facilitates reproduction. J Clin Invest. 2014;124:2550–9.

27. Czaja K, Lakomy M, Sienkiewicz W, Kaleczyc J, Pidsudko Z, Barb CR, Rampacek GB, Kraeling RR. Distribution of neurons containing leptin receptors in the hypothalamus of the pig. Biochem Biophys Res Commun. 2002;298:333–7.

28. Roa J, Vigo E, Garcia-Galiano D, Castellano JM, Navarro VM, Pineda R, Dieguez C, Aguilar E, Pinilla L, Tena-Sempere M. Desensitization of gonadotropin responses to kisspeptin in the female rat: analyses of LH and FSH secretion at different developmental and metabolic states. Am J Physiol Endocrinol Metab. 2008;294:E1088–96.

29. Yu WH, Walczewska A, Karanth S, McCann SM. Nitric oxide mediates leptin-induced luteinizing hormone-releasing hormone (LHRH) and LHRH and leptin-induced LH release from the pituitary gland. Endocrinology. 1997;138: 5055–8.

30. Bauerdantoin AC, Weiss J, Jameson JL. Roles of estrogen, progesterone, and gonadotropin-releasing hormone (GnRH) in the control of pituitary GnRH receptor gene expression at the time of the preovulatory gonadotropin surges. Endocrinology. 1995;136:1014–9.

31. Hersh C, Tsatsanis C, Dermitzaki E, Avgoustinaki P, Malliaraki N, Vasilis V, Margioris AN. The impact of adipose tissue-derived factors on the hypothalamic-pituitary-gonadal (HPG) axis. Hormones. 2015;14:549.

32. Kuang Y, Chen Q, Hong Q, Lyu Q, Ai A, Fu Y, Shoham Z. Double stimulations during the follicular and luteal phases of poor responders in IVF/ICSI programmes (Shanghai protocol). Reprod BioMed Online. 2014;29: 684–91.

33. Zachow RJ, Weitsman SR, Magoffin DA. Leptin impairs the synergistic stimulation by transforming growth factor-beta of follicle-stimulating hormone-dependent aromatase activity and messenger ribonucleic acid expression in rat ovarian granulosa cells. Biol Reprod. 1999;61:1104–9.

34. Zachow RJ, Magoffin DA. Direct intraovarian effects of leptin: impairment of the synergistic action of insulin-like growth factor-I on follicle-stimulating

35. Ghizzoni L, Barreca A, Mastorakos G, Furlini M, Vottero A, Ferrari B, Chrousos GP, Bernasconi S. Leptin inhibits steroid biosynthesis by human granulosa-lutein cells. Horm Metab Res. 2001;33:323–8.

36. Spicer LJ, Francisco CC. Adipose obese gene product, leptin, inhibits bovine ovarian thecal cell steroidogenesis. Biol Reprod. 1998;58:207–12.

37. Kendall NR, Gutierrez CG, Scaramuzzi RJ, Baird DT, Webb R, Campbell BK. Direct in vivo effects of leptin on ovarian steroidogenesis in sheep. Reproduction. 2004;128:757–65.

38. Ahima RS, Dushay J, Flier SN, Prabakaran D, Flier JS. Leptin accelerates the onset of puberty in normal female mice. J Clin Invest. 1997;99:391–5.

39. Barkan D, Hurgin V, Dekel N, Amsterdam A, Rubinstein M. Leptin induces ovulation in GnRH-deficient mice. FASEB J. 2005;19:133–5.

40. Clark BJ, Wells J, King SR, Stocco DM. The purification, cloning, and expression of a novel luteinizing hormone-induced mitochondrial protein in MA-10 mouse Leydig tumor cells. Characterization of the steroidogenic acute regulatory protein (StAR). J Biol Chem. 1994;269:28314–22.

41. Lin D, Sugawara T, Strauss JF 3rd, Clark BJ, Stocco DM, Saenger P, Rogol A, Miller WL. Role of steroidogenic acute regulatory protein in adrenal and gonadal steroidogenesis. Science. 1995;267:1828–31.

42. Sominsky L, Ziko I, Soch A, Smith JT, Spencer SJ. Neonatal overfeeding induces early decline of the ovarian reserve: implications for the role of leptin. Mol Cell Endocrinol. 2016;431:24–35.

43. Daniel SA, Armstrong DT. Involvement of estrogens in the regulation of granulosa cell aromatase activity. Can J Physiol Pharmacol. 1983;61:507.

44. Homer MV, Rosencrantz MA, Shayya RF, Chang RJ. The effect of estradiol on granulosa cell responses to FSH in women with polycystic ovary syndrome. Reprod Biol Endocrinol. 2017;15:13.

45. Thon M, Hosoi T, Yoshii M, Ozawa K. Leptin induced GRP78 expression through the PI3K-mTOR pathway in neuronal cells. Sci Rep. 2014;4:7096.

46. Vaisse C, Halaas JL, Horvath CM, Darnell JE Jr, Stoffel M, Friedman JM. Leptin activation of Stat3 in the hypothalamus of wild-type and Ob/Ob mice but not db/db mice. Nat Genet. 1996;14:95–7.

47. Gautron L, Elmquist JK. Sixteen years and counting: an update on leptin in energy balance. J Clin Invest. 2011;121:2087–93.

48. Gorska E, Popko K, Stelmaszczyk-Emmel A, Ciepiela O, Kucharska A, Wasik M. Leptin receptors. Eur J Med Res. 2010;15(Suppl 2):50–4.

49. Bates SH, Stearns WH, Dundon TA, Schubert M, Tso AW, Wang Y, Banks AS, Lavery HJ, Haq AK, Maratos-Flier E, et al. STAT3 signalling is required for leptin regulation of energy balance but not reproduction. Nature. 2003;421: 856–9.

50. Villanueva EC, Myers MG Jr. Leptin receptor signaling and the regulation of mammalian physiology. Int J Obes. 2008;32(Suppl 7):S8–12.

51. Patterson CM, Villanueva EC, Greenwald-Yarnell M, Rajala M, Gonzalez IE, Saini N, Jones J, Myers MG Jr. Leptin action via LepR-b Tyr1077 contributes to the control of energy balance and female reproduction. Mol Metab. 2012;1:61–9.

52. Ding X, Kou X, Zhang Y, Zhang X, Cheng G, Jia T. Leptin siRNA promotes ovarian granulosa cell apoptosis and affects steroidogenesis by increasing NPY2 receptor expression. Gene. 2017;633:28–34.

24

Frequency of the T307A, N680S, and -29G>A single-nucleotide polymorphisms in the follicle-stimulating hormone receptor in Mexican subjects of Hispanic ancestry

Gabriela García-Jiménez[1][†], Teresa Zariñán[2][†], Rocío Rodríguez-Valentín[3], Nancy R. Mejía-Domínguez[2], Rubén Gutiérrez-Sagal[2], Georgina Hernández-Montes[2], Armando Tovar[4], Fabián Arechavaleta-Velasco[6], Patricia Canto[7], Julio Granados[5], Hortensia Moreno-Macias[8], Teresa Tusié-Luna[9], Antonio Pellicer[1] and Alfredo Ulloa-Aguirre[2]* [iD]

Abstract

Background: *FSHR* SNPs may influence the ovarian sensitivity to endogenous and exogenous FSH stimulation. Given the paucity of data on the *FSHR* c.919A > G, c.2039A > G and − 29G > A SNPs in Hispanic population, we here analyzed their frequency distribution in Mexican mestizo women.

Methods: Samples from 224 Mexican mestizo women enrolled in an IVF program as well as a genotype database from 8182 Mexican mestizo subjects, were analyzed for *FSHR* SNPs at positions c.919, c.2039 and − 29G > A. Association between the genetic variants and reproductive outcomes was assessed.

Results: The c.919 and c.2039 SNPs were in strong linkage disequilibrium and their corresponding genotype frequencies in the IVF group were: AA 46.8%, AG 44.2%, and GG 8.9%, and AA 41.9%, AG 48.2% and GG 9.8%, respectively. For the -29G > A SNP, genotype frequencies were 27% (GG), 50% (GA) and 23% (AA). In normal oocyte donors with the c.2039 GG genotype, the number of oocytes recovered after ovarian stimulation (COS) were significantly ($p < 0.01$) lower than in those bearing other genotypes in this or the -29G > A SNP. Analysis of the large scale database revealed that both allelic and genotype frequencies for the three SNPs were very similar to those detected in the IVF cohort ($p \geq 0.38$) and that female carriers of the c.2039 G allele tended to present lower number of pregnancies than women bearing the AA genotype; this trend was stronger when women with more Native American ancestry was separately analyzed (OR = 2.0, C.I. 95% 1.03–3.90, $p = 0.04$). There were no differences or trends in the number of pregnancies among the different genotypes of the -29G > A SNP.

Conclusions: The frequency of the GG/GG combination genotype for the c.919 and c.2039 SNPs in Mexican hispanics is among the lowest reported. The GG genotype is associated with decreased number of oocytes recovered in response to COS as well as to lower pregnancy rates in Hispanic women from the general population. The absence of any effect of the -29AA genotype on the response to COS, indicates that there is no need to perform this particular genotype testing in Hispanic women with the purpose of providing an individually-tailored COS protocol.

Keywords: Follicle stimulating hormone, Oocyte donation, Ovulation induction, Assisted reproductive techniques, Infertility, Female infertility, FSHR gene SNPs

* Correspondence: aulloaa@unam.mx
[†]Gabriela García-Jiménez and Teresa Zariñán contributed equally to this work.
[2]Red de Apoyo a la Investigación (RAI), Coordinación de la Investigación Científica, Universidad Nacional Autónoma de México (UNAM)-Instituto Nacional de Ciencias Médicas y Nutrición SZ (INCMNSZ), Calle Vasco de Quiroga 15, Tlalpan, 14000 Ciudad de Mexico, Mexico
Full list of author information is available at the end of the article

Background

Follicle-stimulating hormone (FSH), one of the gonado-trophins synthesized by the pituitary gland, plays a pivotal role in reproduction. This gonadotrophin binds its cognate receptor, the follicle-stimulating hormone receptor (FSHR), in the granulosa cells of the ovarian follicles and the Sertoli cells lining the seminiferous tubules of the testes, to regulate an array of biological effects associated with reproductive competence. In the ovary, FSH stimulates follicle growth and maturation, as well as the synthesis of estrogens, whereas in the testes it supports spermatogenesis [1, 2].

Of the nearly 2000 single nucleotide polymorphisms (SNPs) of the FSHR, five are located in exon 10 [3]. Four of these SNPs are non-synonymous and lead to amino acid substitution, resulting in the T307A, R524S, A665T, and N680S FSHR protein variants [4, 5]. The most common and best studied SNPs of this receptor are c.919A > G (rs6165) and c.2039A > G (rs6166), which are inherited in strong linkage disequilibrium [at least in Caucasians and Asians and less in Africans [6]] and whose most common FSHR variants, T307/N680 and A307/S680, are almost equally distributed among Europeans [3, 6–9].

A number of studies indicate that FSHR function is influenced by the p.T307A and p.N680S polymorphisms. In particular, the p.N680S SNP has received special attention because of its association with variations in the sensitivity of the FSHR to its cognate agonist and the ovarian response to FSH stimulation as disclosed by in vitro [10, 11] and in vivo studies [reviewed in [4, 7, 8, 12]]. More specifically, young women with the GG genotype tend to present lower ovarian sensitivity to endogenous FSH, which apparently leads to higher pituitary FSH secretion and longer duration of the menstrual cycle compared to women with the AA genotype [13]. This altered FSHR sensitivity to agonist, frequently makes necessary personalization of the controlled ovarian stimulation (COS) protocol, usually by administering higher FSH doses to overcome the decreased ovarian response provoked by the $N \rightarrow S$ substitution at position 680 of the FSHR [8, 14–17]. Moreover, this particular SNP has been proposed as a predictive biomarker for determining the optimal FSH dose to be used in COS protocols [8, 9, 13, 14, 18]. Apparently, the negative effect of the S680 variant on the FSHR response to agonist decreases with age and fertility status [19–21]. The N680S SNP also has been linked with other abnormalities [22–26], including lower testicular volume in selected North European populations bearing the S680S genotype variant, particularly when it co-exists with the FSHB -211G > A SNP [27].

The less studied –29G > A polymorphism, located in the core promoter region of the FSHR (rs1394205), has been associated with reduced transcriptional activity of the receptor gene in women with the -29AA genotype, as well as to primary or secondary amenorrhea and poor response to exogenous FSH in selected populations [28–31]. The major A allele frequency of this SNP ranges from 50 to 70% in East Asia and Europe [6].

Data on these FSHR SNPs in Hispano-American population are rather scarce, and the only available data comes from the HapMap and the 1000 Genomes Project database obtained in a small cohort of Mexican-American subjects with Mexican origen residing in Los Angeles, CA, USA [32]. In this particular population and according to the HapMap and the 1000 Genomes Project databases, the allele and genotype frequencies of the c.2039 GG SNP variant ranges from 33 to 34.0% and from 6.0 to 7.8%, respectively, whereas for the -29G > A SNP, these data bases indicate frequencies of 26% to 33% for the AA genotype and 49% to 55% for the A allele (http://grch37.ensembl.org), respectively.

The primary objective of the present study was to analyze the frequency distribution of these common FSHR SNPs in Mexican subjects of Hispanic origin, based on data obtained in larger populations than those previously included in reported databases [32]. For this purpose, we analyzed samples and data from three distinctly different groups of subjects in order to obtain the most accurate prevalence values and also to examine the influence of ancestry on the frequency estimates observed in Mexican mestizos. As secondary objectives, we examined the potential associations between the c.2039A > G and -29G > A SNPs genotypes with various outcomes of the COS protocol applied to women belonging to one of the study groups, as well as with some reproductive parameters extracted from the large database used as a reference.

Subjects and methods

Three different groups of Mexican subjects with Hispanic ancestry were included in the study: a cohort of normal and infertile Mexican mestizo women attending a private assisted reproduction clinic in Mexico City (IVF group); a group of 100 normal Mayan mestizo women with low Mayan-Spaniard miscenegation; and a population belonging to a large database of Mexican mestizo subjects in whom data on allelic and genotype frequencies of these SNPs were available.

IVF group

The first study group (IVF group) was conformed by a cohort of 224 Mexican mestizo women [80 normal oocyte donors aged 18 to 29 years (median, 24 years) and 144 infertile patients aged 22–43 years (median, 35 years)] who attended the Instituto Valenciano de Infertilidad-Mexico (IVI) and accepted to participate in the study. All participants in this group were unrelated and of self-reported Mexican mestizo ancestry (at least 3 generations), and both the treating physician and the volunteer were blind to the genotyping results until the end of the study. Women in the donor group were eligible whenever they met the criteria established by the IVI for oocyte donors, including normal karyotype, age between 18 and 30 years, and normal follicular reserve as assessed by intravaginal ultrasound. Inclusion criteria for the infertile group included: *a.* Presence of both ovaries without morphological abnormalities, except when the diagnosis of polycystic ovary syndrome (PCOS) was established [according to the Rotterdam criteria [33]]; *b.* Both ovaries adequately visible by intravaginal ultrasound; *c.* Absence of any endocrinological disease or obesity, except hypothyroidism under treatment or PCOS; and *d.* Any cause of infertility, including tubal factor, endometriosis, male factor, mixed (female/male) factor, and unknown cause.

For COS, women were prepared with an oral contraceptive (OC) (ethynilestradiol 30 μg plus drospirenone 3 mg; Bayer Schering Pharma, Berlin, Germany) for 10–21 days in the cycle preceding the COS cycle and then treated with gonadotrophin-releasing hormone antagonist (GnRHa) and menotropins (highly purified LH/FSH, 1:1; Merapur®, Ferring, Mexico) with or without recombinant human FSH (recFSH; Gonal F®, Merck-Serono, Mexico) as add-on treatment, or with GnRHa and recFSH. All women presented withdrawal bleeding after discontinuation of the OC. Ovarian stimulation was started 5 days after discontinuation of the OC with 150 to 225 IU menotropins, 75 IU menotropins plus 150 IU recFSH, or 150 IU recFSH after establishing ovarian and uterine quiescence by intravaginal ultrasound. Gonadotrophins were administered in a step-up fashion, adjusting the dose every 3 to 4 days depending on the ovarian response and the criteria of the treating physician, following stimulation protocols well established by the IVI. When the mean diameter of the leading follicle reached 14 mm as disclosed by intravaginal ultrasound, daily s.c. injections of 0.25 mg Cetrorelix (Cetrotide; Merck Serono S.A. Mexico) were added to gonadotrophin treatment until one or more follicles reached a mean diameter of 18 mm, time when 250 μg s.c. recombinant human chorionic gonadotrophin (hCG) (Ovidrel®, Merck Serono S.A., Mexico) was administered. Transvaginal ultrasound-guided oocyte retrieval was performed 36 h after hCG injection.

As secondary objective for the IVF study group, the response to COS was recorded and analyzed for differences among women with distinct N680S and -29G/A SNPs. To accomplish this, data containing total FSH and LH administered, serum estradiol [measured by a commercial chemiluminescence immunoassay (Beckman Coulter Life Sciences, Indianapolis, IN, USA)], number of oocytes recovered, and days of stimulus required to reach a mean follicle diameter of 18 mm, were collected from donors and patients who completed the

stimulation cycle until oocyte retrieval. Women who did not complete the COS cycle for any reason (either voluntarily or because of risk of hyperstimulation, poor response in terms of number of growing follicles, low serum E2 levels, and/or asynchrony in follicular growth), as well as patients with the diagnosis of PCOS (a condition that may influence on the ovarian response to COS) were excluded from the secondary analysis. To explore for differences in response among women with different N680S FSHR variants and -29G/A SNP genotypes and to minimize bias in the analysis of the results, we first examined separately in the group of donors and infertile patients who completed the stimulation cycle for homogeneity in the distribution of gonadotrophin treatment, age, and diagnosis (in the infertile group) among the three genotypes of each SNP, and thereafter analyzed within each group the effect of the genotype on the secondary outcomes controlling for gonadotrophin treatment [grouped as follows: *a.* recFSH treatment; *b.* LH/FSH (menotropins) treatment; and *c.* Mixed (menotropins *plus* recFSH) gonadotrophin treatment] and the other parameters.

Mayan mestizo women

The second population group studied was conformed by 100 normal Mayan mestizo women, aged 16 to 37 years (median, 20 years), resulting from the admixture between Mayan and Spaniard population with at least one Mayan surname, and whose DNA was analyzed to determine the frequency of the N680S FSHR variant and the impact of the Spaniard ancestry on the presence of this particular *FSHR* SNP in the Mexican mestizo population. Other *FSHR* SNPs were not analyzed in this group due to insufficient DNA sample available. Data on this particular population has been previously reported [34].

Mexican mestizo subjects from a large database

To compare the allelic and genotype frequency of the *FSHR* SNPs found in the above described groups with those from an open Mexican population, a third group of data (SIGMA cohort) from a large database genotyped using the Illumina OMNI 2.5 array was analyzed. This reference sample was conformed by 8182 Mexican mestizo subjects participants in the Slim Initiative in Genomic Medicine from the Americas (SIGMA) Type 2 Diabetes Consortium [35] [3515 (43%) male and 4667 (57%) female; 4366 (53%) non-diabetic and 3848 (47%) subjects with type 2 diabetes (T2D), all exhibiting Native American and European ancestry as determined by Principal Components Analysis [36]]. Details on the selection criteria, quality control procedure, and estimation of Native American and European ancestry proportions have been reported elsewhere [35]. In our secondary analysis of this reference database, information related with reproductive events such as age at menarche and menopause, and number of pregnancies in a subset of 520 women (aged 34 to 89 years, median 52 years) were extracted from this database (UIDS cohort; [35]) and analyzed for potential associations with the *FSHR* SNPs studied.

FSHR genotyping in samples from the IVF group and the Mayan women

Total DNA was extracted from peripheral blood lymphocytes employing the QIAamp DNA Blood Mini kit (Qiagen Inc., Valencia, CA, USA) and purified using the Wizard Genomic DNA Purification Kit (Promega, Madison, Wisconsin, USA) following the manufacturers' instructions. Analysis of the *FSHR* SNP at position 2039 (N680S) was carried out using a predesigned TaqMan allelic discrimination assay for the StepOne plus system (Applied Biosystems, Inc., Foster City, CA, USA). The results from the TaqMan assay were verified in all samples by PCR-restriction fragment length polymorphism (RFLP) as previously described [37]. In this IVF group, SNPs at positions 919 (T307A) and -29 also were analyzed by PCR-RFLP following the methods and oligonucleotide primers reported by Sudo et al. [37] and Achrekar et al. [28], respectively. For the 3 polymorphisms, the specificity and validity of the TaqMan and RFLP procedures were confirmed in 10% of the PCR products obtained (randomly selected from all samples processed) by direct sequencing. The procedure employed for determining the SNP genotypes in the SIGMA cohort has been described in detail elsewhere [35].

Statistical analysis
Data from the IVF group and Mayan mestizo women
Differences in allelic and genotype frequencies between women included in the IVF group (donors and infertile patients) and Mayan mestizo women were analyzed using the chi-squared test, with Yates' correction for the case of the allelic frequency of the -29G > A SNP.

For the analysis of the secondary objectives in the IVF group and given that the study was not originally designed with the power to evaluate the above described associations among different COS outcomes and genotypes, we first determined whether gonadotrophin treatment and diagnosis (in the case of the group of patients) were homogeneously distributed among the different genotypes and then analyzed for the existence of significant differences in secondary outcomes. To test for homogeneity of gonadotrophin treatment, age, and diagnosis vs genotype, the chi-squared test was employed. Differences in secondary endpoints (dose of gonadotrophins administered, serum E2 levels, days of COS, and number of oocytes retrieved) among genotypes in the donors and infertile patients were then analyzed by a generalized linear mixed model (GLMM), considering genotype as the fixed factor and hormonal treatment, age and diagnosis as random factors [38]. The GLMM test was chosen considering that the study was not originally designed to analyze for differences in secondary outcomes among genotypes and that this test allowed to control simultaneously for age, treatment, and diagnosis (in the case of infertile patients). A GLMM with gamma error was employed to seek for differences in LH doses administered and serum E2 levels, whereas a GLMM with Poison's error was used to calculate for differences in the number of oocytes recovered and days of COS. The Tukey's test was employed as post-hoc test for the effect of the genotype on oocyte number in donors. Although the number of secondary outcomes compared was relatively small, correction for multiple testing was anyway performed employing the Bonferroni's correction procedure [39].

Analysis of data from the SIGMA cohort
Pairedwise proportions test was employed to compare genotype frequencies between the IVF group and SIGMA subjects. Logistic regression models adjusted for ethnicity were employed to explore potential associations between *FSHR* genotypes and some reproductive outcomes such as age at menarche and menopause, and number of pregnancies in the UIDS cohort (see above). When the latter outcome was analyzed, the age was added as covariate in the model.

Linkage disequilibrium in the *FSHR* SNPs variants detected in the IVF group and SIGMA cohort was determined using the Haploview version 4.1 [40], in which $D' = D/Dmax$ (where D is the deviation of the observed from the expected) and r^2 is the correlation coefficient between pairs of loci. The maximum values of D' and r^2 are 1.000, which indicate complete linkage disequilibrium or pairwise correlation between the loci, respectively.

Since the Mayan population studied did not followed Hardy-Weinberg equilibrium for the c2039A > G SNP, and considering that women in the Mexican culture preserve both parents' surnames and that even if married they inherit the parental surnames to their descendants, we further compared the surnames of the Mayan population studied and tested for population equilibrium following the method described by Lasker [41].

Results
Frequency of the T307A, N680S and -29A/G variants in the IVF cohort
The allele and genotype frequency for the T307A and N680S SNPs in the IVF group with 224 women (donors and infertile women) studied are presented in Table 1. As shown, the allelic frequencies for the SNPs at positions 307 and 680 of the FSHR in the donor and patient groups were

Table 1 Allele and genotype frequencies for the single nucleotide polimorphism (SNP) c.919A > G and c.2039A > G of the *FSHR* in the population of normal oocyte donors and infertile Mexican mestizo women

Group	SNP	Allele frequency %	Genotype frequency %
Donors (n = 80)	c.919A > G (p.T307A)	A (T) 68.1[&]	AA (TT) 45.0*
		G (A) 31.8	AG (TA) 46.2
			GG (AA) 8.7
	c.2039A > G (p.N680S)	A (N) 66.8[&&]	AA (NN) 42.5**
		G (S) 33.1	AG (NS) 48.7
			GG (SS) 8.7
Infertile women (n = 144)	c.919A > G (p.T307A)	A (T) 69.4	AA (TT) 47.9
		G (A) 30.5	AG (TA) 43.0
			GG (AA) 9.0
	c.2039A > G (p.N680S)	A (N) 65.6	AA (NN) 41.6
		G (S) 34.3	AG (NS) 48.0
			GG (SS) 10.4
TOTAL (n = 224)	c.919A > G (p.T307A)	A (T) 68.9	AA (TT) 46.8
		G (A)31.0	AG (TA) 44.2
			GG (AA) 8.9
	c.2039A > G (p.N680S)	A (N) 66.0	AA (NN) 41.9
		G (S) 34.0	AG (NS) 48.2
			GG (SS) 9.8

[&]P = 0.930 and [&&]P = 0.987 vs infertile women for the A and G alleles at positions c.919 and c.2039, respectively
*P = 0.897 and **P = 0.922 vs infertile women for the AA, AG, and GG genotypes at positions c.919 and c.2039, respectively

virtually identical. Overall, the allelic frequencies for the A and G alleles at position c.919 (p.T307A) were 69% and 31%, whereas for those at position c.2039 (p.N680S) were 66% and 34%, respectively. Genotype frequencies at position c.2039 were also very similar between the two groups of women: the GG genotype (p.S680 in both alleles) which appears to influence the ovarian response to COS [9] was 8.7% in the donors while in the infertile women it was 10.4% (p = 0.792), yielding a mean frequency of 9.8% in the whole population studied. The frequency distribution of homozygous and heterozygous women for the T307A and N680S SNPs is shown in Fig. 1. As shown in this figure, the frequency distributions of the TT/NN and AA/SS haplotypes in donors and infertile patients were virtually identical [41.25% vs 40.97% (TT/NN), and 8.75% vs 8.33% (AA/SS) in donors and patients, respectively]. Nearly 42% of all women (45% of normal donors and 40% of patients) were heterozygous (TA/NS) for both alleles and the frequency was low for heterozygosity in only one allele (0.44% to 5.8%), with the lowest being the AA/NS haplotype combination, followed by TA/NN, TA/SS, and TT/NS. In this study group, the distribution of the SNPs (including the -29G > A SNP, see below) followed Hardy-Weinberg equilibrium. Analysis of the association between the rs6165 and rs6166 SNPs in the IVF group revealed a strong linkage disequilibrium, with D' = 0.997 (0.970 and 0.918 in donors and patients, respectively) and r^2 = 0.818 (0.889 and 0.781 in

donors and patients, respectively), and minor allele frequencies (MAG) of 0.309 (rs6165, c.919A > G) and 0.339 (rs6166, 2039A > G) for the whole group.

The allelic and genotype frequency for the rs1394205 (−29G > A) SNP as assessed by RFLP (Fig. 2) are shown in Table 2. The frequencies of the G and A alleles and GG and AA genotypes in these groups were almost equally distributed (p = 0.309 and p = 0.296, for the allelic and genotype frequencies, respectively). Although the frequency of the GG genotype (22.5%) tended to be lower than that of the AA genotype (27.5%) in the donor group, and vice versa, the frequency of the latter genotype (20.1%) tended to be lower than that of the former (30.6%) in the group of infertile patients, the differences did not reach statistical significance (p = 0.296). Analysis for linkage disequilibrium of this SNP with those at positions c.919 (p.T307A) and c.2039 (p.N680S) in the total population studied, yielded low values of D' (0.360 and 0.477) and r^2 (0.061 and 0.091) for both the rs6165-rs1394205 and rs6166-rs1394205 SNP pairs, respectively. Similar results were found when the donor and infertile patient groups were analyzed separately.

Response to COS according to the N680S and -29G > A variants in the IVF group

Sixty-nine donors and 125 patients completed the COS cycle, and the data were analyzed to determine

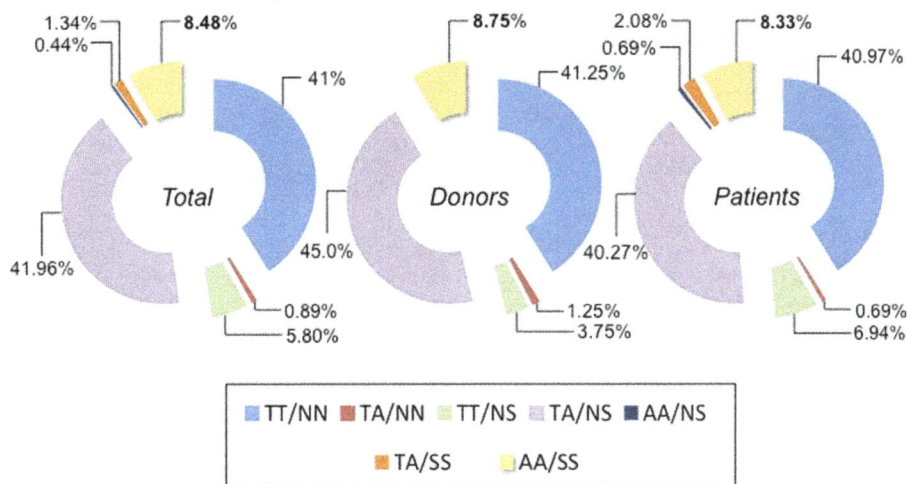

Fig. 1 Frequency distribution of the haplotypes at positions 307 and 680 of the FSHR protein. The homozygous TT/NN and heterozygous TA/NS haplotypes were the two most frequently observed combinations in Mexican mestizo women. The minor homozygous haplotype (AA/SS) was detected in only 8–9% of all women

associations between the response to COS and particular *FSHR* SNP genotypes. All cases included in this secondary analysis exhibited complete linkage disequilibrium between the p.T307A and p.N680S variants. Tables 3 and 4 show the data on secondary outcomes in the oocyte donors and infertile patients grouped according to

the SNPs at positions c.2039 and -29 at the *FSHR*, respectively. Normal donors conformed a quite homogenous group of women similar in age, and the COS protocol received was homogeneously distributed among the three SNP variants in positions c.2039 and -29 at the *FSHR*. Total FSH and LH administered, days

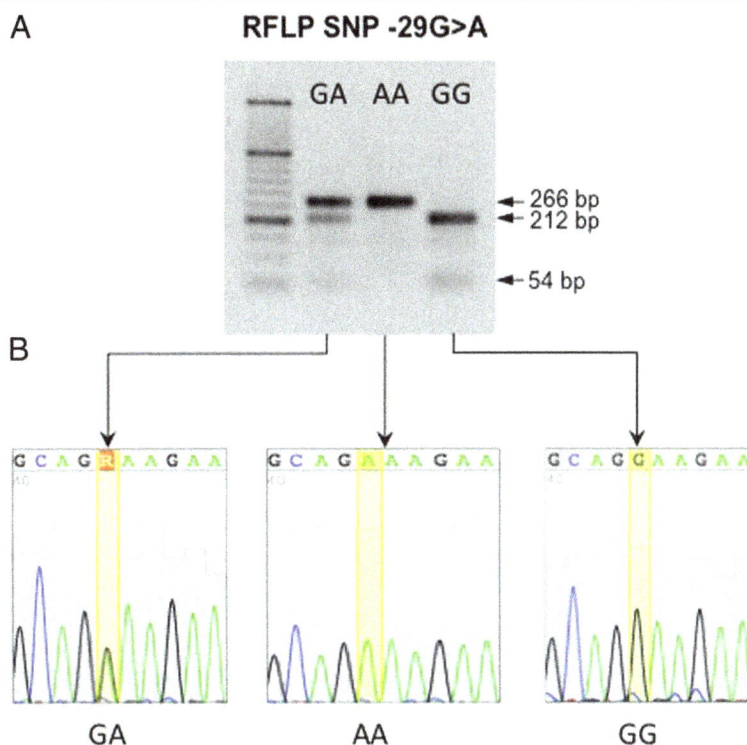

Fig. 2 Restriction fragment length polymorphism (RFLP) analysis of the single nucleotide polymorphism at position − 29 of the *FSHR*. **a** Representative 3% agarose in TBE gel of the digested PCR products showing the migration of the bands corresponding to the GA, AA and GG genotypes. **b** Representative electropherograms obtained after DNA sequencing of the amplified PCR products bearing different genotypes at position − 29

Table 2 Allele and genotype frequencies for the single nucleotide polymorphism (SNP) -29G > A of the *FSHR* in the population of normal oocyte donors and infertile Mexican mestizo women

Group	Allele frequency %	Genotype frequency %
Donors (n = 80)	G 47.5*	GG 22.5**
	A 52.5	GA 50.0
		AA 27.5
Infertile women (n = 144)	G 55.2	GG 30.6
	A 44.7	GA 49.3
		AA 20.1
TOTAL (n = 224)	G 52.4	GG 27.6
	A 47.5	GA 49.5
		AA 22.7

*$P = 0.309$ vs infertile women for the G and A alleles
**$P = 0.296$ vs infertile women for the GG, GA and AA genotypes

of gonadotrophin administration until hCG injection, and serum E2 levels, did not differ significantly among normal women bearing the NN, NS or SS FSHR protein variants (Table 3) ($p \geq 0.122$). Remarkably, the number of oocytes recovered from donors with the S680S variant were significantly lower than in those with the NS and

Table 3 Total gonadotropin dose administered, response to COH in terms of serum estradiol levels and number of oocytes recovered, and stimulation days with gonadotropins until the day of hCG administration in oocyte donors and infertile women undergoing ART, according to the c.2039A > G (N680S) single nucleotide polymorphism at the *FSHR*. Numbers are means ± S.D., unless indicated

Parameter	NN	NS	SS
Oocyte donors (n = 69)			
Number	32	32	5
Age	23.5* (18–29)	24 (20–29)	23 (21–25)
Total FSH (IU)	1673.3 ± 658.2	1888.7 ± 702.4	1791.7 ± 286.7
Total LH (IU)	1887.4 ± 917.4	1796.7 ± 826.4	1275.0 ± 742.5
Estradiol (pg(ml)	2433.6 ± 1094.9	2607.6 ± 1315.9	2431.2 ± 501.8
Oocyte number	13.7 ± 5.1	13.9 ± 5.14	8.8 ± 1.3**
Stimulation days	9.9 ± 1.6	10.3 ± 1.6	10.6 ± 1.1
Infertile women (n = 125)			
Number	54	57	14
Age	35.5* (22–41)	36 (27–43)	34 (25–42)
Total FSH (IU)	2329.7 ± 682.3	2261.2 ± 644.7	2203.4 ± 463.1
Total LH (IU)	857.8 ± 639.9	700.7 ± 394.7	664.2 ± 350.3
Estradiol (pg(ml)	2166.8 ± 1104.1	1977.6 ± 1028.0	2041.1 ± 970.6
Oocyte number	9.2 ± 4.8	8.2 ± 5.7	9.8 ± 6.8
Stimulation days	10.3 ± 1.4	10.2 ± 2.0	9.2 ± 1.8

*Median and range
**$P = 0.005$ vs NN and NS genotypes; the remaining parameters in the donors and all parameters in the infertile group did not differ significantly among genotypes ($P \geq 0.122$ and $P \geq 0.135$, for parameters in donors and infertile women, respectively)

Table 4 Total gonadotropin dose administered, response to COH in terms of serum estradiol levels and number of oocytes recovered, and stimulation days with gonadotropins until the day of hCG administration in oocyte donors and infertile women undergoing ART, according to the -29G > A single nucleotide polymorphism of the *FSHR*. Numbers are mean ± S.D., unless indicated

Parameter	GG	GA	AA
Oocyte donors (n = 69)			
Number	16	37	16
Age*	24 (21–28)	24 (19–29)	23.5 (18–27)
Total FSH (IU)	1874.3 ± 629.9	1681.3 ± 698.2	1921.6 ± 603.9**
Total LH (IU)	1500.0 ± 698.7	1710.4 ± 905.8	2217.8 ± 797.1
Estradiol (pg/ml)	2471.3 ± 1320.2	2445.6 ± 1069.2	2559.1 ± 1156.6
Oocyte number	12.5 ± 4.5	13.9 ± 5.5	13.3 ± 4.5
Stimulation days	10.3 ± 1.4	9.9 ± 1.7	10.5 ± 1.5
Infertile women (n = 125)			
Number	40	59	26
Age*	35 (27–42)	36 (22–43)	35.5 (26–39)
Total FSH (IU)	2367.8 ± 655.95	2178.7 ± 599.05	2395.6 ± 696.4**
Total LH (IU)	802.08 ± 637.9	708.1 ± 431.5	831.3 ± 478.9
Estradiol (pg/ml)	2088.6 ± 1134.9	2116.93 ± 1039.6	1917.8 ± 966.9
Oocyte number	8.8 ± 5.8	8.9 ± 5.4	8.7 ± 5.2
Stimulation days	10.02 ± 1.7	10.0 ± 1.9	10.5 ± 1.5

*Median and range
**None of the parameters analyzed were statistically different among genotypes ($p \geq 0.711$ and $p \geq 0.964$ for parameters in the donor and infertile group, respectively)

NN genotypes (8.8 ± 1.3 vs. 13.9 ± 5.1 and 13.7 ± 5.1, respectively; $p = 0.005$), a difference that was maintained after Bonferroni correction ($P_c = 0.001$). In all cases, the S680S variant associated with lower number of oocytes retrieved corresponded to the combination AA/SS at positions 307/680 of the FSHR (see Fig. 1 for the distribution of this genotype combination).

In the infertile patients from the IVF group the causes of infertility included tubal factor (31.3% of total), endometriosis (9.0%), male factor (14.5%), PCOS with or without male factor (9%), age ≥ 39 years (17.4%), mixed (female/male) factor (0.7%), and unknown cause (18%). In this group of infertile patients, age, COS protocol received and diagnosis also were homogeneously distributed among the different genotypes at positions c.2039 and -29. Nevertheless, and in contrast with the normal group, no significant ($p \geq 0.135$) differences in any of the secondary outcomes analyzed were detected among the three variants at position 680 of the FSHR.

None of the COS response parameters were significantly different among groups of donors ($p = 0.711$) and infertile patients ($p = 0.964$) carrying any of the three genotypes (GG, GA or AA) at position − 29 of the *FSHR* (Table 4).

Frequency of N680S variants in Mayan women with low miscegenation

The frequencies of the A and G alleles of the 2039A > G SNP in this particular population were 65.5% and 34.5%, respectively. The genotype frequency of the minor GG variant was lower (7%) than that detected in the women from the IVF group (9.8%) and the Mexican mestizo population from SIGMA cohort (see below), albeit the difference did not reach statistical significance. Meanwhile, the genotype frequencies of the AA and AG variants in these Mayan women were 38% and 55%, respectively, not significantly different from those found in the other population groups studied ($p = 0.792$ for all three SNP genotypes). Using the surnames as markers for genetic testing, we found that the observed number of homozygous for the Mayan surnames (i.e. Mayan/Mayan paternal and maternal surnames) were lower than those expected by random mating (squared allelic frequencies of Mayan surname = 0.284 and 0.459, observed vs expected, respectively), confirming that the population studied for this particular SNP deviates from Hardy-Weinberg equilibrium as expected by their still preserved low miscegenation [41].

Large database analysis

The large-scale genotype data set from 8182 Mexican mestizo subjects that fall on a cline of Native American and European Ancestry was additionally analyzed [35]. Since the frequency of the three *FSHR* SNPs analyzed was virtually the same between men and women and T2D and non-diabetic subjects, data from all subjects were considered together for the calculation of the allelic and genotype frequencies in these SNPs. The data confirmed the strong linkage disequilibrium between the c.919 and c.2039 SNPs in Mexican subjects (D' = 0.91), and that both allelic and genotype frequencies (Table 5) were very similar to those detected in the IVF cohort, being the frequency of the corresponding GG genotypes 10.0% and 10.8%, respectively [vs 8.9% ($p = 0.59$); and 9.8% ($p = 0.63$) in the IVF population, respectively (see Table 1)]. For the -29G > A SNP, allelic and genotype frequencies were also very similar to those of the IVF cohort (Table 2), with a frequency of 25.6% for the AA genotype [vs 22.7% in the IVI population; ($p = 0.38$)] (Table 5). In subjects with more Native American ancestry (i.e. those falling within the quartile for the highest Native American ancestry as determined by PCA [36]) the frequency of the minor alleles at positions c.919 and c.2039, were lower by 15% and 9%, respectively, than in those with more European ancestry (c.919A > G = 23.0% and c.2039A > G = 28.0%, for subjects with more Native American ancestry vs c.919A > G = 38.0% and c.2039A > G = 37.0%, in subjects with more European ancestry; $p < 0.001$ for differences in both SNPs). Among a subgroup of 520 women in whom data of reproductive parameters was available, those carriers

Table 5 Allele and genotype frequencies for SNPs 307A > G, 680A > G, and -29G > A in an open Mexican mestizo population

SNP	Allele frequency %	Genotype frequency %
c.919A > G (p.T307A)	A (T) 69.2	AA (TT) 48.3
n = 8207	G (A) 30.8	AG (TA) 41.7
		GG (AA) 10.0
c.2039A > G (p.N680S)	A (N) 67.4	AA (NN) 45.6
n = 8182	G (S) 32.6	AG (NS) 43.6
		GG (SS) 10.8
-29G > A	G 50.4	GG 26.5
n = 8195	A 49.6	GA 47.9
		AA 25.6

bearing the G allele at the c.2039 SNP tended to present lower pregnancy frequencies than women bearing the AA genotype, when stratified by either < 3 or ≥ 3 the total number of reported pregnancies per women [OR = 1.3, CI 95% 0.91–1.95 ($p = 0.14$)] (Additional file 1: Table S1)]. This cut-off value was based on data from the National Survey of Demographic Dynamics 2014 in Mexico (http://www.inegi.org.mx/proyectos/enchogares/especiales/enadid/2014/), in which the reported total fertility rate for 15- to 49-year-old Mexican women was 2.21. Further, this trend towards lower number of pregnancies was stronger after analyzing women older than 45 years (who comprised 92.5% of the total women population) separately by the proportion of Native American or European ancestry [OR = 2.0, C.I. 95% 1.03–3.90 ($p = 0.04$) for G allele carriers in the group with more Native American ancestry ($n = 184$ women); OR = 3.25, C.I. 95% 0.90–11.70 ($p = 0.07$) for carriers in the group with more European ancestry ($n = 57$ women] (Additional file 2: Tables S2 and Additional file 3: Table S3). When the models were adjusted for ethnicity, we observed that this factor was not statistically different ($p > 0.05$) between women with ≥3 pregnancies vs those reporting < 3 pregnancies, and thus ethnicity was not a confounder in the association between this outcome and genotypes (Additional file 4: Table S4).

There was no association between the number of pregnancies and the AA genotype at the -29G > A SNP nor between age at menarche or menopause and any of the *FSHR* SNPs analyzed in this large database.

Discussion

In the present study, we determined the frequency of three FSHR/*FSHR* variants (p.T307A, p.N680S and -29G > A), in three groups of Mexican mestizo subjects. These populations, as well as those from other Latin American countries, are particularly unique in that their genetic structure contains an extensive, complex, and variable admixture between Africans, Native Americans, and Europeans (mainly Spaniards) that has significantly contributed to their corresponding phenotypic and genetic makeups [42, 43]. In women from the IVF cohort, we found a higher GG genotype frequency of the *FSHR* c.2039A > G SNP than those previously reported in placental samples from Mexican mestizo women (reported frequency, 5.9%) [23] as well as in the 1000 Genomes Project Phase 3 database [32](http://grch37.ensembl.org/) for a small cohort of Hispanic subjects residing in Los Angeles, CA, USA, of presumptive Mexican ancestry (frequency, 7.8%), but still markedly lower than in Caucasians, in whom the frequency range from ~ 20% to ~ 36% [6] (http://grch37.ensembl.org/). Further, in a population of fertile egg donors from Mediterranean origin residing in Spain, the frequency of this genotype is among the highest reported in Western Europe (42%) [15]. The frequency of the S680S FSHR variant observed in the present study (which was similar in normal oocyte donors and infertile patients), was also lower than that reported in Colombians (~ 14%)(http://grch37.ensembl.org/), in whom the estimated African and European genetic admixture proportions are higher than in Mexicans (11% vs. 5% and 60% vs. 37%, respectively) [42], thus emphasizing on the substantial impact of the admixture with Spaniards on the c.2039A > G *FSHR* SNP in Latin America. The even lower frequency of the GG genotype in Mayan women with low genetic admixture also points towards the genetic influence of Spaniards on the expression of this particular *FSHR* variant in Mexican mestizo women. If this assumption is correct and considering the similar frequency of the heterozygous (AG) genotype in the two populations studied (48% and 55% in the Mexican mestizo and Mayan women, respectively), then one might expect a progressive rise in GG genotype frequency as the admixture with non-Native American individuals increase in this particular Mayan population, which might confirm the Spaniard origin of this SNP in the Mexican mestizo population.

We additionally assessed the ovarian response to COS as well as the time and amount of gonadotrophins required to reach a mean follicle diameter of 18 mm in normal oocyte donors and infertile patients from the IVF group bearing different N680S FSHR variants. Despite the low number of oocyte donors with the GG genotype, we consistently detected an association of this genotype with a lower number of oocytes retrieved after gonadotrophin administration, thus confirming previous studies on the effect of the S680S phenotype on the ovarian sensitivity and response to exogenous FSH administration [6, 7, 15–17, 44–46]. The lower number of oocytes retrieved in donors with the GG genotype was not apparent in the infertile women, finding that may be due to the age-dependent vanishing effect of the N680S polymorphism on the ovarian response to COS, as previously suggested [6].

Another SNP that has been reported to influence the ovarian response to COS is the -29G > A polymorphism [4, 6, 7, 28]. In some studies the AA variant has been associated with reduced transcriptional activity of the *FSHR* and altered level of mRNA and receptor protein expression in vitro [47, 48] as well as with poor ovarian response to FSH during COS [4, 28, 47], although the latter has not been consistently found in other studies [31, 49]. The prevalence of the AA genotype varies depending on the geographic region considered, being relatively low in Caucasians [despite a relatively high frequency of the A allele in some European countries [31]], Africans, and Central-South Asians, and high in East Asians and Americans from both the USA and some Latin America countries [6] (http://grch37.ensembl.org/). In the present study, we found a relatively high prevalence of the AA genotype (~ 20% to 27%) in both donors and infertile patients of the IVF cohort, which was lower than that reported in the 1000 Genomes Project Phase 3 database for Mexican-American residents of the USA (~ 33%) (http://grch37.ensembl.org/). This difference in AA genotype frequency may be due to the relatively low number of samples genotyped and/or the particular genetic structure of the population included in that particular Project database. The frequency of the AA genotype detected in our normal oocyte donors also contrasts with those found in normo-ovulatory and infertile women from India (1% and 14%, respectively) [28], in whom the AA genotype was associated with poor ovarian response to COS as well as with primary and secondary amenorrhea [29]. More vividly, in the population of donors analyzed in the present study, those with the AA genotype did not show any significant difference in response to gonadotrophin administration compared with women exhibiting the GG or GA variants. Coexistence of and interactions with other ethnically-related SNPs at the *FSHR* or other genes involved in the ovarian response to gonadotrophins, may explain these apparent discrepancies among the various studies ([28, 29, 31], and present study).

Data extracted from a large database of SNPs in Mexican individual mestizo confirmed the allelic and genotype frequencies of the *FSHR* SNPs found in samples from the IVF group. Further, data on the number of pregnancies reported by carriers vs no carriers of the G allele at the c.2039A > G SNP, strongly suggests that the fertility potential of carriers of the G allele could be compromised. This might be due to the decreased sensitivity of the S680 FSHR variant to the gonadotrophic stimulus [10, 50] and the failure of the slight to moderate elevations in FSH levels to compensate for the abnormal function of the FSHR S680 variant, particularly in young women [9], as suggested by the longer menstrual cycle length exhibited by women homozygous for the G allele [13, 51]. The finding that the trend to decreased pregnancies in women bearing the G allele persisted even after stratification by the presence of more or less Native American/European ancestry, suggests that the effect of the Ser680 FSHR variant on reproductive potential results from the effect of Ser680 on FSHR function, rather than its interaction with other ethnically-related SNPs at the *FSHR* or other genes implicated in fertility. Overall, the results indicate that the frequency of the c.919A > G and c.2039A > G GG genotypes in Hispanic mestizo subjects are among the lowest reported [6] and remarkably similar to those found in large cohorts of Chinese women [16, 17], and that the presence of the Ser680 FSHR variant may impact on the reproductive potential of women when present in the homozygous state.

A major limitation of the present study is that the sample size in both IVF groups was not sufficiently powered to allow for detection of statistically significant differences in all secondary outcomes as it was not originally designed for this purpose. Nevertheless, we found that age, COS protocols and diagnosis were homogeneously distributed among all genotypes studied and that even after controlling for all these factors the significant difference on the number of oocytes retrieved from donors with the S680S FSHR persisted. Another drawback is that in the IVF groups, ethnicity index was not available and thus models were not adjusted for admixture. Nonetheless, using the UIDS cohort we found that ethnicity was not a confounder in the association between outcomes and genotypes, making valid these findings. Although this is the first large-scale analysis of the fertiliy potential in women with the *FSHR* SNPs analyzed, the information on reproductive events (mainly fertility potential as defined by the number of reported pregnancies) extracted from the large database of hispanic women also should be taken with caution as the questionaire applied was designed to obtain information on several metabolic aspects related to T2D, rather than on reproductive events and parameters that may influence, directly or indirectly, on the reproductive potential of the population studied. Thus, the data on the effect of the G allele at position c.2039 of the *FSHR* on fertility potential in the general population should be confirmed in other populations, particularly in those with a higher prevalence of this particular *FSHR* SNP variant than that reported herein. In this vein, Zilaitiene and colleagues [52] recently reported a significant association between the S680S FSHR variant and lower possibility of natural conception during the first 12 months of planned conception and other fertility parameters in a large population of young Caucasian women.

Conclusions

The allele and genotype frequencies of the *FSHR* SNPs reported in this study add further information to the existing knowledge obtained from other genotyping projects. The frequency of the GG genotype at position c.2039 of the *FSHR* in Mexican mestizo subjects is among the lowest reported in the literature for both

normal and infertile women. In oocyte donors receiving COS, expression of the S680S FSHR phenotype was associated with decreased number of oocytes recovered, whereas in women from the general population this SNP appears to influence on the fertility potential in carriers of the minor allele in terms of pregnancy rate. In contrast, the frequency of the AA genotype in position − 29 of the *FSHR* core promoter region in this particular population is among the highest reported and was not associated with significantly altered ovarian response to COS or particular reproductive events. Considering the absence of any deleterious effect of the − 29 AA genotype on the response to COS in Hispanic women, it is not advisable to perform this particular genotype testing to women from this population with the purpose of designing an individually-tailored protocol of gonadotrophin stimulation.

Additional files

Additional file 1: Table S1. Number of pregnancies (according to < 3 or ≥ 3 pregnancies *per* women) in 52 Mexican mestizo women carriers of the AA genotype or G allele (AG plus GG genotypes) at the c.2039A > G SNP. (DOCX 15 kb)

Additional file 2: Table S2. Number of pregnancies (according to < 3 or ≥ 3 pregnancies *per* women) for each c.2039A > G SNP genotype in 184 Mexican mestizo women with more (4th quartile) Native American ancestry. (DOCX 15 kb)

Additional file 3: Table S3. Number of pregnancies (according to < 3 or ≥ 3 pregnancies *per* women) for each c.2039A > G SNP genotype in 57 Mexican mestizo women with more (4th quartile) European ancestry. (DOCX 15 kb)

Additional file 4: Table S4. ORs of being carrier of minor allele and having < 3 or ≥ 3 pregnancies (*n* = 520 Mexican mestizo women). Logistic regression models adjusted for age. (DOCX 14 kb)

Acknowledgments
The authors thank Ari Kleinberg from the RAI-UNAM for the artwork of Figs. 1 and 2.

Funding
This study was supported by grants from the Consejo Nacional de Ciencia y Tecnología (CONACyT) (grants SALUD-86881 and SEP-240619), and the Coordinación de la Investigación Científica, UNAM. The funding sources had no involvement in study design, collection, analysis, interpretation of data, writing the report or decision to submit the article for publication.

Authors' contributions
GG-J and TZ contributed equally to the study. GG-J Collected data and provided subjects' treatment. TZ Laboratory studies for the T307A and N680S polimorphisms. RR-V Laboratory studies for the -29G/A SNP. NRM-D Statistical analysis of data. FA-V Statistical analysis of data. RG-S Supervised quality control of molecular biology studies and designed RFLP studies. GH-M Analysis of linkage disequilibrium. AT Supervised molecular biology studies (RT-PCR) and trained technician. IPC Provided samples and information on Mayan women. JG

Performed Lasker's analysis for Mayan population. HM-M Extracted and analyzed the database from the SIGMA study. TT-L Provided and analyzed the database from the SIGMA study. AP Study design and wrote the manuscript. AU-A Study design, integration and interpretation of data, wrote the manuscript. All authors read and approved the final manuscript.

Authors' information

Alfredo Ulloa-Aguirre, M.D., D.Sc., is an internationally-recognized authority in FSH and FSHR structure and function, and is currently full Professor and Scientific Director of the Red de Apoyo a la Investigación (RAI) at the UNAM, Mexico.

Antonio Pellicer, M.D., is an internationally-recognized expert in infertility and he is Founder and Co-President of the Instituto Valenciano de Infertilidad, Valencia, Spain.

Competing interests

The authors declare that they have no competing interests

Author details

[1]Instituto Valenciano de Infertilidad (IVINSEMER), Thiers 96, Col. Nueva Anzurez, CP 11590 Mexico City, Mexico. [2]Red de Apoyo a la Investigación (RAI), Coordinación de la Investigación Científica, Universidad Nacional Autónoma de México (UNAM)-Instituto Nacional de Ciencias Médicas y Nutrición SZ (INCMNSZ), Calle Vasco de Quiroga 15, Tlalpan, 14000 Ciudad de Mexico, Mexico. [3]Centro de Investigación en Salud Poblacional, Instituto Nacional de Salud Pública, Av. Universidad 655, CP 62100 Cuernavaca, Mor, Mexico. [4]Department of Physiology of Nutrition, INCMNSZ, Mexico City, Mexico. [5]Department of Transplantation, INCMNSZ, Mexico City, Mexico. [6]Research Unit in Reproductive Medicine, UMAE Hospital de Ginecoobstetricia "Luis Castelazo Ayala", Río de la Magdalena 289, Tizapán San Ángel, Mexico City 01090, Mexico. [7]Facultad de Medicina, UNAM, Ciudad Universitaria, Mexico City, Mexico. [8]Universidad Autónoma Metropolitana-Iztapalapa, Av. San Rafael Atlixco 186, Leyes de Reforma 1ra. Secc., Mexico City 09340, Mexico. [9]Unidad de Biología Molecular y Medicina Genómica, UNAM-INCMNSZ, Mexico City, Mexico.

References

1. Richards JS, Russell DL, Ochsner S, Hsieh M, Doyle KH, Falender AE, et al. Novel signaling pathways that control ovarian follicular development, ovulation, and luteinization. Recent Prog Horm Res. 2002;57:195–220.
2. Huhtaniemi I. A short evolutionary history of FSH-stimulated spermatogenesis. Hormones (Athens). 2015;14:468–78.
3. Laan M, Grigorova M, Huhtaniemi IT. Pharmacogenetics of follicle-stimulating hormone action. Curr Opin Endocrinol Diabetes Obes. 2012;19:220–7.
4. Desai SS, Roy BS, Mahale SD. Mutations and polymorphisms in FSH receptor: functional implications in human reproduction. Reproduction. 2013;146:R235–48.
5. Themmen APN. An update of the pathophysiology of human gonadotrophin subunit and receptor gene mutations and polymorphisms. Reproduction. 2005;130:263–74.
6. Simoni M, Casarini L. Genetics of FSH action: a 2014-and-beyond view. Eur J Endocrinol. 2014;170:R91–107.
7. Casarini L, Santi D, Marino M. Impact of gene polymorphisms of gonadotropins and their receptors on human reproductive success. Reproduction. 2015;150:R175–84.
8. La Marca A, Sighinolfi G, Argento C, Grisendi V, Casarini L, Volpe A, et al. Polymorphisms in gonadotropin and gonadotropin receptor genes as markers of ovarian reserve and response in in vitro fertilization. Fertil Steril. 2013;99:970–8 e971.
9. Perez Mayorga M, Gromoll J, Behre HM, Gassner C, Nieschlag E, Simoni M. Ovarian response to follicle-stimulating hormone (FSH) stimulation depends on the FSH receptor genotype. J Clin Endocrinol Metab. 2000;85:3365–9.
10. Casarini L, Moriondo V, Marino M, Adversi F, Capodanno F, Grisolia C, et al. FSHR polymorphism p.N680S mediates different responses to FSH in vitro. Mol Cell Endocrinol. 2014;393:83–91.
11. Tranchant T, Durand G, Piketty V, Gauthier C, Ulloa-Aguirre A, Crepieux P, et al. N680S SNP of the human FSH receptor impacts on basal FSH and estradiol level in women and modifies PKA nuclear translocation and CREB-dependent gene transcription in vitro. Hum Reprod. 2012;27(Suppl 1):i45–6.
12. Simoni M, Tempfer CB, Destenaves B, Fauser BC. Functional genetic polymorphisms and female reproductive disorders: part I: polycystic ovary syndrome and ovarian response. Hum Reprod Update. 2008;14:459–84.
13. Greb RR, Grieshaber K, Gromoll J, Sonntag B, Nieschlag E, Kiesel L, et al. A common single nucleotide polymorphism in exon 10 of the human follicle stimulating hormone receptor is a major determinant of length and hormonal dynamics of the menstrual cycle. J Clin Endocrinol Metab. 2005; 90:4866–72.
14. Behre HM, Greb RR, Mempel A, Sonntag B, Kiesel L, Kaltwasser P, et al. Significance of a common single nucleotide polymorphism in exon 10 of the follicle-stimulating hormone (FSH) receptor gene for the ovarian response to FSH: a pharmacogenetic approach to controlled ovarian hyperstimulation. Pharmacogenet Genomics. 2005;15:451–6.
15. Lledo B, Guerrero J, Turienzo A, Ortiz JA, Morales R, Ten J, et al. Effect of follicle-stimulating hormone receptor N680S polymorphism on the efficacy of follicle-stimulating hormone stimulation on donor ovarian response. Pharmacogenet Genomics. 2013;23:262–8.
16. Huang X, Li L, Hong L, Zhou W, Shi H, Zhang H, et al. The Ser680Asn polymorphism in the follicle-stimulating hormone receptor gene is associated with the ovarian response in controlled ovarian hyperstimulation. Clin Endocrinol (Oxf). 2015;82:577–83.
17. Yan Y, Gong Z, Zhang L, Li Y, Li X, Zhu L, et al. Association of follicle-stimulating hormone receptor polymorphisms with ovarian response in Chinese women: a prospective clinical study. PLoS One. 2013;8:e78138.
18. Laven JS, Mulders AG, Suryandari DA, Gromoll J, Nieschlag E, Fauser BC, et al. Follicle-stimulating hormone receptor polymorphisms in women with normogonadotropic anovulatory infertility. Fertil Steril. 2003;80:986–92.
19. Anagnostou E, Mavrogianni D, Theofanakis C, Drakakis P, Bletsa R, Demirol A, et al. ESR1, ESR2 and FSH receptor gene polymorphisms in combination: a useful genetic tool for the prediction of poor responders. Curr Pharm Biotechnol. 2012;13:426–34.
20. Genro VK, Matte U, De Conto E, Cunha-Filho JS, Fanchin R. Frequent polymorphisms of FSH receptor do not influence antral follicle responsiveness to follicle-stimulating hormone administration as assessed by the follicular output RaTe (FORT). J Assist Reprod Genet. 2012;29:657–63.
21. Klinkert ER, te Velde ER, Weima S, van Zandvoort PM, Hanssen RG, Nilsson PR, et al. FSH receptor genotype is associated with pregnancy but not with ovarian response in IVF. Reprod BioMed Online. 2006;13:687–95.
22. Wang HS, Cheng BH, Wu HM, Yen CF, Liu CT, Chao A, et al. A mutant single nucleotide polymorphism of follicle-stimulating hormone receptor is associated with a lower risk of endometriosis. Fertil Steril. 2011;95:455–7.
23. Dominguez-Lopez P, Diaz-Cueto L, Arechavaleta-Velasco M, Caldino-Soto F, Ulloa-Aguirre A, Arechavaleta-Velasco F. The follicle-stimulating hormone receptor Asn680Ser polymorphism is associated with preterm birth in Hispanic women. J Matern Fetal Neonatal Med. 2018;31:580–5.
24. Rendina D, Gianfrancesco F, De Filippo G, Merlotti D, Esposito T, Mingione A, et al. FSHR gene polymorphisms influence bone mineral density and bone turnover in postmenopausal women. Eur J Endocrinol. 2010;163:165–72.
25. Qin X, Ma L, Yang S, Zhao J, Chen S, Xie Y, et al. The Asn680Ser polymorphism of the follicle stimulating hormone receptor gene and ovarian cancer risk: a meta-analysis. J Assist Reprod Genet. 2014;31:683–8.
26. Corbo RM, Gambina G, Broggio E, Scacchi R. Influence of variation in the follicle-stimulating hormone receptor gene (FSHR) and age at menopause on the development of Alzheimer's disease in women. Dement Geriatr Cogn Disord. 2011;32:63–9.
27. Tuttelmann F, Laan M, Grigorova M, Punab M, Sober S, Gromoll J. Combined effects of the variants FSHB -211G>T and FSHR 2039A>G on male reproductive parameters. J Clin Endocrinol Metab. 2012;97:3639–47.
28. Achrekar SK, Modi DN, Desai SK, Mangoli VS, Mangoli RV, Mahale SD. Poor ovarian response to gonadotrophin stimulation is associated with FSH receptor polymorphism. Reprod BioMed Online. 2009;18:509–15.

29. Achrekar SK, Modi DN, Meherji PK, Patel ZM, Mahale SD. Follicle stimulating hormone receptor gene variants in women with primary and secondary amenorrhea. J Assist Reprod Genet. 2010;27:317–26.

30. Simoni M, Nieschlag E, Gromoll J. Isoforms and single nucleotide polymorphisms of the FSH receptor gene: implications for human reproduction. Hum Reprod Update. 2002;8:413–21.

31. Wunsch A, Ahda Y, Banaz-Yasar F, Sonntag B, Nieschlag E, Simoni M, et al. Single-nucleotide polymorphisms in the promoter region influence the expression of the human follicle-stimulating hormone receptor. Fertil Steril. 2005;84:446–53.

32. Auton A, Brooks LD, Durbin RM, Garrison EP, Kang HM, Korbel JO, et al. A global reference for human genetic variation. Nature. 2015; 526:68–74.

33. group. REA-SPcw. Revised 2003 consensus on diagnostic criteria and long-term health risks related to polycystic ovary syndrome (PCOS). Hum Reprod. 2004;19:41–7.

34. Canto P, Canto-Cetina T, Juarez-Velazquez R, Rosas-Vargas H, Rangel-Villalobos H, Canizales-Quinteros S, et al. Methylenetetrahydrofolate reductase C677T and glutathione S-transferase P1 A313G are associated with a reduced risk of preeclampsia in Maya-mestizo women. Hypertens Res. 2008;31:1015–9.

35. Williams AL, Jacobs SB, Moreno-Macias H, Huerta-Chagoya A, Churchhouse C, Marquez-Luna C, et al. Sequence variants in SLC16A11 are a common risk factor for type 2 diabetes in Mexico. Nature. 2014;506:97–101.

36. Price AL, Patterson NJ, Plenge RM, Weinblatt ME, Shadick NA, Reich D. Principal components analysis corrects for stratification in genome-wide association studies. Nat Genet. 2006;38:904–9.

37. Sudo S, Kudo M, Wada S, Sato O, Hsueh AJ, Fujimoto S. Genetic and functional analyses of polymorphisms in the human FSH receptor gene. Mol Hum Reprod. 2002;8:893–9.

38. Brown H, Prescott R. Generalised linear mixed models. In: Applied mixed models in medicine. 3rd ed. Chinchester: Jonh Wiley & Sons, Ltd.; 2014.

39. Armstrong RA. When to use the Bonferroni correction. Ophthalmic Physiol Opt. 2014;34:502–8.

40. Barrett JC, Fry B, Maller J, Daly MJ. Haploview: analysis and visualization of LD and haplotype maps. Bioinformatics. 2005;21:263–5.

41. Lasker GW. Surnames in the study of human biology. Am Anthropol. 1980; 82:525–38.

42. Ruiz-Linares A, Adhikari K, Acuna-Alonzo V, Quinto-Sanchez M, Jaramillo C, Arias W, et al. Admixture in Latin America: geographic structure, phenotypic diversity and self-perception of ancestry based on 7,342 individuals. PLoS Genet. 2014;10:e1004572.

43. Moreno-Estrada A, Gignoux CR, Fernandez-Lopez JC, Zakharia F, Sikora M, Contreras AV, et al. Human genetics. The genetics of Mexico recapitulates native American substructure and affects biomedical traits. Science. 2014; 344:1280–5.

44. Tang H, Yan Y, Wang T, Zhang T, Shi W, Fan R, et al. Effect of follicle-stimulating hormone receptor Asn680Ser polymorphism on the outcomes of controlled ovarian hyperstimulation: an updated meta-analysis of 16 cohort studies. J Assist Reprod Genet. 2015;32:1801–10.

45. Casarini L, Pignatti E, Simoni M. Effects of polymorphisms in gonadotropin and gonadotropin receptor genes on reproductive function. Rev Endocr Metab Disord. 2011;12:303–21.

46. Alviggi C, Conforti A, Santi D, Esteves SC, Andersen CY, Humaidan P, et al. Clinical relevance of genetic variants of gonadotrophins and their receptors in controlled ovarian stimulation: a systematic review and meta-analysis. Hum Reprod Update. 2018;24:599–614.

47. Desai SS, Achrekar SK, Pathak BR, Desai SK, Mangoli VS, Mangoli RV, et al. Follicle-stimulating hormone receptor polymorphism (G-29A) is associated with altered level of receptor expression in granulosa cells. J Clin Endocrinol Metab. 2011;96:2805–12.

48. Nakayama T, Kuroi N, Sano M, Tabara Y, Katsuya T, Ogihara T, et al. Mutation of the follicle-stimulating hormone receptor gene 5′-untranslated region associated with female hypertension. Hypertension. 2006;48:512–8.

49. Tohlob D, Abo Hashem E, Ghareeb N, Ghanem M, Elfarahaty R, Byers H, et al. Association of a promoter polymorphism in FSHR with ovarian reserve and response to ovarian stimulation in women undergoing assisted reproductive treatment. Reprod BioMed Online. 2016;33:391–7.

50. Nordhoff V, Sonntag B, von Tils D, Gotte M, Schuring AN, Gromoll J, et al. Effects of the FSH receptor gene polymorphism p.N680S on cAMP and steroid production in cultured primary human granulosa cells. Reprod Biomed Online. 2011;23:196–203.

51. Gromoll J, Simoni M. Genetic complexity of FSH receptor function. Trends Endocrinol Metab. 2005;16:368–73.

52. Zilaitiene B, Dirzauskas M, Verkauskiene R, Ostrauskas R, Gromoll J, Nieschlag E. The impact of FSH receptor polymorphism on time-to-pregnancy: a cross-sectional single-Centre study. BMC Pregnancy Childbirth. 2018;18:272.

Permissions

List of Contributors

Kristina Lasiene and Aleksandras Vitkus
Department of Histology and Embryology, Medical Academy, Lithuanian University of Health Sciences, A. Mickeviciaus str. 9, LT-44307 Kaunas, Lithuania

Donatas Gasiliunas
Kaunas Division of State Forensic Medicine Service, Perlojos str. 28, LT-45305 Kaunas, Lithuania

Nomeda Juodziukyniene
Department of Veterinary Pathobiology, Veterinary Academy, Lithuanian University of Health Sciences, Tilzes str. 18, LT-47181 Kaunas, Lithuania

Li Chen
Department of Reproduction, the Affiliated Changzhou Maternity and Child Health Care, Hospital of Nanjing Medical University, Changzhou 213003, Jiangsu, China
3State Key Laboratory of Reproductive Medicine, Nanjing Medical University, Nanjing 211166, China

Jiangbo Du, Hong Lv, Yifeng Wang, Fang Wu, Feng Liu, Hongxia Ma, Guangfu Jin, Hongbing Shen and Zhibin Hu
Department of Epidemiology, School of Public Health, Nanjing Medical University, Nanjing 211166, China
State Key Laboratory of Reproductive Medicine, Nanjing Medical University, Nanjing 211166, China

Jing Zhao, Mengxi Chen, Xiaojiao Chen, Junqiang Zhang and Xiufeng Ling
State Key Laboratory of Reproductive Medicine, Nanjing Medical University, Nanjing 211166, China.
Department of Reproduction, the Affiliated Nanjing Maternity and Child Health, Hospital of Nanjing Medical University, Nanjing 210004, China

Jingjie Li and Xiaoyan Liang
Center of Reproductive Medicine, the Sixth Affiliated Hospital, Sun Yat-sen University, Guangzhou, China

Lihuan Guan Huizhen Zhang, Yue Gao, Jiahong Sun, Min Huang, Dongshun Li and Huichang Bi
School of Pharmaceutical Sciences in Sun Yat-sen University, 132# Waihuandong Road, Guangzhou, University City, Guangzhou 510006, People's Republic of China

Pan Chen
Pharmacy Department, the First Affiliated Hospital, Sun Yat-sen University, Guangzhou, China

Xiao Gong
School of Public Health, Guangdong Pharmaceutical University, Guangzhou, China

Yanrong Chen, Puyu Yang and Xinyu Zhang
Center for Reproductive Medicine, Department of Obstetrics and Gynecology, Peking University Third Hospital, Beijing 100191, China
National Clinical Research Center for Obstetrics and Gynecology, Beijing 100191, China
Key Laboratory of Assisted Reproductive, Ministry of Education, Beijing 100191, China

Victoria Nisenblat
Center for Reproductive Medicine, Department of Obstetrics and Gynecology, Peking University Third Hospital, Beijing 100191, China
Key Laboratory of Assisted Reproductive, Ministry of Education, Beijing 100191, China

Caihong Ma
Center for Reproductive Medicine, Department of Obstetrics and Gynecology, Peking University Third Hospital, Beijing 100191, China
National Clinical Research Center for Obstetrics and Gynecology, Beijing 100191, China
Key Laboratory of Assisted Reproductive, Ministry of Education, Beijing 100191, China
Beijing, China

Josephine A. Drury
Department of Women's and Children's Health, Institute of Translational Medicine, University of Liverpool, Liverpool, UK

Dharani K. Hapangama
Department of Women's and Children's Health, Institute of Translational Medicine, University of Liverpool, Liverpool, UK
Department of Gynecology, Liverpool Women's Hospital, Liverpool, UK

Asgerally T. Fazleabas
Department of Obstetrics, Gynecology and Reproductive Biology, College of Human Medicine, Michigan State University, Grand Rapids, MI, USA

Kirstin L. Parkin
Department of Obstetrics, Gynecology and Reproductive Biology, College of Human Medicine, Michigan State University, Grand Rapids, MI, USA
Department of Microbiology and Molecular Genetics, Michigan State University, East Lansing, MI, USA.

Emma Giuliani
Department of Obstetrics, Gynecology and Reproductive Biology, College of Human Medicine, Michigan State University, Grand Rapids, MI, USA
Department of Obstetrics and Gynecology, Grand Rapids Medical Education Partners/Michigan State University, Grand Rapids, MI, USA

Lucy Coyne
Department of Gynecology, Liverpool Women's Hospital, Liverpool, UK
Hewitt Fertility Centre; Liverpool Women's Hospital, Liverpool, UK

Shuyu Wang
Department of Reproduction, Beijing Obstetrics and Gynecology Hospital, Capital Medical University, Beijing 100026, China

Yangying Xu
Department of Reproduction, Beijing Obstetrics and Gynecology Hospital, Capital Medical University, Beijing 100026, China
Reproductive Medical Center, Department of Obstetrics and Gynecology, Peking University Third Hospital, Beijing 100123, China
Key Laboratory of Assisted Reproduction, Ministry of Education, Beijing, China.

Victoria Nisenblat, Cuiling Lu, Rong Li, Jie Qiao and Xiumei Zhen
Reproductive Medical Center, Department of Obstetrics and Gynecology, Peking University Third Hospital, Beijing 100123, China
Key Laboratory of Assisted Reproduction, Ministry of Education, Beijing, China

Xuechun Hu, Zhichuan Zou, Yuming Feng, Jinzhao Ma, Xie Ge and Bing Yao
Center of Reproductive Medicine, Nanjing Jinling Hospital, the Medical School of Nanjing University, Nanjing 210002, China

Zhiwei Hong
Center of Reproductive Medicine, Nanjing Jinling Hospital, the Medical School of Nanjing University, Nanjing 210002, China

Department of Urology, Fujian Provincial Hospital, Fuzhou 350000, China

Zheng Ding
Nanjing Jiangning Hospital, the Affiliated Jiangning Hospital of Nanjing Medical University, Nanjing 210000, China

Ruilou Zhu and Chaojun Li
MOE Key Laboratory of Model Animals for Disease Study, Model Animal Research Center and the Medical School of Nanjing University, National Resource Center for Mutant Mice, Nanjing 210061, China

Berthe Youness and Birgitta Messmer
Reproduction Genetics Unit, Department of Gynecological Endocrinology and Fertility Disorders, University Women's Hospital, Heidelberg, Germany

Diego D. Alcoba
Reproduction Genetics Unit, Department of Gynecological Endocrinology and Fertility Disorders, University Women's Hospital, Heidelberg, Germany
Department of Physiology, Institute of Health Sciences, Federal University of Rio Grande do Sul, Porto Alegre, Brazil

Julia Rehnitz
Reproduction Genetics Unit, Department of Gynecological Endocrinology and Fertility Disorders, University Women's Hospital, Heidelberg, Germany
Department of Gynecological Endocrinology and Fertility Disorders, University Women's Hospital, Heidelberg, Germany

Ilma S. Brum
Department of Physiology, Institute of Health Sciences, Federal University of Rio Grande do Sul, Porto Alegre, Brazil

Jens E. Dietrich Alexander Freis, Thomas Strowitzki and Ariane Germeyer
Department of Gynecological Endocrinology and Fertility Disorders, University Women's Hospital, Heidelberg, Germany

Katrin Hinderhofer
Laboratory of Molecular Genetics, Institute of Human Genetics, Heidelberg University, Heidelberg, Germany

Huan Jiang
Department of Reproductive Endocrinology, Longgang District Maternal and Child Healthcare Hospital, 6# Ailong Road, Longgang Central District, Shenzhen City 518172, People's Republic of China

Xiao-Yi Yang and Wei-Jie Zhu
Institute of Reproductive Immunology, College of Life Science and Technology, Jinan University, 601# Huangpu Da Dao Xi, Guangzhou City 510632, People's Republic of China

Ying Wang, Yijie Li, Beibei Zhang and Fuchun Zhang
Xinjiang Key Laboratory of Biological Resources and Genetic Engineering, College of Life Science and Technology, Xinjiang University, 666, Shengli Road, Urumqi 830046, China

Alice Desmarchais, Maeva Durcin, Svetlana Uzbekova and Sebastien Elis
UMR PRC, CNRS, IFCE, INRA, Université de Tours, 37380 Nouzilly, France

Virginie Maillard
UMR PRC, CNRS, IFCE, INRA, Université de Tours, 37380 Nouzilly, France
INRA Centre Val de Loire, Physiologie de la Reproduction et des Comportements, 37380 Nouzilly, France

Yuping Wu, Huihui Zhao, Yuxia Zhou and Liping Wang
Department of Obstetrics and Gynecology, Nanfang Hospital, Southern Medical University, Guangzhou 510515, China.

Congshun Ma
Reproductive Medicine Center, Guangdong Provincial Family Planning Special Hospital, Guangzhou 510699, China

Zhenguo Chen
Department of Cell Biology, School of Basic Medical Sciences, Southern Medical University, Guangzhou 510515, China

Rawad Bassil, Noa Gonen, Jim Meriano, Andrea Jurisicova and Robert F. Casper
Division of Reproductive Sciences, University of Toronto, Lunenfeld-Tanenbaum Research Institute, Mount Sinai Hospital, Toronto, Canada

TRIO fertility partners, 655 Bay St 11th floor, Toronto, ON M5G 2K4, Canada

Jigal Haas
Division of Reproductive Sciences, University of Toronto, Lunenfeld-Tanenbaum Research Institute, Mount Sinai Hospital, Toronto, Canada
TRIO fertility partners, 655 Bay St 11th floor, Toronto, ON M5G 2K4, Canada
Department of Obstetrics and Gynecology, Sheba Medical Center, Sackler School of Medicine, Tel-Aviv University, Tel-Hashomer, Israel

Jun Jing, Li Chen, Yi-Feng Ge, Yuan-Jiao Liang and Bing Yao
The Reproductive Medical Centre, Nanjing Jinling Hospital, Nanjing University School of Medicine, 305 Zhongshan East Road, Nanjing 210002, Jiangsu, China

Jin-Chun Lu
The Reproductive Medical Centre, Nanjing Jinling Hospital, Nanjing University School of Medicine, 305 Zhongshan East Road, Nanjing 210002, Jiangsu, China
Department of Laboratory Science, Nanjing Hospital, Jiangsu Corps, The Armed Police Force, PLA, Nanjing 210028, Jiangsu, China

Rui-Xiang Feng
Department of Laboratory Science, Nanjing Hospital, Jiangsu Corps, The Armed Police Force, PLA, Nanjing 210028, Jiangsu, China

M. C. Inhorn
Department of Anthropology, Yale University, 10 Sachem Street, New Haven, CT 06511, USA

D. Birenbaum-Carmeli
Department of Nursing, University of Haifa, 3498838 Haifa, Israel

J.Birger
Larchmont, USA

L. M. Westphal
Stanford Fertility and Reproductive Medicine Center, Stanford University, 1195 W. Fremont Ave, Sunnyvale, CA 94087, USA

J. Doyle
Shady Grove Fertility, 9600 Blackwell Road, Rockville, MD 20850, USA

N. Gleicher
Center for Human Reproduction, 21 E. 69th Street, New York, NY 10021, USA

D. Meirow and D. Seidman
Department of Obstetrics and Gynecology, Sheba Medical Center, IVF and Fertility Unit, 1 Emek Ha'ella St, 52621 Ramat Gan, Israel

M. Dirnfeld
Division Reproductive Endocrinology-IVF, Department of Obstetrics and Gynecology, Carmel Medical Center, Ruth and Bruce Faculty of Medicine, Technion, 3436212 Haifa, Israel

A. Kahane
9Assuta Medical Center, 13 Eliezer Mazal, 75653 Rishoon Lezion, Israel

P. Patrizio
Yale Fertility Center, Yale University, 150 Sargent Drive, New Haven, CT 06511, USA

Joana Antonela Asensio and María de los Ángeles Sanhueza
1Laboratorio de Fisiopatología Ovárica, Instituto de Medicina y Biología Experimental de Cuyo (IMBECU - CONICET), Mendoza, Argentina

Antonella Rosario Ramona Cáceres and Laura Tatiana Pelegrina
Laboratorio de Fisiopatología Ovárica, Instituto de Medicina y Biología Experimental de Cuyo (IMBECU - CONICET), Mendoza, Argentina
Facultad de Ciencias Veterinarias y Ambientales, Universidad Juan Agustín Maza, Mendoza, Argentina

Myriam Raquel Laconi
Laboratorio de Fisiopatología Ovárica, Instituto de Medicina y Biología Experimental de Cuyo (IMBECU - CONICET), Mendoza, Argentina
Facultad de Ciencias Veterinarias y Ambientales, Universidad Juan Agustín Maza, Mendoza, Argentina
Facultad de Ciencias Médicas, Universidad de Mendoza, Mendoza, Argentina

Leopoldina Scotti and Fernanda Parborell
Laboratorio de Fisiopatología del Ovario, Instituto de Biología y Medicina Experimental (IByME - CONICET), Buenos Aires, Argentina

Giuseppe D'Amato, Anna Maria Caringella, Antonio Stanziano, Clementina Cantatore and Simone Palini
Asl Bari, Department of Maternal and Child Health, Reproductive and IVF Unit, Conversano, BA, Italy

Ettore Caroppo
Asl Bari, Department of Maternal and Child Health, Reproductive and IVF Unit, Conversano, BA, Italy
ASL Bari, PTA "F Jaia", Fisiopatologia della Riproduzione Umana e P.M.A, via de Amicis 30, 70014 Conversano, BA, Italy

Wan Yang, Rui Yang, Mingmei Lin, Yan Yang, Xueling Song, Jiajia Zhang, Shuo Yang, Ying Song, Jia Li, Tianshu Pang, Feng Deng, Ying Wang, Rong Li and Jie Jiao
Center for Reproductive Medicine, Department of Obstetrics and Gynecology, Peking University Third Hospital, 49 N Garden Rd, Haidian District, Beijing 100191, China

Hua Zhang
Research Center of Clinical Epidemiology, Peking University Third Hospital, Beijing, China

Meng Rao, Shuhua Zhao and Li Tang
Department of Reproduction and Genetics, the First Affiliated Hospital of Kunming Medical University, No. 295 Xi Chang road, Kunming 650032, China

Zhengyan Zeng
Department of Neurology, the First Affiliated Hospital of Kunming Medical University, Kunming 650032, China

Majid Dastorani, Esmat Aghadavod and Zatollah Asemi
Research Center for Biochemistry and Nutrition in Metabolic Diseases, Kashan University of Medical Sciences, Kashan, I.R, Iran

Naghmeh Mirhosseini
School of Public Health, University of Saskatchewan, Saskatoon, SK, Canada

Fatemeh Foroozanfard
Department of Gynecology and Obstetrics, School of Medicine, Kashan University of Medical Sciences, Kashan, I.R, Iran

Shahrzad Zadeh Modarres
Laser Application in Medical Science Research Center, Shahid Beheshti University of Medical Sciences, Tehran, Iran

Mehrnush Amiri Siavashani
Taleghani Educational Hospital, IVF Center, Shahid Beheshti University of Medical Sciences, Tehran, Iran

Gabriel Levin and Nathali Guimarães Nóbrega
NUCEL (Cell and Molecular Therapy Center), Internal Medicine Department, Medical School, University of São Paulo, Rua Pangaré, 100, Cidade Universitária, São Paulo, SP 05360-130, Brazil

Tatiane Maldonado Coelho, Marina Trombetta-Lima and Mari Cleide Sogayar
NUCEL (Cell and Molecular Therapy Center), Internal Medicine Department, Medical School, University of São Paulo, Rua Pangaré, 100, Cidade Universitária, São Paulo, SP 05360-130, Brazil
Chemistry Institute, Biochemistry Department, University of São Paulo, São Paulo, SP 05508-000, Brazil

Ana Claudia Oliveira Carreira
NUCEL (Cell and Molecular Therapy Center), Internal Medicine Department, Medical School, University of São Paulo, Rua Pangaré, 100, Cidade Universitária, São Paulo, SP 05360-130, Brazil
Chemistry Institute, Biochemistry Department, University of São Paulo, São Paulo, SP 05508-000, Brazil
Department of Surgery, School of Veterinary Medicine and Animal Science, University of São Paulo, São Paulo, SP 05508-270, Brazil

Chyi-Uei Chern
Department of Obstetrics and Gynecology, Kaohsiung Veterans General Hospital, No.386, Dazhong 1st Rd., Zuoying Dist, Kaohsiung City 81362, Taiwan

Hsiao-Wen Tsai
Department of Obstetrics and Gynecology, Kaohsiung Veterans General Hospital, No.386, Dazhong 1st Rd., Zuoying Dist, Kaohsiung City 81362, Taiwan
Department of Obstetrics and Gynecology, National Yang-Ming University School of Medicine, No. 155, Sec. 2, Li-Nong Street, Pei-Tou, Taipei 112, Taiwan

Kuan-Hao Tsui
Department of Obstetrics and Gynecology, Kaohsiung Veterans General Hospital, No.386, Dazhong 1st Rd., Zuoying Dist, Kaohsiung City 81362, Taiwan
Department of Obstetrics and Gynecology, National Yang-Ming University School of Medicine, No. 155, Sec. 2, Li-Nong Street, Pei-Tou, Taipei 112, Taiwan
Department of Pharmacy and Master Program, College of Pharmacy and Health Care, Tajen University, No.20, Weixin Rd, Yanpu, Township, Pingtung County 90741, Taiwan

Li-Te Lin
Department of Obstetrics and Gynecology, Kaohsiung Veterans General Hospital, No.386, Dazhong 1st Rd., Zuoying Dist, Kaohsiung City 81362, Taiwan
Department of Obstetrics and Gynecology, National Yang-Ming University School of Medicine, No. 155, Sec. 2, Li-Nong Street, Pei-Tou, Taipei 112, Taiwan
Department of Biological Science, National Sun Yat-SenUniversity, 70 Lienhai Rd, Kaohsiung City 80424, Taiwan.

Peng-Hui Wang
Department of Obstetrics and Gynecology, National Yang-Ming University School of Medicine, No. 155, Sec. 2, Li-Nong Street, Pei-Tou, Taipei 112, Taiwan
Department of Obstetrics and Gynecology, Taipei Veterans General Hospital, No. 201, Section 2, Shih-Pai Road, Taipei 112, Taiwan
Department of Medical Research, China Medical University Hospital, No. 2, Yude Road, North District, Taichung City 40447, Taiwan

Salvatore Giovanni Vitale and Antonio Cianci
Department of General Surgery and Medical Surgical Specialties, University of Catania, 95123 Catania, Italy

Zhi-Hong Wen
Department of Marine Biotechnology and Resources, National Sun Yat-sen University, 70 Lienhai Rd, KaohsiungCity 80424, Taiwan

Miao Liu, Jianan Tang, Yu Zhang, Yan Shi and Lin Yu
Key Lab of Reproduction Regulation of NPFPC, SIPPR, IRD, Fudan University, Xietu Road 2140, Xuhui District, Shanghai 200032, China

Xiaoyu Tu
Key Lab of Reproduction Regulation of NPFPC, SIPPR, IRD, Fudan University, Xietu Road 2140, Xuhui District, Shanghai 200032, China
Women's Hospital, School of Medicine, Zhejiang University, Hangzhou, China

Zhaogui Sun
Key Lab of Reproduction Regulation of NPFPC, SIPPR, IRD, Fudan University, Xietu Road 2140, Xuhui District, Shanghai 200032, China
Key Laboratory of Contraceptive Drugs and Devices of NPFPC, Shanghai Institution of Planned Parenthood Research, Xietu Road 2140, Xuhui District, Shanghai 200032, China

Gabriela García-Jiménez and Antonio Pellicer
Instituto Valenciano de Infertilidad (IVINSEMER), Thiers 96, Col. Nueva Anzurez, CP 11590 Mexico City, Mexico

Teresa Zariñán, Nancy R. Mejía-Domínguez, Rubén Gutiérrez-Sagal, Georgina Hernández-Montes and Alfredo Ulloa-Aguirre
Red de Apoyo a la Investigación (RAI), Coordinación de la Investigación Científica, Universidad Nacional Autónoma de México (UNAM)-Instituto Nacional de Ciencias Médicas y Nutrición SZ (INCMNSZ), Calle Vasco de Quiroga 15, Tlalpan, 14000 Ciudad de Mexico, Mexico

Rocío Rodríguez-Valentín
Centro de Investigación en Salud Poblacional, Instituto Nacional de Salud Pública, Av. Universidad 655, CP 62100 Cuernavaca, Mor, Mexico

Armando Tovar
Department of Physiology of Nutrition, INCMNSZ, Mexico City, Mexico

Julio Granados
Department of Transplantation, INCMNSZ, Mexico City, Mexico

Fabián Arechavaleta-Velasco
Research Unit in Reproductive Medicine, UMAE Hospital de Ginecoobstetricia "Luis Castelazo Ayala", Río de la Magdalena 289, Tizapán San Ángel, Mexico City 01090, Mexico

Patricia Canto
Facultad de Medicina, UNAM, Ciudad Universitaria, Mexico City, Mexico

Hortensia Moreno-Macias
Universidad Autónoma Metropolitana-Iztapalapa, Av. San Rafael Atlixco 186, Leyes de Reforma 1ra. Secc., Mexico City 09340, Mexico

Teresa Tusié-Luna
Unidad de Biología Molecular y Medicina Genómica, UNAM-INCMNSZ, Mexico City, Mexico

Index

www.ingramcontent.com/pod-product-compliance
Lightning Source LLC
Chambersburg PA
CBHW061302190326
41458CB00011B/3744